WOUND HEALING

BASIC AND CLINICAL DERMATOLOGY

Series Editors
ALAN R. SHALITA, M.D.
Distinguished Teaching Professor and Chairman
Department of Dermatology
SUNY Downstate Medical Center

Brooklyn, New York

DAVID A. NORRIS, M.D.
Director of Research
Professor of Dermatology
The University of Colorado
Health Sciences Center
Denver, Colorado

WOUND HEALING

Edited by

Anna F. Falabella
University of Miami School of Medicine
Miami, Florida, U.S.A.

Robert S. Kirsner
University of Miami School of Medicine
Miami, Florida, U.S.A.

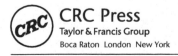

CRC Press
Taylor & Francis Group
Boca Raton London New York

CRC Press is an imprint of the
Taylor & Francis Group, an **informa** business

CRC Press
Taylor & Francis Group
6000 Broken Sound Parkway NW, Suite 300
Boca Raton, FL 33487-2742

First issued in paperback 2019

© 2005 by Taylor & Francis Group, LLC
CRC Press is an imprint of Taylor & Francis Group, an Informa business

No claim to original U.S. Government works

ISBN-13: 978-0-8247-5458-7 (hbk)
ISBN-13: 978-0-367-39233-8 (pbk)

Library of Congress Cataloging-in-Publication Data

Catalog record is available from the Library of Congress

Visit the Taylor & Francis Web site at
http://www.taylorandfrancis.com

and the CRC Press Web site at
http://www.crcpress.com

Series Introduction

During the past 25 years, there has been a vast explosion in new information relating to the art and science of dermatology as well as fundamental cutaneous biology. Furthermore, this information is no longer of interest only to the small but growing specialty of dermatology. Scientists from a wide variety of disciplines have come to recognize both the importance of skin in fundamental biological processes and the broad implications of understanding the pathogenesis of skin disease. As a result, there is now a multidisciplinary and worldwide interest in the progress of dermatology.

With these factors in mind, we have undertaken this series of books specifically oriented to dermatology. The scope of the series is purposely broad, with books ranging from pure basic science to practical, applied clinical dermatology. Thus, while there is something for everyone, all volumes in the series will ultimately prove to be valuable additions to the dermatologist's library.

The latest addition to the series, volume 33, edited by Drs. Anna F. Falabella and Robert S. Kirsner, is both timely and pertinent. The editors are well known authorities in the field of wound healing. We trust that this volume will be of broad interest to scientists and clinicians alike.

Alan R. Shalita
SUNY Downstate Medical Center
Brooklyn, New York, U.S.A.

Preface

Some of the oldest known medical texts in existence, written more than 3000 years ago, describe techniques used by ancient healers to treat wounds. Despite this long history, the art of wound healing did not advance to any significant degree until recent times. Over the past 20 years, our knowledge of the wound healing process has increased dramatically. With this knowledge has come the development of new, exciting technologies that accelerate normal wound healing and counter the pathophysiologic processes that lead to chronic wound formation. From growth factors to bioengineered skin substitutes, the future of wound healing holds great promise. The purpose of this book is to provide its readers with a comprehensive review of the field of wound healing, from the basic principles of wound healing, to assessment and treatment, to promising therapies of the future.

From basic concepts to advanced therapies, this book is the most complete guide for learning in this field. The book is divided into three sections. The first focuses on the basic science of wound healing and describes, in great detail, the pathophysiology of wound healing. The next section concentrates on the general clinical aspects of wound healing, focusing on epidemiology, diagnosis and prevention of wounds. The last section provides an in-depth description of general and specific treatments available for wound healing, and discusses current research issues.

The professionals who have contributed to this text are some of the most experienced clinicians and scientists in the field of wound healing. Readers of the text should come away with an excellent understanding of the wound healing process, the appropriate evaluation of acute and chronic wounds, and management strategies. One should also come away with a better understanding of newer treatment modalities and the principles upon which new therapies are being developed.

Whether particular interests in wound healing involve research or clinical practice, this book should prove to be an invaluable resource for all professionals involved in the field of wound healing.

Anna F. Falabella
Robert S. Kirsner

Contents

Contributors

David G. Armstrong Department of Surgery, Doctor William M. Scholl College of Podiatric Medicine, Rosalind Franklin University of Medicine and Science, Chicago, Illinois, U.S.A.

Meggan R. Banta Department of Dermatology and Cutaneous Surgery, University of Miami School of Medicine, Miami, Florida, U.S.A.

Janice M. Beitz La Salle University School of Nursing, Philadelphia, Pennsylvania, U.S.A.

Ysabel M. Bello Department of Dermatology and Cutaneous Surgery, University of Miami School of Medicine, Miami, Florida, U.S.A.

Brian Berman Department of Dermatology and Cutaneous Surgery, University of Miami School of Medicine, Miami, Florida, U.S.A.

Andrew J. M. Boulton Division of Endocrinology, Diabetes and Metabolism, University of Miami School of Medicine, Miami, Florida, U.S.A. and Department of Medicine, University of Manchester, Manchester, U.K.

A. L. Cazzaniga Department of Dermatology and Cutaneous Surgery, University of Miami School of Medicine, Miami, Florida, U.S.A.

Carlos A. Charles Department of Dermatology and Cutaneous Surgery, University of Miami School of Medicine, Miami, Florida, U.S.A.

Gloria A. Chin Department of Surgery, University of Florida, Gainesville, Florida, U.S.A.

Amy Colwell Department of Surgery, Brigham and Women's Hospital, Boston, Massachusetts, U.S.A.

Ganary Dabiri Albany Medical Center, Center for Cell Biology and Cancer Research, Albany, New York, U.S.A.

S. C. Davis Department of Dermatology and Cutaneous Surgery, University of Miami School of Medicine, Miami, Florida, U.S.A.

Robert H. Demling   Harvard Medical School and Burn Center, Brigham and Women's Hospital, Boston, Massachusetts, U.S.A.

Robert F. Diegelmann   Department of Biochemistry, Medical College of Virginia, Richmond, Virginia, U.S.A.

C. Michael DiPersio   Albany Medical Center, Center for Cell Biology and Cancer Research, Albany, New York, U.S.A.

Celia M. Divino   Division of General Surgery, The Mount Sinai School of Medicine, New York, New York, U.S.A.

Anna Drosou   Department of Dermatology and Cutaneous Surgery, University of Miami School of Medicine, Miami, Florida, U.S.A.

William H. Eaglstein   Miller School of Medicine, University of Miami, Miami, Florida, U.S.A.

George W. Elgart   Department of Dermatology and Cutaneous Surgery, University of Miami School of Medicine, Miami, Florida, U.S.A.

William J. Ennis   Advocate Christ Medical Center Wound Treatment Program, Oak Lawn, Illinois, and Evergreen Healthcare Center, Advanced Wound Care Program, Evergreen Park, Illinois, U.S.A.

Anna F. Falabella   Department of Dermatology and Cutaneous Surgery, University of Miami School of Medicine, Miami, Florida, U.S.A.

Daniel G. Federman   Department of Medicine, Yale University School of Medicine, West Haven, Connecticut, U.S.A.

Caroline E. Fife   Department of Anesthesiology, University of Texas Health Science Center, and Memorial Hermann Center for Wound Healing, Houston, Texas, U.S.A.

David Fivenson   Department of Dermatology, Henry Ford Health System, Detroit, Michigan, U.S.A.

Lawrence E. Gibson   Department of Dermatology, Mayo Clinic and Mayo Foundation, Rochester, Minnesota, U.S.A.

Lauren Grasso   Department of Dermatology, Henry Ford Health System, Detroit, Michigan, U.S.A.

Cathy Thomas Hess   Clinical Operations, Wound Care Strategies, Inc., Harrisburg, Pennsylvania, U.S.A.

Mark D. Hoffman   Department of Dermatology, Rush-Presbyterian-St. Luke's Medical Center, Chicago, Illinois, U.S.A.

Allen Holloway Department of Surgery, Maricopa Medical Center, Phoenix, Arizona, U.S.A.

Harriet W. Hopf Departments of Anesthesia and Surgery, University of California San Francisco, Wound Healing Laboratory, San Francisco, California, U.S.A.

Shasa Hu Department of Dermatology and Cutaneous Surgery, University of Miami School of Medicine, Miami, Florida, U.S.A.

Thomas K. Hunt Departments of Anesthesia and Surgery, University of California San Francisco, Wound Healing Laboratory, San Francisco, California, U.S.A.

Satoshi Itami Department of Dermatology, Osaka University Graduate School of Medicine, Suita, Osaka-fu, Japan

Sarah L. Jensen Department of Dermatology, St. Louis University Hospital, St. Louis, Missouri, U.S.A.

Jonathan Kantor Departments of Dermatology and Biostatistics and Epidemiology, University of Pennsylvania School of Medicine, Philadelphia, Pennsylvania, U.S.A.

Francisco A. Kerdel Chief of Dermatology and Director of Inpatient Services, Cedars Medical Center, Miami, Florida, U.S.A.

Morris D. Kerstein Department of Surgery, Jefferson Medical College, Philadelphia, Pennsylvania and VA Medical and Regional Office Center, Wilmington, Delaware, U.S.A.

Robert S. Kirsner Department of Dermatology and Cutaneous Surgery, University of Miami School of Medicine, Miami, Florida, U.S.A.

Luther C. Kloth Department of Physical Therapy, College of Health Sciences, Marquette University and Department of Plastic Surgery, The Medical College of Wisconsin, Milwaukee, Wisconsin, U.S.A.

Diane L. Krasner Rest Haven—York, York, Pennsylvania, U.S.A.

Jeffrey D. Kravetz Department of Medicine, Yale University School of Medicine, West Haven, Connecticut, U.S.A.

Lawrence A. Lavery Department of Surgery, Scott & White Memorial Hospital, Texas A&M University College of Medicine, Temple, Texas, U.S.A.

Jie Li Department of Dermatology and Cutaneous Surgery, University of Miami School of Medicine, Miami, Florida, U.S.A.

Peggy Lin Department of Dermatology, Boston University School of Medicine, Boston, Massachusetts, U.S.A.

George Tye Liu   Department of Orthopedics, Podiatry Division, The University of Texas Health Science Center, San Antonio, Texas, U.S.A.

Markéta Límová   Department of Dermatology, University of California San Francisco, San Francisco, California, U.S.A.

Michael T. Longaker   Director of Children's Surgical Research, Stanford University Medical Center, Stanford, California, U.S.A.

H. Peter Lorenz   Division of Plastic Surgery, Stanford University Center for Children's Surgical Research, Stanford, California, U.S.A.

John M. MacDonald   Department of Dermatology and Cutaneous Surgery, University of Miami School of Medicine, Miami, Florida, U.S.A.

Antonio Magliaro   Department of Dermatology, University of Pisa, Pisa, Italy

David J. Margolis   Departments of Dermatology and Biostatistics and Epidemiology, University of Pennsylvania School of Medicine, Philadelphia, Pennsylvania, U.S.A.

Lucy K. Martin   Department of Dermatology and Cutaneous Surgery, University of Miami School of Medicine, Miami, Florida, U.S.A.

Harvey N. Mayrovitz   College of Medical Sciences, Nova Southeastern University, Ft. Lauderdale, Florida, U.S.A.

Joseph McCulloch   School of Allied Health Professions, Louisiana State University Health Sciences Center, Shreveport, Louisiana, U.S.A.

Felicia A. Mendelsohn   Department of Internal Medicine, Yale University School of Medicine, New Haven, Connecticut, U.S.A.

Patricia M. Mertz   Department of Dermatology and Cutaneous Surgery, University of Miami School of Medicine, Miami, Florida, U.S.A.

Michael J. Morykwas   Department of Plastic and Reconstructive Surgery, Wake Forest University School of Medicine, Winston-Salem, North Carolina, U.S.A.

George T. Nahass   Department of Dermatology, St. Louis University Hospital, St. Louis, Missouri, U.S.A.

Nicholas Namias   Division of Burns and Department of Surgical Infectious Diseases, University of Miami/Jackson Memorial Medical Center, Miami, Florida, U.S.A.

Peter A. Noseworthy   Dermatology Daycare and Wound Healing Clinic, Sunnybrook and Women's College Health Sciences Centre, Toronto, Ontario, Canada

R. N. Heather Orsted Dermatology Daycare and Wound Healing Clinic, Sunnybrook and Women's College Health Sciences Centre, Toronto, Ontario, Canada

Liza Ovington Ovington & Associates, Inc., Allentown, Pennsylvania, U.S.A.

Wyatt G. Payne Department of Surgery, University of South Florida, Tampa, Florida, U.S.A.

Tania J. Phillips Department of Dermatology, Boston University School of Medicine, Boston, Massachusetts, U.S.A.

Varee Poochareon Department of Dermatology and Cutaneous Surgery, University of Miami School of Medicine, Miami, Florida, U.S.A.

Martin C. Robson Department of Surgery, University of South Florida, Tampa, Florida, U.S.A.

Georgette Rodriguez Department of Dermatology and Cutaneous Surgery, University of Miami School of Medicine, Miami, Florida, U.S.A.

Marco Romanelli Department of Dermatology, University of Pisa, Pisa, Italy

Paolo Romanelli Department of Dermatology and Cutaneous Surgery, University of Miami School of Medicine, Miami, Florida, U.S.A.

Noah A. Rosen Department of Surgery, Boston University Medical Center, Boston, Massachusetts, U.S.A.

Chris B. Ruser Department of Medicine, Yale University School of Medicine, West Haven, Connecticut, U.S.A.

Lawrence A. Schachner Department of Pediatrics, The University of Miami School of Medicine, Miami, Florida, U.S.A.

Stefanie Schluender Department of Surgery, The Mount Sinai Medical Center, New York, New York, U.S.A.

Gregory S. Schultz Department of Obstetrics and Gynecology, University of Florida, Gainesville, Florida, U.S.A.

R. Gary Sibbald Dermatology Daycare and Wound Healing Clinic, Sunnybrook and Women's College Health Sciences Centre, Toronto, Ontario, Canada

Nancy Sims College of Medical Sciences, Nova Southeastern University, Ft. Lauderdale, Florida, U.S.A.

James Spencer Department of Dermatology and Cutaneous Surgery, The Mount Sinai School of Medicine, New York, New York, U.S.A.

John S. Steinberg   Department of Orthopedics, Podiatry Division, The University of Texas Health Science Center, San Antonio, Texas, U.S.A.

Tory P. Sullivan   Department of Dermatology and Cutaneous Surgery, University of Miami School of Medicine, Miami, Florida, U.S.A.

Jennifer T. Trent   Department of Dermatology and Cutaneous Surgery, University of Miami School of Medicine, Miami, Florida, U.S.A.

Isabel C. Valencia   Department of Dermatology and Cutaneous Surgery, The University of Miami School of Medicine, Miami, Florida, U.S.A.

Lia van Rijswijk   La Salle University School of Nursing, La Salle Neighborhood Nursing Center, Newtown and Philadelphia, Pennsylvania, U.S.A.

Adriana Villa   Department of Dermatology and Cutaneous Surgery, University of Miami School of Medicine, Miami, Florida, U.S.A.

Dot Weir   Orlando Regional Healthcare, Lucerne Wound Healing Center, Orlando, Florida, U.S.A.

Esperanza Welsh   Department of Dermatology, University of Miami School of Medicine, Miami, Florida, U.S.A.

Yuji Yamaguchi   Department of Dermatology, Osaka University Graduate School of Medicine, Suita, Osaka-fu, Japan

Sharam Samson Yashar   Department of Dermatology, Henry Ford Health System, Detroit, Michigan, U.S.A.

Kunihiko Yoshikawa   Department of Dermatology, Osaka University Graduate School of Medicine, Suita, Osaka-fu, Japan

1

Historical Aspects of Wound Healing

William H. Eaglstein
Miller School of Medicine, University of Miami, Miami, Florida, U.S.A.

1. ACUTE WOUNDS

The recorded history of Western medicine begins with Greek physicians who created a system of understanding disease as an imbalance in natural substances: blood, phlegm, yellow bile, and black bile. The corresponding descriptive terms now applied to personalities, sanguine, phlegmatic, bilious, and melancholic attest to the durability of this and many other Greek medical constructs and philosophies. One of the major problems of understanding ancient medicine, trying to understand the disease at issue, is not a problem when studying the history of wound care, at least with regard to acute wounds. Wounds inflicted with sharp and blunt instruments, burns, bites, and other such injuries are presumably the same throughout history. With regard to making wounds to treat wounds, Indian medicine, which introduced skin grafting and skin flaps especially to repair noses which were cut off as punishment, was far ahead of western medicine.

Among the medical works predating Greek medicine, we learn from the Smith papyrus (transcriptions of an Egyptian document dating from 3000–2500 B.C.E.) that wound edges were brought together with resin-covered linen strips, that the standard wound salve was made of grease, honey, and lint (functioning much as our current occlusive dressings), and that wounds were categorized as diseased or sick wounds and not sick wounds. Hippocrates in 400 B.C.E. is generally credited with this "discovery." The *Illiad* (approximately 1000 B.C.E.) describes 147 wounds. Although the treatments were holistic—the wounded were carried to a tent, given a seat, told stories, given a cup of wine sprinkled with grated goat cheese and given a barley meal served by a beautiful woman who later washed the wounds with warm water—they were not very effective and the mortality rate was 77.6%. Bleeding probably accounted for most deaths since the only treatment mentioned to check bleeding, beyond skillful bandaging mentioned twice by Homer, was recitation of a charm or singing of a song. Although not mentioned, it is likely based on agriculture records and pottery designs in the shape of poppies that opium was available for the wounded.

Hippocrates (460–370 B.C.E.), whose existence is confirmed by the writing of both Plato and Aristotle, is known through a collection of medical works, none thought to be original but many of which describe his efforts. Hippocrates worked

1

frequently with wounds both at his "office," at home at Kos, and when traveling to treat the ill. Credited with defining first intention healing (i.e., direct healing of closely approximated wound edges without suppuration), he rarely had recourse to this approach. In an era when almost all wounds became infected and in which there was not a distinction between acute wounds, chronic wounds, and ulcers, one of the issues most dealt with by Hippocrates was the issue of pus. The two types of pus he noted would today be described as severe infection and mild infection. The Hippocratic physician was in fact fearful of too little pus believing that: (1) pus which came from liquefaction of dried blood and bruised tissue within the wound produced a needed cleaning of the wound (2); patients unable to swell and produce pus were so sick that they did not survive—thus, no pus = bad, pus = good; (3) good pus prevents bad; and (4) bad humors could be eliminated by ripening and being released as pus.

Greek physicians most often attempted to take the acute wound "rapidly through suppuration," especially if it contained any bruised tissues. Toward this end, the physician deliberately irritated the wound. To prevent suppuration Greek physicians used a class of topicals called Enhemes, which were both dry and wet and usually contained metals such as lead oxide, zinc oxide, copper oxide, and copper sulphate. These are antiseptics but toxic to cells as well as bacteria. Based on Hippocratic teaching, Greek physicians almost always poured wine into wounds and over wound dressings and used sponges with dried wine or vinegar. Studies have indeed demonstrated that wine is bactericidal but the active component is not the 9–12% alcohol (70% is required) but the polyphenol, malvoside. Overall, since Greek physicians chose to induce suppuration we would say that the Greek wound healer found it easier to help infection than to fight it, although infection as we know it was unconceptualized.

Local treatment of the wound was not terribly helpful or harmful. However, the three general treatments of seriously wounded (or ill) patients—bleeding, starving, and purging—were not only harmful but also were long lasting, with bleeding ending only in the eighteenth century.

Bleeding, perhaps the most basic issue in wound care, was as little understood and inadequately dealt with as was infection. The concept of a pump was virtually unknown and blood was not known to circulate. While blood was known to be in veins, arteries were thought to contain air. When a wound was inflamed, it was deemed a problem of excess blood which often was treated by bleeding the patient either from the inflamed wound or from a distant site. Although an occasional wound was sutured to bring the lips together, the idea of tying vessels to stem bleeding was unknown to Hippocrates. However, later Greek physicians, especially the Alexandrians, did discover the value of ligating vessels to stop bleeding. Erasistratos, or his pupils in Alexandria, is credited with the discovery of tying off vessels as well as a faulty but early recognition that blood is pumped peripherally, although circulation was not understood.

The Romans distrusted physicians and Greek physicians in particular. In his compendium of information (and misinformation) known as *Natural History*, Pliny the Elder (23–79 C.E.) states, "Heaven knows, the medical profession is the only one in which anybody professing to be a physician is at once trusted, although nowhere else is an untruth more dangerous. We pay however no attention to the danger, so great for each of us is the seductive sweetness of wishful thinking."

Celsus (14–20 C.E.), who lived in Rome before Pliny, was however a Roman and as Pliny, wrote in Latin rather than Greek. Celsus's book *De Medicina* 1478 C.E.

was the first printed medical book by a medical author. It was "lost" for fourteen centuries, but is the only medical book from Western antiquity to survive in a complete form. Celsus is often credited as the first to differentiate a wound from an ulcer noting that blood comes from a fresh or healing wound while pus comes from an ulcer. Celsus stopped bleeding with compression and if this failed, by ligating the veins, leading to the first description of how to amputate legs. Celsus also described cauterization and cupping a distant site to draw blood as hemostatic methods. For closing acute wounds, he described suturing—a woman's hair was often used—or pins (fibulas). All wounds were to be cleansed with sponges squeezed out of vinegar or wine, while blood, lint, and other foreign materials were to be removed. Neither Celsus nor Pliny was short of topical medical wound treatments. Celsus listed thirty-four ointments and plasters for wounds. All but five contained heavy doses of lead and copper salts, some with mercury and antimony sulfates. The five which did not were meant to induce pus. The carriers were resins, pitch bitumen, wax, oil, and vinegar. Without doubt, Celsus is best known to us as the physician who defined the cardinal signs of acute inflammation—redness, swelling, heat, and pain (rubor, tumor, color, and dolor).

The last great name in medical antiquity, Galen, was born in 13 C.E. in Pergamon. Although he was a Greek who had also studied anatomy in Alexandria, Galen lived most of his adult life in Rome, was the physician to Roman emperors including Marcus Aurelius, wrote hundreds of medical and scientific books and had a wide experience in treating wounds during his three years as a physician to the gladiators. As a scientist, he is credited with opening live arteries to prove that they contained blood, tying the ureters of living animals to prove that urine comes from the kidneys and cutting the spinal cord of animals at various levels to study paralysis. As a wound healer, he pinched, sutured, and twisted vessels to stop bleeding. As an admirer of Hippocrates' works, his local wound care consisted principally of wine- and vinegar-soaked sponges and wound debridement. He famously did not advocate tourniquets, which he believed squeezed and lead to more blood coming out of the wound. Galen strongly advocated the four humors theory of disease, as well as diets we would now call non-nutritious and phlebotomies—bleeding to cure bleeding—as treatment for chronic wounds. Overall, the principal wound healing issues of antiquity seem to have been resolved as follows: bleeding was stopped with compression, vessel ligation, and cautery; inflamed wounds were treated with local or distant bleeding; irritation was used to induce mild suppuration ("laudable pus") and secondary intention healing was favored over primary. These views were expressed in the writings of Galen, who became the ultimate medical authority, and they prevailed throughout the Middle Ages and the Renaissance. However, significant dissent to the doctrine of laudable pus and healing by secondary intention was made by some surgeons, especially by Hugh of Luca the founder of the Bologna School, (1160–1257 C.E.) and his son Theodoric (1205–1296 C.E.). Although Hugh left no written record, through the writings of Theodoric ("Chirurgia, 1267 C.E.) and other followers, including the French surgeon Henri de Mondeville, we know that this group of surgeons advocated primary intention healing; specifically, cleaning the wound, bringing its lips together in the proper anatomical state, and, if necessary, holding them by sutures. They also favored use of an opium-containing soporific sponge applied to the nostrils to induce sleep to allow surgical repair to proceed. Despite such independent thinking, the Galenic view remained dominant through medieval times being followed by the great physicians of the period such as Ambrose Paré. It should be noted that the virtue of open or secondary healing of contaminated wounds was relearned in the World War II and the Korean and the Vietnam wars.

John Hunter the Scottsman (1728–1793), who was an anatomist-turned surgeon, made observations based on animal experimentation and practical war experience which ran counter to the received surgical truths. He described three methods by which wounds healed: by immediate primary union, by implementation with the flow of a cementing "coagulable lymph" or by secondary union (granulation). Using the microscope, he documented that coagulable lymph contained white and red corpuscles, and in contrast to the conclusions of Hippocrates, was not a corrosive fluid derived from the breakdown of devitalized tissue. Hunter's willingness to be guided by direct observation and experimental fact rather than past authority paved the way for the acceptance into medical practice of the scientific advances of the nineteenth century.

Based on their observations that nerves and vessels branched into smaller and smaller units, Greek physicians had developed a concept of "tissue" being composed of invisible strands of nerves and vessels embedded in a material they named interstitia. Greek thinkers are rightly famous for such reasoning, an example of such being their conceptualization of the atom. This technique has been dubbed "the Greek microscope." Having a real microscope, Rudolph Virchow (1821–1902) demonstrated the cellular events of wound healing, especially the key role of the fibroblast. That tissues were composed of cells was an unknown concept in antiquity. It remained for Julius Cohnagin (1839–1884) to show that pus cells are actually blood cells which are allowed to pass into the wound by alteration of the walls of the blood vessels. In the 1860s, the discovery by Louis Pasteur, while working on problems in the silk worm industry, that bacteria played a pivotal role in disease led to dramatic changes in medical thinking. The English surgeon Joseph Lister (1827–1912), noting that simple fractures healed promptly and without suppuration while suppuration and often systemic signs of inflammation were an almost inevitable complication in compound fractures, came to the conclusion that the difference between the two was that the break in the skin allowed micro-organisms into the wound, causing the suppuration in compound fractures. Lister's intuitive conclusions on the applicability of Pasteur's observations to surgical infections as outlined in his 1868 address on the antiseptic approach to surgery, altered operating room behavior rapidly and permanently. The elegant experiments of Robert Koch in the 1870s definitively characterized the etiology of traumatic infected wounds. The role played by the phagocyte host response to bacterial infections was discovered by Elie Metchnikoff (1845–1916).

In 1910, Nobel Prize winner Alexis Carrel divided the stages of wound healing into four periods: quiescent, granulomatous retraction, epidermalization, and cicatricial, based on a series of animal experiments. Hunter had also constructed a time frame for healing but Carrel's work, based on experimental data, was able to assign more precise time limits, and ultimately his work in collaboration with that of others defined some of the effects of diet, temperature, and other factors on the normal wound repair process. The studies of Edward Howes, Joseph Sooy, and Samuel Harvey using tensile strength allowed the study of wounds beyond the skin and led to definition of the influence of aging and vitamin C depletion on the healing of wounds. The introduction of tissue culture techniques by Alexis Carrel and other associates led to many breakthroughs in understanding, including a better appreciation of epidermalization, which was finalized through the work of Shattuck Hartwell and Theodore Gillman. Hartwell in particular noted the considerable difference in the subepithelial healing events between human and animal wounds. In particular, Hartwell pointed out that experimental wounds in animals including the dog, guinea pig, and rabbit, while similar to one another, had histologic findings similar to those seen in human wound healing by secondary intention. Only in domestic swine were the subepithelial events similar to healing by first intention seen in human wounds healing primarily.

The works described provided much of the basis for wound healing as we now understand it. The important role of the fibroblast in generating fibrotic healing characteristic of dermal repair and the key part played by the macrophage (Liebovich and Ross in 1975) were among the many advances of the twentieth century. However, in general, few concerned themselves with or even believed it possible to do more than to optimize the natural healing process. J. E. Dunphy, surgeon and scientist, conducted experiments showing that wounds deliberately reopened and resutured 4–6 days after operation had almost the same tensile strength as a fresh primary that had not been opened at the end of 1 week. Dunphy's postulate of a "wound hormone" to explain these findings led to a search for such a wound hormone and suggested the possibility of speeding healing beyond the natural speed. In 1962, George Winter's studies of occlusive film treatment of superficial swine wounds showed that epithelization could be sped by about 30%. This work was repeated in man by Hinman and Maibach in 1963 showing indeed that in man epithelization could be sped. David Rovee's work showing that occlusion improved scar appearance expanded the concept of controlling wound repair to include dermal as well as epidermal events. In work conducted in the 1960s that ultimately led to a Nobel Prize, Stanley Cohen, observed that submaxillary gland extracts injected into new born mice led to earlier epidermal maturation as manisfested by early eyelid opening and precocious eruption of the incisors. He ultimately isolated EGF as the active principle in studies which reignited the search for agents able to act as "wound hormones."

2. ULCERS

2.1. Venous Ulcer

Although skin ulcers have been noted at different points throughout history, their recognition as specific entities, such as the venous, and the diabetic ulcer have a shorter formal history than acute wounds and injuries. The venous ulcer, most common of the leg ulcers today, is thought to not have been the most common leg ulcer in the 1700s and 1800s. Studies of medical records from that period indicate that leg ulcers were more frequent in men of 20–30 rather than in women and older people as is currently the case. The records suggest that this was related to the frequency of syphilitic, scorbutic, and tuberculous ulcers.

Hippocrates himself is said to have had a large ulcer. In 400 B.C.E., he wrote that "in the case of an ulcer, it is not expedient to stand, especially if the ulcer be situated on the leg." Hippocrates was also aware of the relationship between varicose veins and leg ulcers, as was Celsus. By 400 C.E., leg ulcers were treated by removing the veins which carried "rotten blood." Such "knowledge" notwithstanding, the dominant view of ulcers, especially those on the legs, was that they were portals to discharge unhealthy humors. Although it was considered permissible to improve them, healing ulcers were thought to be dangerous lest the humors ascend to other organs causing more serious disease. In ulcers healing too rapidly, especially in elderly, weak patients were deliberately inflamed with chemicals to stimulate a fresh flow. An alternative was to make a wound elsewhere, most often nearby or on the other leg, and keep it open and flowing with various foreign bodies while allowing the ulcer to heal. The dominance of the humoral theory faded by the early 1800s led by John Bill's teaching. Retardation of circulation and an association with varicose veins was considered an important pathologic factor by the eighteenth century. It was recognized that the valves of varicose veins could not resist high pressure and that their walls were weak. Although vessel ligation and pressure bandages were used by some, at this early date the theory that ulcers were safety valves which should not be compressed as they allowed noxious elements to escape was dominant and precluded widespread use of compression and vessel ligation. Subsequently, medical thought about venous ulcers became dominated by theories and treatment related to retrograde blood flow and stasis of blood flow. Trendelenburg claimed that there was a "private circulatory system" in the varicose veins. Unna believed that there was complete capillary insufficiency. In the mid-1800s, John Gay refuted the relationship between varicose veins and leg ulcers noting varicose ulcers in patients without varicosities and the converse. Hauxhausen's studies of blue dye injected into varicose veins refuted the idea of a private circulatory system and showed considerable flow which was improved with walking. His temperature studies indicated a greater flow in the infected legs. By 1917, Homan recognized the relationship of prior deep vein thrombosis. In the mid-1700s, surgeons recognized the curative effect of bed rest but found that short of constant confinement they recurred. Thomas Brynton of Bristol in 1797 described his method of applying adhesive strips about the limb and over the ulcer to draw the edges together and to support and prevent distention of the veins.

2.2. Diabetic Ulcers

Although Marchal de Cavi clearly described diabetic neuropathy and its relationship to diabetics in 1864 and in 1887, T. Davis Pryce assigned " ...considerable share [of the blame for a perforating foot ulcer] to diabetes and vascular disease." Until the 1930s, diabetes was only credited with causing the painful, dry, or senile gangrene of the foot. Rose and Carless in 1933 recognized in younger diabetic patients a wet gangrene with hot swollen painful foot ulcers under callosities. The link between neuropathies and the deformities as summarized by Charcot was recognized by Lambrinidi in 1937. D.H. Lawrence, himself a diabetic and among the first to use insulin, requested a wedge resection of his metatarsalphalangeal joint and toe leading to the so-called ray amputation, whose healing confirmed the lack of an arteriosclerotic basis for wet gangrene.

2.3. Pressure Ulcers

Pressure ulcers, known also as decubitus ulcers and bed sores, have been recognized throughout much of recorded medical history—bedsores have even been found by contemporary examinations of Egyptian mummies. The therapy recommended by the surgeon Ambrose Paré in his book, *Of Ulcers, Fistulas and Hemorrhoids*, is well illustrated by his description of the case of the Marquis of Auret in 1569. Sent by the French king, Paré found that the wounded Marquis had developed a "buttock bed sore" from "too long a time lying on it...." His treatment included a "rich meat broth ...," " ...a little pillow of down to keep his buttock (wound) in the air without his being supported on it ...," pain killers, a clean, dry, soft bed, and several olive oil-based unguentums for the wound. His approach illustrates a keen appreciation for the role of nutrition, cleanliness, and pressure relief. Although now nearly forgotten, the neurotrophic theory debate was in the mid-1800s centered on the pressure ulcer. Jean-Martin Charcot, whose epinomic foot deformity had also related to a lack of nerve-derived nutritional or trophic factors, supported the idea that both the decubitus acuta, pressure ulcers developing rapidly after paraplegia, and the decubitus chronica, slowly developing pressure ulcers in infirmed and debilitated patients, were strongly if not totally the result of absent neurotrophic factors. He supported his proposal with elaborate drawings of clinical cases and nerve pathways. Ultimately, experimental work in animals by Eduard Brown-Séquard showed that paraplegic animals did not develop ulcers, "... when I took care to prevent any part of their bodies from being in a continued state of compression...." When he allowed ulcers to develop, he cured them by "preventing compression." He also emphasized washing and cleanliness. The debate between Charcot, who dealt with patients, and Brown-Séquard, who studied animals, was heated, with Charcot inscribing above his door the sentence "You will not find a clinic for dogs here." By 1940 Michael Kosiak's now classic and prize-winning paper, Etiology and Pathology of Ischemic Ulcers, showed the inverse relationship between pressure and time and pressure ulcer development. His studies also demonstrated that redness and edema following release of pressure lasted about half as long as the duration of the pressure and that necrosis never occurred before three days. Microscopic pathology was found with as little as 60 mm of mercury for only one hour. The work by J. M. Milholland et al. in 1943 relating low plasma protein to pressure ulcers and showing the therapeutic effect of high protein diet on pressure ulcer healing added considerably to our understanding and ability to treat this still puzzling entity.

3. CONCLUSION

Looking over the history of wound healing, we can appreciate that many strides have been made in understanding and treatment especially of acute wounds. Bleeding can be controlled and infection is understood and in most cases controlled or overcome. Although we are still unable to sufficiently control and improve upon the natural healing of acute wounds, we are able to speed epithelization demonstrating that natural healing can be improved and making improved healing a goal of wound healers. Although our understanding and treatment abilities in the area of ulcers and chronic wounds is less advanced, many of the concepts which inhibited rational thinking about chronic wounds have been overcome and physicians and scientist have joined nurses in their concern for ulcers and chronic wounds.

2

Fetal Wound Repair

Amy Colwell
Department of Surgery, Brigham and Women's Hospital, Boston, Massachusetts, U.S.A.

Michael T. Longaker
Director of Children's Surgical Research, Stanford University Medical Center, Stanford, California, U.S.A.

H. Peter Lorenz
Division of Plastic Surgery, Stanford University Center for Children's Surgical Research, Stanford, California, U.S.A.

1. INTRODUCTION

Scar and fibrosis are the end result of postnatal tissue injury and disease. Remarkably, fetal full-thickness skin wounds heal with restoration of normal epidermal and dermal architecture and not with scar formation. The biology responsible for scarless wound healing, a paradigm for ideal tissue repair, has been actively researched since this discovery.

Despite extensive investigation, the mechanism of fetal wound healing remains largely unknown. We do know that, early in gestation, fetal skin is developing at a rapid pace and the extracellular matrix (ECM) is a loose network facilitating cellular migration. Wounding in this unique environment triggers a cascade of events culminating in a scarless wound phenotype. Comparison between postnatal and fetal wound healing has revealed differences in inflammatory response, cellular mediators, and ECM modulators. Further investigation may reveal novel genes essential to scarless repair and bring us closer to our ultimate goal: elimination of scar.

2. DEVELOPMENT

2.1. Fetal Skin

Since the transition from scarless to scarring wound repair occurs in the context of fetal skin development, an investigation of normal skin maturation is warranted. Development of the epidermis and dermis involves mutual inductive mechanisms between ectoderm and mesoderm. Epidermal primordial cells derived from ectoderm proliferate at 7 weeks gestation forming a squamous layer of periderm and a basal germinative layer. Periderm cells are keritinized, shed, and eventually replaced by the stratum corneum at 21 weeks. The basal germinative layer becomes the stratum germinativum, a source of new cells for dermal appendages and the intermediate layers found in mature skin. The dermis is derived from mesoderm. Mesenchymal cells produce collagen and elastic connective tissue fibers by 11 weeks. Skin maturation with dermal thickening continues into the postnatal period (1).

2.2. Fetal Extracellular Matrix

The fetal ECM is a dynamic layer of collagen, proteoglycans, and glycosaminoglycans which undergoes a series of changes during development. In the past, the ECM was regarded as an inert scaffolding. We now know that it has an important role in cell adhesion, migration, differentiation, and proliferation (2). Fetal ECM differs from adult ECM in collagen composition, hyaluronic acid (HA) content, and proteoglycan ECM modulators. This may have implications in scarless repair.

Type I collagen is the principal component of both adult and fetal ECM. However, fetal skin has a higher ratio of type III to type I collagen than adult skin (3). With maturation, the relative amount of type III collagen in fetal skin diminishes, although the adult phenotype is not seen until the postnatal period (4). Fetal skin contains more HA, the principal glycosaminoglycan of the ECM, than adult skin (5). The net negative charges of HA attract water molecules, thus tissues rich in HA are more "fluid" and facilitate cellular movement (2). Proteoglycan ECM modulators serve a role in collagen synthesis, maturation, and degradation. Decorin, lysyl oxidase, and matrix metalloproteinases (MMPs) increase during fetal skin development while fibromodulin, another modulator of collagen fibrillogenesis, decreases with maturation (6–9).

3. SCARLESS FETAL WOUND REPAIR SPECIFICITY

3.1. Scarless Fetal Wound Phenotype

The developing fetus has the unique ability to heal wounds by regenerating normal epidermis and dermis in contrast to scarring observed in the adult. Fetal wounds are distinguished from adult wounds by differences in collagen deposition and cross-linking patterns, HA content, and differential expression of proteoglycan ECM modulators (6–11).

In scarless fetal wounds, collagen is rapidly deposited in a fine reticular pattern indistinguishable from uninjured skin. In contrast, adult scarring wounds have disorganized thick collagen bundles with more collagen cross-linking (10–12). The HA content of scarless fetal wounds increases more rapidly, is more sustained, and is overall greater than that of adult wounds (5). Fetal wounds have greater HA-stimulating activity and fewer proinflammatory cytokines, such as IL-1 and TNF alpha, that downregulate HA expression (13).

The ECM architecture is influenced by regulators of collagen organization and degradation. Decorin, a modulator of collagen fibrillogenesis, is downregulated in fetal wounds while fibromodulin is upregulated in the fetus (6,9,14). This may prove useful as a marker of wound phenotype—if exogenous factors decrease scarring, they may decrease decorin and increase fibromodulin. Matrix metalloproteinases and tissue-derived inhibitors (TIMPs) function in ECM turnover. Overall, scarless wounds have a higher ratio of MMP to TIMP expression favoring remodeling and less accumulation of collagen (8).

3.2. Scarless Repair Is Intrinsic to Fetal Skin

The capacity for scarless repair was initially attributed to the sterile intrauterine environment. Amniotic fluid is rich in HA and growth factors but devoid of bacteria and inflammatory stimulators. However, early studies demonstrated that the intrauterine environment is neither essential nor sufficient for scarless repair. Fetal marsupials develop outside the uterus in a maternal pouch and heal cutaneous wounds without scar (15). Adult sheep skin transplanted onto the backs of fetal sheep bathed in the amniotic fluid of the intrauterine environment heal incisional wounds with scar (16).

Fetal scarless repair is also organ-specific. At time points early in gestation where fetal skin heals without scar, fetal stomach, intestine, and diaphragm heal with scar formation (17,18). This suggests that certain subpopulations of cells in skin modulate the local wound healing response. Further evidence implicates the fetal fibroblast as the effector cell responsible for scarless repair. Lorenz et al. (19) transplanted human fetal skin from 15–22 weeks gestation subcutaneously and cutaneously onto the backs of athymic adult mice. In this adult system, wounds created in the subcutaneous fetal grafts healed scarlessly with human collagen from fetal fibroblasts. Conversely, wounds made in the gestationally equivalent cutaneous fetal grafts healed with scar composed of mouse collagen from adult fibroblasts.

3.3. Scarless Repair Depends on Gestational Age and Wound Size

Fetal wounds pass from scarless repair to healing with scar formation during gestation. The ontogenetic transition of rat skin has been defined in an organ culture system and confirmed in vivo with confocal microscopic analysis (12,20). This transition point lies between days 16.5 and 18.5 of gestation (Term = 21.5 days). In a human fetal skin model, the transition point occurs after 24 weeks of gestation (19). Wound size modulates the transition point. In fetal lambs, increasing wound size increased the frequency of scarring at a gestational age when smaller wounds healed scarlessly (21). In nonhuman primates, the transition from scarless to scarring repair has been shown to proceed through an intermediate wound phenotype. Fetal monkey lip incisional wounds heal with restoration of normal epidermal appendage and dermal collagen architecture in midgestation. At the start of the third trimester, these wounds do not restore epidermal appendage (hair follicle and sebaceous gland) architecture, but still heal with a normal collagen dermal pattern. Thus, a "transition wound" phenotype occurs. By the mid-third trimester, the wounds heal with a typical scar pattern—no appendages and collagen scar (22).

4. MECHANISMS OF SCARLESS REPAIR

4.1. Wound Healing and Inflammation

The mechanisms underlying fetal wound specificity are under active investigation. In the postnatal animal, tissue injury disrupts the microvasculature of the skin allowing extravasation of blood elements into the wound. Contact with exposed collagen activates platelets causing discharge of their alpha granules and aggregation to form a platelet plug. Adhesion proteins and cytokines, such as platelet-derived growth factor (PDGF) and transforming growth factor-beta (TGF-β), promote additional platelet adhesion and aggregation. These cascades attract macrophages and neutrophils to the postnatal wound, which secrete a plethora of cytokines amplifying the inflammatory response and attracting fibroblasts (23). However, scarless wounds are characterized by a relative lack of inflammation. Furthermore, introduction of inflammation into normally scarless wounds produces dose-dependent increases in wound macrophages, neutrophils, collagen deposition, and scarring (24). This suggests an important role of inflammation in scar formation.

4.2. Cellular Inflammatory Mediators

4.2.1. Platelets and Neutrophils

The absence of an acute inflammatory infiltrate in scarless wounds may be partly explained by decreased fetal platelet degranulation and aggregation. Olutoye et al. (25) measured the aggregatory capabilities of adult and fetal porcine platelets after exposure to collagen and ADP. The fetal platelets responded suboptimally to collagen and showed an age-dependent aggregatory response to ADP exposure corresponding with the transition period for cutaneous scarless to scar-forming wounds. An age-dependent defect in the ability of fetal neutrophils to phagocytose pathogenic bacteria has also been demonstrated in fetal sheep (26).

4.2.2. Fibroblasts

Synthesis and remodeling of the ECM by fibroblasts are essential for wound healing. Adult and fetal fibroblasts are recruited to the site of injury by soluble chemoattractants released by macrophages and neutrophils. Fetal wounds characteristically have less inflammatory cells and cytokine expression yet heal more rapidly than adult wounds. This may be partly explained by intrinsic differences between adult and fetal fibroblasts.

Fetal fibroblasts have a greater ability to migrate into collagen gels than adult fibroblasts. A migration stimulation factor secreted by fetal fibroblasts is purported to be responsible for this enhanced migratory ability (27). Fetal fibroblasts have more surface receptors for HA, which also serves to enhance fibroblast migration (28).

Differences in contractile fibroblasts, termed "myofibroblasts", have also been reported. Wounds made early in gestation have virtually no myofibroblasts. In contrast, scarring fetal and postnatal wounds have progressively more active myofibroblasts, which correlates with contraction and degree of scarring (29).

4.3. Cytokines

4.3.1. Transforming Growth Factor-Beta (TGF-β)

The transforming growth factors were linked to wound healing shortly after their discovery more than 20 years ago. Isoforms TGF-β1 and TGF-β2 are thought to be profibrotic and to promote scar formation because their expression is increased in adult wounds and their exogenous administration to adult wounds increases collagen, protein, and inflammatory cell accumulation (30).

Evidence implicating TGF-β1 as a proscarring cytokine is well established. Scarless wounds in fetal mice have less TGF-β1 staining than neonatal or adult wounds (31). Insertion of PVA sponges containing TGF-β1 into rabbit wounds causes normally scarless wounds to heal with scar (31). Treatment of adult rat wounds with neutralizing antibodies to TGF-β1 and TGF-β2 reduces scar formation (32,33).

Furthermore, the relative proportion of TGF-β isoforms, and not the absolute amount of any one isoform, may determine the wound phenotype. In scarless fetal wounds, TGF-β3 expression is increased while TGF-β1 expression is unchanged. Conversely, TGF-β1 expression is increased and TGF-β3 decreased in scarring fetal wounds (34,35). This suggests the ratio of TGF-β3 to TGF-β1 may determine whether tissue regenerates or forms scar. Treatment of adult rat wounds with exogenous TGF-β3 reduces scar formation (36).

4.3.2. Other Growth Factors

The PDGF and fibroblast growth factor (FGF) are additional profibrotic cytokines. The PDGF, a potent mitogen and chemoattractant for fibroblasts, has prolonged expression during scar formation but disappears by 24 hr in fetal wounds (37). The FGF family of cytokines, including keritinocyte growth factors 1 and 2, has greater expression with increasing gestational age in fetal skin and during adult wounding (38). In contrast, vascular endothelial growth factor (VEGF) increases twofold in scarless wounds while its expression remains unchanged in scarring fetal wounds (39). Thus, an increased stimulus for angiogenesis and vascular permeability may assist in the rapid healing of fetal wounds.

4.3.3. Interleukins

Interleukins are cytokines important in chemotaxis and activation of inflammatory cell mediators. IL-6 stimulates monocyte chemotaxis and macrophage activation while IL-8 attracts neutrophils and stimulates neovascularization. Both IL-6 and IL-8 expression are significantly lower in early fetal fibroblasts at baseline and with PDGF stimulation compared to in adult fibroblasts (40,41). IL-10 has an anti-inflammatory function through decreased production of IL-6 and IL-8. Treating adult mouse wounds with an IL-10 over-expression adenoviral vector reduces inflammation and induces scarless healing (42). This may have potential therapeutic implications in human adult wounds.

4.4. Genetic Controls of Scarless Repair

The mechanistic differences between scarless and scarring repair are likely regulated at the gene expression level. Homeobox genes are transcription factors that are implicated in the patterning and cell type specificiation events during development. Their role in skin embryogenesis and wound healing is being investigated. Human homeobox genes MSX-1, MSX-2, and MOX-1 are differentially expressed in skin development (43). Additionally, human fetal scarless repair is associated with decreased expression of HOXB13 and increased PRX-2 expression (44). Given that scarless repair is inherent to developing skin, it seems likely that coordinated control of groups of genes by transcription factors, such as homeobox genes, has a crucial function during the repair process.

5. SUMMARY

Early in gestation, the fetus heals wounds with regeneration of normal epidermal and dermal architecture. Unique characteristics of fetal extracellular matrix, inflammatory cells, fibroblasts, cytokines, and developmental gene regulation may be responsible for the scarless wound phenotype. The ability to heal scarlessly is independent of the intrauterine environment but dependent upon gestational age and wound size. More research is necessary to unravel the mechanisms underlying scarless repair if we hope to devise more effective therapies for scar reduction and excess fibrosis.

REFERENCES

1. Moore KL. The integumentary system. Moore KL, Persaud TVN, eds. Before We were Born: Essentials of Embryology and Birth Defects. Philadelphia: W.B. Saunders Company, 1998:482–487.
2. Clark RAF. Wound repair: overview and general considerations. Clark RAF, ed. The Molecular and Cellular Biology of Wound Repair. Vol. 23. New York: Plenum Press, 1996:3–50.
3. Merkel JR, DiPaolo BR, Hallock GG, Rice DC. Type I and type III collagen content of healing wounds in fetal and adult rats. Proc Soc Exp Biol Med 1988; 187:493–497.
4. Hallock GG, Merkel JR, Rice DC, DiPaolo BR. The ontogenetic transition of collagen deposition in rat skin. Ann Plastic Surg 1993; 30:239–243.
5. Mast BA, Flood LC, Haynes JH, DePalma RL, Cohen IK, Diegelmann RF, Krummel TM. Hyaluronic acid is a major component of the matrix of fetal rabbit skin and wounds: implications for healing by regeneration. Matrix 1991; 11:63–68.
6. Beanes SR, Dang C, Soo C, Wang Y, Urata M, Ting K, Fohkalsrud EW, Benhaim P, Hedrick MH, Atkinson JB, Lorenz HP. Down-regulation of decorin, a transforming growth factor-beta modulator, is associated with scarless fetal wound healing. J Pediatr Surg 2001; 11:1666–1671.
7. Beanes SR, Dang C, Soo C, Lorenz HP. Ontogenetic transition in the fetal wound extracellular matrix correlates with scar formation. Wound Repair Regen 2001; 9:151.
8. Lorenz V, Soo C, Beanes SR , Dang C, Zhang X, Atkinson JB, Ting K. Differential expression of matrix metalloproteinases and their tissue-derived inhibitors in scarless fetal wound healing. Surg Forum 2001:397–401.
9. Soo C, Hu FY, Zhang X, Wang Y, Beanes SR, Lorenz HP, Hedrick MH, Mackool RF, Plass A, Kim SJ, Longaker MT, Freymiller E, Ting K. Differential expression of fibromodulin, a TGF-β modulator, in fetal skin development and scarless repair. Am J Pathol 2000; 157:423.
10. Longaker MT, Whitby DJ, Adzick NS, Cromblehome TM, Langer JC, Duncan BW, Bradley SM, Stein R, Ferguson MW, Harrison MR. Studies in fetal wound healing. VI. Second and third trimester fetal wounds demonstrate rapid collagen deposition without scar formation. J Pediatr Surg 1990; 25:63–69.
11. Whitby DJ, Ferguson MWJ. The extracellular matrix of lip wounds in fetal, neonatal, and adult mice. Development 1991; 112:651–668.
12. Beanes SR, Hu FY, Soo C, Dang CM, Urata M, Ting K, Atkinson JB, Benhaim P, Hedrick MH, Lorenz HP. Confocal microscopic analysis of scarless repair in the fetal rat: defining the transition. Plast Reconstr Surg 2002; 109:160–170.
13. Kennedy CI, Diegelmann RF, Haynes JH, Yager DR. Proinflammatory cytokines differentially regulate hyaluronan synthase isoforms in fetal and adult fibroblasts. J Pediatr Surg 2000; 35:874–879.
14. Soo C, Beanes S, Dang C, Zhang X, Ting K. Fibromodulin, a TGF-β modulator, promotes scarless fetal repair. Surg Forum 2001; 52:578–581.
15. Armstrong JR, Ferguson MWJ. Ontogeny of the skin and transition from scar free to scarring phenotype during wound healing in the pouch young of *Monodelphis domestica.* Dev Biol 1995; 169:242–260.
16. Longaker MT, Whitby DJ, Ferguson MWJ, Lorenz HP, Harrison MR, Adzick NS. Adult skin wounds in the fetal environment heal with scar formation. Ann Surg 1994; 219:65–72.

17. Longaker MT, Whitby DJ, Jennings RW, Duncan BW, Ferguson MW, Harrison MR, Adzick NS. Fetal diaphragmatic wounds heal with scar formation. J Surg Res 1991; 50:375–385.
18. Meuli M, Lorenz HP, Hedrick MH, Sullivan KM, Harrison MR, Adzick NS. Scar formation in the fetal alimentary tract. J Pediatr Surg 1995; 30:392–395.
19. Lorenz HP, Lin RY, Longaker MT, Whitby DJ, Adzick NS. The fetal fibroblast: the effector cell of scarless wounds repair. Plast Reconst Surg 1995; 96:1251–1259.
20. Ihara S, Motobayashi Y, Nagao E, Kistler A. Ontogenetic transition of wound healing pattern in rat skin occurring at the fetal stage. Development 1990; 110:671–680.
21. Cass DL, Bullard KM, Sylvester KG, Yang EY, Longaker MT, Adzick NS. Wound size and gestational age modulate scar formation in fetal wound repair. J Pediatr Surg 1997; 32:411–415.
22. Lorenz HP, Whitby DJ, Longaker MT, Adzick NS. Fetal wound healing: the ontogeny of scar formation in the non-human primate. Ann Surg 1993; 217:391–396.
23. Singer AF, Clark RAF. Cutaneous wound healing. N Engl J Med 1999; 341(10): 738–746.
24. Frantz FW, Bettinger DA, Haynes JH, Johnson DE, Harvey KM, Dalton HP, Yager DR, Diegelmann RF, Cohen IK. Biology of fetal repair: the presence of bacteria in fetal wounds induces an adult-like healing response. J Pediatr Surg 1993; 28:428–434.
25. Olutoye OO, Alaish SM, Carr ME, Paik M, Yager DR, Cohen IK, Diegelmann RF. Aggregatory characteristics and expression of fetal porcine platelets. J Pediatr Surg 1995; 30:1649–1653.
26. Jennings RW, Adzick NS, Longaker MT, Duncan BW, Scheuenstuhl H, Hunt TK. Ontogeny of fetal sheep polymorphonuclear leukocyte phagocytosis. J Pediatr Surg 1991; 26:853–855.
27. Schor SL, Schor AM, Grey AM, Rushton G. Fetal and cancer patient fibroblasts produce an autocrine migration stimulating factor not made by normal adult fibroblasts. J Cell Sci 1988; 90:391–399.
28. Chen WY, Grant ME, Schor AM, Schor SL. Differences between adult and foetal fibroblasts in the regulation of hyaluronate synthesis: correlation with migratory activity. J Cell Sci 1989; 94:577–589.
29. Estes JM, Vandeberg J, Adzick NS, MacGillirray TE, Desmonliere A, Gabbiani G. Phenotypic and functional features of myofibroblasts in sheep fetal wounds. Differentiation 1994; 56:173–181.
30. Roberts AB, Sporn MB. Transforming growth factor-β. In: Clark RAF, ed. The Molecular and Cellular Biology of Wound Repair. Vol.23. New York: Plenum Press, 1996:275–308.
31. Krummel TM, Michna BA, Thomas Bea. TGF-β induces fibrosis in a fetal wound model. J Pediatr Surg 1988; 23:647–652.
32. Nath RK, LaRegina M, Markham H, Ksander GA, Weeks PM. The expression of transforming growth factor type beta in fetal and adult rabbit skin wounds. J Pediatr Surg 1994; 29:416–421.
33. Shah M, Foreman DM, Gerguson MW. Neutralising antibody to TGF-beta 1,2 reduces cutaneous scarring in adult rodents. J Cell Sci 1994; 107:1137–1157.
34. Hsu M, Peled ZM, Chin GS, Liu W, Longaker MT. Ontogeny of expression of transforming growth factor-beta-1 (TGF-beta-1), TGF-beta-3, and TGF-beta receptors I and II in fetal rat fibroblasts and skin. Plast Reconstr Surg 2001; 107:1787–1794.
35. Dang C, Beanes SR, Soo BC, Hedrick MH, Lorenz HP. A high ratio of TGFß3 to TGFß1 expression in wounds is associated with scarless repair [abstract]. Wound Repair Regen 2001; 9:153.
36. Shah M, Foreman DM, Ferguson MW. Neutralisation of TGF-beta 1 and TGF-beta 2 or exogenous addition of TGF-beta 3 to cutaneous rat wounds reduces scarring. J Cell Sci 1995; 108:985–1002.

37. Whitby DJ, Ferguson MWJ. Immunohistochemical localization of growth factors in fetal wound healing. Dev Biol 1991; 147:207–215.
38. Dang CM, Beanes SR, Soo C, Lorenz HP. Decreased expression of fibroblast and keratinocyte growth factor isoforms and receptors during scarless repair. Plastic Reconstr Surg. In press.
39. Beanes SR, Dang C, Soo C, Lorenz HP. Differential expression of vascular endothelial growth factor in fetal wounds. Wound Repair Regen 2001; 9:154–155.
40. Liechty KW, Adzick NS, Crombleholme TM. Diminished interleukin 6 (IL-6) production during scarless human fetal wound repair. Cytokine 2000; 12:671–676.
41. Liechty KW, Crombleholme TM, Cass DL, Martin B, Adzick NS. Diminished interleukin-8 (IL-8) production in the fetal wound healing response. J Surg Res 1998; 77:80–84.
42. Gordon AD, Karmacharya J, Herlyn M, et al. Scarless wound healing induced by adenoviral-mediated overexpression of interleukin-10. Surg Forum 2001; 52:568–569.
43. Stelnicki EJ, Komuves LG, Holmes D, Clovin W, Harrison MF, Adzick NS, Largman C. The human homeobox genes MSX-1, MSX-2, and MOX-1 are differentially expressed in the dermis and epidermis of fetal and adult skin. Differentiation 1997; 62:33–41.
44. Stelnicki EJ, Arbeit J, Cass DL, Saner C, Harrison M, Largman C. Modulation of the human homeobox genes PRX-2 and HOXB13 in scarless fetal wounds. J Invest Dermatol 1998; 111:57–63.

3

Cellular and Molecular Regulation of Wound Healing

Gloria A. Chin
Department of Surgery, University of Florida, Gainesville, Florida, U.S.A.

Robert F. Diegelmann
Department of Biochemistry, Medical College of Virginia, Richmond, Virginia, U.S.A.

Gregory S. Schultz
Department of Obstetrics and Gynecology, University of Florida, Gainesville, Florida, U.S.A.

1. INTRODUCTION

Acute and chronic wounds share as many physiologic similarities as they do differences. Acute wounds normally heal in an orderly and efficient manner and progress smoothly through the four distinct but overlapping phases of wound healing: hemostasis, inflammation, proliferation, and remodeling (Fig. 1) (1–3). In contrast, chronic wounds will similarly begin the healing process but will have prolonged inflammatory, proliferative, or remodeling phases, resulting in tissue fibrosis and in nonhealing ulcers (4). The process of wound healing is complex and involves a variety of specialized cells such as platelets, macrophages, fibroblasts, and epithelial and endothelial cells. These cells interact with each other and with the extracellular matrix. In addition to the various cellular interactions, healing is also influenced by the action of proteins and glycoproteins such as cytokines, chemokines, growth factors, inhibitors, and their receptors. Each stage of wound healing has certain milestones that must occur in order for normal healing to progress. In order to identify the differences inherent in chronic wounds that prevent healing, it is important to review the process of healing in normal wounds.

2. PHASES OF ACUTE WOUND HEALING

2.1. Hemostasis

Hemostasis occurs immediately following an injury (5). In order to prevent exsanguination, vasoconstriction occurs and platelets undergo activation, adhesion, and aggregation at the site of injury. Platelets become activated when exposed to

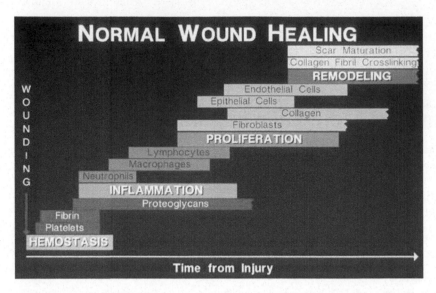

Figure 1 Phases of normal wound healing. Cellular and molecular events during normal wound healing progress through four major, integrated, phases: hemostasis, inflammation, proliferation, and remodeling.

extravascular collagen (such as type I collagen), which they detect via specific integrin receptors, cell surface receptors that mediate a cell's interactions with the extracellular matrix. Once in contact with collagen, platelets will release the soluble mediators (growth factors and cyclic AMP) and adhesive glycoproteins, which signal them to become sticky and aggregate. The key glycoproteins released from the platelet alpha granules include fibrinogen, fibronectin, thrombospondin, and von Willebrand factor. As platelet aggregation proceeds, clotting factors are released resulting in the deposition of a fibrin clot at the site of injury. The fibrin clot serves as a provisional matrix (6). The aggregated platelets become trapped in the fibrin web and provide the bulk of the clot (Fig. 2). Their membranes provide a surface

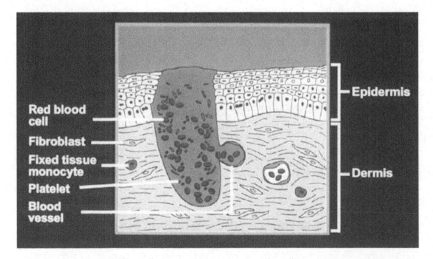

Figure 2 Hemostasis phase. At the time of injury, the fibrin clot forms the provisional wound matrix and platelets release multiple growth factors that initiate the repair process.

on which inactive clotting enzyme proteases are bound, become activated, and accelerate the clotting cascade.

Growth factors are also released from the platelet alpha granules and include platelet-derived growth factor (PDGF), transforming growth factor beta (TGF-β), transforming growth factor alpha (TGF-α), basic fibroblast growth factor (bFGF), insulin-like growth factor-1 (IGF-1), and vascular endothelial growth factor (VEGF). Neutrophils and monocytes are then recruited by PDGF and TGF-β from the vasculature to initiate the inflammatory response. A breakdown fragment generated from complement, C5a, and a bacterial waste product, f-Met-Leu-Phe, also provide additional chemotactic signals for the recruitment of neutrophils to the site of injury. Meanwhile, endothelial cells are activated by VEGF, TGF-α, and bFGF to initiate angiogenesis. Fibroblasts are then activated and recruited by PDGF to migrate to the wound site and begin production of collagen and glycosaminoglycans, proteins in the extracellular matrix that facilitate cellular migration and interactions with the matrix supporting framework. Thus, the healing process begins with hemostasis, platelet deposition at the site of injury, and interactions of soluble mediators and growth factors with the extracellular matrix to set the stage for subsequent healing events (1,2,7).

2.2. Inflammation

Inflammation, the next stage of wound healing, occurs within the first 24 hr after injury and can last for up to 2 weeks in normal wounds and significantly longer in chronic nonhealing wounds (Fig. 3). Mast cells release granules filled with enzymes, histamine, and other active amines, which are responsible for the characteristic signs of inflammation, the *rubor* (redness), *calor* (heat), *tumor* (swelling), and *dolor* (pain)

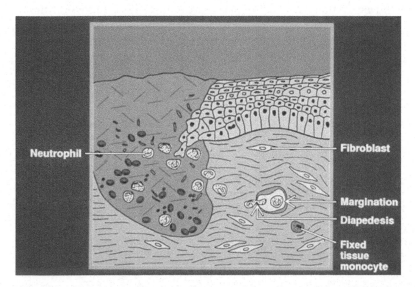

Figure 3 Inflammation phase. Within a day following injury, the inflammatory phase is initiated by neutrophils that attach to endothelial cells in the vessel walls surrounding the wound (margination), change shape and move through the cell junctions (diapedesis), and migrate to the wound site (chemotaxis).

around the wound site. Neutrophils, monocytes, and macrophages are the key cells during the inflammatory phase. They cleanse the wound of infection and debris and release soluble mediators such as proinflammatory cytokines (including IL-1, IL-6, IL-8, and TNF-α) and growth factors (such as PDGF, TGF-β, TGF-α, IGF-1, and FGF) that are involved in the recruitment and activation of fibroblasts and epithelial cell in preparation for the next phase in healing.

2.2.1. Neutrophils

Neutrophils are the first inflammatory cells to respond to the soluble mediators released by platelets and the coagulation cascade. They serve as the first line of defense against infection by phagocytosing and killing bacteria and by removing foreign materials and devitalized tissue. During the process of extravasation of inflammatory cells into a wound, important interactions occur between adhesion molecules [selectins, cell adhesion molecules (CAMs), and cadherins] and receptors (integrins) that are associated with the plasma membranes of circulating leukocytes and vascular endothelial cells (8,9). Initially, leukocytes weakly adhere to the endothelial cell walls via their selectin molecules that cause them to decelerate and begin to roll on the surface of endothelial cells. While rolling, leukocytes can become activated by chemoattractants (cytokines, growth factors, or bacterial products). After activation, leukocytes firmly adhere to endothelial cells as a result of the binding between their integrin receptors and ligands such as VCAM and ICAM that are expressed on activated endothelial cells. Chemotactic signals present outside the venule then induce leukocytes to squeeze between endothelial cells of the venule and migrate into the wounded tissue using their integrin receptors to recognize and bind to extracellular matrix components. The inflammatory cells release elastase and collagenase to help them migrate through the endothelial cell basement membrane and to migrate into the ECM at the site of the wound. Neutrophils also produce and release inflammatory mediators such as TNF-α and IL-1 that further recruit and activate fibroblasts and epithelial cells. After the neutrophils migrate into the wound site, they generate oxygen free radicals, which kill phagocytized bacteria, release high levels of proteases (elastase, neutrophil collagenase, and neutrophil collagenase MMP-8), and remove components of the extracellular matrix that were damaged by the injury. The persistent presence of bacteria in a wound may contribute to chronicity through continued recruitment of neutrophils and their release of proteases, cytokines, and reactive oxygen species. Usually, neutrophils are depleted in the wound after 2–3 days by the process of apoptosis and they are replaced by tissue monocytes.

2.2.2. Macrophages

Activated macrophages play pivotal roles in the regulation of healing, and the healing process does not proceed normally without macrophages. Macrophages begin as circulating monocytes that are attracted to the wound site beginning about 24 hr after injury (Fig. 4). They extravasate by the mechanism described for neutrophils and are stimulated to differentiate into activated tissue macrophages in response to chemokines, cytokines, growth factors, and soluble fragments of extracellular matrix components produced by proteolytic degradation of collagen and fibronectin (10). Similar to neutrophils, tissue macrophages have a dual role in the healing process. They patrol the wound area, ingesting and killing bacteria and removing devitalized tissue through the actions of secreted MMPs and elastase. Macrophages differ from neutrophils in their ability to more closely regulate the proteolytic

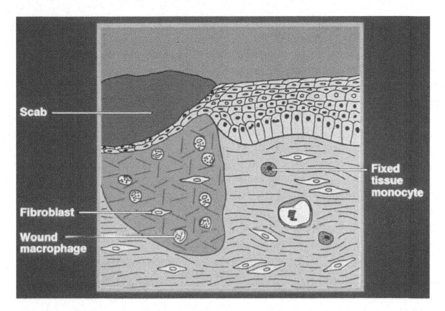

Figure 4 Proliferation phase. Fixed tissue monocytes activate, move into the site of injury, transform into activated wound macrophages that kill bacteria, release proteases that remove denatured ECM, and secrete growth factors that stimulate fibroblast, epidermal cells, and endothelial cells to proliferate and produce scar tissue.

destruction of wound tissue by secreting inhibitors for the proteases. As important as their phagocytic role, macrophages also mediate the transition from the inflammatory phase to the proliferative phase of healing. They release a wide variety of growth factors and cytokines including PDGF, TGF-β, TGF-α, FGF, IGF-1, TNF-α, IL-1, and IL-6. Some of these soluble mediators recruit and activate fibroblasts, which will then synthesize, deposit, and organize the new tissue matrix, while others promote angiogenesis. The absence of neutrophils and a decrease in the number of macrophages in the wound is an indication that the *inflammatory* phase is nearing an end and that the *proliferative* phase is beginning.

2.3. Proliferative Phase

The milestones during the *proliferative phase* include replacement of the provisional fibrin matrix with a new matrix of collagen fibers, proteoglycans, and fibronectin to restore the structure and function to the tissue. Another important event in healing is angiogenesis, the ingrowth of new capillaries to replace the previously damaged vessels and restore circulation. Other significant events in this phase of healing are the formation of granulation tissue and epithelialization. Fibroblasts are the key cells in the *proliferative phase* of healing.

2.3.1. Fibroblast Migration

Fibroblasts migrate into the wound in response to multiple soluble mediators released by initially platelets and later by macrophages (Fig. 4). Fibroblast migration in the extracellular matrix depends on precise recognition and interaction with specific components of the matrix. Fibroblasts in normal dermis are typically quiescent and sparsely distributed, whereas in the provisional matrix of the wound site and in the granulation tissue, they are quite active and numerous. Their migration and accumulation in the wound site requires them to change their morphology and to produce and secrete proteases to clear a path for their movement from the ECM into the wound site.

Fibroblasts begin moving by first binding to matrix components such as fibronectin, vitronectin, and fibrin via their integrin receptors. Integrin receptors attach to specific amino acid sequences (such as R–G–D or arginine–glycine–aspartic acid) or binding sites in these matrix components. While one end of the fibroblast remains bound to the matrix component, the cell extends a cytoplasmic projection to find another binding site. When the next site is found, the original site is released (apparently by local protease activity), and the cell uses its cytoskeleton network of actin fibers to pull itself forward.

The direction of fibroblast movement is determined by the alignment of the fibrils in the ECM and provisional matrix and the gradient of chemotactic growth factors, cytokines, and chemokines. Fibroblasts tend to migrate along these fibrils as opposed to across them. Fibroblasts secrete proteolytic enzymes locally to facilitate their forward motion through the matrix. The enzymes secreted by the fibroblasts include three types of MMPs, such as collagenase (MMP-1), gelatinases (MMP-2 and MMP-9) that degrade gelatin substrates, and stromelysin (MMP-3) that has multiple protein substrates in the ECM.

2.3.2. Collagen and Extracellular Matrix Production

The collagen, proteoglycans, and other components that comprise granulation tissue are synthesized and deposited primarily by fibroblasts. PDGF and TGF-β are two of the most important growth factors that regulate fibroblast activity. PDGF, which predominantly originates from platelets and macrophages, stimulates a number of fibroblast functions including proliferation, chemotaxis, and collagenase expression. TGF-β, also secreted by platelets and macrophages, is considered to be the master control signal that regulates extracellular matrix deposition. Through the stimulation of gene transcription for collagen, proteoglycans, and fibronectin, TGF-β increases the overall production of matrix proteins. At the same time, TGF-β downregulates the secretion of proteases responsible for matrix degradation and also stimulates synthesis of tissue inhibitor of metalloproteinases (TIMP), to further inhibit breakdown of the matrix. Recent data indicate that a new growth factor, named connective tissue growth factor, mediates many of the effects of TGF-β on the synthesis of extracellular matrix (11).

Once the fibroblasts have migrated into the matrix, they again change their morphology, settle down, and begin to proliferate and to synthesize granulation tissue components including collagen, elastin, and proteoglycans. Fibroblasts attach to the cables of the provisional fibrin matrix and begin to produce collagen. At least 20 individual types of collagen have been identified to date. Type III collagen is initially synthesized at high levels, along with other extracellular matrix proteins and proteoglycans. After transcription and processing of the collagen messenger ribonucleic acid (mRNA), it is attached to polyribosomes on the endoplasmic reticulum, where the new collagen chains are produced. During this process, there is an important step involving hydroxylation of proline and lysine residues. Three protein chains associate and begin to form the characteristic triple helical structure of the fibrillar collagen molecule, and the nascent chains undergo further modification by the process of gly-cosylation. Hydroxyproline in collagen is important because it plays a major role in stabilizing the triple helical conformation of collagen molecules. Fully hydroxylated collagen has a higher melting temperature. When levels of hydroxyproline are low, for example in vitamin C-deficient conditions (scurvy), the collagen triple helix has an altered structure and denatures (unwinds) much more rapidly at lower tempera-tures. To ensure optimal wound healing, wound care specialists should be sure that patients are receiving good nutritional support with a diet with ample protein and vitamin C.

Finally, procollagen molecules are secreted into the extracellular space, where they undergo further processing by proteolytic cleavage of the short, nonhelical seg-ments at the N- and C-termini. The collagen molecules then spontaneously associate in a head-to-tail and side-by-side arrangement forming collagen fibrils, which associ-ate into larger bundles that form collagen fibers. In the extracellular spaces, an important enzyme, lysyl oxidase, acts on the collagen molecules to form stable, cova-lent, cross-links. As the collagen matures and becomes older, more and more of these intramolecular and intermolecular cross-links are placed in the molecules. This important cross-linking step gives collagen its strength and stability, and the older the collagen, the more the occurrence of cross-link formation.

Dermal collagen on a per weight basis approaches the tensile strength of steel. In normal tissue, it is a strong molecule and highly organized. In contrast, collagen fibers formed in scar tissue are much smaller and have a random appearance. Scar tissue is always weaker and will break apart before the surrounding normal tissue.

2.3.3. Angiogenesis

Damaged vasculature must be replaced to maintain tissue viability. The process of angiogenesis is stimulated by local factors of the microenvironment including low oxygen tension, low pH, and high lactate levels (12). In addition, certain soluble mediators are potent angiogenic signals for endothelial cells. Many of these are pro-duced by epidermal cells, fibroblasts, vascular endothelial cells, and macrophages and include bFGF, TGF-β, and VEGF. It is now recognized that oxygen levels in tissues directly regulate angiogenesis by interacting with oxygen sensing proteins that regulate the transcription of angiogenic and antiangiogenic genes. For example, synthesis of VEGF by capillary endothelial cells is directly increased by hypoxia through the activation of the recently identified transcription factor, hypoxia-inducible factor (HIF), which binds oxygen (13). When oxygen levels surrounding capillary endothelial cells drop, levels of HIF increase inside the cells. HIF-1 binds to specific DNA sequences and stimulates transcription of specific genes, such as VEGF, that promote angiogenesis. When oxygen levels in wound tissue increase, oxygen binds to HIF, leading to the destruction of HIF molecules in cells and decreased synthesis of angiogenic factors. Regulation of angiogenesis involves both stimulatory factors like VEGF and antiangiogenic factors like angiostatin, endo-statin, thrombospondin, and pigment epithelium-derived factor.

Binding of angiogenic factors causes endothelial cells of the capillaries adjacent to the devascularized site to begin to migrate into the matrix and then proliferate to form buds or sprouts. Once again, the migration of these cells into the matrix requires the local secretion of proteolytic enzymes, especially MMPs. As the tip of the sprouts extends from endothelial cells and encounters another sprout, they develop a cleft that subsequently becomes the lumen of the evolving vessel and complete a new vascular loop. This process continues until the capillary system is sufficiently repaired and the tissue oxygenation and metabolic needs are met. It is these new capillary tuffs that give granulation tissue its characteristic bumpy or granular appearance.

2.3.4. Granulation

Granulation tissue is a transitional replacement for normal dermis, which eventually matures into a scar during the remodeling phase of healing. It is characterized from unwounded dermis by an extremely dense network of blood vessels and capillaries, elevated cellular density of fibroblasts and macrophages, and randomly organized collagen fibers. It also has an elevated metabolic rate compared with normal dermis, which reflects the activity required for cellular migration and division and protein synthesis.

2.3.5. Epithelialization

All dermal wounds heal by three basic mechanisms: contraction, connective tissue matrix deposition, and epithelialization. Wounds that remain open heal by contraction; the interaction between cells and matrix results in the movement of tissue toward the center of the wound. As previously described, matrix deposition is the process by which collagen, proteoglycans, and attachment proteins are deposited to form a new extracellular matrix. Epithelialization is the process where epithelial cells around the margin of the wound or in residual skin appendages, such as hair follicles and sebaceous glands, lose contact inhibition and by the process of *epiboly* begin to migrate into the wound area. As migration proceeds, cells in the basal layers begin to proliferate to provide additional epithelial cells.

Epithelialization is a multistep process that involves epithelial cell detachment and change in their internal structure, migration, proliferation, and differentiation (14). The intact mature epidermis consists of five layers of differentiated epithelial cells ranging from the cuboidal basal keratinocytes nearest the dermis up to the flattened, hexagonal, tough keratinocytes in the uppermost layer. Only the basal epithelial cells are capable of proliferation. These basal cells are normally attached to their neighboring cells by intercellular connectors called desmosomes and to the basement membrane by hemidesmosomes. When growth factors such as EGF, keratinocyte growth factor (KGF), and TGF-α are released during the healing process, they bind to receptors on these epithelial cells and stimulate migration and proliferation. The binding of the growth factors triggers the desmosomes and hemidesmosomes to dissolve so that the cells can detach in preparation for migration. Integrin receptors are then expressed, and the normally cuboidal basal epithelial cells flatten in shape and begin to migrate as a monolayer over the newly deposited granulation tissue, following along collagen fibers. Proliferation of the basal epithelial cells near the wound margin supply new cells to the advancing monolayer apron of cells (cells that are actively migrating are incapable of proliferation). Epithelial cells in the leading edge of the monolayer produce and secrete proteolytic enzymes (MMPs) that enable the cells to penetrate scab, surface necrosis, or eschar. Migration continues until the epithelial cells contact other advancing cells to form a confluent sheet. Once this contact has been made, the entire epithelial monolayer enters a proliferative mode and the stratified layers of the epidermis are re-established and begin to mature to restore barrier function. TGF-β is one growth factor that can speed up the maturation (differentiation and keratinization) of the epidermal layers. The intercellular desmosomes and the hemidesmosome attachments to the newly formed basement membrane are also re-established. Epithelialization is the clinical hallmark of healing, but it is not the final event—remodeling of the granulation tissue is yet to occur.

2.4. Remodeling

Remodeling is the final phase of the healing process in which the granulation tissue matures into scar and tissue tensile strength is increased (Fig. 5). The maturation of granulation tissue involves a reduction in the number of capillaries via aggregation into larger vessels and a decrease in the amount of glycosaminoglycans and the water associated with the GAGs and proteoglycans. Cell density and metabolic activity in the granulation tissue decrease during maturation. Changes also occur in the type, amount, and organization of collagen, which enhance tensile strength. Initially, type III collagen was synthesized at high levels, but it becomes replaced by type I collagen, the dominant fibrillar collagen in skin. The tensile strength of a newly epithelialized wound is only about 25% of normal tissue. Healed or repaired tissue is never as strong as normal tissues that have never been wounded. Tissue tensile strength is enhanced primarily by the reorganization of collagen fibers that were deposited randomly during granulation and increased covalent cross-linking of collagen molecules by the enzyme, lysyl oxidase, which is secreted into the ECM by fibroblasts. Over several months or more, changes in collagen organization in the repaired tissue will slowly increase the tensile strength to a maximum of about 80% of normal tissue.

Finally, in the process of collagen remodeling, collagen degradation occurs. Specific collagenase enzymes in fibroblasts, neutrophils, and macrophages clip the molecule at a specific site through all three chains and break it down to characteristic three-quarter and one-quarter pieces. These collagen fragments undergo further denaturation and digestion by other proteases.

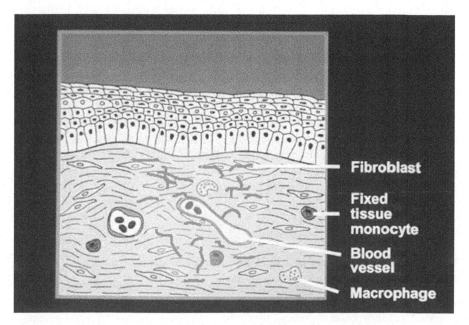

Figure 5 Remodeling phase. The initial, disorganized scar tissue is slowly replaced by a matrix that more closely resembles the organized ECM of normal skin.

2.5. Summary of Acute Wound Healing

Four phases of wound healing are as follows:

- Hemostasis—Establishes the fibrin provisional wound matrix, and platelets provide initial release of cytokines and growth factors in the wound.
- Inflammation—Mediated by neutrophils, and macrophages remove bacteria and denatured matrix components that retard healing and are the second source of growth factors and cytokines. Prolonged, elevated inflammation retards healing due to excessive levels of proteases and reactive oxygen that destroy essential factors.
- Proliferation—Fibroblasts, supported by new capillaries, proliferate and synthesize disorganized ECM. Basal epithelial cells proliferate and migrate over the granulation tissue to close the wound surface.
- Remodeling—Fibroblast and capillary density decreases, and initial scar tissue is replaced by ECM that is more similar to normal skin.

Cellular functions during the different phases of wound healing are regulated by key cytokines and growth factors. Cell actions are also influenced by interaction with components of the ECM through their integrin receptors and adhesion molecules. MMPs produced by epidermal cells, fibroblasts, and vascular endothelial cells assist in the migration of the cells, whereas proteolytic enzymes produced by neutrophils and macrophages remove denatured ECM components and assist in remodeling of initial scar tissue.

3. COMPARISON OF ACUTE AND CHRONIC WOUNDS

3.1. Normal and Pathological Responses to Injury

Pathological responses to injury can result in nonhealing wounds (ulcers), inadequately healing wounds (dehiscence), or in excessively healing wounds (hypertrophic scars and keloids). Normal repair is the response that re-establishes a functional equilibrium between scar formation and scar remodeling and is the typical response that most humans experience following injury. The pathological responses to tissue injury stand in sharp contrast to the normal repair response. In excessive healing, there is too much deposition of connective tissue that results in altered structure, and thus, loss of function. Fibrosis, strictures, adhesions, keloids, hypertrophic scars, and contractures are examples of excessive healing. Contraction is part of the normal process of healing, but if excessive, it becomes pathologic and is known as a contracture. Deficient healing is the opposite of fibrosis. It occurs when there is insufficient deposition of connective tissue matrix and the tissue is weakened to the point where scars fall apart under minimal tension. Chronic nonhealing ulcers are examples of severely deficient healing.

3.2. Biochemical Differences in the Molecular Environments of Healing and Chronic Wounds

The healing process in chronic wounds is generally prolonged, incomplete, and unco-ordinated, resulting in a poor anatomic and functional outcome. Chronic, nonhealing ulcers are a prime clinical example of the importance of the wound cytokine profile and the critical balance necessary for normal healing to proceed. As cytokines, growth factors, proteases, and endocrine hormones play key roles in regulating acute wound healing, it is reasonable to hypothesize that alterations in the actions of these molecules could contribute to the failure of wounds to heal normally. Several methods are used to assess differences in molecular environments of healing and chronic wounds. The mRNA and protein levels can be measured in homogenates of wound biopsies. The proteins in wounds can be immunolocalized in histological sections of biopsies. Wound fluids collected from acute surgical wounds and chronic skin ulcers are used to analyze the molecular environment of healing and chronic wounds. From these studies, several important concepts have emerged from the molecular analyses of acute and chronic wound environments.

The first major concept to emerge from wound fluid analysis is that the molecular environments of chronic wounds have reduced mitogenic activity compared with the environments of acute wounds (4). Fluids collected from acute mastectomy wounds, when added to cultures of normal human skin fibroblasts, keratinocytes, or vascular endothelial cells, consistently stimulated DNA synthesis of the cultured cells. In contrast, addition of fluids collected from chronic leg ulcers typically did not stimulate DNA synthesis of the cells in culture. In addition, when acute and chronic wound fluids were combined, the mitotic activity of acute wound fluids was inhibited. Similar results were reported by several groups of investigators who also found that acute wound fluids promoted DNA synthesis, whereas chronic wound fluids did not stimulate cell proliferation (15–17).

The second major concept to emerge from wound fluid analysis is the elevated levels of proinflammatory cytokines observed in chronic wounds when compared with the molecular environment of acute wounds. The ratios of two key inflammatory cytokines, TNF-α and IL-1β, and their natural inhibitors, P55 and IL-1 receptor antagonist, in mastectomy fluids were significantly higher in mastectomy wound fluids than in chronic wound fluids (Fig. 3). Trengove et al. (18) also reported high levels of the inflammatory cytokines IL-1, IL-6, and TNF-α in fluids collected from venous ulcers of patients admitted to the hospital. More importantly, levels of the cytokines significantly decreased in fluids collected 2 weeks after the chronic ulcers had begun to heal. Harris et al. (17) also found that cytokine levels were generally higher in wounds fluids from nonhealing ulcers than healing ulcers. These data suggest that chronic wounds typically have elevated levels of proinflammatory cytokines, and that the molecular environment changes to a less proinflammatory cytokine environment, as chronic wounds begin to heal.

The third important concept that emerged from wound fluid analysis was the elevated levels of protease activity in chronic wounds compared with acute wounds (4,19,20). For example, the average level of protease activity in mastectomy fluids determined using the general MMP substrate, Azocoll, was low (0.75 µg collagenase equivalents/mL, $n = 20$) with a range of 0.1–1.3 µg collagenase equivalents/mL (21). This suggests that protease activity is tightly controlled during the early phase of wound healing. In contrast, the average level of protease activity in chronic wound fluids (87 µg collagenase equivalents/mL, $n = 32$) was ~116-fold higher ($p < 0.05$) than in mastectomy fluids. In addition, the range of protease activity in chronic wound fluids is rather large (from 1 to 584 µg collagenase equivalents/mL). More importantly, the levels of protease activity decrease in chronic venous ulcers 2 weeks after the ulcers begin to heal (21). Yager et al. (22) also found 10-fold higher levels of MMP-2 protein, 25-fold higher levels of MMP-9 protein, and 10-fold higher collagenase activity in fluids from pressure ulcers when compared with surgical wound fluids using gelatin zymography and cleavage of a radioactive collagen substrate.

Other studies using immunohistochemical localization observed elevated levels of MMPs in granulation tissue of pressure ulcers, along with elevated levels of neutrophil elastase and cathepsin-G (23). The TIMP-1 levels were found to be decreased while MMP-2 and MMP-9 levels were increased in fluids from chronic venous ulcers when compared with mastectomy wound fluids (24). Recently, Ladwig et al. (25) reported that the ratio of active MMP-9/TIMP-1 was closely correlated with healing outcome of pressure ulcers treated by a variety of protocols (Fig. 6).

It is interesting to note that the major collagenase found in nonhealing chronic pressure ulcers was MMP-8, the neutrophil-derived collagenase. Thus, the persistent influx of neutrophil-releasing MMP-8 and elastase appears to be a major underlying mechanism resulting in tissue and growth factor destruction and thus impaired healing. This suggests that chronic inflammation must decrease if pressure ulcers are to heal.

Other classes of proteases also appear to be elevated in chronic wound fluids. It has been reported that fluids from skin graft donor sites or breast surgery patients contained intact α1-antitrypsin, a potent inhibitor of serine proteases, very low levels of neutrophil elastase activity, and intact fibronectin (26). In contrast, fluids from the chronic venous ulcers contained degraded α1-antitrypsin, 10-fold to 40-fold higher levels of neutrophil elastase activity, and degraded fibronectin. Chronic leg ulcers were also found to contain elevated MMP-2 and MMP-9, and that fibronectin degradation in chronic wounds was dependent on the relative levels of elastase, α1-proteinase inhibitor, and α2-macroglobulin (27,28).

Besides being implicated in degrading essential extracellular matrix components like fibronectin, proteases in chronic wound fluids have also been reported to degrade exogenous growth factors in vitro such as EGF, TGF1-α, or PDGF (1,21,29,30). In contrast, exogenous growth factors were stable in acute surgical

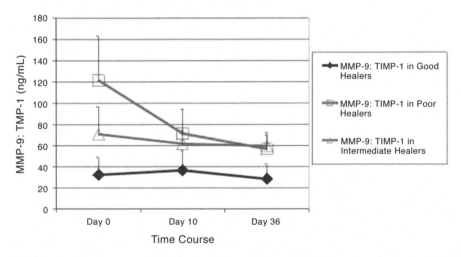

Figure 6 Low protease/inhibitor ratios correlate with healing. Low values of the ratio of MMP-9/TIMP-1 in wound fluids from patients with chronic pressure ulcers correlate with healing of chronic pressure ulcers over 36 days of treatment, supporting the concept that high protease/inhibitor ratios prevent healing of chronic wounds.

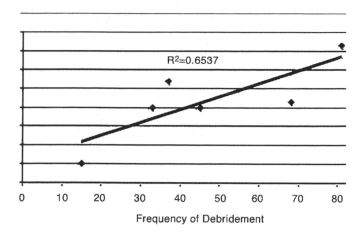

Figure 7 Frequency of wound debridement correlates with improved healing. There was a strong correlation between frequency of debridement and healing of chronic diabetic foot ulcers, supporting the concept that the abnormal cellular and molecular environment of chronic wounds impairs healing.

wound fluids in vitro. Supporting this general concept of increased degradation of endogenous growth factors by proteases in chronic wounds, the average immunoreactive levels of some growth factors such as EGF, TGF-β, PDGF were found to be lower in chronic wound fluids than in acute wound fluids, whereas PDGF-AB, TGF-α, and IGF-1 were not lower (29,31).

In general, these results suggest that many chronic wounds contain elevated MMP and neutrophil elastase activities. The physiological implications of these data are that elevated protease activities in some chronic wounds may directly contribute to the failure of wounds to heal by degrading proteins that are necessary for wound healing, such as extracellular matrix proteins, growth factors, their receptors, and protease inhibitors. Interestingly, Steed et al. (32) reported that extensive debridement of diabetic foot ulcers improved healing in patients treated with placebo or with recombinant human PDGF (Fig. 7). It is likely that frequent sharp debridement of diabetic ulcers helps to convert the detrimental molecular environment of a chronic wound into a pseudo-acute wound molecular environment.

3.3. Biological Differences in the Response of Chronic Wound Cells to Growth Factors

The biochemical analyses of healing and chronic wound fluids and biopsies have suggested that there are important molecular differences in the wound environments. However, these data only indicate half of the picture. The other essential component is the capacity of the wound cells to respond to cytokines and growth factors. Interesting new data are emerging, which suggest that fibroblasts in skin ulcers, which have failed to heal for many years, may not be capable of responding to growth factors and divide as fibroblasts in healing wounds. Agren et al. (33) reported that fibroblasts from chronic venous leg ulcers grew to lower density than fibroblasts from acute wounds from uninjured dermis. In addition, fibroblasts from venous leg ulcers that had been present > 3 years grew more slowly and responded more poorly to PDGF than fibroblasts from venous ulcers that had been present for < 3 years. These results suggest that fibroblasts in ulcers of long duration may approach senescence and have a decreased response to exogenous growth factors.

4. FROM BENCH TO BEDSIDE

4.1. Role of Endocrine Hormones in the Regulation of Wound Healing

Classical endocrine hormones are molecules that are synthesized by a specialized tissue and secreted into the blood stream, which are then carried to distant target tissue where they interact with specific cellular receptor proteins and influence the expression of genes that ultimately regulate the physiological actions of the target cell. It has been known for decades that alterations in endocrine hormones can alter wound healing. Diabetic patients frequently develop chronic wounds due to multiple direct and indirect effects of the *inadequate insulin action* on wound healing. Patients receiving anti-inflammatory *glucocorticoids* for extended periods are also at risk of developing impaired wound healing due to the direct suppression of collagen synthesis in fibroblasts and the extended suppression of inflammatory cell function. The association of *estrogen* with healing was recently reported by Ashcroft et al. (34) when they observed that healing of skin biopsy sites in healthy, postmenopausal women was significantly slower than in healthy premenopausal women. Molecular analyses of the wound sites indicated that TGF-β protein and mRNA levels were dramatically reduced in postmenopausal women in comparison with sites from premenopausal women. However, the rate of healing of wounds in postmenopausal women taking estrogen replacement therapy occurred as rapidly as in premenopausal women. Furthermore, molecular analyses of wounds in postmenopausal women treated with estrogen replacement therapy demonstrated elevated levels of TGF-β protein and mRNA that were similar to levels in wounds from premenopausal women. Aging was also associated with elevated levels of MMPs and decreased levels of TIMPs in skin wounds, which were reversed by estrogen treatment (35,36). The beneficial effects of estrogen on wound healing could be achieved with topical estrogen and were also observed in healthy aged men (37). These data indicate the significant interactions that can occur between endocrine hormones and growth factors in the regulation of wound healing.

4.2. Molecular Basis of Chronic Nonhealing Wounds

Conditions that promote chronic wounds are repeated trauma, foreign bodies, pressure necrosis, infection, ischemia, and tissue hypoxia. These wounds share a chronic inflammatory state characterized by an increased number of neutrophils, macrophages, and lymphocytes that produce inflammatory cytokines such as TNF-α, IL-1, and IL-6. In vitro studies have shown that TNF-α and IL-1 induce the expression of MMPs in a variety of cells including macrophages, fibroblasts, keratinocytes, and endothelial cells. They are also involved in the downregulation of TIMP expression. Although there may be a relative excess of MMPs in the wound, they are secreted as proenzymes that require activation for matrix degradation to occur. Serine proteinases will degrade matrix components and activate MMPs, and neutrophil elastase, also present in increased concentrations in chronic wounds, is important in orchestrating matrix-degrading events (4,19,22,30). Although the inflammatory

MOLECULAR ENVIRONMENT OF WOUNDS

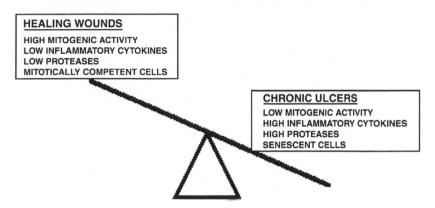

Figure 8 Comparison of the molecular and cellular environments of healing and chronic wounds. Elevated levels of cytokines and proteases in chronic wounds reduce mitogenic activities and response of wound cells, impairing healing.

profile differs in the various types of chronic ulcers, the general relationship is an increase in inflammatory cytokines that lead to the activation of proteinases and MMPs and a decrease in tissue inhibitors resulting in a degradative state and wound chronicity. Nwomeh et al. (20). further describe this common pathway as a selfperpetuating environment of oxygen metabolites and degradative enzymes that overwhelm the equilibrium to destroy the endogenous protease inhibitors to establish a chronic wound.

On the basis of these biochemical analyses of the molecular environments of acute and chronic human wounds, it is possible to propose a general model of differences between healing and chronic wounds. As shown in Fig. 8, the molecular environment of healing wounds promotes mitosis of cells and has low levels of inflammatory cytokines, low levels of proteases, and high levels of growth factors and cells capable of rapid division. In contrast, the molecular environments of chronic wounds generally have the opposite characteristics, i.e., not promote mitosis of cells, elevated levels of inflammatory cytokines, high levels of proteases, and low levels of growth factors and cells that are approaching senescence (38,21,18). If these general concepts are correct, then it may be possible to develop new treatment strategies that would re-establish in chronic wounds the balance of cytokines, growth factors, proteases, their natural inhibitors, and competent cells found in healing wounds.

4.3. Chronic Venous Stasis Ulcers

Mechanisms involved in the creation and perpetuation of chronic wounds are varied and depend on the individual wounds. In general, the inability of chronic venous stasis ulcers to heal appears to be related to impairment in wound epithelialization. The wound edges show hyperproliferative epidermis under microscopy, even though further immunohistochemical studies revealed optimal conditions for keratinocyte recruitment, proliferation, and differentiation. The extracellular matrix and the expression of integrin receptors by keratinocytes that allow it to translocate play an important regulatory role in epithelialization. After receiving the signal to migrate, epidermal cells begin by disassembling its attachments from basement membrane and neighboring cells. They then travel over a provisional matrix containing fibrinogen, fibronectin, vitronectin, and tenascin and stop when they encounter laminin. During this process, keratinocytes are producing fibronectin and continue to do so until the epithelial cells contact, at which time they again begin manufacturing laminin to regenerate the basement membrane.

There is evidence that the interaction between the integrin receptors on keratinocytes with the ECM will transform resting cells to a migratory phenotype. Integral in this transformation is the alteration in the pattern of integrin receptors expressed. After epithelialization is completed, integrin expression reverts back to the resting pattern. To further complicate this process, growth factors are involved in mediating keratinocyte activation, integrin expression, and in alterations in the matrix. Growth factors are able to differentially affect these processes; for example, TGF-β is able to promote epithelial migration while inhibiting proliferation. Although TGF-β induces the necessary integrin expression for migration, the cells behind those at the leading edge have little proliferative ability and so epithelial coverage of the wound is inhibited. Some chronic wounds may be deficient in TGF-β and its receptor (39).

4.4. Pressure Ulcers

Chronic wounds have also been demonstrated to have elevated matrix-degrading enzymes and decreased levels of inhibitors for these enzymes. Pressure ulcers , unlike chronic venous stasis ulcers, appear to have difficulty in healing related to impairment of ECM production. Studies have indicated that neutrophil elastase present in chronic wounds can degrade peptide growth factors and is responsible for degrading fibronectin. Pressure ulcers have also shown an increase in matrix metalloproteinases and in plasminogen activators in tissue. Chronic wound fluids demonstrate increased levels of gelatinases MMP-2 and MMP-9. Levels of MMP-1 and MMP-8 were also found to be higher in pressure ulcers and in venous stasis ulcers than in acute healing wounds. In addition, several of the endogenous proteinase inhibitors were shown to be decreased in chronic wounds. Proteinase inhibitors serve a regulatory role in matrix degradation by containing the matrix-degrading enzymes. Factors that promote MMP production or activation could counteract the effectiveness of proteinase inhibitors, for example, the destruction of TIMP by neutrophil elastase. The tissue inhibitor level to MMP ratio may indicate an imbalance that contributes to the wound chronicity.

4.5. Future Concepts for the Treatment of Chronic Wounds

Although the etiologies and the physical characteristics for the various types of chronic wounds are different, there is a common trend in their biochemical profiles. The precise pattern of growth factor expression in the different types of chronic wounds is not yet known, but it has been determined that there is generally a decreased level of growth factors and their receptors in chronic wound fluids. The absolute levels of growth factors may not be as important as the relative concentrations necessary to replace the specific deficiencies in the tissue repair processes. For the treatment of chronic wounds, Robson (40) proposed that growth factor therapy be tailored to the deficiency in the repair process. Therefore, the effectiveness of the therapy is predicated on adequate growth factor levels and the expression of their receptors balanced against receptor degradation by proteases and the binding of growth factors by macromolecules such as macroglobulin and albumin.

Studies that evaluated topical growth factor treatment of chronic wounds, such as PDGF in diabetic foot ulcers and EGF in chronic venous stasis ulcers, have shown an improvement in healing. These findings have led us to hypothesize that altering the cytokine profile of chronic wounds through the use of MMP inhibitors, addition of growth factors, and the elimination of inflammatory tissue and proteases by debridement would shift the wound microenvironment towards that of an acute wound, thereby improve healing.

Current treatment strategies are being developed to address the deficiencies (growth factor and protease inhibitor levels) and excesses (MMPs, neutrophil elastase, and serine protease levels) in the chronic wound microenvironment. Although the more specific and sophisticated treatments remain in the lab at this time, such as the new potent, synthetic inhibitors of MMPs and the naturally occurring protease inhibitors, TIMP-1 and α1-antitrypsin, available by recombinant DNA technology, the use of gene therapy in the treatment of chronic diabetic foot ulcers is currently being evaluated in a clinical trial. A phase III clinical trial is underway to determine the efficacy of KGF-2 in the treatment of chronic venous stasis ulcers. The treatment strategy to add growth factor to a chronic wound has been in place for the past several years. Regranex®, human recombinant platelet-derived growth factor (PDGF-BB), has been available for the treatment of diabetic foot ulcers and demonstrated ~20% improvement in healing compared with controls (41). In keeping with the strategy to restore a deficient wound environment, Dermagraph® and Apligraf®, engineered tissue replacements, have been applied to chronic diabetic ulcers (42,43). Although Apligraf® is no longer available, both tissue replacements have proven to be effective in selected types of ulcers. Other approaches to the treatment

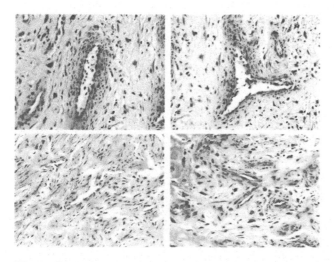

Figure 9 Oral doxycycline reduced inflammation in chronic pressure ulcer. Top panels show pressure before oral doxycycline treatment (100 mg, bid, 7 days). Note a large number of inflammatory cells (neutrophils) around inflamed vessels and reduced matrix (faint pink staining). Bottom panels show biopsies from the same patient following doxycycline treatment. Note reduced inflammation and increased matrix (intense pink staining).

of chronic wounds have been to remove the increased protease levels. This is, in part, the strategy of a vacuum-assisted negative pressure wound dressing (44) and in the recent development of dressings that bind and remove MMPs from the wound fluid, such as Pomogram® (45,46).

Another strategy is the use of a protease inhibitor to decrease MMPs and protease levels in the wound environment. Using an oral doxycycline (100 mg, bid, for 7 days), an MMP inhibitor, suggests some improvement in the healing of chronic wounds (Fig. 9). Low dose doxycycline (20 mg, bid) has been proven to be beneficial in other pathologic states such as periodontitis that are characterized by chronic, neutrophil-driven inflammation, and matrix destruction (47). In the future, treatment of chronic wounds may require the use of specific growth factors or inhibitors unique to the type of ulcer or use of combinations of selective inhibitors of proteases, growth factors, and tissue replacements to act synergistically to promote healing.

As previously described, endocrine hormones such as insulin, glucocorticoids, and estrogen have a regulatory role in wound healing. Although no current therapy exists that specifically addresses the molecular deficits created by inadequate insulin levels or to insulin intolerance, the treatment is directed at the local wound microenvironment. For patients who have been receiving long-term corticosteroids, the use of vitamin A has facilitated wound healing. There are studies at this time to determine the efficacy of topical estrogen applications on skin aging.

5. CONCLUSION

The molecular environment of chronic wounds contains elevated levels of inflammatory cytokines and proteases, low levels of mitogenic activity, and cells that often respond poorly to growth factors compared with acute, healing wounds. As chronic wounds begin to heal, this molecular pattern shifts to one that resembles a healing wound. As we continue to develop new information about the unique biochemical profiles associated with normal and pathologic wound healing responses, then the better prepared will be to develop new strategies to treat these costly clinical problems.

REFERENCES

1. Bennett Neil T, Schultz Gregory S. Growth factors and wound healing: part II. Role in normal and chronic wound healing. Am J Surg 1993; 166:74–81. 3–16–1995.
2. Bennett Neil T, Schultz Gregory S. Growth factors and wound healing: biochemical properties of growth factors and their receptors. Am J Surg 1993; 165:728–737. 3–16–1995.
3. Lawrence WT. Physiology of the acute wound. Clin Plast Surg 1998; 25:321–340.
4. Mast BA, Schultz GS. Interactions of cytokines, growth factors, and proteases in acute and chronic wounds. Wound Rep Reg 1996; 4:411–420.
5. Schultz GS. Molecular regulation of wound healing. In: Bryant RA, ed. Acute and Chronic Wounds: Nursing Management. 2nd ed. Philadelphia: Mosby, 2000:413–429.
6. Gailit J, Clark RAF. Wound repair in context of extracellular matrix. Curr Opin cell Biol 1994; 6:717–725.
7. Rumalla VK, Borah GL. Cytokines, growth factors, and plastic surgery. Plast Reconstr Surg 2001; 108:719–733.

8. Frenette PS, Wagner DD. Adhesion molecules, blood vessels and blood cells. N Engl J Med 1996; 335:43–45.

9. Frenette PS, Wagner DD. Molecular medicine, adhesion molecules. N Engl J Med 1996; 334:1526–1529.

10. Diegelmann RF, Cohen IK, Kaplan AM. The role of macrophages in wound repair: a review. Plast Reconstr Surg 1981; 68:107–113.

11. Duncan MR, Frazier KS, Abramson S, Williams S, Klapper H, Huang X, Grotendorst GR. Connective tissue growth factor mediates transforming growth factor beta-induced collagen synthesis: down-regulation by cAMP. FASEB J 1999; 13:1774–1786.

12. Bhushan M, Young HS, Brenchley PE, Griffiths CE. Recent advances in cutaneous angiogenesis. Br J Dermatol 2002; 147:418–425.

13. Semenza GL. HIF-1 and tumor progression: pathophysiology and therapeutics. Trends Mol Med 2002; 8:S62–S67.

14. O'Toole EA. Extracellular matrix and keratinocyte migration. Clin Exp Dermatol 2001; 26:525–530.

15. Bucalo B, Eaglstein WH, Falanga V. Inhibition of cell proliferation by chronic wound fluid. Wound Rep Reg 1993; 1:181–186.

16. Katz MH, Alvarez AF, Kirsner RS, Eaglstein WH, Falanga V. Human wound fluid from acute wounds stimulates fibroblast and endothelial cell growth. J Am Acad Dermatol 1991; 25:1054–1058.

17. Harris IR, Yee KC, Walters CE, Cunliffe WJ, Kearney JN, Wood EJ, Ingham E. Cytokine and protease levels in healing and non-healing chronic venous leg ulcers. Exp Dermatol 1995; 4:342–349.

18. Trengove NJ, Bielefeldt-Ohmann H, Stacey MC. Mitogenic activity and cytokine levels in non-healing and healing chronic leg ulcers. Wound Repair Regen 2000; 8:13–25.

19. Yager DR, Nwomeh BC. The proteolytic environment of chronic wounds. Wound Repair Regen 1999; 7:433–441.

20. Nwomeh BC, Yager DR, Cohen IK. Physiology of the chronic wound. Clin Plast Surg 1998; 25:341–356.

21. Trengove NJ, Stacey MC, Macauley S, Bennett N, Gibson J, Burslem F, Murphy G, Schultz G. Analysis of the acute and chronic wound environments: the role of proteases and their inhibitors. Wound Repair Regen 1999; 7:442–452.

22. Yager DR, Zhang LY, Liang HX, Diegelmann RF, Cohen IK. Wound fluids from human pressure ulcers contain elevated matrix metalloproteinase levels and activity compared to surgical wound fluids. J Invest Dermatol 1996; 107:743–748.

23. Rogers AA, Burnett S, Moore JC, Shakespeare PG, Chen WYJ. Involvement of proeolytic enzymes-plasminogen activators and matrix metalloproteinases-in the pathophysiology of pressure ulcers. Wound Repair Regen 1995; 3:273–283.

24. Bullen EC, Longaker MT, Updike DL, Benton R, Ladin D, Hou Z. Tissue inhibitor of metalloproteinases-1 is decreased and activated gelatinases are increased in chronic wounds. J Invest Dermatol 1995; 104:236–240.

25. Ladwig GP, Robson MC, Liu R, Kuhn MA, Muir DF, Schultz GS. Ratios of activated matrix metalloproteinase-9 to tissue inhibitor of matrix metalloproteinase-1 in wound fluids are inversely correlated with healing of pressure ulcers. Wound Repair Regen 2002; 10:26–37.

26. Rao CN, Ladin DA, Liu YY, Chilukuri K, Hou ZZ, Woodley DT. Alpha 1-antitrypsin is degraded and non-functional in chronic wounds but intact and functional in acute wounds: the inhibitor protects fibronectin from degradation by chronic wound fluid enzymes. J Invest Dermatol 1995; 105:572–578.

27. Wysocki AB, Staiano-Coico L, Grinnell F. Wound fluid from chronic leg ulcers contains elevated levels of metalloproteinases MMP-2 and MMP-9. J Invest Dermatol 1993; 101:64–68.

28. Grinnel F, Zhu M. Fibronectin degradation in chronic wounds depends on the relative levels of elastase, α1-proteinase inhibitor, and α2-macroglbulin. J Invest Dermatol 1996; 106:335–341.

29. Tarnuzzer RW, Schultz GS. Biochemical analysis of acute and chronic wound environments. Wound Repair Regen 1996; 4:321–325.

30. Yager DR, Chen SM, Ward SI, Olutoye OO, Diegelmann RF, Cohen IK. Ability of chronic wound fluids to degrade peptide growth factors is associated with increased levels of elastase activity and diminished levels of proteinase inhibitors. Wound Repair Regen 1997; 5:23–32.

31. Baker EA, Leaper DJ. Proteinases, their inhibitors, and cytokine profiles in acute wound fluid. Wound Repair Regen 2000; 8:392–398.

32. Steed DL, Donohoe D, Webster MW, Lindsley L. Effect of extensive debridement and treatment on the healing of diabetic foot ulcers. J Am Coll Surg 1996; 183:61–64.

33. Agren MS, Eaglstein WH, Ferguson MW, Harding KG, Moore K, Saarialho-Kere UK, Schultz GS. Causes and effects of the chronic inflammation in venous leg ulcers. Acta Derm Venereol Suppl (Stockh) 2000; 210:3–17.

34. Ashcroft GS, Dodsworth J, van Boxtel E, Tarnuzzer RW, Horan MA, Schultz GS, Ferguson MW. Estrogen accelerates cutaneous wound healing associated with an increase in TGF-beta1 levels. Nat Med 1997; 3:1209–1215.

35. Ashcroft GS, Horan MA, Herrick SE, Tarnuzzer RW, Schultz GS, Ferguson MW. Age-related differences in the temporal and spatial regulation of matrix metalloproteinases (MMPs) in normal skin and acute cutaneous wounds of healthy humans. Cell Tissue Res 1997; 290:581–591.

36. Ashcroft GS, Herrick SE, Tarnuzzer RW, Horan MA, Schultz GS, Ferguson MW. Human ageing impairs injury-induced in vivo expression of tissue inhibitor of matrix metalloproteinases (TIMP)-1 and -2 proteins and mRNA. J Pathol 1997; 183:169–176.

37. Ashcroft GS, Greenwell-Wild T, Horan MA, Wahl SM, Ferguson MW. Topical estrogen accelerates cutaneous wound healing in aged humans associated with an altered inflammatory response. Am J Pathol 1999; 155:1137–1146.

38. Trengove NJ, Langton SR, Stacey MC. Biochemical analysis of wound fluid from nonhealing and healing chronic leg ulcers. Wound Repair Regen 1996; 4:234–239.

39. Cowin AJ, Hatzirodos N, Holding CA, Dunaiski V, Harries RH, Rayner TE, Fitridge R, Cooter RD, Schultz GS, Belford DA. Effect of healing on the expression of transforming growth factor beta(s) and their receptors in chronic venous leg ulcers. J Invest Dermatol 2001; 117:1282–1289.

40. Robson MC. The role of growth factors in the healing of chronic wounds. Wound Repair Regen 1997; 5:12–17.

41. Smiell JM, Wieman TJ, Steed DL, Perry BH, Sampson AR, Schwab BH. Efficacy and safety of becaplermin (recombinant human platelet-derived growth factor-BB) in patients with nonhealing, lower extremity diabetic ulcers: a combined analysis of four randomized studies. Wound Repair Regen 1999; 7:335–346.

42. Falanga V, Margolis D, Alvarez O, Auletta M, Maggiacomo F, Altman M, Jensen J, Sabolinski M, Hardin-Young J. Rapid healing of venous ulcers and lack of clinical rejection with an allogeneic cultured human skin equivalent. Human Skin Equivalent Investigators Group. Arch Dermatol 1998; 134:293–300.

43. Kirsner RS, Falanga V, Eaglstein WH. The development of bioengineered skin. Trends Biotechnol 1998; 16:246–249.

44. Argenta LC, Morykwas MJ. Vacuum-assisted closure: a new method for wound control and treatment: clinical experience. Ann Plast Surg 1997; 38:563–576.

45. Cullen B, Smith R, McCulloch E, Silcock D, Morrison L. Mechanism of action of PROMOGRAN, a protease modulating matrix, for the treatment of diabetic foot ulcers. Wound Repair Regen 2002; 10:16–25.

46. Veves A, Sheehan P, Pham HT. A randomized, controlled trial of Promogran (a collagen/oxidized regenerated cellulose dressing) vs. standard treatment in the management of diabetic foot ulcers. Arch Surg 2002; 137:822–827.

47. Golub LM, McNamara TF, Ryan ME, Kohut B, Blieden T, Payonk G, Sipos T, Baron HJ. Adjunctive treatment with subantimicrobial doses of doxycycline: effects on gingival fluid collagenase activity and attachment loss in adult periodontitis. J Clin Periodontol 2001; 28:146–156.

4

Extracellular Matrix and Wound Healing

Jie Li and Robert S. Kirsner

Department of Dermatology and Cutaneous Surgery, University of Miami School of Medicine, Miami, Florida, U.S.A.

1. INTRODUCTION

The extracellular matrix (ECM) components play important roles in every step of wound healing processes by providing both scaffold support and signaling roles. They promote cell adhesion and migration during wound repair. They mediate the interactions between cells, cells and matrices, as well as matrix proteins. They also serve as reservoir and modulator for growth factors. For example, shortly after tissue injury, inflammatory cells need to interact with and migrate through the basement membrane ECM of the blood vessels to come to the site of the injury. During the reepithelialization, the ECM provides tracks and signals for epithelial keratinocytes to migrate on the wound surface matrix and reestablish the skin cover. ECM proteins play critical roles in the granulation tissue formation, including angiogenesis and matrix formation, which contribute to the reestablishment of dermis. Most remarkably, the formation of functional basement membrane in dermal–epidermal junction, by ECM protein interactions, is essential for connecting epidermis to dermis and is crucial to restore the integrity and function of the skin.

For past decade, there has been enormous progress that has shed light on the structural and biological functions of these ECM components. There are some major general properties of ECM that define some mechanisms of their actions. Each molecule consists of a series of structural and functional subdomains for binding to cells, as well as to other ECM molecules. Extracellular matrix binds cells through specific cell surface receptors, of which integrins are the major receptors for ECM proteins. The sequence Arg-Gly-Asp (RGD) has been found frequently to be the major recognition sequence for cell surface integrin receptors. Most of molecules have repetitive structural units such as epidermal growth factor (EGF) - or fibronectin-like repeats that can be specialized for different functions. These molecules can form homo- or hetero-dimers or polymers, often by formation of disulfide bonds between two chains or sometimes by noncovalent association. Each family of closely related proteins consists of number of members generated from different genes or from the same gene by alternative splicing or gene duplication. In human skin, fibroblasts are the major resource for ECM synthesis and deposition, keratinocytes and endothelial cells also produce some ECM component, such as collagen type IV, VII and laminins that present in basement membranes. The expression and function of these ECM proteins and their receptors are highly regulated spatially and temporally during wound healing and tissue remodeling. Inappropriate deposition of ECM components will impair the normal healing and function of the tissues. Due to page limitation, in this chapter, we will only discuss some of ECM components and their roles in wound repair.

2. COLLAGEN

Collagens are the most abundant ECM proteins in the tissue. Collagen family proteins are homo- or hetero-trimeric glycoproteins. Each collagen is composed of three α chains that can be identical or different. A structural feature of each collagen α chain polypeptide sequence is the repetitive motif of (Gly-X-Y)n, where every third amino acid is a glycine and X and Y represent amino acids other than glycine. This sequence structure allows three collagen α chains fold into a triple helix. The collagen superfamily now includes 20 collagen types with more than 38 genetically distinct collagen α chains (1,2). According to their structures, collagens can be roughly divided into two supergroups, fibril-forming (types I, II, III, V, and XI) and non-fibrillar collagens. Integrins α1β1, α2β1, α3β1, α10β1, and α11β1 are the major cell surface receptors for collagens, while α2β1 binds much better with fibrillar collagens of I–III and α1β1 binds preferentially collagens IV and VI (3). In normal adult human skin, collagens comprise about 80% of dry weight of the dermis. During wound healing, impaired balance of collagen deposition and degradation leads to healing defects or the development of fibrosis. In addition to their structural scaffold roles, collagens promote cell attachment and migration. The non-collagen domains in many collagens also have some important functions that are distinct from those of the collagen domains, such as endostatin, a 22-KDa C-terminal fragment of type XVIII collagen is a potent endogenous inhibitor of angiogenesis and tumor growth by specifically inhibits endothelial cell proliferation (4). Mutations in collagen genes have been identified pathogenic in several human diseases, such as collagens I, III, and V in Ehlers–Danlos syndrome (EDS), collagen VII and collagen XVII in epidermolysis bullosa (EB) (1, Table 1).

2.1. Type I and Type III Collagens in Dermis

Type I and type III collagens constitute the major interstitial fiber-forming collagens in normal human dermis. Both type I and type III collagens are present in the same fiber structure. Type I collagen comprises 80% of the total collagen and is predominant in normal human dermis, while type III collagen, which comprises 10% of the total dermal collagen, provides additional tensile strength to the skin. Type I collagen has been shown strongly to promote keratinocyte attachment and migration. During wound healing, collagen III and fibronectin are deposited in the initial phase, and later on, collagen III is gradually replaced by collagen I. An in situ hybridization analysis detected spatial distribution of collagen I mRNA in granulation tissue in a rat wound model (5). Twenty-four hours after injury, type I collagen mRNA expression was found in the deep layers of granulation tissue. At day 6, strong expression of collagen I mRNA was found in most fibroblasts evenly

Table 1 Major Collagens Identified in the Skin

Location	Type	Function/structure	Related skin disease
BMZ			
Dermal-epidermal	IV	Major component of lamina densa	
	VII	Anchoring fibrils	Dystrophic EB
	XVII	Transmembrane, 180-kD bullous pemphigoid antigen	Atrophic EB
	XVIII	Multiplexin	
	XIX	FACIT	
Dermal vascular	IV	Major collagen component	
	VIII	Hexagonal network, vascular endothelium	
	XV	Multiplexin	
	XVIII	Multiplexin	
	XIX	FACIT	
Dermis	I	Major fibrils	EDS
	III	Major fibrils	EDS
	V	Fibrils associated into type I/III co-polymers	EDS
	VI	Microfibrils	
	XII	FACIT	
	XIV	FACIT	

Abbreviations: BMZ, basement membrane zone; FACIT, fibril-associated collagens with interrupted triple helix; Multiplexin, collagen protein with multiple triple-helix domains and interruptions; EB, epidermolysis bullosa; EDS, Ehlers-Danlos syndrome.
Note: See text for references.

distributed throughout the tissue. At day 13, the transcripts were found mainly in the upper layers of the tissue. After 4 weeks, only weak labeling was detected in restricted area of upper dermis. A similar time course has been found for collagen III mRNA expression (6).

2.2. Skin Basement Membrane Collagens

Collagens IV, VII, and XVII are the major collagen components in the basement membrane zone (BMZ) of dermo-epidermal junction (Fig. 1), with collagen IV the most abundant. Collagen IV forms a three-dimensional lattice-network within the lamina densa of the BMZ. In addition, collagen IV is also predominant collagen in the BMZ of dermal blood vessels. Collagen VII proteins, also called anchoring fibrils, span from the lamina densa of dermal–epidermal BMZ to the upper papillary dermis where they form a structure known as anchoring plaque that also contains collagen IV. Anchoring fibril loops are also associated with interstitial collagens of primarily types I and III collagens. Collagen XVII, also known as bullous pemphigoid antigen (BPAG-2 or BP180), is a 180-KDa trans-membrane protein located on hemidesmosome complex of basal keratinocytes. Collagen XVII has a short N-terminus inside cell and a long triple helix collagenous extracellular domains at its C-terminus that associate with anchoring filaments at lumina lucida of cutaneous basement membrane (1).

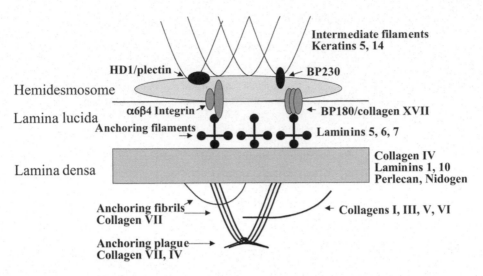

Figure 1 The schematic structure of dermal–epidermal basement membrane zone.

3. LAMININ

Laminins are the major non-collagenous glycoproteins of ECM present in a wide range of basement membranes within human tissues. All laminins are large, extracellular, heterotrimeric glycoproteins composed of α, β, and γ chain each, which form an asymmetric cross-shaped structure. To date, five α, three β, and three γ chains have been reported and shown to be distinct gene products, and total of 15 laminins have been identified (Table 2). Tissue specificity of laminin functions is achieved through the diversity of different combinations of three laminin chains. While the amino-terminus of laminin chains interact with underlying basement membrane, their carboxyl-terminal regions, notably the globular G domains of the long arm α

Table 2 Nomenclature of Currently Identified Laminins

Name	Chain composition	Main tissue distribution
Laminin 1	$\alpha1,\beta1,\gamma1$	Wide range
Laminin 2	$\alpha2,\beta1,\gamma1$	Muscle, nerve
Laminin 3	$\alpha1,\beta2,\gamma1$	Neuro-muscular junction
Laminin 4	$\alpha2,\beta2,\gamma1$	Ligaments
Laminin 5	$\alpha3,\beta3,\gamma2$	Epithelium
Laminin 6	$\alpha3,\beta1,\gamma1$	Epithelium
Laminin 7	$\alpha3,\beta2,\gamma1$	Epithelium
Laminin 8	$\alpha4,\beta1,\gamma1$	Blood vessels
Laminin 9	$\alpha4,\beta2,\gamma1$	ND
Laminin 10	$\alpha5,\beta1,\gamma1$	Epithelium, blood vessels
Laminin 11	$\alpha5,\beta2,\gamma1$	ND
Laminin 12	$\alpha2,\beta1,\gamma3$	ND
Laminin 13	$\alpha3,\beta2,\gamma3$	ND
Laminin 14	$\alpha4,\beta2,\gamma3$	ND
Laminin 15	$\alpha5,\beta2,\gamma3$	ND

Abbreviation: ND, not determined.
Note: See text for references.

chains, contain cell-binding sites and interact with cell surface receptors. Integrins $\alpha1\beta1$, $\alpha2\beta1$, $\alpha3\beta1$, $\alpha6\beta1$, $\alpha7\beta1$, $\alpha6\beta4$, $\alpha v\beta3$ and $\alpha v\beta5$ are reported major receptors for laminins. As it has recently been appreciated that laminins affect tissue morphogenesis and function by influencing the proliferation, migration, and differentiation of various types of cells (7). The biomedical importance of laminins is underscored by the discovery of gene mutations in the laminin chains in human diseases. For example, mutations found in laminin $\alpha2$ chain lead to some form of congenital muscular dystrophy. Deficiencies of laminin 5 have been linked to a severe and often lethal blistering disease called junctional EB (8,9).

3.1. Laminins in the Basement Membrane of Dermal–Epidermal Junctions

Several laminins have been reported present in the basement membrane of dermal–epidermal junction. Laminin 1, which is the prototype of laminin family, was the first reported present in the lamina densa. Three $\alpha3$ chain containing laminins, 5 ($\alpha3\beta3\gamma2$, previously named kalinin, epiligrin, nicein, BM600), 6 ($\alpha3\beta1\gamma1$, previously called k-laminin), and 7 ($\alpha3\beta2\gamma1$), are found within the lamina lucida. They are the integral components of the anchoring filaments traversing from the hemidesmosome across the lamina lucida to the lamina densa and involved in the attachment of epidermal keratinocytes to the basement membrane (10). Evidence that laminins are involved in skin wound repair mainly comes from studies of laminin 5. In response to wound, the leading keratinocytes in the outgrowing front-edge deposit laminin 5, which serves as a track to allow following keratinocytes to migrate and spread (11). Recently, a new member of laminin family, laminin 10 ($\alpha5\beta1\gamma1$), has been located within the lamina densa (12). It is also found a major laminin of dermal microvascular blood vessels. The laminin 10 showed strong promoting effects on human keratinocyte attachment. Laminin 10 knockout mouse skin exhibited discontinuity in BMZ lamina densa, hyper- and hypo-keratosis in the epidermis and fibrosis in the dermis, indicating its role in wound healing although its function and the mechanisms remain unclear (13).

3.2. Dermal Microvascular Laminins

It was long believed that blood vessel endothelial cells produced only one form of laminin, laminin 1 ($\alpha1\beta1\gamma1$). Until recently, it was found that the laminin $\beta1$ and $\gamma1$, but not $\alpha1$, transcripts were expressed by newly formed capillaries, indicating that laminin 1 is not present (14). Two newly identified laminins, 8 ($\alpha4\beta1\gamma1$) and 10 ($\alpha5\beta1\gamma1$), have been found as the major laminins produced by human skin dermal microvascular endothelial cells (HDMECs). Laminin 8 $\alpha4$ chain was found to promote HDMEC attachment, migration and microvascular capillary tubule formation, which could be blocked by antibodies directed against $\beta1$ or/and $\alpha v\beta3$ integrins (15). Antibody to the $\alpha4$ chain of laminin 8 inhibited endothelial cell branching (16), further suggesting a role of laminin 8 in angiogenesis. Monoclonal antibody 4C7, which is specifically directed against the $\alpha5$ chain of laminin 10, detected high expression of laminin 10 in HDMEC cells and stained strong positive in newly formed blood vessels of dermal granulation tissue in human skin wound, indicating an important role in wound angiogenesis (15).

4. BASEMENT MEMBRANE IN WOUND HEALING

The dermal–epidermal BMZ forms an attachment structure that its upper part serves as an attachment site for epidermal basal keratinocytes through the formation of hemidesmosome-anchoring filament complex, while the lower portion stabilizes the attachment to the underlying dermis by anchoring fibrils (Fig. 1, see Sec. 2 and 3 for details). The formation of intact functional BMZ is critical to reestablish the integrity of the skin during wound repair. The importance of individual BMZ proteins in providing skin integrity is evidenced by a group of inherited blistering diseases known as epidermolysis bullosa (EB), such as the mutations of hemidesmosome component collagen XVII in atrophic EB, defects of laminin 5 of major anchoring filaments in junctional EB, and deficiency of collagen VII anchoring fibrils in dystrophic EB.

5. FIBRONECTIN

Fibronectin is a large multifunctional glycoprotein found in blood plasma, fibrin clots, and ECM in various tissues. It comprises three general types of structural homologous repeating units, called types I, II, and III, which are organized into multiple structural domains with a variety of binding sites for cells and for other ECM molecules. Most cells can bind to fibronectin via $\alpha 3 \beta 1$, $\alpha 5 \beta 1$, or $\alpha v \beta 5$ integrin receptor at its central primary cell-binding domain that consists of an RGD (Arg-Gly-Asp) site and a synergy site. A second cell-binding site is located in an alternative splice region termed CS or V region containing a LDV (Leu-Asp-Val) sequence and an independent REDV (Arg-Glu-Asp-Val) sequence specific for $\alpha 4 \beta 1$ integrin receptor (17). In addition to the cell-binding, fibronectin functions through its specific binding sites interacting with other ECM components, such as fibrin, heparin, and collagen. It also contains the site for binding to another fibronectin molecule that leads to the assembly of the fibronectin into fibrils and matrices. Fibronectin is a key component of the provisional matrix during wound repair (18). It promotes cell migration and granulation tissue formation by providing scaffolding for contact guidance, a reservoir for cytokines and growth factors, and signals to cells through integrin receptors (19,20). During wound repair, human keratinocytes were found migrating on fibronectin via $\alpha 5 \beta 1$ integrin (21), while fibroblasts via $\alpha 3 \beta 1$ and $\alpha 5 \beta 1$ integrin receptors (22).

6. VITRONECTIN

Vitronectin, also called serum spreading factor, S-protein, and epibolin, is another glycoprotein of plasma and ECM. Vitronectin molecule is a 75 KDa monomer that can be proteolytically cut into two chains, of 65 KDa and 10 KDa, and linked by a disulfide bond. It has a cell-binding site with RGD sequence and a heparin-binding domain. The expression of vitronectin is not detectable in the normal skin of children. In normal adult skin, vitronectin is found at the periphery of dermal elastic fibers and accumulates as skin aging (23). Vitronectin is also a major component of provisional matrix, colocalized with fibronectin in fibrin clot, promotes cell adhesion and migration during wound healing. It has been demonstrated that keratinocytes bind vitronectin via $\alpha v \beta 5$ receptor (24). Keratinocytes from homozygous β5 integrin null mouse exhibited impaired migration on and adhesion to vitronectin (25). Attachment of fibroblasts to vitronectin is mediated by the integrin receptors, including αvβ1, αvβ3, αvβ5, and αIIbβ3 (26). In skin wound, vitronectin expression from day 7 was found increased in granulation tissue similar to the expression pattern of αv integrin and decreased in scar dermis by day 27 (27).

7. MATRICELLULAR PROTEINS

Matricellular proteins are referred to a group of secreted extracellular proteins that act contextually to modulate cell–matrix interactions, such as thrombospondin 1 and 2, SPARC, Tenascin C, and osteopontin. These macromolecules act as adapters by interacting with cell surface specific receptors, ECM, growth factors, and/or proteases but do not serve structural roles like other ECM molecules (28). They are expressed primarily in developing embryo tissues, adult tissues with continued turnover, such as skin, and in response to tissue injury.

7.1. Thrombospondins

To date, five thrombospondin (TSP) members have been identified. TSP consists of an NH2-terminal heparin-binding domain, a site for inter-chain disulfide bonding linking each subunit into a trimer, a linear domain in the center with a number of fibronectin-like repeats, and a COOH-terminal calcium binding domain. TSP1 and TPS2 are trimeric glycoproteins; each composed three identical subunits with molecular weight of 145 KDa. TSP1 is found in neural tube, head mesenchyme, platelets, and megakaryocytes. TSP2 expression is also found in megakaryocytes but not platelets, and confined to connective tissue and myoblasts. CD36 is a major cell surface receptor for TSP1-2, while some cells use integrins αIIbβ3 and avβ3 as well as integrin-associated protein (IAP) (28). TSP1-2 have some functions in common, such as modulating platelets function, cell adhesion, and migration, deposition of fibronecin, organization of collagen fibrils, and inhibition of angiogenesis (29). However, they are spatially and temporally regulated and exert some distinct roles during wound healing. Expression of both TSP proteins is induced in response to injury with inductions of TSP1 in early and TSP2 in late phase (30,31). The primary source of the TSP1 mRNA within wounds is from platelets and macrophage-like cells in the inflammatory infiltrate, while the major source of TSP2 is from fibroblasts. TSP1 has been shown to activate latent TGF-β in vitro (32). TSP1 null mice exhibited prominent inflammation responses possibly due to the deficiency of activated TGF-β.

7.2. Tenascins

Three tenascin family members have been described in mammalian system, tenascin-C (TNC, cytotactin), tenascin-R (TNR, restrictin, only found in the central nerve system), and Tenascin-X (TNX). They share a modular structure consisting of an NH2-terminal sequence responsible for oligomerization, a variable number of EGF-like repeats, fibronectin type III-like repeats, and a COOH-terminal fibrinogen-like globular domain. Tenascins exert pro- and counter-adhesive activities depending on their binding to other ECM proteins and to cell surface receptors. TNC, which exists predominantly as a hexamer with six subunits of 190–230 kDa linked by disulfide bonds, is widely expressed around motile cells, at proliferation site, in developing nervous system, blood vessels, cartilage, tendons, and skin. Tenascin-C was also shown increased expression at the margin of wounds, keloids and in the tumor stroma (33). Tenascin-C knockout mice exhibited defects in structure and repair of neuromuscular junctions, and in recovery from chemically induced dermatitis. There is significant decrease of fibronectin expression in the wounds of skin and corneas, indicating a role in regulating the expression or retention of fibronectin. In addition, keratinocytes are absent in corneal wound, suggesting a role in keratinocyte migration or survival (34). Tenascin-X is highly expressed in connective tissue of developing muscle, around tendons, ligaments, and in skin. Recent development identified the association between TNX gene deficiency and human disease Ehlers–Danlos syndrome (EDS), with typical skin and joint hyper-extensibility and easy bruising due to tissue fragility through alteration of collagen deposition (35,36).

7.3. SPARC (Secreted Protein Acidic and Rich in Cysteine)

Quite different from other matricellular proteins, SPARC consists of three modular domains representing different activities, an N-terminal acidic domain, a follistatin-like domain, and a C-terminal E-C domain. SPARC has potential roles in organization of ECM in connective tissue and basement membrane, due to the fact that SPARC binds to several ECM molecules including TSP1, vitronectin, nidogin, and collagen types I–V. SPARC is expressed in a variety of developing tissues and in adult tissue that undergo constantly turnover or in sites of wounds. SPARC exerts negative effects in vitro on cell proliferation, adhesion, and migration but positive effect on angiogenesis (37). In SPARC knockout mouse skin wound, there is a decrease of fibronectin (38,39).

REFERENCES

1. Myllyharju J, Kivirikko KI. Collagens and collagen-related diseases. Ann Med 2001; 33:7–21.
2. Tomono Y, Naito I, Ando K, Yonezawa T, Sado Y, Hirakawa S, Arata J, Okigaki T, Ninomiya Y. Epitope-defined monoclonal antibodies against multiplexin collagens demnstrate that type XV and XVIII collagens are expressed in specialized basement membranes. Cell Struct Funct 2002; 27:9–20.
3. Mercurio AM. Lessons from the α2 integrin knockout mouse. Am J Pathol 2002; 161: 3–6.
4. O'Reilly MS, Boehm T, Shing Y, Fukai N, Vasios G, Lane WS, Flynn E, Birkhead JR, Olsen BR, Folkman J. Endostatin: an endogenous inhibitor of angiogenesis and tumor growth. Cell 1997; 88:277–285.
5. Scharffetter K, Kulozik M, Stolz W, Lankat-Buttgereit B, Hatamochi A, Sohnchen R, Krieg T. Localization of collagen alpha 1(I) gene expression during wound healing by in situ hybridization. J Invest Dermatol 1989; 93:405–412.
6. Oono T, Specks U, Eckes B, Majewski S, Hunzelmann N, Timpl R, Krieg T. Expression of type VI collagen mRNA during wound healing. J Invest Dermatol 1993; 100:329–334.
7. Jones JC, Dehart GW, Gonzales M, Goldfinger LE. Laminins: an overview. Microsc Res Tech 2000; 51:211–213.
8. McGowan KA, Marinkovich MP. Laminins and human disease. Microsc Res Tech 2000; 51:262–279.
9. Uitto J, Pulkkinen L, McLean WH. Epidermolysis bullosa: a spectrum of clinical phenotypes explained by molecular heterogeneity. Mol Med Today 1997; 3:457–465.

10. Carter WG, Kaur P, Gil SG, Gahr PJ, Wayner EA. Distinct function for integrins $\alpha 3\beta 1$ in focal adhesion and $\alpha 6\beta 3$/bullous pemphigoid antigen in a new stable anchoring contact (SAC) of keratinocytes: relation to hemidesmossomes. J Cell Biol 1990; 111: 3141–3154.

11. Nguyen BP, Ryan MC, Gil SG, Carter WG. Deposition of laminin 5 in epidermal wounds regulates integrin signaling and adhesion. Curr Opin Cell Biol 2000; 12:554–562.

12. Miner JH, Cunningham J, Sanes JR. Roles for laminin in embryogenesis: exencephaly, syndactyly, and placentopathy in mice lacking the laminin alpha5 chain. J Cell Biol 1998; 143:1713–1723.

13. Li J, Tzu J, Chen Y, Zhang YP, Nguyen N, Gao J, Keene DR, Oro A, Miner JH and Marinkovich MP. Laminin 10 is essential for hair follicle development. EMBO J 2003; 22:2400–2410.

14. Sephel GC, Kennedy R, Kudravi S. Expression of capillary basement membrane components during sequential phases of wound angiogenesis. Matrix Biol 1996; 15:263–279.

15. Li J, Zhang YP and Kirsner RS. Angiogenesis in wound repair: Angiogenic growth factors and the extracellular matrix. Microsc Res Tech 2003; 60:107–114.

16. Gonzales M, Weksler B, Tsuruta D, Goldman RD, Yoon KJ, Hopkinson SB, Flitney FW, Jones JC. Structure and function of a vimentin-associated matrix adhesion in endothelial cells. Mol Biol Cell 2001; 12:85–100.

17. Huhtala P, Humphries MJ, McCarthy JB, Tremble PM, Werb Z, Damsky CH. Cooperative signaling by alpha 5 beta 1 and alpha 4 beta 1 integrins regulates metalloproteinase gene expression in fibroblasts adhering to fibronectin. J Cell Biol 1995; 129:867–879.

18. Greiling D, Clark RA. Fibronectin provides a conduit for fibroblast transmigration from collagenous stroma into fibrin clot provisional matrix. J Cell Sci 1997; 110:861–870.

19. Miyamoto S, Katz BZ, Lafrenie RM, Yamada KM. Fibronectin and integrins in cell adhesion, signaling, and morphogenesis. Ann NY Acad Sci 1998; 857:119–129.

20. Pereira M, Simpson-Haidaris PJ. Fibrinogen modulates gene expression in wounded fibroblasts. Ann NY Acad Sci 2001; 936:438–443.

21. Kim JP, Zhang K, Chen JD, Wynn KC, Kramer RH, Woodley DT. Mechanism of human keratinocyte migration on fibronectin: unique roles of RGD site and integrins. J Cell Physiol 1992; 151:443–450.

22. Xu J, Clark RA. Extracellular matrix alters PDGF regulation of fibroblast integrins. J Cell Biol 1996; 132:239–249.

23. Hintner H, Dahlback K, Dahlback B, Pepys MB, Breathnach SM. Tissue vitronectin in normal adult human dermis is non-covalently bound to elastic tissue. J Invest Dermatol 1991; 96:747–753.

24. Kim JP, Zhang K, Chen JD, Kramer RH, Woodley DT. Vitronectin-driven human keratinocyte locomotion is mediated by the alpha v beta 5 integrin receptor. J Biol Chem 1994; 269:26926–26932.

25. Huang X, Griffiths M, Wu J, Farese RV Jr, Sheppard D. Normal development, wound healing, and adenovirus susceptibility in beta5-deficient mice. Mol Cell Biol 2000; 20:755–759.

26. Clark RAF. Fibrin and wound healing. Ann NY Acad Sci 2001; 936:355–367.

27. Noszczyk BH, Klein E, Holtkoetter O, Krieg T, Majewski S. Integrin expression in the dermis during scar formation in humans. Exp Dermatol 2002; 11:311–318.

28. Bornstein P. Thrombospondins as matricellular modulators of cell function. J Clin Invest 2001; 107:929–934.

29. Streit M, Velasco P, Riccardi L, Spencer L, Brown LF, Janes L, Lange-Asschenfeldt B, Yano K, Hawighorst T, Iruela-Arispe L, Detmar M. Thrombospondin-1 suppresses wound healing and granulation tissue formation in the skin of transgenic mice. EMBO J 2000; 19:3272–3282.

30. DiPietro LA, Nissen NN, Gamelli RL, Koch AE, Pyle JM, Polverini PJ. Thrombospondin 1 synthesis and function in wound repair. Am J Pathol 1996; 148:1851–1860.

31. Kyriakides TR, Tam JW, Bornstein P. Accelerated wound healing in mice with a disruption of the thrombospondin 2 gene. J Invest Dermatol 1999; 113:782–787.

32. Murphy-Ullrich JE, Poczatek M. Activation of latent TGF-beta by thrombospondin-1: mechanisms and physiology. Cytokine Growth Factor Rev 2000; 11:59–69.

33. Jones PL, Jones FS. Tenascin-C in development and disease: gene regulation and cell function. Matrix Biol 2000; 19:581–596.

34. Mackie EJ, Tucker RP. The tenascin-C knockout revisited. J Cell Sci 1999; 112: 3847–3853.

35. Burch GH, Gong Y, Liu W, Dettman RW, Curry CJ, Smith L, Miller WL, Bristow J. Tenascin-X deficiency is associated with Ehlers–Danlos syndrome. Nat Genet 1997; 17:104–108.

36. Mao JR, Taylor G, Dean WB, Wagner DR, Afzal V, Lotz JC, Rubin EM, Bristow J. Tenascin-X deficiency mimics Ehlers–Danlos syndrome in mice through alteration of collagen deposition. Nat Genet 2002; 30:421–425.

37. Bradshaw AD, Sage EH. SPARC, a matricellular protein that functions in cellular differentiation and tissue response to injury. J Clin Invest 2001; 107:1049–1054.

38. Basu A, Kligman LH, Samulewicz SJ, Howe CC. Impaired wound healing in mice deficient in a matricellular protein SPARC (osteonectin, BM-40). BMC Cell Biol 2001; 2:15.

39. Bradshaw AD, Reed MJ, Sage EH. SPARC-null mice exhibit accelerated cutaneous wound closure. J Histochem Cytochem 2002; 50:1–10.

5

Matrix Metalloproteinases (MMPs)

Ganary Dabiri and C. Michael DiPersio
Albany Medical Center, Center for Cell Biology and Cancer Research,
Albany, New York, U.S.A.

1. PROTEOLYTIC REMODELING OF THE EXTRACELLULAR MATRIX DURING CUTANEOUS WOUND HEALING

The cutaneous extracellular matrix (ECM) is compartmentalized into the collagen-rich connective tissue matrix of the dermis and a specialized laminin-rich basement membrane that separates the epidermis from the underlying dermis. While both types of ECM are rich in various glycoproteins and proteoglycans, there are differences in the chemical composition and physical properties of the basement membrane and the dermal matrix. The cutaneous basement membrane is rich in laminins (i.e., laminins 5, 10/11), non-fibrillar collagens (i.e., collagen type IV) and proteoglycans (i.e., entactin, perlecan) and forms a sheet-like structure to which the basal keratinocyte layer of the stratified epidermis is attached (1,2). In contrast, the ECM of the dermis consists of layer of loose connective tissue adjacent to the basement membrane, and a deeper layer of dense connective tissue below the loose connective tissue. The dermal ECM consists of fibrillar collagens (i.e., collagens type I, II, III), non-collagenase proteins (i.e. fibronectin, elastin, fibrillin), and proteoglycans such as aggrecan, that are covalently linked to glycosaminoglycans (GAGs) such as hyaluronin (2,3).

Despite these differences in composition, the epidermal basement membrane and the dermal ECM have several important functions in common. A major function of both ECMs is to physically compartmentalize cellular and molecular components of the epidermis and the dermis and prevent cell invasion and movement of macromolecules between these two tissue compartments (3). In addition, resident cells of the skin bind to individual matrix proteins via integrins, the major family of cell adhesion receptors, as well as via other cell surface receptors such as syndecans (4,5). These interactions regulate cell attachment and migration during embryonic development and morphogenesis of skin, as well as during wound healing in postnatal skin (6). In addition to serving as a scaffold for cell adhesion and a barrier between tissue compartments, the ECM is a reservoir for many growth factors, cytokines, and proteases that are bound to matrix proteins in latent form. As discussed below, release and/or activation of ECM-bound factors by extracellular proteases can influence a number of cell functions important for tissue remodeling processes, including migration, angiogenesis, proliferation, and survival.

When the integrity of skin is compromised during wounding, both the dermal ECM and the epidermal basement membrane undergo extensive remodeling. These ECM remodeling events are tightly regulated by extracellular proteases that are expressed and secreted by the various cell types within both the epidermal and dermal compartments of the skin, including keratinocytes, melanocytes, and dendritic cells in the epidermis, and fibroblasts, macrophages, lymphocytes, and endothelial cells in the dermis and vasculature . One of the major enzyme families responsible for the proteolysis of the ECM is the matrix metalloproteinases (MMPs) (2,3,7). Although many different types of proteolytic enzymes are expressed during cutaneous wound healing, MMPs clearly play a key role in regulating cell migration, ECM degradation and assembly, and cell proliferation in the skin (8).

2. STRUCTURE AND FUNCTION OF MMPs

To date roughly 23 members of the MMP family have been discovered, and they can be divided into several groups based on their substrate specificity, domain organization, and/or sequence similarity. These groups are the collagenases, the gelatinases, the matrilysins, the membrane type MMPs (MT-MMP), and other MMPs (9). Here we will briefly describe some general characteristics of MMP structure and activation, with a focus on MMPs that are implicated in wound healing. A comprehensive and detailed description of the MMP family can be found in several excellent reviews that have been published in recent years (3,9–12). Most MMPs share an N-terminus signal peptide followed by a pro-peptide domain that inhibits protease activity by shielding the catalytic domain. This pro-peptide domain must be proteolytically cleaved by another MMP or protease for the MMP to be activated. Many MMPs contain a hemopexin domain, which modulates substrate recognition and specificity and is involved in binding to TIMPs (see the following sections). MT-MMPs differ from other MMPs in that they are anchored to the cell surface through a type I transmembrane domain, or interactions with glycosylphosphatidylinositol (GPI) anchored proteins. Transmembrane anchoring of MT-MMPs is important in that it restricts ECM proteolysis to the pericellular environment, and also scaffolds and nucleates multi-protein complexes that initiate protease cascades (discussed in the following sections). Some MMPs also contain a furin cleavage site necessary for their intracellular cleavage. MMP-2 and MMP-9 contain type II fibronectin repeats which contribute to substrate binding through interactions with gelatin, elastin and collagen (13).

3. REGULATION OF MMP EXPRESSION AND FUNCTION

MMPs are expressed and secreted as inactive pro-enzymes by a wide variety of cell types found in the wound environment, including fibroblasts and other dermal cells, epidermal keratinocytes, and inflammatory cells, and it is clear that MMP expression can be regulated at multiple levels within each of these cell types. There have been numerous studies describing the regulation of MMP gene expression (for reviews of this subject, see Ref. 14) (12,14). Collectively, these studies have shown that MMP gene expression can be induced by a wide variety of extracellular stimuli present in the wound environment, including growth factors, cytokines, and interactions of integrins with ECM (15). While the majority of this regulation occurs at the level of transcriptional regulation (12,16), an increasing number of studies in recent years have indicated an important role for post-transcriptional regulation of mRNA stability in the regulation of several MMPs (17–20). Both transcriptional and post-transcriptional mechanisms have been shown to involve mitogen-activated protein kinase (MAP kinase) signaling pathways. Transforming growth factor beta (TGFβ) and tumor necrosis factor alpha (TNFα) each induce MMP-9 expression in keratinocytes via the MAP kinases p38 and ERK (21,22). Similarly, epidermal growth factor (EGF) and hepatocyte growth factor (HGF) each induce MMP-9 in keratinocytes via an ERK pathway (23). In addition to gene regulation, a number of studies have shown that some MMPs can be regulated post-translationally at the level of protein secretion (18,19).

Activation of the pro-enzyme can occur in three different regulated processes; stepwise activation by other proteases, cell surface activation by another MMP, or intracellularly (9,13,24,25). *Stepwise activation* involves other proteinases such as plasmin. For example, during wound healing, plasmin-mediated cleavage of the pro-peptide may lead to the activation of certain MMPs, such as MMP-1, -2, and -9 (9,24,26). *Cell surface activation* can be mediated by MT-MMPs. For instance, MT1-MMP activates ProMMP-13 (27) and ProMMP-2 (13) through the formation of multi-meric complexes on the cell surface that involve interactions with TIMPs and/or the hemopexin domain (9). Finally, many MMPs, such as MT-MMPs, are activated *intracellularly* by Golgi-associated proteinases such as furin; these MMPs contain a furin cleavage site between the pro-peptide domain and the catalytic domain and are secreted in an active form (28).

Once MMPs are secreted and activated, their proteolytic activities can be further regulated through binding interactions with inhibitory proteins, such as members of the tissue inhibitor of matrix metalloproteinase (TIMP) family. To date, at least four TIMPs have been described; TIMP-1,-2,-3, and TIMP-4. TIMP-1 and TIMP-2 inhibit a broad range of MMPs. TIMP-3 preferentially inhibits MMP-1, -3,-7, and 13, and TIMP-4 inhibits MMP-2 and MMP-9 (3). TIMPs bind tightly to activated MMPs at the active site cleft, thereby competing for substrate binding and inhibiting MMP-mediated proteolysis (9). Therefore, even under conditions in which activated MMPs are present in the tissue microenvironment, the ratio of TIMP levels to MMP levels is a major factor in determining the extent of ECM degradation/remodeling that occurs (29).

4. ROLES FOR SPECIFIC MMPs IN CUTANEOUS WOUND HEALING

Generally speaking, once MMPs are expressed and exposed to the extracellular environment, their activity is restricted to the pericellular environment through binding to cell surface receptors, or by anchoring through the transmembrane domain in the case of the MT-MMPs (7). Importantly, there is enormous potential for different cell types in the wound environment to bind and utilize MMPs that are produced by other cell types and released into the extracellular environment. This sort of cross-talk between distinct cell types within the wound environment is likely to be important for the coordinated regulation of different aspects/stages of wound repair.

A number of individual MMP genes have now been knocked-out in mice, including MT1-MMP, and MMPs-2,-3,-7,-9, and -12. MT1-MMP-deficient mice showed a marked defect in turnover of collagen during wound healing (30). However, wound healing studies with other MMP-null mice have failed to identify necessary roles for individual MMPs, raising the possibility that different MMPs, or MMPs and other proteases, have overlapping or compensatory functions during wound repair. Consistent with this notion, while plasminogen-deficient mice showed impaired keratinocyte migration (31), treatment of these mice with an MMP inhibitor completely inhibited keratinocyte migration (32), suggesting that plasmin and MMPs play overlapping roles in re-epithelialization during wound healing. Despite the results of genetic studies with knockout mice, histological studies and cell culture studies of individual cell types from the wound environment strongly support important roles for specific MMPs in wound healing, as discussed below.

During wound healing, MMPs regulate the proteolytic degradation of existing basement membrane and dermal ECM, as well as the synthesis, deposition, and proteolytic processing of new ECM as the wound is repaired. However, the potential roles for MMPs clearly extend well beyond proteolysis of matrix proteins and ECM degradation (11). As outlined in Figure 1, additional functions of MMPs include proteolytic activation of other extracellular proteases and initiation of protease cascades, release of cryptic peptides or ECM-bound growth factors that promote cell migration, and activation of mitogenic factors, all of which can impact

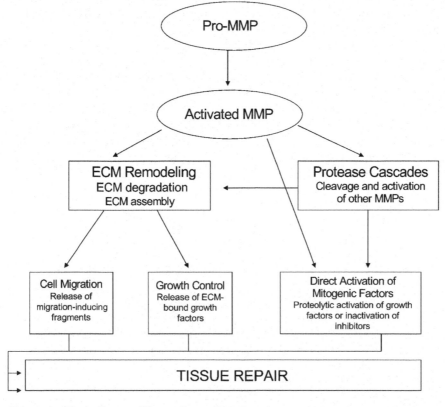

Figure 1   Flow diagram illustrating various functions and consequences of MMP activation that can impact tissue repair.

distinct cellular events that are important for tissue repair. Indeed, MMP-mediated degradation of the ECM leads to the release of growth factors and cryptic ECM ligands that can promote the proliferation, migration, and survival of various cell types involved in different aspects of wound healing including keratinocytes during re-epithelialization (15), inflammatory cells (33), endothelial cells during angiogenesis (34–36), and fibroblasts and other dermal cells during wound contraction (24). (See Table 1 for a list of MMPs and their putative roles in cutaneous wound healing.)

Some MMPs have been shown to directly or indirectly activate various growth factors during wound healing or other tissue remodeling processes. For example, the small proteoglycan decorin binds to TGFβ1 and serves as a reservoir for TGFβ1 in the ECM that is sequestered from cell surface receptors. It has been shown that degradation of decorin by MMP-2, -3, and -7 liberates ECM-bound TGFβ1 and promotes its bioavailability (10). Similarly, MMP-1 and MMP-3 can degrade the proteoglycan perlecan to release ECM-bound FGF (37), and MMP-9 has been shown to facilitate the release of ECM-bound vascular endothelial growth factor (VEGF) in some tumor models (38). MMPs can also directly activate mitogenic factors. For example, MMP-2 and MMP-9 can activate latent TGFβ1 by cleaving its latent associated peptide (LAP) (39).

During wound re-epithelialization keratinocytes express MMPs, some of which degrade ECM to expose cryptic ligands that promote migration. For example, basal keratinocytes bind to collagen in the provisional ECM of the wound via integrin α2β1, leading to induction of MMP-1 expression. MMP-1 then degrades collagen, which promotes cell migration and re-epithelialization of the wound (40). MMP-3 and MMP-10 are also expressed by migrating keratinocytes at the wound boundary in both normal and chronic wounds (29). MMP-2 and MT1-MMP have each been shown to cleave the basement membrane protein laminin-5, generating cleavage products that provide new cell adhesion ligands and induce epithelial cell migration (41,42). MMP-9 is also expressed in activated keratinocytes in response to both soluble factors and integrins and it is thought to promote wound re-epithelialization (22,43,44). TIMPs may also influence keratinocyte migration during wound healing, since in normal healing wounds TIMP-1 is expressed in wound edge keratinocytes, TIMP-2 is localized under the migrating epithelial tongue, and TIMP-3 is expressed in the proliferating epidermis of a wound (29).

Neutrophils, lymphocytes, and macrophages are recruited during wound healing to clear the wound site of debris (45). During the initial stages of wound healing, macrophages produce MMP-1; however, several days after re-epithelialization is complete they begin to express MMP-12 (15). Early in the inflammatory phase, MMP-9 that is stored in macrophages and in neutrophil granules is released into the microenvironment (33). Neutrophils also store and release MMP-8 (collagenase 2) (46).

MMPs play important roles in the angiogenic response during wound healing, as they facilitate vascular migration by dissolving the tissue in front of the sprouting vessel tip; i.e. as the vessel extends the surrounding tissue is remodeled (47). Several studies have identified interactions between integrin αVβ3 on endothelial cells and specific MMPs that regulate endothelial cell function and angiogenesis. For example, proteolysis of collagen type IV by MMP-2 exposes a cryptic binding site for αVβ3 that promotes angiogenesis (34,36). On the other hand, proteolysis of collagen type IV by MMP-2 or MMP-9 can liberate the peptide fragment tumstatin, which can interact with αVβ3 to inhibit integrin signaling and angiogenesis (35). Similarly, MMP-7 and MMP-9 can each cleave plasminogen to generate angiostatin, another

Table 1 MMPs Involved in Wound Repair

MMP number	Enzyme	Secreted by (cell type)	Substrates	Biological effects in wound healing
MMP-1	Collagenase 1	Keratinocytes, dermal cells, inflammatory cells	Type I collagen, fibronectin, MMP-2; MMP-9	Platelet aggregation, keratinocyte migration and re-epithelialization, dermal cell migration, reduced cell adhesion and spreading, bioavailability of IGF1 and cell proliferation
MMP-2	Gelatinase A	Dermal cells	Fibronectin, laminins	Dermal cell migration, epithelial cell migration, reduced cell adhesion and spreading, increased bioavailability of TGFβ1
MMP-3	Stromelysin 1	Keratinocytes, dermal cells	Fibronectin, perlecan, collagens (III, IV), decorin, laminin, plasminogen, IL-1beta; MMP-2/TIMP-2, MMP-7, MMP-8, MMP-9, MMP-13	Cell migration, bFGF release, reduced cell adhesion and spreading, increased bioavailability of TGFβ1, generation of angiostatin
MMP-7	Matrilysin 1	Dermal cells	Decorin, collagens IV fibronectin, laminin, plasminogen, Beta4-integrin; MMP-1, MMP-2, MMP-9, MMP-9/TIMP-1	Increased bioavailability of TGFβ1, generation of angiostatin
MMP-8	Collagenase 2	Inflammatory cells	Type I collagen, fibronectin	Neutrophil infiltration
MMP-9	Gelatinase B	Keratinocytes, inflammatory cells	Collagen IV, fibronectin, plasminogen, IL-1beta	Generation of angiostatin, anti- and pro-inflammatory
MMP-10	Stromelysin 2	Keratinocytes	Collagen III, MMP-1, MMP-8	Reduced IL-2 response
MMP-12	Macrophage elastase	Inflammatory cells	Collagen IV, fibronectin, vitronectin, laminin, fibrinogen fibrin, plasminogen	Generation of angiostatin
MMP-13	Collagenase 3	Dermal cells	Collagen III, plasminogen, fibronectin, MMP-9	Release of bFGF, anti-inflammatory
MMP-14	MT1-MMP	Dermal cells	Collagens (I-III), fibronectin, laminin, vitronectin, proteoglycans, MMP-2, MMP-13	Cell migration, anti-inflammatory

Source: Information in this table was compiled from several review articles (Refs. 9,15).

inhibitor of angiogenesis (10). Endothelial cells also express TIMP-1 and TIMP-3, which may contribute to the regulation of stromal remodeling and angiogenesis in the wound bed (29).

Fibroblasts play a key role in the formation of granulation tissue during wound healing (45). As activated growth factors stimulate fibroblasts from the intact dermis to migrate into the wound bed, MMPs facilitate this migratory process (45,48). For example, MMP-2 has been shown to colocalize with WAVE1 (WASP family verprolin-homologous proteins which activate Arp2/3 complex at the leading edge of lamellipodia) in dorsal ruffles, which may localize ECM proteolysis and promote fibroblast migration (49). MMP3 has also been shown to be important in wound contraction (50), since MMP-3-null mice fail to upregulate actin in dermal fibroblasts (51). TGFβ1 and connective tissue growth factor coordinately stimulate migrating fibroblasts to synthesize and secrete MMP-2 and MMP-9 that are necessary for ECM assembly and wound contraction (52).

5. IMBALANCES BETWEEN MMPs and TIMPs CONTRIBUTE TO PATHOLOGICAL WOUND HEALING

An imbalance between MMPs and TIMPs is frequently associated with pathological processes such as chronic wounds and autoimmune skin blistering diseases (15,53,54). For example, in chronically healing wounds such as pressure ulcers, MMP-8 is secreted at higher levels than in normal wounds. Similarly, while expression of TIMP-1 and -3 mRNAs was found in proliferating keratinocytes in normal healing epidermis, no epidermal expression of these TIMPs was detected in chronic ulcers. Reduced TIMP-2 expression near the migrating epithelial wound edge might contribute to uncontrolled activity of MMP-2 in chronic ulcers (29). MMP-13 is expressed abundantly by fibroblasts deep in the chronic ulcer bed, where it most likely plays a role in the remodeling of collagenous matrix (55,56). Increased TGFβ activity is associated with increased levels of MMP-2 in patients with chronic venous insufficiency, which leads to venous ulcers (18). There is also increased expression of MMP-2 and MMP-3 in dermal fibroblasts isolated from diabetic patients, which could contribute to the risk of non-healing foot ulceration in these patients (57).

In contrast with chronic wounds, fibrotic wounds such as severe burn trauma or hypertrophic scars (HTS) show increased levels of TIMP-1 expression (58) accompanied by decreases in MMP-1 and MMP-3, which may contribute to excessive accumulation of collagen in HTS (59). The mechanisms whereby these imbalances in MMPs and TIMPs arise remain unclear. However, there is evidence that MMP-1 expression in dermal fibroblasts is suppressed in response to platelet-derived growth factor (PDGF) through intracellular signaling pathways that activate the MAPK p38, which may contribute to the pathogenesis of cutaneous fibrosis (60). The underlying mechanisms leading to imbalances in MMP and TIMP expression need to be taken into consideration in the development of effective strategies for treatment of chronic and fibrotic wounds.

In summary, the diverse functions of MMPs are important during each stage of wound healing. Environmental or genetic factors that alter the expression and/or activities of MMPs or TIMPS can cause defects in the wound healing process, and imbalances in the relative expression levels of MMPs and TIMPs lead to the development of chronic or fibrotic wounds. Identification of factors that alter the expression or function of MMPs and TIMPs, and characterization of the molecular mechanisms whereby these factors lead to changes in MMP function, will greatly facilitate therapeutic approaches towards restoring normal wound healing in patients with chronic or fibrotic wounds. In addition, further characterization of specific roles for individual MMPs at distinct stages, or within distinct tissue compartments, of the wound healing process should contribute to the development of anti-MMP therapies. Topical therapies that are targeted specifically towards reducing local levels of MMPs in chronic non-healing wounds have recently entered into clinical trials. Despite the clearly important roles of MMPs in cutaneous wound healing, a more clear elucidation of their regulation needs to be addressed in vivo in order to fully understand their roles in tissue remodeling and wound repair.

REFERENCES

1. Burgeson RE, Christiano AM. The dermal–epidermal junction. Curr Opin Cell Biol 1997; 5:651–658.
2. Bosman FT, Stamenkovic I. Functional structure and composition of the extracellular matrix. J Pathol 2003; 200:423–428.
3. Stamenkovic I. Extracellular matrix remodelling: the role of matrix metalloproteinases. J Pathol 2003; 200:448–464.
4. Hynes RO. Integrins: bidirectional, allosteric signaling. Cell 2002; 110(6):673–687.
5. Couchman JR, Woods A. Syndecans, signaling, and cell adhesion. J Cell Biochem 1996; 61(4):578–584.
6. Wehrle-Haller B, Imhof BA. Integrin-dependent pathologies. J Pathol 2003; 200:481–487.
7. Werb Z. ECM and cell surface proteolysis: regulating cellular ecology. Cell 1997; 91(4):439–442.
8. Kahari VM, Saarialho-Kere U. Matrix metalloproteinases in skin. Exp Dermatol 1997; 6(5):199–213.
9. Visse R, Nagase H. Matrix metalloproteinases and tissue inhibitors of Metalloproteinases: structure, function, and biochemistry. Circ Res 2001; 92:827–839.
10. Vu TH, Werb Z. Matrix metalloproteinases: effectors of development and normal physiology. Genes Dev 2000; 14:2123–2133.
11. McCawley LJ, Matrisian LM. Matrix metalloproteinases: they're not just for matrix anymore!. Curr Opin Cell Biol 2001; 13(5):534–540.
12. Westermarck J, Kahari VM. Regulation of matrix metalloproteinase expression in tumor invasion. FASEB 1999; 13(8):781–792.
13. Woessner JF, Nagase H. Matrix Metalloproteinases and TIMPs. Oxford: Oxford University Press, 2000.
14. Vincenti MP. The matrix metalloproteinase (MMP) and tissue inhibitor of metalloproteinase (TIMP) genes. Transcriptional and posttranscriptional regulation, signal transduction and cell-type-specific expression. Methods Mol Biol 2001; 151:121–148.
15. Parks WC. Matrix metalloproteinases in repair. Wound Repair Regen 1999; 7:423–432.
16. Borden P, Heller RA. Transcriptional control of matrix metalloproteinases and the tissue inhibitors of matrix metalloproteinases. Crit Rev Eukaryot Gene Exp 1997; 7(1–2): 159–178.
17. Sehgal I, Thompson TC. Novel regulation of type IV collagenase (matrix metalloproteinase-9 and -2) activities by transforming growth factor-beta1 in human prostate cancer cell lines. Mol Biol Cell 1999; 10(2):407–416.
18. Saito S, Trovato MJ, You R, et al. Role of matrix metalloproteinases 1, 2, and 9 and tissue inhibitor of matrix metalloproteinase-1 in chronic venous insufficiency. J Vasc Surg 2001; 34(5):930–938.

19. Tamai K, Ishikawa H, Mauviel A, Uitto J. Inteferon-gamma coordinately upregulates MMP-1 and MMP-3 but not TIMP-1 expression in cultured keratinocytes. J Invest Dermatol 1995; 104(3):384–390.

20. Hieta N, Impola U, Lopez-Otin, et al. Matrix metalloproteinase-19 expression in dermal wounds and by fibroblasts in culture. J Invest Dermatol 2003; 121:997–1004.

21. Holvoet S, Vincent C, Schmitt D, Serres M. The inhibition of MAPK pathway is correlated with down-regulation of MMP-9 secretion induced by TNF-alpha in human keratinocytes. Exp Cell Res 2003; 290:108–119.

22. Johansson N, Ala-aho R, Uitto V, et al. Expression of collagenase-3 (MMP-13) and collagenase-1 (MMP-1) by transformed keratinocytes is dependent on the activity of p38 mitogen-activated protein kinase. J Cell Sci 2000; 113:227–235.

23. Zeigler ME, Chi Y, Schmidt T, Varani J. Role of ERK and JNK pathways in regulating cell motility and matrix metalloproteinase 9 production in growth factor-stimulated human epidermal keratinocytes. J Cell Physiol 1999; 180(2):271–284.

24. Wong TTL, Sethi C, Daniels JT, et al. Marix metalloproteinases in disease and repair processes in the anterior segment. Surv of Ophthalmol 2002; 47:239–256.

25. Murphy G, Gavrilovic J. Proteolysis and cell migration: creating a path. Curr Opin Cell Biol 1999; 11(5):614–621.

26. Monea S, Lehti K, Keski-Oja J, Mignatti P. Plasmin activates pro-matrix metalloproteinase-2 with a membrane-type 1 matrix metalloproteinase-dependent mechanism. J Cell Physiol 2002; 192(2):160–170.

27. Knauper V, Bailey L, Worley JR, et al. Cellular activation of pro-MMP-13 by MT1-MMP depends on the C-terminal domain of MMP-13. FEBS Let 2002; 532:127–130.

28. Santavicca M, Noel A, Angliker H. Characterization of structural determinants and molecular mechanisms involved in pro-stromelysin-3 activation by 4-aminophenyl-mercuric acetate and furin-type convertases. Biochem J 1996; 315:953–958.

29. Gomez DE, Alonso DF, Yoshiji H, Thorgeirsson UP. Tissue inhibitors of metalloproteinases: structure, regulation, and biological functions. Eur J Cell Biol 1997; 74:111–122.

30. Holmbeck K, Bianco P, Caterina J, et al. MT1-MMP deficient mice develop dwarfism, osteopina. Cell 1999; 99:81–92.

31. Romer J, Bugge TH, Pyke C. Impaired wound healing in mice with a disrupted plasminogen gene. Nat Med 1996; 2:287–292.

32. Lund LR, Romer J, Bugge TH. Functional overlap between two classes of matrix-degrading proteases in wound healing. EMBO J 1999; 18:4645–4656.

33. Kjeldsen L, Sengelov H, Lolike K. Isolation and characterization of gelatinase granules from human nuetrophils. Blood 1994; 83:1640–1649.

34. Silletti S, Kessler T, Goldburg J, et al. Disruption of matrix metalloproteinase 2 binding to integrin alphaV beta3 by an organic molecule inhibits angiogenesis and tumor growth in vivo. Proc Natl Acad Sci 2001; 98(1):119–124.

35. Kalluri R. Discovery of type IV collagen non-collagenous domains as novel integrin ligands and endogenous inhibitors of angiogenesis. Cold Spring Symp Quant Biol 2002; 67:255–266.

36. Xu J, Rodriguez D, Petitclere E, et al. Proteolytic exposure of a cryptic site within collagen type IV is required for angiogenesis and tumor growth in vivo. J Cell Biol 2001; 154(5):1069–1079.

37. Whitelock JM, Murdoch AD, Iozza RV, Underwood PA. The degradation of human endothelial cell derived perlecan and release of bound basic fibroblast growth factor by stromelysin, collagenase, plasmin, and heparanases. J Biol Chem 1996; 271:10079–10086.

38. Bergers G, Brekken R, McMahon G, et al. Matrix metalloproteinase-9 triggers the angiogenic switch during carcinogenesis. Nat Cell Biol 2000; 2(10):734–744.

39. Yu Q, Stamenkovic I. Cell surface-localized matrix metalloproteinase-9 proteolytically activates TGF-beta and promotes tumor invasion and angiogenesis. Genes Dev 2000; 14:163–176.

40. Pilcher BK, Dumin JA, Sudbeck BD, et al. The activity of collagenase-1 is required for keratinocyte migration on a type 1 collagen matrix. J Cell Biol 1997; 137(6):1445–1457.

41. Koshikawa N, Giannelli G, Cirulli V, et al. Role of cell surface metalloprotease MT1-MMP in epithelial cell migration over laminin-5. J Cell Sci 2000; 148(3):615–624.

42. Giannelli G, Falk-Marziller J, Schiraldi O. Induction of cell migration by matrix metalloprotienases-2 cleavage of Laminin-5. Science 1997; 277:225–258.

43. Larjava H, Lyons JG, Salo T, et al. Anti-integrin antibodies induce type IV collagenase expression in keratinocytes. J Cell Physiol 1993; 157(1):190–200.

44. DiPersio CM, Shao M, Di Costanzo L, Kreidberg JA, Hynes RO. Mouse keratinocytes immortalized with large T antigen acquire alpha3beta1 integrin-dependent secretion of MMP-9/gelatinase B. J Cell Sci 2000; 113(Pt 17):2909–2921.

45. Singer AJ, Clark RAF. Cutaneous wound healing. N Engl J Med 1999; 341(10):738–746.

46. Nwomeh BC, Liang HX, Cohen K, Yager DR. MMP-8 is the predominant collagenase in healing wounds and nonhealing ulcers. J Surg Res 1999; 81:189–195.

47. Li WW, Li VW. Angiogenesis in wound healing. Contemp Surg 2003:1–35.

48. Pilcher BK, Wang M, Qin Xj. Role of matrix metalloproteinases and their inhibition in cutaneous wound healing and allergic contact hypersensitivity. Ann NY Acad Sci 1999; 878:12–24.

49. Suetsugu S, Yamazaki D, Kurisu S, Takenawa T. Differential roles of WAVE1 and WAVE2 in dorsal and peripheral ruffle formation for fibroblast cell migration. Dev Cell 2003; 4:595–609.

50. Bullard KM, Mudgett J, Scheuenstuhl H, Hunt TK, Banda MJ. Stromelysin-1 deficient fibroblasts display impaired contraction in vitro. J Surg Res 1999; 84:31–34.

51. Bullard KM, Lund L, Mudgett JS, et al. Impaired wound contraction in stromelysin-1 deficient mice. Ann Surg 1999; 230:260–265.

52. Daniels JT, Schultz GS, Blalock TD, et al. Mediation of transforming growth factor beta-1 stimulated matrix contraction by fibroblasts: a role for connective tissue growth factor in contractile scarring. Am J Pathol 2003; 163(5):2043–2052.

53. Chakraborti S, Mandal M, Das S, et al. Regulation of matrix metalloproteinases: an overview. Mol Cell Biochem 2003; 253:269–285.

54. Vaalamo M, Leiva T, Saarialho-Kere U. Differential expression of tissue inhibitors of metalloproteinases (TIMP-1,-2,-3, and -4) in normal and abberrant wound healing. Hum Pathol 1999; 30:795–802.

55. Kere-Saarialho K. Patterns of matrix metalloproteinase and TIMP expression in chronic ulcers. Arch Dermatol Res 1998; 290:S47–S54.

56. Vaalamo M, Mattila L, Johansson N, et al. Distinct populations of stromal cells express collagenase-3 (MMP-13) and collagenase-1 (MMP-1) in chronic ulcers but not in normally healing wounds. J Invest Dermatol 1997; 109:96–101.

57. Wall SJ, Sampson MJ, Levell N, Murphy G. Elevated matrix metalloproteinase-2 and -3 production from human diabetic dermal fibroblasts. Br J Dermatol 2003; 149:13–16.

58. Ulrich D, Noah EM, Heimburg D, Pallua N. TIMP-1, MMP-2, MMP-9, and PIIINP as serum markers for skin fibrosis in patients following severe burn trauma. Plast Reconstr Surg 2003; 111(4):1423–1431.

59. Dasu MR, Hawkins HK, Barrow RE, et al. Gene expression profiles from hypertrophic scar fibroblasts before and after IL-6 stimulation. J Pathol 2004; 202(4):476–485.

60. Endo H, Utani A, Shinkai H. Activation of p38 MAPK suppresses matrix metalloproteinase-1 gene expression induced by platelet-derived growth factor. Arch Dermatol Res 2003; 294(12):552–558.

6

Comprehensive Wound Assessment and Treatment System

William J. Ennis
*Advocate Christ Medical Center Wound Treatment Program, Oak Lawn, Illinois,
and Evergreen Healthcare Center Advanced Wound Care Program, Evergreen Park,
Illinois, U.S.A.*

1. INTRODUCTION

The workup of a patient with a nonhealing wound can be complicated and, at times, all consuming. In an effort to be thorough, many unnecessary laboratory and diagnostic tests are frequently ordered. The differential diagnosis of a patient with a leg ulcer includes disease states ranging from common conditions to esoteric syndromes. How can the wound care clinician navigate through this maze and arrive at a timely, accurate, cost-effective diagnosis and treatment plan?

As the business of healthcare becomes entwined with the practice of medicine, theoretical constructs from the business world can be borrowed to assist the clinician. One such concept is known as medical manufacturing. At first pass, this term offends the practicing clinician. "I am caring for a patient not building a widget," "no two patients are alike," "you can't practice medicine with a cookbook," and "my patients are the sickest" are just a few of the comments overheard when this topic is introduced to the clinical staff. In fact, common things are common. On average, 70% of all leg ulcers evaluated in an outpatient wound clinic are venous in origin (1). If the wound clinician adopts a systematic approach to all patients with nonhealing wounds, regardless of etiology, the workup becomes routine and fewer subtle signs, symptoms, and diagnoses will be overlooked. Medical error rates and hospital-based complications are becoming more common, and the general public is more aware of treatment inconsistencies (2,3) Standardizing a clinical approach to wound care can help limit a missed diagnosis or a delay in treatment.

It was thought that the creation of guidelines and protocols would eliminate practice variability and begin to standardize the practice of medicine. Failure of guideline implementation has severely thwarted those efforts (4,5). In this chapter, the author outlines a "work in progress" known as the comprehensive wound assessment and treatment system (CWATS), which we have utilized over the past 10 years. This system, which includes a concept known as the "Least common denominator model" (LCD model), attempts to take the patient workup from the organism to the cellular level (6). Recently, some of the concepts from the CWATS system were incorporated with those of other wound care clinicians in a round table consensus meeting held in Hamburg, Germany, sponsored by Johnson and Johnson Wound Management Worldwide. The result of that meeting was the generation of a visual aide called the "Core Healing Principles," a guideline for wound care clinicians to use when approaching the wound care patient (Fig. 1) (7).

2. CWATS

The physician who deals with a recalcitrant wound must be skilled in communication, negotiation, and change management in order to co-ordinate an interdisciplinary team of specialists focused on a unified objective. The physician must possess an awareness and understanding of surgical concepts and treatment outcomes in plastic, orthopedic, vascular, and general surgery in order to make appropriate, timely

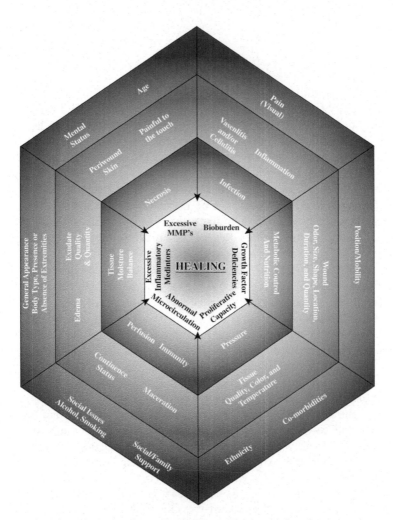

Figure 1 Core healing principles as developed by the consensus panel, wound healing meeting, Ethicon Surgical Institute, Hamburg, Germany, October 2003 (From Ref. 7.)

referrals during the continuum of care. Regardless of the physician's primary background, the wound clinician must incorporate knowledge and skills from both surgical and medical fields. The physician must also command a knowledge of dermatology, rheumatology, endocrinology, and general medicine in order to integrate the management of chronic systemic disease states into local wound care therapy. Communication with patients and family is paramount. An awareness of the social, psychological, spiritual, or existential concerns that are often involved with the possibility of limb loss and/or loss of independence and functionality is required to approach the wound patient in a holistic way. Many times, a patient has already received conflicting therapeutic recommendations from other health care professionals leading to frustration that can easily be misdirected towards the wound physician. Given the broad base of knowledge and skills required coupled with a paucity of clinical experience most physicians have in wound care, the practice of wound management is as challenging, demanding, and complex as that of any other field in medicine. Clinical training programs need to be developed at medical school and postgraduate levels in order to address these deficits (8).

Much information can be obtained by simply watching the patient walk into the clinic. Information concerning general appearance, body type, age, absence of a limb, ethnicity, and mobility can all be evaluated before the formal exam begins. The patient may deny pain verbally, but their body position and facial expressions may indicate otherwise. The formal process begins with a comprehensive history and review of systems. Wound care is not unlike other specialties, in that, for a majority of cases, a working diagnosis can be achieved with a thorough history. Past medical history is important because many comorbid illnesses exist in a complex wound care patient. Most patients with rheumatoid arthritis (RA) and a leg ulcer on the medial side of the leg for example, will be venous in origin, but the knowledge that the patient has RA will allow the clinician to consider a vasculitic wound in the differential diagnosis (9). A history of coronary disease in a patient with a venous ulcer should alert the clinician to the possibility of peripheral vascular disease and a mixed etiology for the leg ulcer. This has implications for the workup, expected time to healing, and the level of therapeutic compression to be used (10).

The social history will address confounding variables such as alcohol use, tobacco use, illicit drug use, occupational history, and level of activities. The patient must be questioned about the presence of any allergies to medications, environmental factors and foods. A detailed list of all medications taken by the patient is also important. With an increasing number of patients using herbals, vitamins, homeopathics, and supplements, it is important to emphasize to the patient that all medications should be listed. It is well known that steroid use can negatively impact healing, but more recently, the commonly prescribed cox-2 inhibitors, ace inhibitors, and calcium channel blockers have been implicated in slowing angiogenesis, a necessary component for normal healing (11,12). A family history will help identify risk factors and might shed light onto the patient's diagnosis, as often times the patient will not recognize the correlation between a disease in their family history and their own current problem.

A complete past surgical history is important. Patients with prior venous surgery are known to have wounds that are harder to heal (13). Knowledge of this fact might influence the clinician to utilize more advanced technologies earlier in the treatment regimen to provide appropriate care beyond that considered standard of care for that wound type (14).

The patient and their families' desired outcomes from the treatment program should be thoroughly understood and agreed upon from the onset of treatment.

For example, an elderly female with a highly exudative venous ulcer may be most concerned with controlling the drainage. Although the patient might like the wound to heal, their primary concern for exudate management might explain why the patient became more noncompliant as the treatment program progressed and "their" outcome was reached. In addition, there is a growing population of patients in whom by choice, terminal illness or chronic condition wounds have reached a steady state and are not able to achieve healing. This group of patients might be better served with a palliative wound protocol that emphasizes the surrogate endpoints of pain control, exudates and odor management, infection control, and quality of life outcomes rather than total healing (15).

Finally, a history of present illness (wound history) should be recorded. This part of the history needs to occur after all of the previously mentioned information has been gathered. If the interview begins with the wound history, an inordinate amount of time will be utilized. The subsequent shorter overall comprehensive history can frequently overlook potentially important details. The wound history should include the timing of the ulcer occurrence, location, prior ulcer history, current and past treatments, size and appearance, complications, procedures performed, drainage, and pain.

After the history the clinician should begin a physical examination. Vital signs, pain scale score, height, weight, and comment on general appearance should be recorded. The blood pressure should be taken in both arms and legs at the initial visit in order to calculate an ankle brachial index. A thorough exam should be conducted using appropriate documentation as described in the CPT manual for evaluation and management coding (16). A complete exam frequently uncovers findings that aid in the final diagnosis but also ensure appropriate documentation and reimbursement for your work. After the complete history and physical is performed, the clinician should turn their attention to the wound itself. It is important to let the patient know that the clinician intends to conduct a complete exam at the onset. Many patients assume they will simply have to remove their bandage and show the clinician their wound. They occasionally will become angry if much time is spent on what they perceive as "unnecessary" components to the office consultation. Frequently, they do not understand how important it is to get a complete medical picture before embarking on a wound treatment program. It is useful to send the patients a welcome packet describing the entire process either to their home prior to the visit or on arrival to the waiting area. The patient should fill in information concerning prior history and medications, which will expedite the visit and start them thinking about their wound on a more systemic level.

The examination of the wound takes into account the important issues of wound location, drainage quality and quantity, surrounding skin condition, quality of wound bed tissue (granular, fibrinous, eschar, etc.), pain, odor, condition of wound perimeter (i.e., presence of undermining, etc.), as well as standard measurements (length, width, and depth).

The wound workup next focuses on what has been termed "the LCD model" (6). Composed of six subsections (tissue perfusion/oxygenation, infection, nutrition/immune status, psychosocial, pressure/neuropathy, and wound bed), this model ensures that the clinician consider all factors that impact healing for a wound of any etiology. Although nutrition and psychosocial aspects have been covered in the history and physical exam, these concepts are now revisited as they specifically relate to the wound and the potential for healing.

The most important aspect of the LCD model is the adequacy of tissue perfusion/oxygenation. It is imperative that tissue perfusion is analyzed within the paradigm of both macro- and microvascular status. The initial evaluation focuses on the macrocirculation with the palpation of peripheral pulses. Ankle pulses are, however, not sufficient to detect impaired arterial circulation, and additional testing is frequently required for the patient with leg ulcerations (17). Performing an ankle arm index is useful not only for wound healing prediction, but also as an overall marker for cardiovascular health (18). Only about 10% of patients presenting to an outpatient wound clinic will have isolated arterial disease as an etiology for their leg ulcer (19). Arterial duplex scans, segmental pressures including toe pressures, pulse volume recordings, and magnetic resonance angiography, and rapid sequence CT scans are other noninvasive macrocirculation studies that may be ordered. An interventional angiogram is still considered the gold standard at this time, although many facilities are utilizing MRA as an alternative. After a complete assessment of the macrocirculation, the clinician's attention must be turned to the status of the microcirculation. Adequacy of macrovascular flow does not ensure the occurrence of healing.

There are several tests that can evaluate the status of the microcirculatory system. Intravital capillaroscopy is a noninvasive technique that utilizes a microscope to identify nutrient capillaries (20). $TcPO_2$, also called transcutaneous oximetry, is a technique widely used to detect the skin oxygen tension. A dime-sized Clarke type solid-state polarographic electrode, containing a platinum cathode with a reference electrode of silver chloride, is housed in a probe tip along with a heater and a thermistor (21). This procedure indirectly evaluates total microcirculation without the ability to differentiate nutritive from the non-nutritive flow. Nutritive flow refers to the flow that relies on the perpendicular capillary flow towards the skin surface but not on the parallel flow that is seen in the dermis and functions mainly as a shunt for thermoregulation.

Laser Doppler perfusion imaging is a recently developed technique that utilizes a low intensity laser (Helium–Neon) light (22). The device measures the backscattering created by moving red blood cells over a specific rectangular area analyzing up to 4096 individual points. The wavelength of this monochromatic light is 670 nm with a maximum accessible power of 1 mW. Two parameters of the returning laser light from the skin are analyzed. The first is the number of shifted photons, which relates to the concentration of moving red blood cells. The second is the mean Doppler shift of these photons, which relates to the blood cell velocity. These Doppler shift results are accumulated and translated into numeric values expressed in volts and in an image colored map. Colors range from dark blue to burnt red and indicate minimum and maximum perfusion, respectively. The laser Doppler flux is a value that results from the multiplication of these two parameters and is expressed in arbitrary units (au) (23). The penetration of the laser beam reaches 500 μn when applied to intact skin. However, penetration can reach 2.5 times greater in other nonskin tissues like granulation tissue (24). The shallow penetration of the laser beam allows for a closer approximation of nutritive flow and may allow for the quantification of the angiogenesis process in granulation tissue (25).

Other tests for microcirculation include positron emission tomography, nuclear magnetic resonance spectroscopy, xenon washout, and near infrared spectroscopy (26–29).

If a patient has a leg ulcer and abnormal macrovascular flow studies and if physiological studies (i.e., transcutaneous oximetry) indicate adequate values for healing, then a trial of aggressive local wound care is warranted. If after a 4-week treatment course there is no significant improvement either in wound dimensions or in quality of tissue, then further invasive studies followed by revascularization might be necessary. Approaching the wound patient in this manner will avoid unnecessary high risk procedures, and the limited treatment time will minimize potential harmful outcomes. If the microcirculatory studies are abnormal, then a trial of treatments aimed at enhancing the microcirculation (i.e., electrical stimulation, growth factors, bioengineered tissue, and therapeutic ultrasound) could be used along with aggressive wound care for a short course. Systemic therapy, along with life style modifications, should also be employed (30,31).

The second component of the LCD model refers to the determination of infection. Bacteria are present in all chronic wounds. There is a natural balance between the quantity of bacteria present (bioburden) and the host's immune status. When equilibrium is reached there is no clinical infection. If the innoculum of bacteria is increased ($> 10^5$organism/g tissue) or the host suffers a decrease in immunity, clinical infection occurs (32). Many examples are cited in the literature describing the failure of skin grafts, delayed closures, and overall wound healing problems when the bacterial bioburden exceeds 10^5. This value is accepted by many as the quantitative definition of infection except in the presence of beta-hemolytic streptococcus where the value is somewhat lower (10^3) (33). The bacteria compete for nutrients and oxygen with host repair cells in the granulating bed. Bacterial byproducts of metabolism can be toxic to the host's normal cellular functioning. The presence of necrotic debris, foreign body, and the desiccation of the wound bed enhances bacterial growth. The concept of colonization (the mere presence of organisms) and infection (the invasion of organisms into the tissue) can usually be determined by the physical exam (34). The cardinal signs of inflammation—erythema, pain, swelling, and increased temperature—may be clues to impending infection. Many patients are clinically unable to mount an inflammatory response, and in those patients, the use of quantitative culturing, along with clinical intuition, is necessary. There are numerous ways to obtain cultures of a wound, but the quantitative biopsy remains the gold standard (35). Wound bioburden and infection must be thought of as a continuum and not a point in time when a specific number of organisms are present. This concept is important to emphasize because the presence of granulation tissue depends on the presence of some bacteria (36).

Recently, the theoretical concept of "critical colonization" has been proposed as a point where colonization falls below classical quantitative values for infection but can negatively impact on the patient's ability to heal by competing for nutrients and the release of toxic metabolic endproducts (37).

The third category within the LCD model focuses on the immunological state of the patient. Malnutrition is a major factor to consider here. Although the literature fails to provide us with statistically significant relationships between healing and nutritional status, it is obvious that a patient needs to be repleted nutritionally in order to maximize their chances for healing. Patients are not considered for surgical wound closure until they have achieved nutritional support and lab testing confirms success (i.e., prealbumen level, serum transferrin level, total lymphocyte count, albumen level, etc.). Every attempt is made to support patients with multivitamins, minerals, and enteral or parenteral support. Patients should be evaluated for other forms of immunosuppression such as use of steroids, antimetabolic agents, overwhelming infection, and chronic disease states such as diabetes and HIV.

Psychosocial issues were discussed earlier in the paper but should be re-examined at this point. Chronic depression has been shown to affect healing, and many wound patients suffer from psychiatric conditions if the clinician carefully probes during the history (38). Pain can exacerbate underlying psychiatric issues and can delay healing in and of itself through the psychoneuroimmunological connections (39). As society ages and more patients live with chronic diseases, we will be faced with patients in whom healing options are limited and in whom maintenance of the wound bed, prevention of infection, exudate management, odor control, and wound pain issues will take priority over healing (40).

The LCD next addresses pressure on the wound and surrounding tissues. Pressure must be offloaded in order to maximize healing. This seems obvious when dealing with classic pressure ulcers located on the trunk but applies to pressure from wheelchair leg rests, bed railings, oxygen tubing, and improperly fitting shoe-gear. There are many products available to offload the patient, such as mattresses, orthotics and prosthetics, and foam padding for wheelchairs and beds.

The wound bed is the last aspect of the LCD model. The periwound tissue should be assessed first. The skin can be painful to the touch, erythematous, macerated, dry and cracked, or edematous. A patient's continence status may play a pivotal role in wound healing and should be noted in the record. The wound bed must be assessed for the state of moisture balance, presence of necrotic tissue, and quality of granulation tissue. If the wound has been present for > 6 months to 1 year and/or has an abnormal appearance, then strong consideration should be given to performing a biopsy. Histology can help achieve a diagnosis, rule out malignancy, or provide confirmation to a clinical suspicion. The threshold for biopsy should be low, as many wounds do not demonstrate classical features on presentation. After a "macroscopic" view of the wound bed, the clinician should consider microenvironmental issues. The microcirculation has already been reviewed and those results need to be documented in the patient's record as well. The biochemistry of the wound is becoming more important to wound healing, as new concepts in healing have been elucidated. A hostile wound environment with excess matrix metalloproteases can lead to the destruction of both endogenous and exogenous growth factors leading to delayed healing (41,42). The bioburden of the wound can lead to the presence of metabolic waste products in the wound bed. Inflammatory mediators and cytokines can create an environment that does not allow for proliferation to occur. Interestingly, this situation can develop with adequate macrovascular flow. Consider the patient with a venous ulcer, palpable pulses, but severe lipodermatosclerosis and relative dermal tissue hypoxia. The previously described wound would be difficult to heal and might require modifying the biochemical composition of the wound bed to accelerate healing (43).

The differential diagnosis of leg ulcers is long and covers diverse disease states. By systematically performing a history and physical and then considering all the features from the LCD model, the clinician should be able to narrow the list down to a provisional diagnosis and two to three potential confounding conditions. At this point, laboratory testing can help arrive at a diagnosis and a treatment plan prescription. The patient should be seen weekly from weeks 1 through 4. If after the fourth visit there is little change in either wound dimensions or quality of wound tissue, then the diagnosis should be reconsidered and the patient should cycle back through the process again. This will ensure nothing is missed and minimize any time spent on an ineffective treatment protocol. Using this system, the author has been able to achieve similar healing rates at a community hospital and a tertiary care facility. There has been no statistically significant differences in healing rates amongst the various wound etiologies in either site of care (44).

3. SUMMARY

In this chapter, the author have attempted to identify the essential components of a wound workup, regardless of wound etiology. By systematically evaluating all patients with the same "pathway," fewer mistakes will be made. Clearly, not all initial diagnoses and treatment plans will be accurate, but by limiting the time any given treatment is utilized without observing clinical improvements, the less likely the clinician is to delay appropriate care. Wound care has become complicated and clinically diverse. Our practice includes patients with acute trauma, postoperative wound complications from orthopedic, vascular, general, neurosurgical, and obstetrical services. Chronic wounds from all etiological categories are referred along with the frail, elderly nursing home patients and the complex spinal cord patients as well. The scope and variety of these cases necessitates a consistent, reproducible approach to care. The advent of the electronic medical record has recently given the clinician the potential to gather information about the patient across a continuum of care from a single office-based clinic.

REFERENCES

1. Valencia IC, Falabella A, Kirsner R, Eaglstein WH. Chronic venous insufficiency and venous leg ulceration. J Am Acad Dermatol 2001; 44(3):401–421.
2. Institute of Medicine. to Err is Human Building a Safer Health Care System. Washington, DC: National Academy Press, 1999.
3. Meyer G, Lewin G, Eisenberg D. To err is preventable: medical errors and academic medicine. Am J Med 2001; 110(7):597–603.
4. Leaper L. Adherence to practice guidelines: the role of specialty society guidelines. Am Heart J 2003; 145(1):19–26.
5. Ward MM. Physician knowledge, attitudes, and practices regarding a widely implemented guideline. J Eval Clin Pract 2002; 8(2):155–162.
6. Ennis WJ, Meneses P. Clinical evaluation: outcomes, benchmarking, introspection and quality improvement. Buzz words for business, soon the language of wound care. Ostomy Wound Management 1996; 42,10A, (suppl):40S–47S.
7. Consensus panel Hamburg, Germany, Vicci Driver DPM, William J Ennis DO, Ian Gordon MD, Michael Maier DPM. Johnson and Johnson Wound Care Worldwide.
8. Ennis WJ, Valdes W, Meneses P. Specialty training. Wound Repair Regen 2004.
9. Magro CM, Crowson AN. The spectrum of cutaneous lesions in rheumatoid arthritis: a clinical and pathological study of 43 patients. J Cutan Pathol 2003; 30(1):1–10.
10. Vowden K, Vowden P. Mixed aetiology ulcers. J Wound Care 2001; 10(1):520.
11. Masferrer J. Approach to angiogenesis inhibition based on cyclo-oxygenase-2. Cancer J 2001; 7(3):S144–S150.
12. Qiu JG, Factor S, Chang TH, Knighton D, Nadel H, Levenson SM. Wound healing: captopril, an angiogenesis inhibitor, and Staphylococcus aureus peptidoglycan. J Surg Res 2000; 92(2):177–185.
13. Margolis D. Risk factors associated with the failure of a venous leg ulcer to heal. Arch Dermatol 1999; 135(8):920–926.
14. Ennis WJ, Meneses P. Standard, appropriate and advanced care and medical-legal considerations: part one. Venous Wounds 2003; 15(4):107–122.
15. Alvarez O, Meehan M, Ennis WJ, et al. Chronic wound management: palliative medicine for the frail population Wounds 2002; 14(8):5s–27s.
16. AMA Press CPT 2004 Professional ISBN-1-57947-421-7.
17. Moffat C. Ankle pulses are not sufficient to detect impaired arterial circulation in patients with leg ulcers. J Wound Care 1995; 4(3):134–138.

18. Newman AB, Shemanski L, Manolio TA, Cushman M, Mittelmark M, Polak JF, Powe NR, Siscovick D. Ankle-arm index as a predictor of cardiovascular disease and mortality in the cardiovascular health study. Arterioscler Thromb Vase Biol 1999; 19:538–545.

19. Hafner J, Schaad I, Schneider E, Seifert B, Burg G, Cassina PC. Leg ulcers in peripheral arterial disease (arterial leg ulcers): impaired wound healing above the threshold of chronic critical limb ischemia. J Am Acad Dermatol 2000; 43(6):1001–1008.

20. Pazos-Moura CC, Moura EG, Bouskela E, Torres Filho IP, Breitenbach MMD. Nail-fold capillaroscopy in non-insulin dependent diabetes mellitus: blood flow velocity during rest and post-occlusive reactive hyperaemia. Clin Physiol 1990; 10:451–461.

21. Sheffield PJ. Measuring tissue oxygen tension: a review. Undersea Hyper Med 1998; 25(3):179–188.

22. Kernick DP, Shore AC. Characteristics of laser Doppler perfusion imaging in vitro and in vivo. Physiol Meas 2000; 21:333–340.

23. Coleridge Smith PD. The microcirculation in venous hypertension. Vasc Med 1997; 2:203–213.

24. Kolarova H, Dritichova D, Wagner J. Penetration of laser light into the skin in vitro. Lasers Surg Med 1999; 24:231–235.

25. Christ F, Bauer A, Brugger D. Different optical methods for clinical monitoring of the microcirculation. Eur Surg Res 2002; 34:145–151.

26. Hopkins NF, Spinks TJ, Rhodes CG, et al. Positron emission tomography in venous ulceration and liposclerosis study of regional tissue function. Br J Med 1983; 286: 333–336.

27. Ennis WJ, Driscoll DM, Meneses P. A preliminary study on 31 P NMR spectroscopy: a powerful tool for wound analysis using high energy phosphates. Wounds 1994; 6:166–173.

28. Neufield GR, Galante SR, Whang JM, DeVries D, Baumgardner JE, Graves DJ, Quinn JA. Skin blood flow from gas transport: helium xenon and laser Doppler compared. Microvasc Res 1988; 35(2):143–152.

29. Scheufler O, Andressen R. Tissue oxygenation and perfusion in inferior pedicle reduction mammaplasty by near-infra red reflection spectroscopy and color coded duplex sonography. Plast Reconstr Surg 2003; 111(3):1131–1146.

30. Hiatt WR. Pharmacologic therapy for peripheral arterial disease and claudication. J Vasc Surg 2002; 36:1283–1291.

31. Dean SM, Vaccaro PS. Successful pharmacologic treatment of lower extremity ulcerations in 5 patients with chronic critical limb ischemia. J Am Board Fam Pract 2002; 15(1):55–62.

32. Robson MC. Infection in the surgical patient: an imbalance in the normal equilibrium. Clin Plastic Surg 1979; 6:493.

33. Robson MC, et al. Wound healing alterations caused by infection. Clin Plastic Surg 1990; 17:485.

34. Field CK, Kerstein MD. Overview of wound healing in a moist environment. Am J Surg 1994; 167(suppl 1A):2S.

35. Stotts NA. Determination of bacterial burden in wounds. Adv Wound Care 1995; 8:28.

36. Burke JF. Effects of inflammation on wound repair. J Dent Res 1971; 50:296.

37. Kingsley A. The wound infection continuum and its application to clinical practice. Ostomy Wound Management 2003; 49(suppl 7A):1–7.

38. Cole-King A. Psychological factors and delayed healing in chronic wounds. Psychosom Med 2001; 63(2):216–220.

39. Tournier JN. Neuro-immune connections: evidence for a neuro-immunological synapse. Trends Immunol 2003; 24:114–115.

40. Ennis WJ. Healing: can we? must we? should we? Ostomy Wound Management 2001; 47(9):6–8.

41. Zu W-H, Guo X, Villaschi S. Regulation of vascular growth and regression by matrix metalloproteinases in the rat aorta model of angiogenesis. Lab Invest 2000; 80(4): 545–550.
42. Ovington L, Cullen B. Matrix metalloproteinases and growth factor protection. Wounds 2002; 14(5):2–13.
43. Cullen B, Smith R, McCulloch E, Sllcock D, Morrison L. Mechanism of action of promogran a protease modulating matrix for the treatment of diabetic foot ulcers. Wound Repair Regeneration 2002; 10:16–25.
44. Ennis WJ, Meneses P. Issues impacting wound healing at a local level: the stunned wound. Ostomy Wound Management 2000; 46(suppl 1A):39S–48S.

7

Approach to Diagnosis of a Patient with a Lower Extremity Ulcer

Peggy Lin and Tania J. Phillips
Department of Dermatology, Boston University School of Medicine, Boston, Massachusetts, U.S.A.

1. INTRODUCTION

Chronic leg ulcers are open wounds, often below the knee, which are a significant problem in contemporary society, and are a source of frustration for approximately 2.5 million people in the United States (1). Medical costs of nonhealing wounds approach 1.5–3.5 billion dollars a year (1) and an estimated 2 million workdays per year are lost secondary to leg ulcers (1). The incidence and prevalence of these problems increase as the population ages (3). A key step in the appropriate management of a lower extremity ulcer is an accurate and prompt diagnosis. A complete history, followed by a thorough physical exam, and then finally any necessary ancillary investigations should be performed. An approach to the diagnosis of the lower extremity ulcer will be emphasized in this chapter. The most common causes of leg ulcers will be discussed, followed by a brief discussion of less common causes of leg ulcers. Please refer to Table 1 for common and uncommon causes of leg ulcers.

2. BASIC ASSESSMENT OF THE LOWER EXTREMITY ULCER

2.1. General History: An Aid for Developing a Differential Diagnosis

Pertinent parts of the history include: the number, duration, location, and prior treatments of previous ulcers, if any. The patient should be asked about his or her ulcer-related and recent symptoms of general health. Any topical and systemic medications should be recorded since they may provide clues to the pathogenesis of the ulcer. They may be the cause of a hypersensitivity vasculitis or may be part of the therapy regimen for the systemic disease contributing to the ulcer. A familial history of leg ulcers may be present and significant. Social history may help in deciding whether the patient will need visiting nurse services.

Table 1   Causes of Leg Ulcers

I. Vascular diseases
  A. Venous
  B. Arterial
    1. Atherosclerosis
    2. Arteriovenous malformation
    3. Cholesterol embolism
  C. Vasculitis
    1. Small vessel
      a. Hypersensitivity vasculitis
      b. Rheumatoid arthritis
      c. Lupus erythematosus
      d. Scleroderma
      e. Sjogren's syndrome
      f. Behcet's disease
      g. Atrophie blanche
    2. Medium and large vessel
      a. Polyarteritis nodosa
      b. Nodular vasculitis
      c. Wegener's granulomatosis
  D. Lymphatics
  E. Lymphedema
II. Neuropathic
  A. Diabetes
  B. Tabes dorsalis
  C. Syringomyelia
III. Metabolic
  A. Diabetes
  B. Gout
  C. Prolidase deficiency
  D. Gaucher's disease
IV. Hematologic diseases
  A. Red blood cell disorders
    1. Sickle cell anemia
    2. Hereditary spherocytosis
    3. Thalassemia
    4. Polycythemia rubra vera
  B. White blood cell disorders
  C. Dysproteinemias

V. Trauma
  A. Pressure
  B. Cold injury (frostbite, pernio)
  C. Radiation dermatitis
  D. Burns (thermal, chemical)
  E. Factitia
VI. Neoplastis
  A. Epitheliomas
    1. Squamous cell carcinoma
    2. Basal cell carcinoma
  B. Sarcoma (e.g., Kaposi's sarcoma)
  C. Lymphoproliferative
    1. Lymphoma
    2. Cutaneous T-cell lymphoma
  D. Metastatic tumors
VII. Infection
  A. Bacterial
    1. Furuncle
    2. Ecthyma
    3. Ecthyma gangrenosum
    4. Septic emboli
    5. Gram-negative infections
    6. Anaerobic infections
    7. Mycobacterial (typical and atypical)
    8. Spirochetal
  B. Fungal
    1. Majocchi's granuloma
    2. Deep fungal infections
  C. Protozoal
  D. Leishmania
  E. Infestations and bites
VIII. Panniculitis
  A. Weber–Christian disease
  B. Pancreatic fat necrosis
  C. Necrobiosis lipoidica
IX. Pyoderma gangrenosum

Source: From Ref. 1.

3.   COMMON CAUSES OF LEG ULCERS

Although leg ulcers can have various etiologies (see Table 1), most (72%) are due to venous insufficiency, 6% are due to pure arterial disease, and 22% are secondary to mixed venous/arterial etiology (1,3). Neuropathic ulcers are a common cause of lower extremity ulcers, principally occurring on the feet. Diabetes is the major contributor of neuropathic foot ulcers (4).

Table 2 Comparison of Clinical Findings in Common Leg Ulcers

	Venous	Arterial	Neuropathic/ diabetic
Location	Malleolar regions	Pressure sites Distal points (toes) Bony prominences	Pressure sites (foot)
Morphology	Irregular borders	Necrotic base "Punched out," deep	"Punched out" Undermined edge

Surrounding skin	Hemosiderin
	  pigmentation
	Lipodermatosclerosis
		Shiny atrophic skin
		  with hair loss
			Thick callus

Other physical
  examination
  findings
	Varicosities
	Leg/ankle edema
	± Eczema
	± Lymphedema
		Weak/absent peripheral
		  pulses
		Prolonged capillary refill
		  time
		Pallor on leg elevation
			Neuropathy with
			  insensitivity
			Charcot joints
			Hammertoes

Source: Adapted from Kanj LF, Phillips TJ. Management of leg ulcers. Fitzpatrick's J Clin Dermatol 1994; 52–60.

3.1. Venous Ulcers

There are an estimated 600,000–2.5 million venous leg ulcers in the United States (2). Most (85%) of the affected patients are over 65 years old (5). There is a slight female predominance (1.6:1) (6). Patients with chronic venous insufficiency (CVI) are older, obese, male, with a history of phlebitis, and a history of severe leg injury. This suggests that prior deep vein thrombosis, either clinical or subclinical, may be a predisposing factor for CVI (3). Factors predicting poor healing include large wound area, long ulcer duration, fibrin covering over 50% of the wound surface, a low ankle-brachial pressure index (<0.8), and a history of venous stripping or ligation and a history of hip or knee replacement surgery (7).

Common complaints of venous disease include limb heaviness and aching that is accompanied by swelling and exacerbated by standing. Lower extremity swelling is usually worse at the end of the day, and often is alleviated with leg elevation (1). Patients may complain of odor, copious drainage, and pruritic surrounding skin. The majority of patients with venous ulcers complain of pain, which can significantly diminish their quality of life. The size of the ulcer does not correlate with the amount of pain, small ulcers in a background of atrophie blanche can often be extremely painful. Allergy to a wide variety of topical medications may also be present in the history (8).

3.2. Arterial Ulcers

The age-adjusted prevalence of peripheral arterial disease is approximately 12% (9). Major risk factors for peripheral arterial disease include cigarette smoking, diabetes mellitus, hyperlipidemia, and age over 40 years (9). Patients are usually middle-aged to elderly and men are often affected more frequently than women. Other risk factors for the development of an arterial ulcer include sedentary lifestyle, hypertension, hyperhomocysteinemia, atherosclerosis, thrombosis, trauma, vasospastic diseases, and a family history of arterial ulcers or premature ischemic heart disease (9). Arterial ulcers are usually severely painful. A history of intermittent claudication in one or both legs, defined as severe pain, numbness, or paresthesia with walking or other activity and relieved with rest may be present. These symptoms usually affect the calves, but can occur anywhere on the leg (including the thighs or buttocks). In more advanced arterial disease, patients may suffer from rest pain, especially in the distal foot and toes. The pain is usually aggravated by elevation and relieved by dependency (9).

3.3. Neuropathic Ulcers

The most common etiology of neuropathic foot ulcers in the United States is diabetes. Of the 16 million affected diabetic patients in the United States, it is estimated that 20% will develop an ulcerated foot during their lifetime (10). Of patients affected by a diabetic neuropathic foot ulcer, 14–24% will require an amputation (11). Diabetes is the primary cause (85%) of nontraumatic lower extremity amputations in the United States (12).

A history that includes symptoms of neuropathy in the feet (burning, numbness, tingling, needlelike pain and/or paresthesias) should make one consider the diagnosis of diabetes. However, neuropathic ulcers are often asymptomatic (1). More rare, non-diabetic causes of neuropathy include spinal cord lesions, alcohol, and leprosy.

If the patient is diabetic, one should inquire about the quality of control of his or her diabetic disease. HbA_{1C} levels are a good indicator of glycemic control over the previous 90 days. Well-controlled diabetics have HbA_{1C} levels between 7% and 8%. Progressive neuropathic and nephropathic changes are associated with HbA_{1C} levels $> 9\%$. (13). Wound healing and infection control are impaired when HbA_{1C} levels approach over 12%, since leukocytic functions such as chemotaxis, adherence, phagocytosis, and intracellular bactericidal activity are altered (14). Risk factors for diabetic foot ulcers include a long history (> 10 years) of uncontrolled or poorly controlled diabetes, which may be associated with impaired vision or blindness, neuropathy, nephropathy, peripheral vascular disease, history of previous foot ulcers, structural foot abnormalities, poorly fitting footware, poor foot hygiene, a history of amputation, noncompliance, and male gender (4,12,15).

4. VARIOUS ATYPICAL CAUSES OF LEG ULCERS

4.1. Lymphedema

Ulceration can be difficult to manage when associated with lymphedema. Lymphatic channels which usually run parallel to venous channels become damaged secondary to repeated tissue injury from venous ulcers and lipodermatosclerosis. Lymph fluid accumulates in the tissues and the high protein constituents cause inflammation and tissue fibrosis. Lymphedema is classified into primary and secondary types. The age of presentation further classifies primary lymphedema into three groups: (1) congenital, which is present from birth to within 2 years old; (2) lymphedema praecox, which usually presents at the time of puberty; and (3) lymphedema tarda, which usually presents after 35 years (16). Lymphedema is often seen in association with venous insufficiency.

4.2. Hypercoagulable States

In young patients with venous thrombosis or venous ulceration, especially where there is a family history, prothrombotic states such as Factor-V-Leiden mutation prothrombin gene mutation, protein C, and protein S deficiency, and/or antiphospholipid antibody syndrome should be excluded. Other causes of hypercoagulable state to consider include pregnancy, oral contraceptive use, Buerger's disease, Behcet's disease, malignancy, intravenous catheters, and intravenous drug use (17).

4.3. Pyoderma Gangrenosum

The history of progression of the ulcer can be an important aid to diagnosis. For example, if the ulcer began as a painful pustule, one should consider pyoderma gangrenosum on the differential diagnosis, especially if the patient gives a history of associated chronic systemic disease such as diseased small- or large-bowel (i.e., Crohn's disease, ulcerative colitis, and diverticulosis), Behcet's syndrome, chronic active hepatitis, paraproteinemias, myeloproliferative disorders, or rheumatoid arthritis. It is important to note, however, up to 50% of cases of pyoderma gangrenosum can occur without these associations (18,19). The patient may state that the ulcers may extend slowly or rapidly and that new ones develop as older lesions heal. Diagnosis is often made on the clinical appearance of the ulcer and exclusion of other potential causes for the ulcer.

4.4. Hematologic Disorders That May Be Associated with Lower Extremity Ulcers

Please refer to Table 1 for a list of hematological disorders that may be associated with ulcers. An important part of obtaining a thorough medical history is to uncover underlying systemic disease, which may be the cause of or contributing to the prognosis of the ulcer. These include sickle cell anemia, thalassemia, hereditary spherocytosis, Felty's syndrome, polycythemia vera, essential thrombocythemia, coumadin necrosis (associated with protein C deficiency), and heparin-induced necrosis (18).

4.5. Vasculitic Syndromes

Chronic leg ulcers may be associated with vasculitis. Clinically, palpable purpura, livedo reticularis, and multiple ulcers may be seen. Vasculitic syndromes can be associated with other systemic conditions, such as infections (i.e., hepatitis B, hepatitis C), hypersensitivity to oral medications (i.e., penicillins, sulfonamides), and chronic medical conditions, such as myeloproliferative disorders, cryoglobulinemia and other paraproteinemias, collagen vascular diseases (i.e., rheumatoid arthritis and systemic lupus erythematosus), and renal carcinoma. Medium and large vessels can be affected in vasculitic syndromes and may present with leg ulcers associated with systemic manifestions (18).

4.6. Malignancy

In ulcers of long duration which have not responded to standard therapy and ulcers with atypical presentation, biopsy should be performed to rule out malignancy. The commonest ulcerated neoplasms include basal cell carcinoma, and squamous cell carcinoma. Lymphoma, leukemia, Kaposi's sarcoma, malignant melanoma, epithelioid sarcoma, and reticulosarcoma are seen rarely (18).

5. PHYSICAL EXAM AND ANCILLARY INVESTIGATIONS AS TOOLS TO AID DIAGNOSIS

Global assessment should include an assessment of the general appearance of the patient. Does the patient have a butterfly rash of lupus erythematosus? Does the patient have scleroderma-like changes in the skin? Is the patient in cardiac failure? Where is the ulcer located? Is it in the gaiter or nongaiter area? If it is in the gaiter area, a venous ulcer is high on the differential list. If the ulcer is located on the foot, a venous ulcer is less likely and the diagnosis of arterial or neuropathic ulcer is more likely. Do the ulcers occur singly or multiply? If the answer is multiple, a vasculitis is more likely. The appearance of the wound edges can also be clues to the diagnosis. If the edges are sharply demarcated, this points more to an arterial ulcer than a venous ulcer. If the border is violaceous and undermined, one should consider pyoderma gangrenosum. A hyperkeratotic thick callus around the ulcer edge suggests meuropathic ulcer.

Is the skin cool, shiny, and hairless, suggesting arterial disease? The lower extremities should be closely examined. Are the peripheral pulses present? Is there evidence of neuropathy? Are there signs of venous disease such as varicose veins, peripheral edema, hemosiderin pigmentation, or lipodermatosclerosis? Are there signs of venous eczema?

The ulcer-specific evaluation of the wound begins with wound cleansing in order to examine appearance of the wound bed and to appreciate the length, width, and depth of the wound, and any presence of undermining sinus tracts. Tracings of the wound onto sterile acetate or clear pieces of plastic, as well as photography, aid documentation of the wound size over time.

The color of the wound bed and the appearance of the wound edges and its surrounding skin should be noted. Approximate percentages of granulation tissue, necrotic tissue, fibrin, eschar, and exudates should be recorded.

5.1. Venous Ulcer Physical Exam

Venous ulcers are usually located in the gaiter area, i.e., between the lower calf and the lower malleolus along the most superficial course of the saphenous vein. They may be single or multiple, usually shallow in depth, and with an irregular border. Healthy granulation tissue at the wound base is often revealed once the normally moderate-to-heavy fibrinous exudate is debrided. Venous ulcers are usually larger than non-venous ulcers and may involve the entire circumference of the leg (1,6).

Brown-yellow hyperpigmentation due to hemosiderin deposition (secondary to extravasated red blood cells and hemosiderin within macrophages) can be seen on the leg. The skin may be dry and pruritic secondary to venous dermatitis. In long-standing venous insufficiency, the skin becomes indurated and "woody" feeling (lipodermatosclerosis). In advanced disease, an "inverted-champagne-bottle" shape is seen in the leg, with proximal leg swelling and induration and fat necrosis around the ankle. Mild-to-severe varicosities may be present anywhere on the leg. Atrophie blanche characterized by white, atrophic, and waxy-appearing skin speckled with tiny telangiectatic vessels may occur in both venous disease and in arterial disease. Pulses are usually normal, although venous and arterial disease can coexist (Figs. 1 and 2).

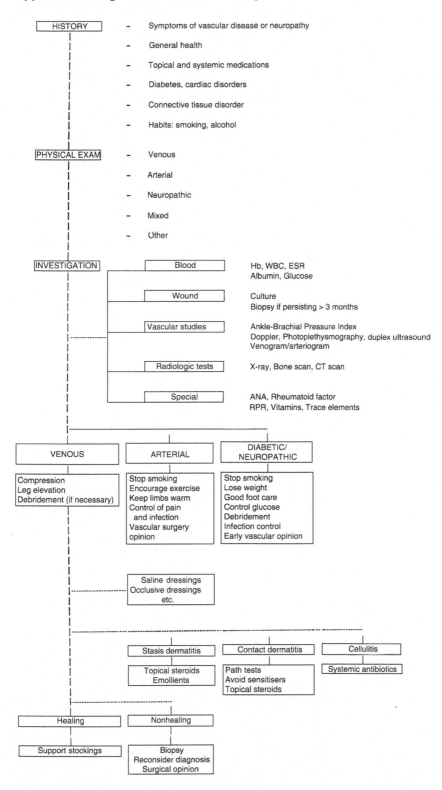

Figure 1 Venous ulcer physical exam protocol.

5.2. Physical Exam for Arterial Ulcers

In patients with arterial disease, peripheral pulses (femoral, popliteal, dorsalis pedis, and/or posterior tibial) may be decreased or absent. The limb is often cool and skin may be shiny and hairless. Capillary refilling time is prolonged to more than 3–4 sec. This is determined by blanching the skin of the great toes with fingertip pressure, releasing the finger and measuring the time taken to return to normal color. Elevation of an ischemic leg to 45° for 1 min. may result in a pallor of the extremity. The leg is then placed in a dependent position and delayed rubor occurs originating in the feet and spreading proximally until the leg becomes bright pink or red in color. It is believed the degree of arterial insufficiency is correlated with a more intense and extensive rubor (1).

Arterial ulcers usually occur over bony prominences on areas subject to trauma or rubbing of footwear, such as the tips of the toes, between the toes, over the phalangeal heads, and ankle. The shapes of arterial ulcers vary, but may follow the outline of traumatic pressure. Arterial ulcers typically are round, sharply demarcated, and with a pale, deep wound bed that is usually devoid of granulation tissue and with minimal exudate. The base may be covered by a dry, thick eschar of necrotic debris. Exposure of tendons or deep tissues also suggests an arterial etiology and usually indicates more severe disease. Surrounding skin may appear normal or may be dry, cold, shiny, and hairless. There may be loss of subcutaneous tissue, muscle wastage, and atrophic skin over the lower calf and foot. Toenails may be coarse and thickened. Audible bruits may be present over the femoral artery and the distal vessels, although peripheral pulses may be diminished or absent (1).

The ABPI is the ratio of the systolic pressure at the ankle compared to the systolic pressure in the arm. In the absence of arterial occlusive disease, the ABPI is slightly greater than or equal to one, since the ankle pressure should be equal to the arm pressure. The ABPI in those with calcified vessels, i.e., diabetics, can be misleadingly high. Occlusive arterial disease may be indicated by an ABPI between 0.5 and 0.9. Severe obstructive occlusive disease is usually demonstrated when the ABPI is < 0.5. These patients often have pain at rest. When necessary, Doppler segmental pressures can be used to identify the presence, location, and severity of arterial occlusive disease. Those with evidence of inadequate arterial blood flow should be referred to a vascular surgeon (9).

5.3. Physical Exam of Neuropathic Ulcers

Sensory neuropathy results in loss of the protective sensation of pain to pressure and temperature. Thus, patients with sensory neuropathy are unaware of foot trauma from ill-fitting shoes, improper nail trimming, immersion of feet in hot water, or penetration of foreign bodies into their feet. Repetitive stress on feet can cause callus buildup and subsequent ulceration. Cutaneous perception is confirmed with the Semmes–Weinstein monofilament test. The patient is considered to have lost protective sensation if a 5.07 monofilament, which is equated to 10 g of linear pressure, cannot be detected, since a 4.17 monofilament, which is equated with 1 g of linear pressure, is normally felt in a person with intact sensation (15).

Motor neuropathy progresses to impaired motor nerve function and failure of the small muscles of the foot to keep proper tension and tone in the foot muscles. Foot deformities occur when tendons fail to keep proper alignment and muscles fail to balance each other. Examples of common foot deformities include Charcot's foot, hammertoes (Fig. 3), and claw toes. Foot deformities result in altered distribution of

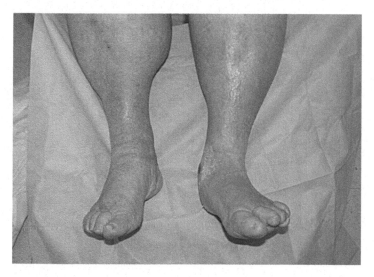

Figure 2 Typical venous ulcer over medial malleolus. Note lipodermatosclerosis which gives the leg a "champagne bottle" deformity.

weight, progressing to increased focal pressure and formation of callus (15). Ulceration may lead to infection, osteomyelitis, and possibly gangrene. Diabetic foot ulcers are often round, punched out and deep, with a thick, elevated rim of callus surrounding the ulcer. Autonomic neuropathy can result in dryness and fissuring of skin. Wound exudate is usually low to moderate, unless there is infection. Figure 4 shows a diabetic neuropathic foot ulcer.

Diabetic neuropathic ulcers are usually located on over bony prominences, i.e., the plantar aspects of the foot (beneath the metatarsal heads), over metatarsal heads, and under the heel. Ulcers between the toes may be a cause by shoes that are too

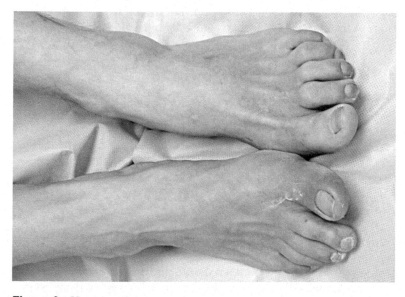

Figure 3 Hammertoes.

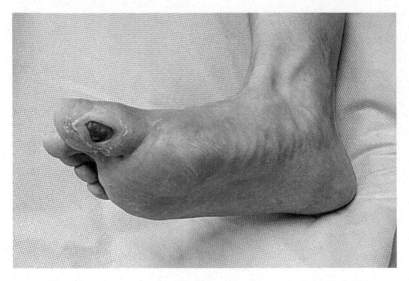

Figure 4 Diabetic neuropathic foot ulcer.

narrow. Ulcers under the metatarsal heads may be secondary to a claw deformity making the metatarsal heads more prominent. Ulcers in the middle of the weight-bearing surface beneath the arch suggest Charcot's deformity. Diabetic foot ulcers should be probed with a metal instrument. If bone can be palpated, osteomyelitis is highly likely.

Pulses in diabetic patients are altered secondary to medial calcification of arteries and severity of arterial disease in the diabetic patient is often underestimated by noninvasive vascular studies. Tibial and peroneal arterial occlusion is common, resulting in an ischemic foot with a strong popliteal pulse (20). Therefore, arteriography should be performed if ischemic disease is suspected (15). Atherosclerosis should be suspected if there is a history of claudication and if on physical exam there is delayed toe capillary refill, limb pallor with elevation, and rubor with dependency. Additional suggestions of arterial disease include shiny atrophic skin and thickened toenails (1).

6. OTHER IMPORTANT CONSIDERATIONS

6.1. Infection

Indications of infection include delayed healing, rapid wound enlargement, darker color of granulation tissue, cellulitis, increased friability and bleeding, pain, persistently malodorous wound even after cleansing, purulent discharge, and $> 10^5$ organisms per gram of wound tissue. Some of these signs and symptoms may be altered in immunocompromised patients.

Biopsy or curettage of the ulcer for tissue samples for culture is preferred to tissue swab in helping to differentiate between colonization vs. infection ($> 10^5$ organisms/gm tissue) (8,18). Bacterial culture with sensitivities may guide antibiotic therapy in cellulitis or sepsis. Systemic antibiotics should not be used as they do not improve healing time of noninfected wounds and may select for resistant microorganisms.

6.2. Debridement

Indications for debridement include presence of necrotic tissue in the presence of adequate circulation, severe infection, and deep eschar with viable tissue underneath. Diabetic foot ulcers should be debrided of callus, down to bleeding tissue. Debridement is contraindicated in noninfected wounds and in wounds free of fibrin and foreign matter. One should also be cautious with patients with poor circulation, i.e., patients with arterial disease requiring surgical evaluation, and pyoderma gangrenosum.

6.3. Laboratory Investigations

Routine bloodwork such as a complete blood count and glucose may help diagnose infection, anemia, polycythemia, and diabetes. Nutritional deficiencies may be disclosed by obtaining serum albumin, prealbumin, vitamin A, vitamin C, iron, transferrin levels, and zinc (1). Other laboratory tests to consider include, but are not limited to, erythrocyte sedimentation rate, cryoglobulins, cryofibrinogen, rheumatoid factor, antinuclear antibodies, lupus anticoagulant, antithrombin III, protein C, protein S, hepatitis A and C antibodies, and/or hepatitis B surface antigen (8,21). If the ulcer fails to heal after 3–6 months of treatment, biopsy may help exclude malignancy or vasculitis. Mycobacterial and fungal cultures should also be considered.

6.4. Noninvasive vs. Invasive Studies

Investigations begin with the physical examination of the pulses, followed by an ABPI. An ABPI should be performed by dividing the systolic pressure at the ankle (dorsalis pedis or posterior tibialis) by the higher of the systolic blood pressures of both arms. The importance of doing an ABPI is to rule out arterial disease, which is indicated by values < 0.9. It is essential to document a medical history of diabetes, as the ABPI can be inaccurate in these patients. In diabetics, the toe brachial index can give a more accurate indication of arterial status.

A duplex ultrasound of the lower extremities can diagnose venous reflux disease. Noninvasive vascular studies can provide information about the superficial, communicating, and deep venous systems, as well as information about arterial systems. They may measure degree of venous reflux, and provide data about the efficiency of the calf muscle pump. Examples of simple noninvasive tests include the color duplex ultrasound (considered the gold standard for diagnosing venous insufficiency), photoplethysmography (PPG), and air plethysmography (APG). Invasive phlebography studies such as venography are generally only recommended as an investigation prior to valvular surgery (8,6).

If osteomyelitis is suspected, one should consider an x-ray, bone scan, computed tomography scan, gallium scan, and/or bone biopsy to confirm the diagnosis. Patients with chronic leg ulcers commonly have allergic contact dermatitis to topical creams and ointments containing antibacterial agents such as neomycin and bacitracin, lanolin, and preservatives such as parabens and should undergo patch testing (18).

7. CONCLUSION

Proper management of chronic lower extremity ulcers begins with the appropriate diagnosis achieved by history, physical examination, and appropriate diagnostic tests. Once the underlying pathology has been correctly identified, treatment can be initiated. Briefly, in venous disease, the primary treatment is leg elevation and compression therapy (stockings, bandages, orthotics, and/or pneumatic compression) with consideration of skin substitutes or surgery for hard-to-heal ulcers. In arterial disease, the main goal of therapy is the re-establishment of an adequate arterial supply. Therefore, referral should be made to a vascular surgeon for assessment and possible revascularization (13,22). Neuropathic ulcers must be aggressively debrided, infection treated, and pressure relieved (23). For ulcers, which look or behave atypically, or fail to respond to treatment, alternative diagnoses should be considered.

In addition to the above, general principles should be applied. For example, constant monitoring for infection and sensitization to topical agents can help prevent complications. Consider biopsy if the ulcer fails to heal after 3–6 months of appropriate therapy to rule out malignancy. Local wound care such as maintaining a moist wound environment, cleansing, debridement, and the selection of an appropriate dressing are important. Novel therapies including biologic skin substitutes and growth factors may be appropriate (1).

ACKNOWLEDGMENTS

I would like to acknowledge Amy Ramos, CCRC for her generous assistance in obtaining figures for this chapter.

REFERENCES

1. Phillips TJ, Dover JS. Leg ulcers. J Am Acad Dermatol 1991; 25:965–987.
2. Phillips TJ. Chronic cutaneous ulcers: etiology and epidemiology. J Invest Dermatol 1994; 102(suppl 6):38S–41S.
3. Scott TE, LaMorte NW, Gorin DR, Menzoian JO. Risk factors for chronic venous insufficiency: a dual case-control study. J Vasc Surg 1995; 22:622–628.
4. Caputo GM, Cavanagh PR, Ulbrecht JS. Assessment and management of foot disease in patients with diabetes. New Eng J Med 1994:854–860.
5. Nelzen O, Bergquist D, Lindhagen A, et al. Chronic leg ulcers: an underestimated problem in primary health care among elderly patients. J Epidemiol Community Health 1991; 45:184–187.
6. Valencia IC, Falabella A, Kirsner RS, Eaglstein WH. Chronic venous insufficiency and venous leg ulceration. J Am Acad Dermatol 2001; 44:401–42.
7. Margolis DM, Berlin JA, Strom BL. Risk factors associated with the failure of a venous ulcer to heal. Arch Dermatol 1999; 135:920–926.
8. Ongenae KC, Phillips TJ. Leg ulcer management. Emergency Med 1993; 45–53.
9. Hiatt WR. Medical treatment of peripheral arterial disease and claudication. New Eng J Med 2001; 344(2).
10. Pham HT, Rich J, Veves. Wound healing in diabetic foot ulceration: A review and commentary. Wounds 2000; 12(4):79–81.
11. American Diabetes Association. Consensus Development Conference on Diabetic Foot Wound Care: 7–8 April 1999, Boston, MA.
12. Browne AC, Sibbald RG. The diabetic neuropathic ulcer: an overview. Ostomy/Wound Manage 1999; 45(1A) (suppl):6S–20S.
13. Phillips TJ. Successful methods of treating leg ulcers. Postgrad Med 1999; 105(5):159–178.
14. Menzoian JO, Arbid EJ, Phillips TJ, Bhawan J, LaMorte WW. Venous system of the lower extremities: physiology and pathophysiology. In: Sidawy AN, Sumpio BE,

Depalma RG, eds. The Basic Science of Vascular Disease. Armonk, NY: Futura Publishing Company, Inc., 1997:385–406.

15. Sumpio BE. Foot ulcers. Primary Care 343(11):787–793.
16. Rockson SG. Lymphedema. Am J Med 2001; 110(4):288–295.
17. Samlaska CP, James WD. Superficial thrombophlebitis II. Secondary hypercoagulable states. J Am Acad Dermatol 1990; 23(1):1–18.
18. Oahes N, Phillips TJ. Leg ulcers. Curr Probl Dermatol 1995; 7:109–142.
19. Hickman JG, Lazarus GS. Pyoderma gangrenosum: a reappraisal of associated systemic disease. Br J Dermatol 1980; 102:235–237.
20. Phillips TJ, Stanton B, Provan A, et al. A study of the impact of leg ulcers on quality of life: financial, social, and psychological implications. J Am Acad Dermatol 1994; 31: 49–53.
21. Bello YM, Phillips TJ. Management of venous ulcers. J of Cut Med Surg 1998; 3(suppl 1): S1–S6–S1–S12.
22. Margolis DJ. Venous leg ulcer: incidence and prevalence in the elderly. J Am Acad Dermatol 2002; 46:381–386.
23. Miller OF, Phillips TJ. Leg ulcers. J Am Acad Dermatol 2000; 43:91–95.
24. Baker SR, Jopp-McKay AG, Hoskin SE, Thompson PJ. Epidemiology of chronic venous ulcers. Br J Surg 1991; 78:864–867.
25. Callum MF, Ruckley CV, Harper DR, et al. Chronic ulceration of the leg: extent of the problem and provision of care. Br Med J 1985; 290:1855–1857.
26. Bello YM, Phillips TJ. Therapeutic dressings. Adv Dermatol 2000; 16:253–270.
27. McGovern, TW, Enzenauer RJ, Fitzpatrick JE. Treatment of recalcitrant leg ulcers in cryoglobulinemia type I and II with plasmapheresis. Arch Dermatol 1996; 132(5): 498–500.
28. Beightler E, Diven DG, Sanchez RL, Solomon AR. Thrombotic vasculopathy associated with cryofibrinogenemia. J Am Acad Dermatol 1991; 24:342–345.
29. Klein AD. Purpura and recurrent ulcers on the lower extremities. Arch Dermatol 1991; 127:113–118.
30. Bello YM, Khachemoune A , Stefanato CM, Phillips TJ. Diagnostic Dilemmas (Cryofibrinogenemia). Wounds 2000; 12(4):76–78.
31. De Villez RL, Roberts ML. Acroangiodermatitis of Mali. Southern Med J 1984; 77(2):255–258.
32. Lyle WG, Given KS. Acroangiodermatitis (Pseudo-Kaposi's sarcoma) associated with Klippel–Trenaunay syndrome). Ann Plast Surg 1996; 37(6):654–656.
33. Phillips TJ. Current approaches to venous ulcers and compression. Dermatol Surg 2001; 27:611–621.

8
Wound Microbiology and the Use of Antibacterial Agents

Lucy K. Martin, Anna Drosou, and Robert S. Kirsner
Department of Dermatology and Cutaneous Surgery, University of Miami School of Medicine, Miami, Florida, U.S.A.

1. INTRODUCTION

Cutaneous wound healing is a well-orchestrated cascade of events. These events lead to repair when the underlying dermis is compromised, while alternatively leading to regeneration when only the epidermis is injured. This process, should it occur in a timely fashion, is termed "acute wound healing" typically with restoration of skin integrity occurring a period of days to weeks. Classically, acute wound healing is considered to occur in three overlapping phases termed the inflammatory, proliferative, and remodeling phases, respectively (1). Conversely, when this process is disrupted and healing is prolonged, delayed or does not occur, the wound is termed a "chronic wound" (2). An exact time does not exist when acute wound healing becomes chronic but is rather dependent upon variables such as patient age and comorbid conditions and wound related variables such as the location of the wound, the size, depth and shape of the wound, or by what method the wound was created.

The most common types of chronic wounds include the venous leg ulcers, diabetic foot ulcers secondary to neuropathy, pressure ulcers, and ulcers secondary to vascular disease. A chronic wound may take months to heal or may not show a tendency to heal at all. This unfortunately is not rare, as less than 25% of diabetic foot ulcers enrolled in the standard of care arm in recent clinical trials healed during the study period and less than half of diabetic foot ulcers heal in clinical practice (3,4). Significant attention has focused on chronic wounds, especially those that have failed to heal, as they are associated with significant cost in both human and financial terms. Among the many factors suggested being causal in retarding healing is an abnormal microbiologic environment of the wound. Therefore, knowledge of wound microbiology is essential.

There are a number of ways in which wound microbiology affects healing. Bacteria may be present in abundant numbers, the criteria for and the definition of "abundant" may depend upon the type and virulence of the bacteria and host characteristics as well. For example, the abnormal presence of bacteria in wounds prolongs the inflammatory phase of wound healing, which may delay the process in which wounds start to heal. Bacteria present in wounds consume glucose and oxygen and therefore may lead to tissue anoxia. Cell lysis is promoted by a low pH and tissue anoxia (5).

While it is possible for acute wounds to lack bacteria, most, but not all, chronic wounds contain bacteria and this bacterial presence has been termed "bioburden." Bioburden refers to the metabolic load imposed by bacteria (6). Often, it is the relation between the resident bacteria and the host whereby the balance between the bioburden and the host defenses determine if infection or detriment to healing will occur (6,7). While, some authors believe density of microorganisms is the critical factor in determining whether a wound is likely to heal (8–12), others believe specific pathogens are of primary importance in delayed healing (13–18). However, not all are convinced the importance of bacteria in delayed healing (19–25). This chapter focuses on bacteria in wounds and attempts to eradicate those bacteria to correct any healing detriment they may possess.

2. BIOFILMS AND PLANKTONIC BACTERIA

Bacteria grow in various forms. Best known are free floating or planktonic bacteria. An alternative method in which bacteria may grow is in biofilms. Biofilms are complex communities of bacteria (as well as other microorganisms) that adhere to solid surfaces (26). The microorganisms in biofilms are embedded in an extracellular polysaccharide matrix or glycocalyx (27). Bacterial biofilms are known to be in a sessile or in an adherent form, which differs from the planktonic or free-living form of bacteria. These biofilms have been implicated in chronic infections and are known to be resistant to antimicrobial agents (26). The ways in which biofilms are resistant to different antimicrobial agents include an inability of the antimicrobial agent to penetrate the depth of the biofilm, slower rate of growth of the biofilm bacteria due to nutrient limitation (28) or an adoption of a distinct phenotype of bacteria as a response to growth on a surface (29).

Reports of evidence supporting the presence of biofilms on the surface of chronic human wounds as well as in animal models involving partial thickness wounds are relatively new (30,31). As tight attachment is among the hallmark features of biofilms, theoretically, attempts to treat biofilms with agents that prevent attachment or promote the detachment of biofilms would be advantageous (27). Biofilms have the ability to survive in hostile environments. They contain different structures including channels in which circulation of nutrients can occur, cells in different areas of the biofilm exhibit diverse patterns of gene expression (32,33). It is believed that an acylated homoserine lactone (acyl-HSL) is responsible for the maturation of the biofilm (34). One special characteristic that biofilms have is known as quorum sensing. Quorum sensing is the way bacteria communicate and this process allows bacteria to survive without consuming all of their nutrients and allows biofilms to dispose their waste products (35).

Biofilms can be caused by a single organism or in combination with a variety of different species of bacteria (or other microorganisms including fungi) (27). The same species of bacteria that cause biofilms can occur at the same time as planktonic bacteria. Due to factors mentioned above related to resistance, antibiotic therapy destroys planktonic cells without harming the biofilm (36). It should be mentioned that much of the information learned about bacteria and wounds is from studies of planktonic bacteria. Much more needs to be and will be learned about the role of biofilm bacteria in healing and wounds.

3. THE IMPORTANCE OF BACTERIA WITHIN WOUNDS

It is important to distinguish between colonization and infection. Some acute wounds and virtually all chronic wounds contain bacteria and many heal. Occlusive dressings, have been used as part which speed healing, reduce pain and scarring, in fact, encourage microbial proliferation in wounds (22,37), yet the infection rate is lower under occlusive dressings than under conventional dry dressings (38,39). Therefore, the mere presence of bacteria is not necessarily bad. Whether faster healing using occlusive dressings is related to the increased number of bacteria is under investigation.

When clinical signs of infection, such as pain and tenderness, redness, warmth, and swelling in the surrounding and adjacent tissue as seen in patients experiencing cellulitis, or lymphangitis, the clinical importance of a microbiologic findings of bacteria is obvious (39). These features and perhaps wound histology may be used to distinguished infection from colonization. Histology may be useful as by definition, infection involves invasion of viable tissue by pathogens (40). On the other hand, colonization refers to the presence of multiplying bacteria without immunological reaction or clinical symptoms (41).

However, another situation is when clinical signs of infection are not present or are blunted by patient characteristics (diabetes, age concomitant medications, etc.), yet a wound has increased exudate, odor or simply fails to heal. This situation represents an intermediate site on the spectrum from colonization to infection and may represent situations where normal healing is altered without tissue invasion. It is this situation that is the focus of many clinicians involved with chronic wound care.

4. MICROBIOLOGY OF WOUNDS

The effect of specific types of microorganisms on wound healing has been widely published. The majority of wounds are polymicrobial, involving both aerobes and anaerobes, aerobic pathogens such as *Staphylococcus aureus, Pseudomonas aeruginosa*, and beta-hemolytic *Streptococci* have been most frequently cited as the cause of delayed wound healing and infection (15,17,18,42–47). A consensus meeting of the European Tissue Repair Society and the European Wound Management Association in 1998, a general opinion was that the presence of beta-hemolytic (group A) *Streptococci* or *P. aeruginosa* in a chronic wound was an indicator of the need for antimicrobial therapy.

However, it may be that the polymicrobial bacteriology may play a role in healing. In a study of the bacteriology of chronic leg ulcers in 52 patients, Trengove et al. (25) reported that no single microorganism or group of microorganisms was more detrimental to wound healing than any other (inclusive of *S. aureus, P. aeruginosa*, beta-hemolytic *Streptococci*, anaerobes, and coliform bacteria). However, a significantly lower probability of healing was observed if four or more bacterial groups were present in any ulcer (25), and this indicates that microbial interactions may have induced an enhanced pathogenic effect. Similarly, Bowler and Davies (48) reported a greater diversity of microorganisms in infected leg ulcers than in noninfected leg ulcers (means of 5.1 and 3.6 isolates per wound, respectively). These observations support an earlier view of Kingston and Seal (49), who argued that all species associated with a microbial disease should be considered potentially synergistic, rather than a single species being causative, as is commonly perceived. Additionally, certain organisms make the identification of other bacteria difficult. For example, Proteus species, which has a high incidence in venous ulcers, has a swarming characteristic hiding the presence of other organisms. Alternative culture conditions or methods may help obviate this (50).

In addition to type of bacteria in 1964, Bendy et al. (51) described effect of bacterial number on healing of decubitus ulcers and found healing progressed only when the bacterial load was $< 10^6$ CFU/mL of wound fluid. In that study, quantification was determined by using superficial wound swab samples. Similar observations, using counts from tissue biopsy specimens, with skin graft survival in experimental wounds (52), pressure ulcer healing (53), and delayed closure of surgical wounds (54). Work from Robson and Heggers, among others, suggests acute or chronic wound infection exists when the microbial load is $> 10^5$ CFU/g of tissue.

However, Pruitt et al. (55) reported quantitative cultures incapable of differentiating between burn wound colonization and infection, and they described histological analysis as being the most effective and rapid method for determining invasive burn wound infection.

Keep in mind that immuno-compromised patients can have infection at less than 10^5 colonies (5). While classically one thinks of an immunocompromised patientas someone with HIV infection, having or being treated for cancer or a transplant recipient, a broader definition including diabetics, the elderly and infermed may be worthwhile. It is also important to consider that certain organisms (less than 10^5 organisms/g) are known to cause infection at lower concentration even in the immuno-competent such as group A beta-hemolytic *Streptococcus* (6,53,56).

5. SAMPLING TECHNIQUES

Identifying wound bacteria is essential in the treatment of wounds. In addition to delayed to healing, bacteria present in wounds can lead to cellulitis, osteomyelitis, bacteremia, or sepsis, therefore proper identification and management should be addressed (5). Several methods exist with the two major methods of identifying bacteria being tissue biopsy and swab culture. Both methods have the common goal of identifying bacteria both in a qualitative and quantitative fashion. The gold standard used to determine bacterial bioburden is tissue biopsy (36). This is because using this technique, one may be able to identify both the type and quantity of bacteria reliably.

The acquisition of deep tissue during biopsy following initial debridement and cleansing of superficial debris is recognized as being the most useful method for determining the microbial load and the presence of invasive pathogens (57–59). Tissue is obtained aseptically and is then weighed, homogenized, serially diluted, and cultured on selective and nonselective agar media under aerobic and anaerobic conditions to provide quantitative and qualitative information. It is rationalized that determining the bacteria in tissue as opposed to the surface of a wound may have greater clinical significance. Tissue biopsies, however, are not always performed due to various reasons (60). These include the high cost, pain, damage to healing tissue, unavailability of materials used to process tissue biopsies, and the need for expertise in obtaining a sample.

Additionally, the relative delay in obtaining results from this techniques have suggested other possibilities including a rapid Gram stain technique, which may reliably predict a microbial load of $> 10^5$ CFU/g of tissue if a single microorganism was seen on the slide preparation (9,12). However, in diabetic foot infections and burn wounds, both of which involve complex microbial ecosystems, a poor correlation between Gram stain and culture results from deep tissue biopsy specimens have been reported (61). Regarding the speed of obtaining culture results, it appears culture results serve different needs dependent upon the situation taken. For acute infections, culture results serve to confirm the choice of empiric therapy prescribed. In this case, the clinician does not have the luxury to wait for culture results prior to prescribing therapy. For chronic wounds, where antimicrobial is being considered to reverse the inhibitory effect of bacteria within the wound, the clinician can await the results prior to instituting therapy.

The swab culture is a relatively simple procedure and has been recommended without the above mentioned disadvantages (62). Wound swabbing most frequently involves the use of a cotton-tipped swab to sample superficial wound fluid and tissue debris, and this enables a semiquantitative and qualitative analysis of the wound microflora. An alginate-tipped swab can also be used to perform a fully quantitative analysis, since the swab will dissolve and release all associated microorganisms when transferred to an appropriate diluent.

Swab sampling has been challenged on the basis that the superficial microbiology does not reflect that of deeper tissue (63,64) and that subsequent cultures do not correlate with the presence of pathogenic bacteria (65). Also, if a swab sample is taken inappropriately (i.e., prior to wound cleansing and removal of devitalized superficial debris), the resulting culture has been considered to reflect only surface contamination (66) and provide misleading or useless information (57). However, since the majority of wounds are contaminated with endogenous microorganisms from the external environment, any microorganisms present in deeper tissue are also likely to be present in the superficial debris. Consequently, it is most likely that superficial wound fluid and tissue debris display a full spectrum of the wound aerobic and anaerobic microflora, some of which may be involved in pathogenesis and some of which may not be.

Regarding anaerobes, anaerobes are not regarded as being detrimental to normal wound healing (18,20,21,67). Compared with aerobic and facultative microorganisms, the culture, isolation, and identification of anaerobic bacteria is more time-consuming, labor-intensive, and expensive and is often deemed to be too demanding for many diagnostic microbiology laboratories. This concept has recently been challenged (68).

Several studies have demonstrated a correlation between surface cultures and tissue biopsy cultures. Levine et al. (69) demonstrated a close correlation between quantitative swab and tissue biopsy specimen counts in open burn wounds, and Armstrong et al. (70) observed no difference in the isolation rate of microorganisms from deep tissue and superficial curettage in 112 diabetic foot ulcer infections. Using an experimental rat model, Bornside and Bornside (71) demonstrated tissue counts of 10^5 CFU/g were equivalent to a 10^3 CFU/mL count obtained from a moist swab. Similarly, Thomson (59) demonstrated a correlation between a semiquantitative surface swab count (1+ to 4+) and a fully quantitative biopsy specimen count in burn wounds; 1+ growth from a swab correlated with a tissue count of 10^2 to 10^3

CFU/g, and 4+ correlated with a tissue count of approximately 10^7 CFU/g. Other studies (24,48) also demonstrated a close correlation between the isolation of microorganisms in superficial and deep tissue.

Rudensky et al. (66) compared wound swab cultures, tissue aspiration, and tissue biopsies and found that tissue biopsies were the most effective method. However, it is possible the results are altered due to surface colonization in devitalized tissue. Proper swab culture technique is required with prior cleansing of the surface tissue before obtaining swab cultures in addition to pressure application to exude fluid from the wound tissue (36,69). Once again it should be highlighted that proponents of the equivalency of wound swabs point out that wound contamination most often occurs from sources external to the wound. Thus, superficial tissue is likely to harbor a diversity of microorganisms, one or more of which may invade deeper tissue, and it is highly unlikely that superficial tissue will be "sterile" while deeper tissue is "infected." Most wounds are colonized with microorganisms, and a failure to isolate them is more likely to be a consequence of poor microbiological technique.

As technology expands new techniques in bacteriologic identification emerge. Examples include certain fluorescent stained microbes visualized under ultraviolet light. DNA analysis using gene probes, DNA finger-printing, and DNA amplification are other examples (72,73). Serologic analysis can also be used to identify microbes, providing information on antigenic determinants in bacterial cell walls, capsules, and flagella.

6. WHEN TO CULTURE A WOUND

Routine culturing of wound is not indicated but should be reserved for wounds that are either clinically infected or those that have no clinical signs of infection but are deteriorating or failing to heal. In the former situation, a surface swab sample can provide useful data regarding the presence of potential pathogens, the diversity of microorganisms involved, and, direct antimicrobial therapy. In the latter situation, optimally a tissue culture for qualitative and quantitative analysis should be obtained or if not available a swab vulture may suffice. A swab sample can also provide a semiquantitative estimation of the microbial load (e.g., light growth to heavy growth, or $> 10^5$ CFU/mL), which is considerably easier to perform than a fully quantitative analysis. A correlation between semiquantitative swab data and quantitative biopsy data has previously been demonstrated (59,69–71,74,75). Although wound cleansing is considered necessary to avoid the pointless exercise of sampling superficial devitalized tissue (63–66), Hansson et al. (23) observed no difference in the qualitative and quantitative microbiology of leg ulcers, whether or not they were cleansed prior to sampling with absorbent disks.

7. MANAGEMENT OF BACTERIA IN WOUNDS

Although systemic antibiotic therapy is essential for advancing cutaneous infections and those that involve deeper tissues, wounds that exhibit only localized signs of infection or are failing to heal but do not have clinical signs of infection (having a clinical important bioburden) may initially be treated with topical agents. Topical antimicrobial agents include both antiseptics and antibiotics.

In support of this concept are recent guidelines on the treatment of pressure ulcers issued by the European Pressure Ulcer Advisory Panel that recommended that systemic antibiotics not be required for pressure ulcers that exhibit only clinical signs of local infection (76). Since leg ulcers and foot ulcers often exhibit a similar microflora to pressure ulcers, such advice could probably be extended to cover a wider variety of chronic wound types. In the absence of advancing cellulitis, bacteremia, fever, or pain, topical antimicrobial agents (antibiotics or antiseptics) may offer the most useful first line of treatment. This section focuses on the use of antiseptics for nonhealing ulcers.

8. ANTISEPTICS

Antiseptics are agents that destroy or inhibit the growth and development of micro-organisms, in or on living tissue. Unlike antibiotics that act selectively on a specific target, antiseptics have multiple targets and a broader spectrum of activity, which include bacteria, fungi, viruses, protozoa, and even prions (77,78). Several antiseptic categories exist including alcohols (ethanol), anilides (triclocarban), biguanides (chlorhexidine), bisphenols (triclosan), chlorine compounds, iodine compounds, silver compounds, peroxygens, and quaternary ammonium compounds. Among the most commonly used products in the clinical practice today are povidone iodine, chlorhexidine, alcohol, acetate, hydrogen peroxide, boric acid, silver nitrate, silver sulfadiazine (SSD), and sodium hypochlorite.

Several antiseptic agents focus on cleansing intact skin and are used for preparing patients preoperatively, prior to injections or venous punctures, pre- and post-operative scrubbing in the operating room and hand washing by medical personnel. Some contain a detergent, which renders them too harsh for use on the non-intact skin (79). The usefulness of antiseptics on intact skin is well established and broadly accepted (19). However, the use of antiseptics as prophylactic anti-infective agents for open wounds such as lacerations, abrasions, burns, and chronic ulcers, has been an area of intense controversy for several years.

Two official guidelines have been released concerning antiseptic use on wounds. Povidone iodine has been FDA approved for short-term treatment of superficial and acute wounds (80). The statement includes that povidone-iodine has not been found to either promote or inhibit wound healing. On the other hand, guidelines for the treatment of pressure ulcers by the U.S. Department of Health and Human Services strongly discourage the use of antiseptics and promote the use of normal saline for cleansing pressure ulcers (81).

The main rationale for using antiseptics on open wounds is prevention of infection, and therefore increased rate of the healing process. It is well established that infections can delay healing, cause failure to healing and even wound deterioration (82). Consequently, although creation of an optimal environment for the wound healing process is currently the primary objective of wound care, prevention of infection still plays a critical role in wound management. Another argument for the use of antiseptics is that antiseptics are considered preferable to topical antibiotics with regard to development. Antiseptics work by eliminating all pathogenic bacteria of the wound, while antibiotics are effective only to the certain bacteria that are sensitive to them. Although resistance towards antiseptics has been reported it is significantly lesser than reported with antibiotic usage (83). According to McDonnell and Russell (77) some acquired mechanisms of resistance (especially to heavy metals) have been shown to be clinically significant, but in most cases the results have been speculative. Moreover, development of resistance against povidone iodine, which is the most commonly used antiseptic today, in practice does not exist (84). Payne et al.

(85) state that the sensible use of antiseptics could help decrease the usage of antibiotics, preserving their advantage for clinically critical situations.

Antiseptics are also considered superior to topical antibiotics when their rates of causing contact sensitization are compared. Aminoglycosides, especially neomycin, have a much higher sensitization rate compared to povidone-iodine (86). Moreover, patients allergic to one antibiotic may acquire cross-allergy to other antibiotics as well. The sensitization rate to povidone-iodine, the most commonly used antiseptic, has been found to be only 0.73% (86,87).

A main concern prior to applying a topical agent on a wound is to assure it is safe. Agents that are cytotoxic or cause delay on wound healing are regarded with reservation. The strongest argument against the use of antiseptics on wounds is the fact that antiseptics have been found, mainly in in vitro models, to be cytotoxic to cells essentials for the wound healing process, such as fibroblasts, keratinocytes, and leukocytes (88–90). However, this cytotoxicity seems to be concentration dependent since several antiseptics in low concentrations are not cytotoxic while they keep their antibacterial activity in vitro (86). Since the in vitro results are not always predictive of what may happen in vivo, numerous studies have been conducted on animal and human models. The results of these studies are conflicting and will be presented below.

A second reason against the use of antiseptics on open wounds, first stated by Fleming in 1919 (91), is that antiseptics are not as effective against bacteria that reside in wounds as they are against bacteria in vitro. The presence of exudate, serum or blood seems to decrease their activity. However, several bacteriological studies show that antiseptics may decrease the bacterial counts of wounds (92,93).

9. IODINE COMPOUNDS

Since the first discovery of the natural element iodine in 1811 by the chemist Bernard Courtois, iodine and its compounds have been broadly used for prevention of infection and treatment of wounds (94). However, molecular iodine can be very toxic for tissues, so formulations composed by combination of iodine with a carrier that decreases iodine availability, were developed. Povidone-iodine (PVP-I) results from the combination of molecular iodine and polyvinylpyrrolidone. Povidone-iodine is available in several forms (solution, cream, ointment, and scrub). The scrub form contains detergent and should be used only on intact skin. Cadexomer iodine consists of spherical hydrophilic beads of cadexomer-starch which contain iodine, is highly absorbent, and release iodine slowly in the wound area. It is available as an ointment and as a dressing. Numerous studies have been conducted in order to determine the safety and efficacy of iodine compounds on wound healing.

9.1. Effects of Iodine Compounds on the Bacterial Load of Wounds
9.1.1. Povidone Iodine (PVP-I)
Several animal studies have been done examining the effects of PVP-I on the bacterial load of wounds. These results have not proven the efficacy of PVP-I; however, the results of numerous clinical trials show that it is effective in reducing the bacterial load of wounds. Rodeheaver et al. (95) found povidone iodine solutions significantly reduce bacterial load 10 min after the application of the antiseptic, this effect did not persist as there was no decreased rate of infection or decreased bacteria number, four days after a single PVP-I application. Another study (96) that evaluated contami-

nated 12-hour old lacerations in a guinea pig model failed to find any decrease of wound bacterial counts after irrigation with PVP-I in comparison to normal saline.

However, most of the human trials performed prove the efficacy of PVP-I in clinical situations. In an uncontrolled study, Georgiade et al. (97) showed PVP-I that controlled bacterial growth in 50 patients. Gravett et al. (98) found 1% PVP-I solution reduced the incidence of infection in sutured lacerations in 395 patients. In a recent study (99) on venous leg ulcers, the combination of PVP-I with hydrocolloid dressing was shown to reduce the bacterial load and increase the healing rate in comparison to the hydrocolloid dressing alone.

Viljanto (100), in surgical wounds in 294 pediatric patients, found a 5% PVP-I aerosol, increased infection, which they related to excipients (glycerol, citrate–phosphate buffer, polyoxyethylated nonylphenol) in the aerosol. Follow-up experiments found the 5% aerosol caused pronounced leukocyte migration, a 5% solution without excipients caused slighter inhibition, while the 1% solution was practically no different to the control (saline). Subsequently, spraying wounds with a 1% PVP-I solution had no effect on wound healing while significantly decreased infection rate, and increased bactericidal activity is found at lower concentrations (101).

Conversely, some studies have not confirmed those previously mentioned results. PVP-I soaking was not found to significantly decrease bacterial counts in acute traumatic contaminated wounds that required debridement, while saline soaking caused increased counts. PVP-I solution was not found to be an effective substitute to wound cleaning and debridement (102).

9.1.2. Cadexomer Iodine

The efficacy of cadexomer iodine has been shown in both animal and human models. Using a porcine model, Mertz et al. (103) found daily cadexomer iodine significantly reduced MRSA and total bacteria in the wounds, in comparison to no treatment control and vehicle (cadexomer) at all time points. Danielsen et al. (104) found negative culture results in an uncontrolled series treating ulcers with cadexomer iodine that were colonized with *P. aeruginosa* in 65% and 75% of patients after 1 and 12 weeks treatment, respectively.

9.2. Effects of Iodine Compounds on Wound Healing Process
9.2.1. PVP-I

Literature regarding the effect of PVP-I on wound healing in animal wound models is conflicting. Briefly, in some studies, PVP-I was found to cause no inhibition on wound re-epithelialization (105,106), while in others it retarded healing (107). Similarly, conflicting results regarding effect on tensile strength has been reported with PVP-I causing increased tensile strength (108), reduced tensile strength (109), or having no effect (110). It has also been found to have no effect on collagen (109) and granulation tissue production or nonsignificant reduction (111). Moreover, it has been shown to increase revascularization (112).

Clinical studies evaluating the influence of PVP-I in wound healing are numerous. Most of them showed no decrease in wound healing rate from the use of PVP-I. The aforementioned study by Viljanto (100) found no effect on wound healing when a 1% solution is used. Niedner (79) concluded that neither suction blister healing (113) nor healing after Moh's surgery (114) or burns (115) is negatively influenced by PVP-I.

Piérard-Franchimont et al. (99) examined the effect of PVP-I in combination with hydrocolloid dressing on venous leg ulcers and found healing rate was accelerated. Lee et al. (116) in a noncontrolled study, found reduction of infection and promotion of healing in patients with long standing (6 months to 16 years) decubitus and venous ulcerations. In a review of in vivo studies, Mayer and Tsapogas (117) summarized the data by concluding PVP-I was not found to negatively influence wound healing in comparison to the control group or to other treatments.

9.2.2. Cadexomer Iodine

In animal models, cadexomer iodine has been reported to increase epidermal regeneration and epithelialization in both partial thickness and full thickness wounds (92,118). However, cadexomer iodine appears to have no effect on granulation tissue formation, neovascularization, or wound contraction (79).

Cadexomer iodine has also been the subject of many clinical studies. In these studies, cadexomer iodine has been found to effective and beneficial to wound healing. Nine clinical trials comparing the effects of cadexomer iodine with other treatments on chronic venous ulcers showed enhancement of wound healing. The other treatments compared to cadexomer iodine included "standard treatment" (cleansing with diluted hydrogen peroxide or diluted potassium permanganate baths and covering with either a zinc paste dressing or nonadherent dressings, mainly paraffin-impregnated or saline dressings, or saline wet-to-dry compressive dressings, or gentian violet and polymyxin-bacitracin ointment, or support bandaging/stocking and a dry dressing) (119–124), dextranomer (125) and hydrocolloid dressing or paraffin gauze dressings (126). In one study, no control group was used since the main purpose of the study was to examine the safety of cadexomer iodine as far as the development of sensitivity is concerned (127). In several of these studies, the ulcers had been recalcitrant or non-responding to previous treatments. All these studies found cadexomer iodine not only not inhibit healing, but also accelerate it. Moreover, observations of other positive effects included reduction of pain, removal of pus, debris, and exudate, and stimulation of granulation tissue formation were made (128). As an example, Moberg et al. (129) in a randomized trial compared cadexomer iodine with standard treatment in patients with decubitus ulcers. Cadexomer iodine significantly accelerated the healing rate and reduced pus, debris, and pain of the ulcers.

Summarizing the review of numerous in vivo studies of iodine compounds we can conclude that in humans PVP-I and cadexomer iodine do not have a negative effect healing, while cadexomer iodine possibly accelerates it in chronic human wounds. Both can be effective in reducing bacteria number and decreasing infections. Results of animal studies depend on many variables and should be interpreted with caution. The studies of PVP-I rendered more conflicting results, especially on the animal models and have caused concern on many clinicians. Nevertheless, the results from the studies evaluating cadexomer iodine are clear and leave no doubt that this newer iodine compound is effective without having any negative influence on wound healing rate; instead, an acceleration of wound healing has been observed.

10. SILVER COMPOUNDS

Silver compounds have widely been used as wound antiseptics, mainly in burns. Silver sulfadiazine (SSD) and silver nitrate ($AgNO_3$) are among the most commonly used. Silver sulfadiazine is the most broadly used treatment for the prevention of infection in patients with burn wounds (130,131). Combinations of SSD with cerium nitrate (132) and nanocrystalline silver releasing systems (Acticoat dressing) (133) have been developed in order to increase its efficacy and/or reduce its toxicity. The newer silver formulations, such as Acticoat, seem to increase the rate and degree of microbial killing, decrease exudate formation and can remain active for days (134).

Animal studies examining the effects of SSD and $AgNO_3$ on wounds have showed no significant effect (107) on epithelialization rate. Silver sulfadiazine was also found to increase the rate of neovascularization. In another study in rats, silver compounds were found to promote wound healing, reduce the inflammatory and granulation phases of healing and influence metal ion binding (135). Moreover, Geronemus et al. (105) found increased re-epithelialization rate in domestic pigs with the use of SSD. However, Leitch et al. (136) found SSD to cause inhibition of wound contraction in an acute wound rat model. Likewise, Niedner and Schopf (111) found a slight, nonsignificant reduction of granulation tissue formation with the use of $AgNO_3$.

Little controversy exists over the role of silver products in burn wounds, however, the use of sliver in other wound is less widely accepted. Kucan et al. (137) examined the effects of SSD on bacterial counts in patients with infected chronic pressure ulcers. They found SSD to be effective in decreasing the bacteria below 10^5 per gram tissue in all the ulcers treated. In a randomized, trial with venous ulcers, SSD 1% cream statistically reduced the ulcer size compared to the placebo (138), while in another study it found well tolerated, and effective on wound cleansing and granulation tissue formation (139). Livingstone et al. (140) studied the effect of $AgNO_3$ and an antibiotic solution (neomycin plus bacitracin) on reducing autogenous skin graft loss due to infection in patients with thermal injury. They found both medications to be effective in comparison to the control group (Ringer's lactate solution), but the antibiotic solution was associated with the rapid emergence of drug-resistant organisms, while $AgNO_3$ was not.

Summarizing, it appears that silver compounds have no negative effect on wounds, and maybe they can accelerate wound healing clinically. Their in vivo antimicrobial activity is not in question.

11. OLD AND EMERGING ANTI-MICROBIALS

Many essential oils possess anti-microbial properties, and tea tree oil in particular (derived from the Australian native plant *Melaleuca alternifolia*) has been recognized for its efficacy against methicillin-resistant *S. aureus* and has consequently been considered as an alternative treatment for mupirocin-resistant methicillin-resistant *S. aureus* (140). Additional work regarding safety and clinical efficacy data needs to be generated.

Honey is an ancient remedy gaining renewed popularity as an alternative treatment for antibiotic-resistant bacteria. Both honey and sugar (in a paste form) are considered useful as topical antimicrobial agents, primarily as a consequence of their high osmolarity and ability to minimize water availability to bacteria (141). Although the dilution of honey in the presence of wound fluid is likely to reduce the efficacy of its osmotic effect, the slow and sustained production of hydrogen peroxide by some types of honey (e.g., manuka honey) is capable of maintaining an antimicrobial effect at a concentration approximately 1000-fold lower (and less toxic) than that commonly used in antiseptics (i.e., 3%) (142). Also, components of manuka honey such as flavonoids and aromatic acids, demonstrate antimicrobial properties (143). Honey may also serve as a wound deodorizing agent, and attributed to the glucose that is metabolized by bacteria as opposed to proteinaceous necrotic tissue, resulting in the production of lactic acid and not the malodorous compounds generated by protein degradation. Honey's use in infected wounds has been attributed to the high glucose content and low pH both which stimulate macrophages (144).

Prior to antibiotics, larvae (maggots) as a wound debridement strategy (145,146) was routine. Biosurgical debridement has played a minor role in wound management during the last 50 years, its popularity has gradually increased again during the 1990s as alternative treatments have been sought in an attempt to combat the surge in infections caused by antibiotic-resistant bacteria. Larval therapy is currently being used in the treatment of a variety of infected acute and chronic wounds, including those colonized by resistant bacteria such as methicillin-resistant *S. aureus* (147,148). The fly maggots of *Lucilia sericata* are capable of physically and enzymatically degrading devitalized tissue in a safe, effective manner. During this process, potentially pathogenic bacteria may be destroyed as part of the natural feeding process, but endogenous antimicrobial secretions are also considered to play an important role in microbial elimination (147,148). Additional data suggest that fly larvae may stimulate fibroblast proliferation in vitro (158).

12. CONCLUSION

Appreciation of the role of bacteria in healing is critical. Bacteria may be a detriment to patients by causing infection or prolonging or preventing healing. To fully recognize the effect of bacteria upon healing for any given patient, the way in which bacteria live, the number and type of bacteria and characteristics of the host are all important. In addition to planktonic form, bacteria may live in a tightly adherent and resistant colonies as biofilms. For planktonic bacteria, studies suggest that greater than 10^5 CFU of bacteria per gram of tissue is detrimental to healing but certain bacteria and in certain patients, lower levels may be important as well. Both qualitative and quantitative cultures will assist in evaluating problematic but random cultures of patients with wounds are not recommended. To appropriately treat an abnormal bacterial burden and to decrease the development of host resistance, a variety of topical treatment options may be utilized including the use of novel agents.

REFERENCES

1. Kirsner RS, Bogensberger G. The wound healing process. In: McColluch JM, Kloth LC, Feedar JA, eds. Wound Healing Alternatives in Management. 3rd ed. Philadelphia: F.A. Davis Company, 2001.
2. Schultz GS, Sibbald RG, Falanga V, Ayello EA, Dowsett C, Harding K, Romanelli M, Stacey MC, Teot L, Vanscheidt W. Wound bed preparation: a systematic approach to wound management. Wound Repair Regen 2003; 11(suppl 1):S1–S28.
3. Margolis DJ, Kantor J, Berlin JA. Healing of diabetic neuropathic foot ulcers receiving standard treatment. A meta-analysis. Diab Care 1999; 22:692–695.
4. Margolis DJ, Kantor J, Santanna J, Strom BL, Berlin JA. Effectiveness of platelet releasate for the treatment of diabetic neuropathic foot ulcers. Diab Care 2001; 24:483–488.

5. Corum GM. Characteristics and prevention of wound infection. J Et Nurs 1993; 20: 21–25.

6. Stotts, NA, Whotney JD. Identifying and evaluating wound infection. Home Healthc Nurse 1999; 17(3):159–164.

7. Robson MC. Wound infection: a failure of wound healing caused by an imbalance of bacteria. Surg Clin N Am 1977; 77(3):637–650.

8. Heggers JP. Defining infection in chronic wounds: does it matter? J Wound Care 1998; 7:389–392

9. Heggers JP, Robson MC, Doran ET. Quantitative assessment of bacterial contamination of open wounds by a slide technique. Trans R Soc Trop Med Hyg 1969; 63: 532–534.

10. Mangram AJ, Horan TC, Pearson ML, Silver LC, Jarvis WR. Guideline for prevention of surgical site infection. Am J Infect Control 1999; 27:97–134.

11. Raahave D, Friis-Moller A, Bjerre-Jespen K, Thiis-Knudsen J, Rasmussen LB. The infective dose of aerobic and anaerobic bacteria in postoperative wound sepsis. Arch Surg 1986; 121:924–929.

12. Robson MC. Lessons gleaned from the sport of wound watching. Wound Rep Regen 1999; 7:2–6.

13. Danielsen LE, Balslev G, Döring N, Høiby SM, Madsen M, Ågren M, Thomsen HK, Fos HHS, Westh H. Ulcer bed infection. Report of a case of enlarging venous leg ulcer colonised by *Pseudomonas aeruginosa*. APMIS 1998; 106:721–726.

14. Lavery LA, Harkless LB, Felder-Johnson K, Mundine S. Bacterial pathogens in infected puncture wounds in adults with diabetes. J Foot Ankle Surg 1994; 33:91–97.

15. Madsen SM, Westh H, Danielsen L, Rosdahl VT. Bacterial colonisation and healing of venous leg ulcers. APMIS 1996; 104:895–899.

16. Pallua N, Fuchs PC, Hafemann B, Völpel U, Noah M, Lütticken R. A new technique for quantitative bacterial assessment on burn wounds by modified dermabrasion. J Hosp Infect 1999; 42:329–337.

17. Schraibman IG. The significance of beta-haemolytic streptococci in chronic leg ulcers. Ann R Coll Surg Med 1990; 7292:123–124.

18. Sehgal SC, Arunkumar BK. Microbial flora and its significance in pathology of sickle cell disease leg ulcers. Infection 1992; 20:86–88.

19. Annoni F, Rosina M, Chiurazzi D, Ceva M. The effects of a hydrocolloid dressing on bacterial growth and the healing process of leg ulcers. Int Angiol 1989; 8:224–228.

20. Eriksson G, Eklund AE, Kallings LO. The clinical significance of bacterial growth in venous leg ulcers. Scand J Infect Dis 1984; 16:175–180.

21. Gilchrist B, Reed C. The bacteriology of chronic venous ulcers treated with occlusive hydrocolloid dressings. Br J Dermatol 1989; 121:337–344.

22. Handfield-Jones SE, Grattan CEH, Simpson RA, Kennedy CTC. Comparison of a hydrocolloid dressing and paraffin gauze in the treatment of venous ulcers. Br J Dermatol 1988; 118:425–427.

23. Hansson C, Hoborn J, Moller A, Swanbeck G. The microbial flora in venous leg ulcers without clinical signs of infection. Acta Dermatol Venereol (Stockh) 1995; 75:24–30.

24. Sapico FL, Witte JL, Canawati HN, Montgomerie JZ, Bessman AN. The infected foot of the diabetic patient: quantitative microbiology and analysis of clinical features. Rev Infect Dis 1984; 6:171–176.

25. Trengove NJ, Stacey MC, McGechie DF, Mata S. Qualitative bacteriology and leg ulcer healing. J Wound Care 1996; 5:277–280.

26. Bello YM, Falabella AF, DeCaralho H, Nayyar G, Kirsner RS. Infection and wound healing. Wounds 2001; 13(4):127–131.

27. Costerton JW, Lewandowski Z, Caldwell DE, Korber DR, Lappin-Scott HM. Microbial biofilms. Annu Rev Microbiol 1995; 49:711–745.

28. Bowler PG, Davies BJ. The microbiology of infected and noninfected leg ulcers. Int J Dermatol 1999; 38:101–106.

29. Costerton JW, Stewart PS, Greenberg EP. Bacterial biofilms: a common cause of persistent infections. Science 1999; 284:1318–1322.
30. Serralta VW, Harrison-Balestra C, Cazzaniga AL, Davis SC, Mertz PM. Lifestyles of bacteria in wounds: presence of biofilms? Wounds 2001; 13(1):29–34.
31. Bello YM, Falabella AF, Cazzaniga AL, Harrison-Balestra C, Mertz PM. Are biofilms present in human chronic wounds? Symposium on Advanced Wound Care and Medical Research Forum on Wound Repair in Las Vegas, NV, April 30–May 3, 2001.
32. DeBeer D, Stoodley P, Lewandowski Z. Biotech Bioeng 1994; 44:636.
33. Davies DG, Chakrabarty AM, Geesey GG. Appl Environ Microbiol 1993; 59:1181.
34. Kolter R, Losick R. One for all and all for one. Science 1998; 280:226–227.
35. Brown MRW, Allison DG, Gilbert P. Resistance of bacterial biofilms to antibiotics: a growth-rate related effect? J Antimicrob Chemother 1988; 22:777.
36. Marrie TJ, Nelligan J, Costerton JW. Circulation 1982; 66:1399.
37. Lance George W. Other infections of skin, soft tissue, and muscle. In: Finegold SM, Lance George W, eds. Anaerobic Infections in Humans. San Diego, California: Academic Press, Inc., 1989:1491–1492.
38. Boulton AJM, Meneses P, Ennis WJ. Diabetic foot ulcers: a framework for prevention and care. Wound Rep Regen 1999; 7:7–16.
39. Hutchinson JJ, Lawrence JC. Wound infection under occlusive dressings. J Hosp Infect 1991; 17:83–94.
40. Bucknall TE. Factors affecting healing. In: Bucknall TE, Ellis H, eds. Wound Healing for Surgeons. London: Bailliere-Tindall, 1984:42–74.
41. White RJ, Cooper R, Kingsley A. Wound colonization and infection: the role of topical antimicrobials. Br J Nurs 2001; 10(9):563–578.
42. Brook I. Aerobic and anaerobic microbiology of necrotising fasciitis in children. Pediatr Dermatol 1996; 13:281–284.
43. Daltrey DC, Rhodes B, Chattwood JG. Investigation into the microbial flora of healing and non-healing decubitus ulcers. J Clin Pathol 1981; 34:701–705.
44. Gilliland EL, Nathwani N, Dore CJ, Lewis JD. Bacterial colonisation of leg ulcers and its effect on the success rate of skin grafting. Ann R Coll Surg Engl 1988; 70:105–108.
45. Halbert AR, Stacey MC, Rohr JB, Jopp-McKay A. The effect of bacterial colonisation on venous ulcer healing. Australas J Dermatol 1992; 33:75–80.
46. MacFarlane DE, Baum KF, Serjeant GR. Bacteriology of sickle cell leg ulcers. Trans R Soc Trop Med Hyg 1986; 80:553–556.
47. Twum-Danso K, Grant C, Al-Suleiman SA, Abdel-Khaders S, Al-Awami MS, Al-Breiki H, Taha S, Ashoor AA, Wosornu L. Microbiology of postoperative wound infection: a prospective study of 1770 wounds. J Hosp Infect 1992; 21:29–37.
48. Bowler PG, Davies BJ. The microbiology of infected and non infected leg ulcers. Int J Derm 1999; 38:72–79.
49. Kingston D, Seal DV. Current hypotheses on synergistic microbial gangrene. Br J Surg 1990; 77:260–264.
50. Cooper R, Lawrence JC. The isolation and identification of bacteria from wounds. J Wound Care 1996; 5(7):335–340.
51. Bendy RH, Nuccio PA, Wolfe E, Collins B, Tamburro C, Glass W, Martin CM. Relationship of quantitative wound bacterial counts to healing of decubiti. Effect of topical gentamicin. Antimicrob Agents Chemother 1964; 4:147–155.
52. Krizek TJ, Robson MC, Kho E. Bacterial growth and skin graft survival. Surg Forum 1967; 18:518–519.
53. Robson MC, Heggers JP. Bacterial quantification of open wounds. Mil Med 1969; 134:19–24.
54. Robson MC, Heggers JP. Delayed wound closures based on bacterial counts. J Surg Oncol 1970; 2:379–383.
55. Pruitt BA Jr, McManus AT, Kim SH, Goodwin CW. Burn wound infections: current status. World J Surg 1998; 22:135–145.

56. Kerstein MD. Wound infection: assessment and management. Wounds: A Compendium Clin Res Prac. 1996; 8:141–144.

57. Fowler E. Wound infection: a nurse's perspective. Ostomy Wound Manage 1998; 44:44–53.

58. Neil JA, Munro CL. A comparison of two culturing methods for chronic wounds. Ostomy Wound Manage 1997; 43:20–30.

59. Thomson.

60. Bill T, Ratliff C, Donovan A, Knox L, Morgan R, Rodeheaver G. Quantitative swab culture vs. tissue biopsy: a comparison in chronic wounds. Ostomy Wound Manage 2001; 47(1):34–37.

61. Taddonio TE, Thomson PD, Tait MJ, Prasad JK, Feller I. Rapid quantification of bacterial and fungal growth in burn wounds: biopsy homogenate Gram stain vs. microbial culture results. Burns 1988; 14:180–184.

62. Stotts NA. Determination of bacterial bioburden in wounds. Adv Wound Care 1995; 8:46–52.

63. Gradon J, Adamson C. Infections of pressure ulcers: management and controversies. Infect Dis Clin Pract 1995; 1:11–16.

64. Perry CR, Pearson RL, Miller GA. Accuracy of cultures of material from swabbing of the superficial aspect of the wound and needle biopsy in the preoperative assessment of osteomyelitis. J Bone Joint Surg 1991; 73A:745–749.

65. Brown DJ, Smith DJ. Bacterial colonization/infection and the surgical management of pressure sores. Ostomy Wound Manage 1999; 45:119s–120s.

66. Rudensky B, Lipschits M, Isaacsohn M, Sonnenblick M. Infected pressure sores: comparison of methods for bacterial identification. South Med J 1992; 85:901–903.

67. Majewski W, Cybulski Z, Napierala M, Pukacki F, Staniszewski R, Pietkiewicz K, Zapalski S. The value of quantitative bacteriological investigations in the monitoring of treatment of ischaemic ulcerations of lower legs. Int Angiol 1995; 14:381–384.

68. Bowler PG, Duerden BI, Armstrong DG. Wound microbiology and associated approaches to wound management. Clin Microbiol Rev 2001; 14:244–269.

69. Levine NS, Lindberg RB, Mason AD, Pruitt BA. The quantitative swab culture and smear: a quick simple method for determining the number of viable bacteria on open wounds. J Trauma 1976; 16:89–94.

70. Armstrong DG, Liswood PJ, Todd WF. Prevalence of mixed infections in the diabetic pedal wound. A retrospective review of 112 infections. J Am Podiatr Med Assoc 1995; 85:533–537.

71. Bornside GH, Bornside BB. Comparison between moist swab and tissue biopsy methods for quantitation of bacteria in experimental incisional wounds. J Trauma 1979; 19:103–105.

72. Van Belkum A. DNA fingerprinting of medically important micro-organisms by use of PCR. Clin Microbiol Rev 1994; 7:174–184.

73. Hogg SJ, Cooper RA, Harding K. Genotypic variability in streptococci from venous leg ulcers. In: Cherry GW, Gottrup F, Lawrence JC, et al. eds. Proceedings of the 5th European Conference on Advances in Wound Management, London, Macmillan magazines, 1996, 243–245.

74. Lawrence JC. The bacteriology of burns. J Hosp Infect 1985; 6:3–17.

75. European Pressure Ulcer Advisory Panel. Guidelines on treatment of pressure ulcers. EPUAP Rev 1999; 1:31–33.

76. Vindenes H, Bjerknes R. Microbial colonisation of large wounds. Burns 1995; 21:575–579.

77. McDonnell, Russell AD. Antiseptics and disinfectants: activity, action and resistance. Clin Microbiol Rev 1999; 12:147–179.

78. Taylor DM. Inactivation of unconventional agents of the transmissible degenerative encephalopathies. In: Russell AD, Hugo WB, Ayliffe GAJ, eds. Principles and Practice

of Disinfection, Preservation and Sterilization. 3rd ed. Oxford, England: Blackwell Science.

79. Niedner R. Cytotoxicity and sensitization of povidone iodine and other frequently used anti-infective agents. Dermatology 1997; 195(suppl 2):89–92.

80. 56 Federal Register 33644 at 33662.

81. Bergstrom N, Bennet MA, Carlson CE, et al. Clinical Practice Guideline No 15: Treatment of Pressure Ulcers. Rockville, Maryland: Agency for Health Care Policy and Research, Public Health Service, US Department of Health and Human Services, 1994. AHCPR Publication 95–0652.

82. Dow G, Browne A, Sibbald RG. Infection in chronic wounds: controversies in diagnosis and treatment. Ostomy Wound Manage 1999; 45:23–40.

83. Eriksson G, Eklund A, Kallings L. The clinical significance of bacterial growth in venous leg ulcers. Scand J Infect Dis 1984; 16:175–180.

84. Fleischer W, Reimer K. Povidone-iodine in antisepsis: state of the art. Dermatology 1997; 195(suppl 2):3–9.

85. Payne DN, Gibson SAW, Lewis R. Antiseptics: a forgotten weapon in the control of antibiotic resistant bacteria in hospital and community settings. J Roy Soc Health 1998; 118:18–22.

86. Drosou A, Falabella AF, Kirsner RS. Antiseptics on wounds: an area of controversy. Wounds 2003; 15:149–166.

87. Kirsner RS. Infection and intervention. Wounds 2003; 15:127–128.

88. Lineaweaver W, Howard R, Soucy D, et al. Topical antimicrobial toxicity. Arch Surg 1985; 120:267–270.

89. Greenberg L, Ingalls JW. Bactericide/leukocide ratio: a technique for the evaluation of disinfectants. J Am Pharm Assoc 1958; XLVII:531–533.

90. Cooper ML, Laxer JA, Hansbrough JF. The cytotoxic effects of commonly used topical antimicrobial agents on human fibroblasts and keratinocytes. J Trauma 1991; 31(6):775–784.

91. Fleming A. The action of chemical and physiological antiseptics in a septic wound. Br J Surg, 1919; 7:99–129.

92. Mertz PM, Davis S, Brewer L, Franzen L. Can antimicrobials be effective without impairing wound healing? The evaluation of a cadexomer iodine ointment. Wounds 1994; 6(6):184–193.

93. Skog E, Amesjo B, Troeng T, et al. A randomized trial comparing cadexomer iodine and standard treatment in the outpatient management of chronic venous ulcers. Br Med J 1983; 109:77–83.

94. Fleischer W, Reimer K. Povidone iodine in antisepsis—state of art. Dermatology 1997; 195(suppl 2):3–9.

95. Rodeheaver G, Bellamy W, Kody M, et al. Bactericidal activity and toxicity of iodine-containing solutions in wounds. Arch Surg 1982; 117:181–185.

96. Howell JM, Stair TO, Howell AW, et al. The effect of scrubbing and irrigation with normal saline, povidone iodine, and cefazolin on wound bacterial counts in a guinea pig model. Am J Emerg Med, 1993; 11:134–138.

97. Georgiade NG, Harris WA. Open and closed treatment of burns with povidone iodine. Plast Reconst Surg 1973; 52:640–644.

98. Gravett A, Sterner S, Clinton JE et al. A trial of povidone iodine in the prevention of infection in sutured lacerations. Ann Emerg Med 1987; 16(2):167/47–171/51.

99. Piérard-Franchimont C, Paquet P, Arrese JE, et al. Healing rate and bacterial necrotizing vasculitis in venous leg ulcers. Dermatology 1997; 194:383–387.

100. Viljanto J. Disinfection of surgical wounds without inhibition of wound healing. Arch Surg 1980; 115:253–256.

101. Berkelman RL, Holland BW, Anderson RL. Increased bactericidal activity of dilute preparations of povidone iodine solutions. J Clin Microbiol 1982; 15:635–639.

102. Lammers RL, Fourré M, Calahan ML, et al. Effect of povidone iodine and saline soaking on bacterial counts in acute, traumatic, contaminated wounds. Ann Emerg Med 1990; 19:709/155–714/160.

103. Mertz PM, Oliveira-Gandia MF, Davis SC. The evaluation of a cadexomer iodine wound dressing on methicillin resistant Staphylococcus aureus in acute wounds. Dermatol Surg 1999; 25:89–93.

104. Danielsen L, Cherry GW, Harding K, Rollman O. Cadexomer iodine in ulcers colonized by *Pseudomonas aeruginosa*. J Wound Care 1997; 6:169–172.

105. Geronemus RG, Mertz PM, Eaglstein WH. Wound healing: the effects of topical antimicrobial agents. Arch Dermatol 1979; 15:1311–1314.

106. Gruber RP, Vistnes L, Pardoe R. The effect of commonly used antiseptics on wound healing. Plast Reconst Surg 1975; 55:472–476.

107. Kjolseth D, Frank JM, Barker JH et al. Comparison of the effects of commonly used wound agents on epithelialization and neovascularization. J Am Coll Surg 1994; 179:305 312.

108. Menton DN, Brown M. The effects of commercial wound cleansers on cutaneous wound healing in guinea pigs. Wounds 1994; 6:21–27.

109. Mulliken JB, Healey NA, Glowacki J. Povidone iodine and tensile strength of wounds in rats. J Trauma 1980; 20:323–324.

110. Kashayap A, Beezhold D, Wiseman J, Beck WC. Effect of povidone-iodine dermatologic ointment on wound healing. Am Surg 1995; 61:486–491.

111. Niedner R, Schopf E. Inhibition of wound healing by antiseptics. Br J Dermatol 1986; 115(suppl 31):41–44.

112. MacRae SM, Brown B, Edelhauser HF. The corneal toxicity of presurgical antiseptics. Am J Ophthalmol 1984; 97:221–232.

113. Hopf K, Grandy R, Stahl-Bayliss C, Fitzmartin R. The effect of betadine cream vs. silvadene cream on reepithelialization in uninfected experimental wounds. Proc Burn Assoc 1991; 23:166.

114. Robins P, Day CL Jr, Lew RA. A multivariate analysis of factors affecting wound healing time. Dermatol Surg Oncol 1984; 10:219–222.

115. De Kock M, van der Merwe AE, Swarts C. A comparative study of povidone iodine cream and silver sulfadiazine in the topical treatment of burns. In: Selwyn S, ed. Proceedings of The First Asian/Pacific Congress Of Medicine Services. London: Royal Society of Medicine Services, 1998:65–71.

116. Lee BY, Trainor FS, Thoden WR. Topical application of povidone-iodine in the management of decubitus and stasis ulcers. J Am Geriatr Soc 1979; 27:302–306.

117. Mayer DA, Tsapogas MJ. Povidone-iodine and wound healing: a critical review. Wounds 1993; 5:14–23.

118. Lamme EN, Gustafsson TO, Middelkoop E. Cadexomer iodine shows stimulation of epidermal regeneration in experimental full thickness wounds. Arch Dermatol Res 1998; 290:18–24.

119. Laudanska H, Gustavson B. In-patient treatment of chronic varicose venous ulcers. A randomized trial of cadexomer iodine versus standard dressings. J Int Med Res 1988; 16:428–435.

120. Hillstrom L. Iodosorb compared to standard treatment in chronic venous ulcers—a multicenter study. Acta Chir Scand1988(suppl 544):53–56.

121. Skog E, Arnesjo B, Troeng T, et al. A randomized trial comparing cadexomer iodine and standard treatment in the out-patient management of chronic venous ulcers. Br J Dermatol 1983; 109:77–83.

122. Holloway GA, Johansen KH, Barnes RW, Pierce GE. Multicenter trial of cadexomer iodine to treat venous stasis ulcers. West J Med 1989; 151:35–38.

123. Ormiston MC, Seymour MTJ, Venn GE, Cohen RI, Fox JA. Controlled trial of iodosorb in chronic venous ulcers. Br Med J 1985; 291:308–310.

124. Harcup JW, Saul PA. A study of the effect of cadexomer iodine in the treatment of venous leg ulcers. Br J Clin Pract 1986; 40:360–364.

125. Tarvainen K. Cadexomer iodine (iodosorb) compared with dextranomer (debrisan) in the treatment of chronic leg ulcers. Acta Chir Scand 1988; (suppl 544):57–59.

126. Hansson C, et al. The effects of cadexomer iodine paste in the treatment of venous leg ulcers compared with hydrocolloid dressing and paraffin gauze dressing. Int J Dermatol 1998; 37:390–396.

127. Floyer C, Wilkinson JD. Treatment of venous leg ulcers with cadexomer iodine with particular reference to iodine sensitivity. Acta Chir Scand 1988; (suppl 544):60–61.

128. Apelqvist J, Ragnarson Tennvall G. Cavity foot ulcers in diabetic patients: a comparative study of cadexomer iodine and standard treatment. An economic analysis along side a clinical trial. Acta Derm Venereol 1996; 76:231–235.

129. Moberg S, Hoffman L, Grennert ML, Holst A. J Am Geriat Soc 1983; 31:462–465.

130. Klasen HJ. A historical review of the use of silver in the treatment of burns. II. Renewed interest for silver. Burns 2000; 26:131–138.

131. Monafo WW, West MA. Current treatment recommendations for topical burn therapy. Drugs 1990; 40:364–373.

132. de Gracia CG. An open study comparing topical silver sulfadiazine and topical silver sulfadiazine–cerium nitrate in the treatment of moderate and severe burns. Burns 2001; 27:67–74.

133. Tredget EE, Shankowsky HA, Groeneveld A, Burrell R. A matched-pair, randomized study evaluating the efficacy and safety of Acticoat silver-coated dressing for the treatment of burn wounds. J Burn Care Rehabil 1998; 19:531–537.

134. Demling RH, DeSanti L. Effects of silver on wound management. Wounds 2001; 13: 5–15.

135. Lansdown AB, Sampson B, Laupattarakasem P, Vuttivirojana A. Silver aids healing in the sterile skin wound: experimental studies in the laboratory rat. Br J Dermatol 1997; 137:728–735.

136. Leitch IO, Kucukcelebi A, Robson MC. Inhibition of wound contraction by topical antimicrobials. Aust N Z J Surg 1993; 63:289–293.

137. Kucan JO, Robson MC, Heggers JP, et al. Comparison of sliver sulfadiazine, povidone iodine and physiologic saline in the treatment of pressure ulcers. J Am Geriatr Soc 1981; XXIX:232–235.

138. Bishop JB, Phillips LG, Mustoe TA, VanderZee AJ, Wiersema L, Roach DE, Heggers JP, Hill DP Jr, Taylor EL, Robson MC. A prospective randomized evaluator-blinded trial of two potential wound healing agents for the treatment of venous stasis ulcers. J Vasc Surg 1992; 16:251–257.

139. Ouvry PA. A trial of silver sulfadiazine in the local treatment of venous ulcer. Phlebologie 1989; 42:673–679.

140. Livingstone DH, Cryer HG, Miller FB, et al. A randomized prospective study of topical antimicrobial agents on skin grafts after thermal injury. Plast Reconst Surg 1990; 86:1059–1064.

141. Carson CF, Riley TV, Cookson BD. Efficacy and safety of tea tree oil as a topical antimicrobial agent. J Hosp Infect 1998; 40:175–178.

142. Molan PC. The role of honey in the management of wounds. J Wound Care 1999; 8: 415–418.

143. Cooper RS, Molan PC. Honey in wound care. J Wound Care 1999; 8:340.

144. Moch D, Fleischmann W, Russ M. The BMW (biosurgical mechanical wound treatment) in diabetic foot. Zentralbl Chir 1999; 124(suppl 1):69–72.

145. Mumcuoglu KY, Ingber A, Gilead L, Stessman J, Friedmann R, Schulman H, Bichucher H, Ioffe-Uspensky I, Miller J, Galun R, Raz I. Maggot therapy for the treatment of intractable wounds. Int J Dermatol 1999; 38:623–627.

146. Thomas S, Andrews A, Jones M. Maggots are useful in treating infected or necrotic wounds. Br Med J 1999; 318:807.

147. Thomas S, Jones M. The use of larval therapy in wound management. J Wound Care 1998; 7:521–524.
148. Prete PE. Growth effects of *Phaenicia sericata* larval extracts on fibroblasts: mechanism for wound healing by maggot therapy. Life Sci 1997; 60:505–510.

9

Venous Ulcers: Pathophysiology and Epidemiology

Allen Holloway
Department of Surgery, Maricopa Medical Center, Phoenix, Arizona, U.S.A.

1. INTRODUCTION

Chronic leg ulcers, which may have a variety of causes, are unfortunately common, particularly in the older population. The majority of these fit into the categories of arterial, diabetic, pressure, and venous ulcers. The incidence and prevalence of each of these depends upon the population that is being examined. In an elderly nursing home population, pressure sores may be the more common, whereas in a younger more active population with a high incidence of diabetes, diabetic ulcers may predominate. However, if one explores larger population groups, ulcers that are attributed to problems with the venous system are usually the most common. In wound care centers, it is said that one-half to three-fourths of the ulcers are venous in origin. These ulcers can occur in any age group and are commonly associated with significant long-term morbidity. Furthermore, from an individual as well as societal perspective, this type of ulcer is costly both in terms of the expense of treatment and lost productivity from absenteeism from work. It is the purpose of this chapter to explore both the pathophysiology and epidemiology of this type of chronic ulcer.

2. DEFINITION

What defines a "venous ulcer" is neither clear nor specific. It is generally accepted that it is an ulcer caused by venous insufficiency but what part of the venous system is abnormal and to what degree cannot be standardized to any individual case. In an attempt to better classify venous insufficiency, the CEAP classification was devised (1). Venous disease in an individual patient can be classified according to a combination of clinical, etiologic, anatomic, and pathophysiologic characteristics which describes the status of the venous system and any ulcers that may be present. This system is quite inclusive, but is somewhat difficult to use clinically and because of that, has not been widely utilized by wound healing practitioners. Here, we will use the general definition that it is an ulcer caused by malfunction of some aspect of the lower extremity venous system.

3. NORMAL VENOUS ANATOMY

To better understand the abnormal venous system, we need to first understand the normal lower extremity venous system. There are basically two venous systems that coexist and interconnect in the legs. The deep system consists of single or duplicate veins that accompany the major arterial system throughout the extremity. In the thigh, a companion vein accompanies the common, deep, and superficial femoral as well as the popliteal arteries. Below the popliteal space, the veins continue to accompany the major tibial and peroneal arteries down into the foot but are usually duplicate or even triplicate. The deep system by definition runs in the deep spaces in the leg and is contained within compartments surrounded by dense, non-compliant fascia. The superficial system, in contrast, runs within the softer fatty subcutaneous tissue and has a much less regular anatomy. The greater saphenous vein which runs medially down the leg beginning at the groin, and the lesser saphenous vein which runs laterally down the calf beginning in the popliteal space are the largest and most anatomically predictable of these veins. They join the deep system draining into the common femoral vein in the groin at the sapheno-femoral junction and into the popliteal vein in the popliteal space at the lesser saphenous–popliteal junction, respectively. The deep and superficial systems are also connected along the medial and, to a lesser extent, lateral aspects of the calf by the so-called perforating veins which pass through perforations in the fascia. These are multiple and are located at relatively predictable anatomic locations particularly along the lower half of the medial calf.

Veins differ anatomically from arteries by being thin walled and having valves which prevent the reflux of blood. The valves are very thin membranous structures which are only several cell layers thick at their ends, and are more common the more distal the vein. By virtue of their thin structure, they are easily damaged.

4. NORMAL VENOUS PHYSIOLOGY

There are two elements which are involved in the normal function of the venous system, particularly in the lower extremity. These are an intact venous anatomy and a normally functioning venous pump. The deep venous system is the main conduit for the return of blood to the heart. When in the recumbent position, this is a function of gravity. However, when sitting or standing, blood pools in the leg veins and it is muscular contraction in the calf which compresses these deep veins and expels the blood toward the heart. Valves, of which there are more in distal segments, prevent blood from refluxing back into the just emptied segments. Blood flows into this deep system from the superficial system through the direct connections between the lesser saphenous and popliteal veins and the greater saphenous and femoral veins, as well as through the medial, and to some degree, lateral perforating veins. This occurs when the calf pump relaxes decreasing the pressure in the deep veins and allowing blood from the superficial system to flow into this now low pressure system. Valves in both the superficial and perforating veins prevent the blood from refluxing back into the superficial system in the normal patient.

Pressure in the lower extremity veins varies markedly depending upon the position of the individual. When in the supine position, resting venous pressure is approximately 10 mmHg. However, in the sitting and standing positions, a column of blood from the level of the heart pushes down resulting in pressures from 80 to

100 mmHg in the lower legs and feet at rest, and increases in veins within the muscles to 200 mmHg with muscle contraction. This pressure is decreased to 0–10 mmHg transiently after muscle contraction ceases which allows blood from the superficial system to flow down the pressure gradient into the deep system (2). The valves are not able to maintain their seal continuously under these pressures, and when the muscles are not contracting, the venous pressure gradually increases to the level induced by the gravitational effects of the column of blood.

5. PATHOPHYSIOLOGY OF VENOUS ULCERS

Why do patients develop venous ulcers? It is recognized that some form of abnormality of the venous system is a contributing factor but this does not explain the whole problem. Abnormal physiology in the lower extremity venous system can be due to abnormal function of the venous pump, or obstruction or insufficiency of one or more segments of the venous system or any combination of these elements. The important factor is that these can lead to venous hypertension which is the basic element in the causation of venous ulcers (Fig. 1).

5.1. Venous Pump

The venous pump is basically a function of walking and contraction of the calf muscles. In patients who are non-ambulatory the pump is essentially non-functional and venous return is markedly reduced. Venous hypertension is the end result. We can see the effect of this in individuals who sit or stand for long periods of time and develop foot and calf edema as, for example, after a long plane flight. Nursing home

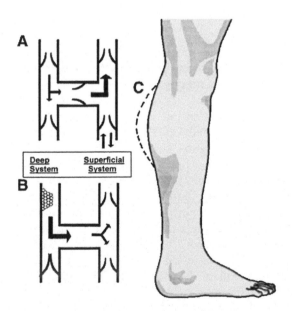

Figure 1 Pathophysiologic mechanisms in venous ulceration. (A) Superficial and/or communicating and/or deep system insufficiency. (B) Deep venous outflow obstruction (i.e., thrombus formation). (C) Muscle dysfunction and calf muscle pump failure.

patients who sit motionless in chairs for long intervals can develop very severe edema that can subsequently ulcerate.

5.2. Venous Obstruction and Insufficiency

When veins are obstructed, venous return is hindered and venous pressure increases. The same end result is seen when the competency of venous valves is lost and blood flows back into the segments from which it was just pumped despite a normally functioning venous pump. Obstruction most often occurs following an episode of deep venous thrombosis (DVT) where the veins are occluded by the process and do not, or only partially recanalize after the process subsides. However, other processes, such as compression by lymph nodes or other masses, can also cause obstruction.

Venous insufficiency is due to reflux at one or more levels of the deep or superficial venous system. It is not completely agreed upon as to which system is more important. Weingarten et al. (3) determined that venous ulceration was significantly associated with reflux in multiple venous segments as opposed to reflux in isolated venous segments. Labropoulos looked at the superficial system and noted that of 255 limbs in 217 patients with superficial venous insufficiency and normal perforating and deep veins, 48.2% had reflux confined to the greater saphenous system, 32.6% had reflux confined to the short saphenous system, and 19.2% had reflux in both long and short saphenous system (4). He also looked at perforating veins and demonstrated that the number as well as diameter of both competent and incompetent veins was related to chronic venous disease (5). The most common underlying cause associated with these venous disorders is DVT in the deep system or thrombophlebitis in the superficial system. The valves, as indicated above, are very thin and easily destroyed by the process which consists of blood coagulation and a greater or lesser degree of inflammation.

5.3. Venous Hypertension

The end result of these three problems is increased venous pressure. This may be present at rest even in the recumbent position, but is worsened by the legs being in the dependent position or by a normally functioning venous pump working against an obstructed or leaking venous system.

The mechanism by which the venous hypertension causes the changes of chronic venous stasis and ulceration is not well understood. However, there are several theories proposed to explain the sequence of events. The first of these was proposed by Browse and Burnand who noted pericapillary fibrin "cuffs" in patients with venous hypertension in areas of lipodermatosclerosis (2). They suggested that these were due to capillary dilation and subsequent leakage into the tissues of large molecules including fibrinogen which would then form fibrin. This would produce a barrier to diffusion of nutrients and oxygen as fibrin was deposited in the tissues. Several authors have demonstrated that there is excess leakage of fibrinogen into the tissues (6,7). However, other studies have suggested that although fibrin is present, it may not, by itself, be adequate to explain the end result. The fibrin cuffs have been noted to be discontinuous as well as not evenly distributed in capillaries and capillary groups (8). Additionally, the degree of lipodermatosclerosis has not been shown to correlate well with the amount of fibrin deposited in the tissues (9).

A second hypothesis was proposed by Falanga and Eaglstein in 1993 (10). They suggested that the fibrin cuffs could serve as a "trap" for growth factors and other cytokines which were necessary to maintain tissue integrity both to maintain the status quo as well as to repair tissue damage which would occur secondary to trauma or other events. No additional data have been published that has either strongly refuted or supported this theory.

A third theory proposed by Dormandy and coworkers in 1988 (11) noted that leukocytes aggregated in capillaries with decreased flow and between 5% and 20% of these could accumulate in the legs of normal individuals in the dependent position. In patients with venous disease, this percentage was noted to be even higher, especially in the dependent position. They proposed that this "trapping" of leukocytes together with sluggish erythrocyte flow resulted in plugging of the capillaries. This resulted in localized ischemia in the surrounding tissue leading to necrosis. These leukocytes were also postulated to liberate various cytokines and other toxic substances which would lead to worsening of the ischemia and necrosis.

Nicolaides examined 236 limbs in 220 patients with venous problems and measured several variables including ambulatory venous pressure. Of these, 83 patients had ulcers. It was noted that when the ambulatory venous pressure was less than 30 mmHg, ulceration did not occur. However, when the pressure was greater than 90 mmHg, ulceration was inevitable (12).

6. EPIDEMIOLOGY OF VENOUS ULCERS

6.1. Incidence and Prevalence

As indicated above, venous disease is one of the main causes of ulcerations in the lower extremity. In wound clinics or other settings which see a variety of different types of ulcers, approximately one half to three fourths of these may be diagnosed as having a venous etiology (13–17). However, as we have also touched on, this diagnosis is dependent upon exactly how "venous etiology" is defined as well as who is making the diagnosis and from what information. Does the patient have a non-functioning or poorly functioning venous pump, venous obstruction, venous insufficiency, or a combination of these? Is the deep system, superficial system, or both involved? Or is there a single incompetent perforating vein entering the base of the ulcer?

The incidence and prevalence of venous disease and venous ulcers are also not well defined due to similar problems. Different populations in different geographical sites have been examined in the few studies looking at this problem. Cherry et al. (18) have reviewed the literature looking at venous leg ulcers in Europe and found that prevalence ranged from 0.1% to 1.02% in studies from four different countries. The Alexander House consensus paper of venous leg ulcers found a prevalence ranging from 0.18% to 1.3% (19). Baker et al. (13) noted an overall prevalence of 0.62% in a metropolitan population from Perth, WA but found that this increased to 3.3% in the population aged 60 and older. Cesarone et al. (20) looking at 30,000 subjects in eight villages in central Italy showed a prevalence of 0.48% of venous ulcers. Cornwall et al. (21) examined a regional Health District in the United Kingdom with a populations of 198,900 and found the overall prevalence to be 0.18% but increased to 0.38% in the population over 40 years of age. The incidence of venous ulcers as determined from the medical records of patients in Olmstead County, MN, USA was looked at by Heit et al. (22) who estimated the incidence of chronic venous insufficiency and venous ulcers to be 0.076% per year. Margolis et al. (23) studied the General Practice Research Database in the United States and estimated the annual prevalence of venous leg ulcers among the elderly to be 1.69, with an incidence rate of 0.76 for men and 1.42 for women, whereas Nelzen, in a Swedish population of 270,000, found a point prevalence of 0.16 % (16). In the Mid-Western Health Board region of Ireland, O'Brien found the prevalence to be 0.12% overall, but it increased to 1.03% in patients over age 70. Other studies have looked at the prevalence and incidence in other smaller population groups and have found generally the same results. From these studies, we can surmise that roughly 1–2% of the general population is afflicted with venous ulcers and that the prevalence does increase with age, especially in the older age groups.

6.2. Costs

Trying to estimate the cost of venous ulcers is even more difficult. Again the definition of what we include in "cost" will markedly change this estimate. To be considered is cost of treatment of the ulcer to the individual, to insurance payers and to the government as well as less tangible costs which would include loss of productivity. A few studies from different political and geographic areas have attempted to do this. Ohlsson et al. (24) looked at comparative costs for gauze vs. hydrocolloid dressings in 30 patients in a primary health care clinic in Sweden and estimated the total treatment cost in the former as SEK 4126 ($US 528) compared to SEK 1565 ($US 200) for the latter. Cherry et al. (18) in their review arrived at the cost of £ 342–6741 ($US 520–10,230) for a 12-week treatment course in the United Kingdom, $US 480–581 for a 12-week treatment in Sweden. Marston et al. (25) in an outpatient clinic in the Eastern United States determined the cost of a 10-week treatment at $US 1444–2711. From this, it is seen that there is a wide variation in costs as we might expect, and more accurate determinations will have to depend on future studies. It is apparent, however, that treatment of these ulcers is expensive. Additionally, it is well recognized that the recurrence rates for these ulcers are also high, and that the long-term costs will include recurrent treatments with significantly greater costs. Phillips et al. (26) attempted to assess the financial, social, and psychologic implications of leg ulcers. Interviews were obtained with 73 patients with leg ulcers. Most of the patients had "moderate to severe" symptoms, especially pain, and felt that their mobility was limited. Financial and loss of work were also noted to be significant problems.

6.3. Risk Factors

Various risk factors have been stated to be important for both initial and recurrent venous ulcers and multiple references mention these but very few studies are found which examine this. There is not room in this chapter to evaluate these in detail. Previous DVT, clotting disorders, age, and obesity are some of the factors implicated in this problem and depend to some degree on whether the deep, superficial or both systems are involved. Eberth-Willershausen and Marshall (14) specifically looked at this question in a population from Germany and commented upon several factors which were seen to be associated with venous ulcers in that population. Scott et al. (27) performed a case–control study to examine some of the factors and stated that many of the previously suggested associations found with CVI are in reality due to greater age, and that patients with chronic venous insufficiency are older, male, obese, have a history of phlebitis, and have a history of serious leg injury. Taylor et al. (28) looked at factors likely to predict non-healing of ulcers and showed that a history of previous leg ulceration, "quite wet" ulcer exudate, high body mass index, large initial total ulcer area, increasing age and male gender in this group of 325 patients were all correlated with ulcers that did not heal. There are obviously many factors which are felt to be associated with the risk of sustaining a venous ulcer, risk of recurrence of a venous ulcer and, as shown in this last study, risk of not healing a venous ulcer. Further studies are indicated to identify which of these factors are actually valid for prediction in the clinical setting.

7. SUMMARY

In this chapter, we have looked at the anatomy and physiology of the lower extremity venous system in the normal individual. This can be seen to relate to the problem of venous ulcers through action of the venous pump as well as venous obstruction, venous insufficiency or both in the deep system or venous insufficiency in the perforating or superficial systems. The end result is venous hypertension which is shown to be directly related to the presence of venous ulcerations. How this might cause these ulcers is then looked at in terms of the several proposed theories which include fibrin cuffing, leukocyte trapping, cytokine trapping, or a combination of these. The epidemiology of venous ulcers was then examined and looked at in terms of incidence, prevalence as well as direct cost to the system and indirect costs in terms of lost productivity and personal suffering.

Chapter 10 covers the clinical presentation of these ulcers.

REFERENCES

1. Kistner RL. Definitive diagnosis and definitive treatment in chronic venous disease: a concept whose time has come. J Vasc Surg 1996; 24:703–710.
2. Browse NL. The pathogenesis of venous ulceration: a hypothesis. J Vasc Surg 1988; 7: 468–472.
3. Weingarten MS, Branas CC, Czeredarczuk M, Schmidt JD, Wolferth CC Jr. Distribution and quantification of venous reflux in lower extremity chronic venous stasis disease with duplex scanning. J Vasc Surg 1993; 18:753–759.
4. Labropoulos N, Leon M, Nicolaides AN, Giannoukas AD, Volteas M, Chan P. Superficial venous insufficiency: correlation of anatomic extent of reflux with clinical symptoms and signs. J Vasc Surg 1994; 20:953–958.
5. Labropoulos N, Mansour MA, Kang SS, Gloviczki P, Baker WH. New insights into perforator vein incompetence. Eur J Vasc Endovasc Surg 1999; 18:228–234.
6. Speiser DE, Bollinger A. Microangiopathy in mild chronic venous incompetence (CVI): morphological alterations and increased transcapillary diffusion detected by fluorescence videomicroscopy. Int J Microcirc: Clin Exp 1991; 10:55–66.
7. Bollinger A, Jager K, Geser A, Sgier F, Seglias J. Transcapillary and interstitial diffusion of Na-fluorescein in chronic venous insufficiency with white atrophy. Inter J Microcirc Clin Exp 1982; 1:5–17.
8. Pardes JD, Tonneson MG, Falanga V, Eaglstein WH, Clark RA. Skin capillaries surrounding chronic venous ulcers demonstrate smooth muscle hyperplasia and increased laminin type IV collagen. J Invest Dermatol 1990; 94:563.
9. Mani R, White JE, Barrett DF, Weaver PW. Tissue oxygenation, venous ulcers and fibrin cuffs [see comments]. J R Soc Med 1989; 82:345–346.
10. Falanga V, Eaglstein WH. The trap hypothesis of venous ulceration. Lancet 1993; 341:1006–1008.

11. Coleridge-Smith PD, Thomas P, Scurr JH, Dormandy JA. Causes of venous ulceration: a new hypothesis. Br Med J 1988; 296:1726–1727.

12. Nicolaides AN, Hussein MK, Szendro G, Christopoulos D, Vasdekis S, Clarke H. The relation of venous ulceration with ambulatory venous pressure measurements. J Vasc Surg 1993; 17:414–419.

13. Baker SR, Stacey MC, Jopp-McKay AG, Hoskin SE, Thompson PJ. Epidemiology of chronic venous ulcers. Br J Surg 1991; 78:864–867.

14. Eberth-Willershausen W, Marshall M. Prevalence, risk factors complications of peripheral venous diseases in the Munich population. Hautarzt 1984; 35:68–77.

15. Oien RF, Hakansson A, Ovhed I, Hansen BU. Wound management for 287 patients with chronic leg ulcers demands 12 full-time nurses. Leg ulcer epidemiology and care in a well-defined population in southern Sweden. Scand J Prim Health Care 2000; 18:220–225.

16. Nelzen O, Bergqvist D, Lindhagen A. Venous and non-venous leg ulcers: clinical history and appearance in a population study. Br J Surg 1994; 81:182–187.

17. Baker SR, Stacey MC, Singh G, Hoskin SE, Thompson PJ. Aetiology of chronic leg ulcers. Eur J Vasc Surg 1992; 6:245–251.

18. Cherry GW, Price P, Kronin K, Avdic A. The burden of leg ulcers in Europe: a review of the literature [abstr], Symposium on Advanced Wound Care, Baltimore, Maryland, USA, 2002. HMP Communications.

19. Consensus paper on venous leg ulcer. The Alexander House Group. J Dermatol Surg Oncol 1992; 18:592–602.

20. Cesarone MR, Belcaro G, Nicolaides AN, et al. "Real" epidemiology of varicose veins and chronic venous diseases: the San Valentino Vascular Screening Project. Angiology 2002; 53:119–130.

21. Cornwall JV, Dore CJ, Lewis JD. Leg ulcers: epidemiology and aetiology. Br J Surg 1986; 73:693–696.

22. Heit JA, Rooke TW, Silverstein MD, Mohr N, Lohse CM, Petterson TM, O'Fallon WM, Melton LJ. Trends in the incidence of venous stasis syndrome and venous ulcer: a 25-year population-based study. J Vasc Surg 2001; 33:1022–1027.

23. Margolis DJ, Bilker W, Santanna J, Baumgarten M. Venous leg ulcer: incidence and prevalence in the elderly. J Am Acad Dermatol 2002; 46:381–386.

24. Ohlsson P, Larsson K, Lindholm C, Moller M. A cost-effectiveness study of leg ulcer treatment in primary care. Comparison of saline-gauze and hydrocolloid treatment in a prospective, randomized study. Scand J Prim Health Care 1994; 12:295–299.

25. Marston MA, Carlin RE, Passman MA, Farber MA, Keagy BA. Healing rates and cost efficacy of outpatient compression treatment for leg ulcers associated with venous insufficiency. J Vasc Surg 1999; 30:491–498.

26. Phillips T, Stanton B, Provan A, Lew R. A study of the impact of leg ulcers on quality of life: financial, social, and psychologic implications. J Am Acad Dermatol 1994; 31:49–53.

27. Scott TE, LaMorte WW, Gorin DR, Menzoian JO. Risk factors for chronic venous insufficiency: a dual case–control study. J Vasc Surg 1995; 22:622–628.

28. Taylor RJ, Taylor AD, Smyth JV. Using an artificial neural network to predict healing times and risk factors for venous leg ulcers. J Wound Care 2002; 11:101–105.

10

Venous Leg Ulcer Clinical Presentation and Differential Diagnosis

R. Gary Sibbald, R. N. Heather Orsted, and Peter A. Noseworthy
Dermatology Daycare and Wound Healing Clinic, Sunnybrook and Women's College Health Sciences Centre, Toronto, Ontario, Canada

1. INTRODUCTION

Case Study: A 53-year-old woman presents with a large shallow ulcer on the medial aspect of the calf (measuring 4×1 cm) of 6 months duration. She complains of diffuse pain in her legs and sharp pain in the skin surrounding the ulcer. She has had swelling in her ankles in the evenings for the last four years. She had a varicose vein stripping procedure 19 years ago for severe varicosities following the birth of her third child. On examination, she is overweight, with a height of 5'2" and a weight of 200 lbs (BMI $33 \, kg/m^2$ with ideal BMI of fat below $20 \, kg/m^2$). Her legs are swollen and firm below the knee. There is a dark calf and shin discoloration. The legs and feet have palpable dorsalis pedis, posterior tibial, and popliteal pulses bilaterally. There is also a good capillary refill time with no distal rubor or decreased temperature on palpation.

Leg ulcers are a common health problem, affecting 1% of the adult population and 3.6% of people over 65 years old (1). Venous leg ulcers are most common in women (female:male ratio = 2:3) in their seventh or eighth decade of life but occur in individuals of all ages and of both sexes. The average duration of a venous ulcer is typically more than one year (2). These ulcers tend to be painful, slow healing, and cause considerable morbidity. The treatment of venous ulcers demands constant monitoring of healing status, adjustment of therapy, and compensatory interventions to decrease associated morbidity.

2. ETIOLOGY

2.1. Risk Factors

Patients are at increased risk of developing leg ulcers if they are obese, have had multiple pregnancies, coexisting exacerbating diseases, or spend a large amount of time standing or sitting. A history of venous surgery such as varicose vein stripping or sclerotherapy is associated with an increase incidence of venous ulcers. Younger

111

patients are more likely to have a positive family history of venous reflux, previous surgery, or a coagulation defect (3). Previous trauma such as broken bones, stab or gunshot wounds, or crush injury may damage the venous valves and predispose the patients to developing venous ulceration in the future. Similarly, previous deep vein thrombosis may result in ulceration or appear as a well-established pathophysiologic phenomenon known as postphlebitic syndrome. Some patients have a hereditary predisposition to develop venous ulceration. Recurrent thrombophlebitis in younger adults (less then 50) may alert clinicians to an underlying coagulopathy such as a deficiency in factor V (Leiden), protein C, or protein S or a congenital predisposition to valvular dysfunction. Most socioeconomic factors have not been shown to relate to the risk of venous ulceration, however, the lack of medical insurance has been shown to be a risk factor in the United States (4).

3. PATHOGENESIS

In order to outline the pathogenesis of venous leg ulcers, a conceptual model of the vascular anatomy of the leg is important. The venous system of the leg consists of three components, the deep system, the superficial system, and the perforating veins that connect these two compartments. This system can be illustrated by an analogy to a ladder (the deep and superficial systems forming the sides and the perforators forming the rungs—see Fig. 1). In healthy individual, blood drains from the superficial system through the perforating veins into the deep compartment. This movement is driven by action of the calf muscle pump to maintain flow through the deep system and the presence of valves to prevent retrograde flow. A patient is at increased risk of developing ulceration if there is a breakdown at any of these steps.

The first stage in the pathogenesis of leg ulceration is venous hypertension. Venous hypertension arises when there is decreased flow though the veins of the leg due to either valvular dysfunction (inherited valve destruction with previous infection or post-traumatic), obstruction of venous return (e.g., deep vein thrombosis), or failure of the calf muscle pump (e.g., decreased activity, paralysis, joint deformity, and decreased range of motion). The increased pressure in the venous system causes distention of the capillaries and leakage of intravascular fluid into the interstitium. The mechanism of the resultant ulceration is unclear and may be multifactorial; however, several hypotheses have been proposed to explain the cellular and molecular events leading to ulceration. More detail is presented in subsequent chapters.

3.1. Fibrin Deposition Hypothesis

One hypothesis proposes that ulceration results from fibrin deposition in the dermal and subcutaneous tissues (5). When venous hypertension is sustained, the capillaries become distended and leak fluid and macromolecules such as fibrinogen into the surrounding tissue. The deposited fibrinogen polymerizes to form fibrin cuffs that may create a barrier to the diffusion of oxygen and nutrients and, over time, induce ulceration. This hypothesis is supported by histologic studies that show the presence of fibrin cuffs in ulcer biopsies (6), and by in vitro studies that demonstrate that fibrin sheets create a physical barrier to oxygen diffusion (7). However, the link between fibrin cuffs and ulceration may not be conclusive. More recent studies have shown that fibrin cuffs are discontinuous and form only partial diffusion barriers (8),

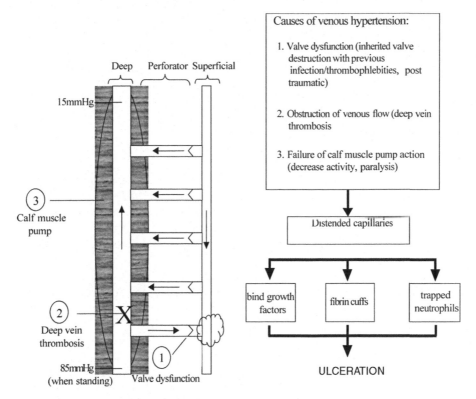

Figure 1   Mechanism of venous ulceration.

and that the amount of fibrin deposition does not directly correlate to the severity of the ulceration (9). Rather than creating a physical barrier, fibrin may induce molecular events that cause or potentate ulceration. For example, fibrin has been shown to decrease the synthesis of procollagen I and may hinder wound healing in this manner (8). It is likely that fibrin deposition is one component of a complex physical and molecular process that results in skin ulceration.

3.2. Neutrophil Trapping Hypothesis

An additional hypothesis is that neutrophils become entrapped in the leg capillaries. As venous hypertension develops, the pressure gradient between the arterial and venous systems is reduced, resulting in decreased blood flow. This decrease in blood flow may cause neutrophils to become trapped in the capillaries where they cause blockage and local ischemia. This capillary plugging has been observed in histologic sections of lipoderosclerotic tissue (10). Furthermore, the persistence of white cells in the tissue may cause the release of inflammatory mediators and proteolytic enzymes that increase vascular permeability creating chronic inflammation and hindering wound healing (11).

3.3. Growth Factor Trapping Hypothesis

In addition to creating a physical barrier and inducing local inflammation, the leakage of serum proteins into the interstitial space may bind growth factors and render them ineffective in the healing process (12). For instance, alpha 2-macroglobulin a well-established growth factor scavenger, has been shown to colocalize with transforming growth factor beta (TGF-beta) in the fibrin cuffs of ulcerated tissue (13). These hypotheses likely represent convergent physical and molecular components of the complex pathogenesis of venous ulceration.

4. CLINICAL PRESENTATION

4.1. History

The clinical history can be divided into predisposing and precipitating factors. Important factors that predispose to leg ulcers include prolonged standing, obesity, multiple pregnancies, and history of leg trauma or surgery (vein stripping, hip surgery, and knee surgery). Ankle joint mobility is critical to activation of the calf muscle pump function and normal gait (14). Hereditary ankle deformity, previous trauma, or disease (arthritis, charcot joint, etc.) will predispose to a dysfunctional ankle joint and interfere with calf muscle pump function. Trauma, infection, or a worsening of existing venous disease and edema may precipitate the occurrence of leg ulcers.

Patients may present with a range of symptoms. Contrary to commonly held beliefs, venous leg ulcers are often painful. As many as 64% of patients report pain as a chief complaint, however, the surface area of the ulcer does not correlate with the presence of pain (3,15). Deep ulcers or those surrounded by atrophy blanche have a high-level local pain. A careful pain history is critical because severe pain may indicate an underlying infection, coexisting arterial disease, or other inflammatory disorder. Inflammation of the veins, superficial or deep phlebitis or an acute inflammation of collagen may also cause severe pain (acute lipodermosclerosis) (Figs. 2 and 3, Table 1).

Most patients will report swelling in the ankles associated with a feeling of heaviness. Their edema is worse at the end of day and improves on recumbency. In addition, patients may report foul odor, exudate, and pruritus in the area surrounding the ulcer. Medical management of venous disease requires support stockings for life (16). Patients who do not adhere to the treatment protocol are more susceptible to develop venous ulceration.

4.2. Physical Examination

Leg ulcers typically occur on the medial aspect of the leg over the medial malleolus (Fig. 4) (17). This distribution overlies the great saphenous vein which is often the first vein affected by venous hypertension. The great saphenous vein may be prone to develop disease because of its abrupt curvature and propensity to develop valvular damage due to its superficial location. For this reason, venous ulcers are uncommon on the foot or above the mid-calf. If the ulceration occurs outside the usual distribution, the clinicians should consider other etiologies.

Venous ulcers usually have a granulation tissue base, or typically moist and do not usually have necrotic debris. Early venous ulcers may have a firm yellow base that serves as the scaffold for mature granulation at later stages (17). This should be differentiated from arterial ulcers that have a characteristic "punched-out" appearance and are frequently associated with slough in the base and black discoloration or areas of necrosis (Fig. 5) (18).

Table 1 Differential Diagnosis of Venous Pain

Diagnosis	Clinical/investigation	Treatment	Comments
Pitting edema	Dull ache at end of day. Press thumb into skin and note degree of depression Grade 1+ to 4+	Compression bandaging; support stockings; ambulation, exercise improve calf muscle pump	Nonelastic stockings or compression bandaging may initially be preferred as they are less likely to cause pain at rest
Superficial phlebitis	Pain and tenderness along affected vein—usually saphenous	Compression; ambulation; NSAID therapy	Risk of associated underlying DVT is low, especially if affected area is below the knee
Deep phlebitis (DVT)	Acute, red, tender, swollen calf—almost too painful to touch. Doppler necessary to confirm diagnosis	ASA, unfractionated heparin Warfarin Low-molecular weight heparin Bed rest	Suspect a DVT in patients with a sudden increase in calf pain, with risk factors such as immobilization, recent surgery, oral contraceptives, etc.
Acute lipodermosclerosis	Diffuse, purple-red, swollen leg resembling cellulitis; aching and tenderness is common	Compression bandaging; support stockings; NSAID	Usually bilateral, though may be more prominent on one leg; compression therapy essential
Chronic lipodermosclerosis	Diffuse brown sclerotic pigmentation with widespread chronic pain	Same as with acute lipodermosclerosis but with topical steroids and lubricants pentoxifylline	Support stockings may have to be custom made to accommodate for leg shape
Wound infection	Change in pain character associated with other clinical signs of infection	Topical antimicrobial agents and oral antibiotics, if indicated	Maintain bacterial balance, and watch for increase in pain, size, exudate, odor or changes in granulation tissue as signs of infection
Cellulitis	Diffuse bright red, hot leg; usually unilateral associated with tenderness and often fever	Oral antibiotics, with i.v. antibiotics needed for severe episodes or with low-host resistance	Venous ulcers may make individuals more prone to cellulitis
Atrophie blanche	Pain, stellate, white, scar-like areas associated with pain at rest and standing	NSAID therapy; other analgesics	May be seen in association with scars of healed ulcers, or may be an independent clinical feature
Acute contact dermatitis	Itching, burning red areas on leg corresponding to area of use of topical product	Remove the allergen; apply topical steroids	Lanolin, colophony, latex, neomycin are some of the more likely agents involved

Venous ulceration typically follows a progression of skin changes that makes it possible to assess the duration of the disease and the prognosis. These characteristic processes can be divided into early, intermediate, and late changes. It is important that not all patients will progress through each of these stages and some patients may have atypical presentations.

4.3. Early Changes

The first sign of venous disease is often dilation of the long saphenous vein on the medial aspect of the calf. Varicose veins may be present and range from a mild submalleolar flare (Fig. 1) to prominent venous vessel dilation (23). At this initial stage, mild pitting edema may be evident around the ankle toward the end of the day. The skin may be slightly warm and dusky in color, however, there are usually no major changes in the skin texture or pigmentation.

4.4. Intermediate Changes

As the severity of the venous disease progresses, the edema becomes marked and persists throughout the day. With time, red blood cells leak through dilated capillary beds depositing hemosiderin and promoting melanin deposition giving the skin a characteristic dark and mottled appearance. In addition, if the vascular permeability is high, purpura and echymoses may be present in the lower leg. Patients may often display a classic submalleolar flare with dilated prominent small veins on the dorsum of the foot extending to the leg below the ankle.

At this stage, changes in the texture and composition of the skin appear. Atrophy blanche may develop on the ankle or foot forming ivory-white atrophic plaques and small telangiectasias. Although atrophy blanche is common in venous disease occurring in 38% of patients with chronic venous disease (3), it is a nonspecific finding indicating a number of vascular and systemic conditions including various types of vasculitis.

Redness, scale, and pruritus are common in chronic venous disease and may represent the inflammatory changes of venous dermatitis. Factors such as frequent dressing changes, the use of many topical preparations, and the breakdown of the epidermis are associated with increased rates of contact irritant and contact allergic dermatitis. A marked scale and diffuse erythema should alert the clinician to an underlying sensitivity to the topical preparation applied to the wound site. Common allergens include lanolin, perfumes, colophony (including pentolin H in some hydrocolloids) formaldehyde releasing preservatives, neomycin, and bacitracin (19).

4.5. Late Changes

If the edema is longstanding, an "inverted champagne bottle" appearance may develop where the edema is greatest through the calf and tapers abruptly at the ankle. With chronic venous stasis, the surrounding tissue is typically nonpitting and sclerotic (woody fibrosis) resulting from deposition of fibrin in the edematous tissue. The skin is often atrophic and may show loss of hair follicles and sweat glands. With time, regions of hyperpigmentation and hypopigmentation interspersed with telangiectasias may develop. These characteristic changes are collectively referred to as atrophy blanche. The dermal collagen also becomes woody due to extravasated collagen and the skin becomes hard and woody losing its flexibility.

This collagen change is referred to as lipodermosclerosis. When areas of lipodermosclerosis become inflamed, they may present with painful deep red erythema that may mimic cellulites (20).

4.6. Course of Illness

Venous leg ulcers typically last less than 1 year, but frequently recur. In the most difficult cases, the ulcers can last for several years. Margolis et al. (21) have identified several factors that are predictive of poor healing rates. The most important risk factor is previous stripping of varicose veins. Patients who underwent vein-stripping procedures were 4.58 times more likely to have a nonhealing wound at 12 weeks than the normal venous leg ulcer population. Other prognostic indicators that are more likely to make the ulcers difficult to heal include previous hip/knee surgery (odds ratio = 3.53), yellow fibrin greater than 50% of the ulcer base (odds ratio = 3.42), larger size (odds ratio = 1.19), and longer duration of the ulcer (odds ratio = 1.09).

Recent studies indicate that a decrease in ulcer site during the first 4 weeks of treatment is predictive of the healing rate after 12 weeks (22). The ulcer size should be 30% smaller after 4 weeks of intensive treatment for a high probability of healing at 12 weeks. If the ulcer is not healing at the expected rate, the clinician needs to reassess the underlying cause and the treatment.

5. DIFFERENTIAL DIAGNOSIS

Although the majority of leg ulcers are venous (58–76%), there are other underlying conditions that have similar clinical presentations and may initially be misdiagnosed as venous leg ulcers (23). The absence of signs of ulcer healing in 4 to 12 weeks despite adequate treatment should alert the clinician to biopsy the edge for unsuspected diagnosis (22). The differential diagnosis of leg ulcers is summarized in Table 2.

5.1. Arterial Insufficiency

Arterial ulcers have a characteristic "punched-out" appearance, and often occur on the dorsum of the foot or over bony prominences. However, trauma may localize the ulcer to more proximal areas and lead to confusion with venous ulcers. Patients often report pain made worse by elevating the leg (pallor), and resolving on dependency (leading to rubor). Similarly, claudication may be present, with pain on exertion and dissipating in a few minutes of rest. The tissue may feel cool to the touch, and pulses may be absent. Trophic changes occur over time and hair loss on the distal leg with a shiny appearance and loss of nail luster may indicate arterial disease.

If the clinician suspects arterial disease, a holistic assessment including a clinical exam, an ankle brachial index (ABI) should be calculated. An ABI < 0.5 indicates severe arterial disease and the patient should be referred to a vascular surgeon for surgical assessment. An ABI 0.5–0.8 indicates moderate arterial disease, and treatment should be adjusted accordingly. Arterial and venous disease may exist concurrently.

5.2. Neuropathic

Neuropathic ulcers are most often localized to the weight-bearing surface of the feet especially over bony prominences. They may occur in insensate areas on the lower

Table 2 Differential Diagnosis of Venous Leg Ulcers

Cause	History	Physical/assessment	Management
Venous	Pitting edema at the end of the day, obesity, multiple pregnancies, previous surgeries	Venous varicosities, pitting edema, pigment, woody fibrosis serpiginous ulcer often around the medial malleolus, granulation tissue base	High compression Venous surgery in selected cases
Arterial insufficiency	Claudication, ± smoker, rest pain	Punched out lesions, distal gangrene, ABI < 0.5	Pain control, vascular surgery
Neuropathic	Associate diabetes or other cause of neuropathy	Usually occurs on the foot or areas of callus, persisting high pressure	Pressure redistribution
Lymphedema	Bilateral, chronic swelling	Woody hardness, nonpitting edema, uniform diameter from foot to knee, ABI > 0.8	Prevent infection
Pyoderma gangrenosum	Rapidly enlarging ulcer, pain, underlying condition	Red tender nodules/ pustules with bluish edge, biopsy	High dose steroids, ± immunosuppression
Vasculitis	Pain	Palpable purpuric lesions, ± necrosis, bilateral, biopsy edge	Systemic treatment of underlying cause
Infection	History of trauma	Local lymphadenopathy, nodules/pustules prior to ulceration, swab or biopsy	Antimicrobial agents
Malignancy	Long standing, slowly expanding	Atypical location, biopsy	Surgical removal if indicated

legs. The ulcers can often be localized through elastic compression wraps on the skin overlying the malloli. Treatment should be aimed at relieving pressure. If edema coexists locally, nonelastic short stretch bandaging is preferred to decrease the local pressure at rest.

5.2.1. Lymphedema

Lymphedema can occur alone or as a consequence of longstanding (venolymphedema) of venous disease. It is characterized by a woody hardness of tissue with surface hyperkeratosis similar to changes seen with warts or verrucae. The skin becomes darkened and often has multiple fissures predisposing the leg to infection. Lymphedema is nonpitting and typically affects the dorsum of the foot and the leg. In contrast to the inverted champagne bottle appearance of long-standing venous disease, a uniform swelling of the entire leg and foot usually characterizes lymphedema. Stemmer's sign is often useful in the diagnosis of lymphedema. Because the skin on the dorsal surface of the great toe loses its elasticity, it cannot be pinched, indicating a positive Stemmer's sign of lymphedema as opposed to the other causes of leg swelling.

Treatment of lymphedema is difficult and often requires very high compression bandaging (> 40 mmHg). Prior to initiating high compression therapy it is critical to evaluate arterial status including clinical assessment and the ABI to ensure that there is adequate arterial supply. In addition, because lymphedema predisposes to infection, good hygiene is critical to prevent lymphadenitis, cellulites, or osteomyelitis. If recurrent infection becomes a problem, prophylactic oral antibiotics should be considered.

5.2.2. Pyoderma Gangrenosum

Pyoderma gangrenosum (PG) is a destructive, necrotizing ulceration of the skin. It can occur anywhere in the body but often occurs on the calves, buttocks, thighs, or face and often follows minimal trauma. The lesions start as papules or pustules and evolve into tender hot, erythematous nodules that rapidly enlarge and ulcerate. The lesions typically have a bluish raised and rolled margin with an overhanging or undermining edge and a cribriform base. Approximately half of PG is associated with an underlying condition, most commonly rheumatoid arthritis, inflammatory bowel disease, or hematologic malignancies. If no associated disease is detected within the first 6 months of diagnosis, the disease is likely idiopathic (24). The diagnosis of PG is difficult and is often a diagnosis of exclusion. Tissue biopsy is useful for excluding other pathology, but is not sufficient for diagnosis without a compatible clinical presentation.

6.2.3. Vasculitis

Leg ulcers may be a feature of and underlying vasculitis. Palpable purpura in the skin surrounding the ulcer should alert the clinician to investigate for leukocytoclastic or other vasculitis. Ulcers associated with vasculitis are often multiple and start as painful, pruritic, and necrotic lesions. The ulcers are most common in the lower leg where stasis is most severe, trauma is most frequent, and the leg is the coolest. Furthermore, the basement membrane is thickest in the lower leg and is thus most prone to collect immune complexes. Many vasculitides have other organ involvement, and commonly affect the joints, liver, kidney, and gastrointestinal system. Vasculitis less frequently affects the brain, heart, and lungs. Drugs and infectious agents can cause or exacerbate vasculitis. The diagnosis of vasculitis requires an exhaustive inquiry into systemic manifestations. A skin biopsy detects the level of superficial or deep dermal vessel involvement as well as the type of cell attacking the vessel wall. This information is required to help diagnose the condition accurately, to establish the prognosis, and to institute appropriate treatment.

Cryoproteinemias and antiphospholipid syndrome often presents with a net-like of livedo reticularis pattern to the vasculature over the lower legs. Skin biopsy may show clotting of the small venules with very little in the way of diagnostic inflammatory infiltrates seen in skin biopsies from other vasculitides.

5.3. Infection

Osteomyelitis and cellulitis are a common cause of nonhealing wounds (25). The early clinical detection of these problems is paramount to the prevention of long-term damage and the prevention of amputation.

Ulcers that probe to bone should be considered as having osteomyelitis until proven otherwise (26). Antimicrobial treatment should begin immediately while superficial swabs and ulcer biopsies are preformed (25). Osteomyelitis is usually painful and x-rays will confirm the diagnosis in most cases. When the diagnosis is not clear, more sophisticated studies may be done. White blood cell scans are preferable to bone or gallium scans for the diagnosis of osteomyelitis.

Cellulitis typically presents as a hot, tender, and painful swelling. Cellulitis is most common in patients with lymphedema but can occur anytime there is a break in the continuity of the skin (as occurs with a ulceration or fissures). If a patient is immunosuppressed, they are more likely to acquire deep tissue infection from a loss of skin surface integrity. In the context of coexisting venous disease, cellulitis can be difficult to distinguish from severe contact or statis dermatitis, deep vein thrombosis or acute lipodermosclerosis. However, in contrast to venous related dermatitis, cellulitis typically has a rapid onset and is not pruritic.

Deep fungal or atypical mycobacterial infections may start as nodular growths that ulcerate. Diagnosis is based on biopsy for histology and culture. A more detailed discussion is presented in Chapter 5 on topical and systemic treatment of infection.

5.4. Malignancy

Cutaneous malignancies can be mistaken for other causes of leg ucleration. The clinician should suspect an underlying malignancy when the ulcer is not healing despite adequate treatment or if the ulcer occurs in an unusual location. Although most malignant ulcers are the result of a primary malignancy, some noncancerous ulcers may develop premalignant and malignant change with time (27).

Basal cell carcinomas (BCC) occur in about 1/7 of Caucasians and can be a source of diagnostic confusion. They start as a pearly translucent papule with surface telagiectasias. When the lesion reaches a critical size, it ulcerates forming a local destructive lesion referred to as a rodent ulcer. If it is not removed, it will grow insidiously until it takes on the appearance of a nonhealing expanding ulcer. Careful examination for telangiectasias on the thin translucent raised ulcer border can make the diagnosis of BCC. However, most often the diagnosis is made based on biopsy. Although these malignancies do not typically metastasize, they can be locally disfiguring. Small lesions can be managed conservatively with curettage. A large lesion may require radiotherapy or excision and skin grafting.

Squamous cell carcinomas (SCC) are less common than BCC but are still an important cause of malignant ulceration. They typically start as a keratotic papular cutaneous horn with an irregular base. With time, these lesions ulcerate and can mimic other causes of ulceration. Squamous cell carcinomas occur most commonly in areas of chronic sun exposure, but can occur in areas of chronic inflammation or scarring. They may be associated with local pain while basal cell carcinomas are often painless.

Malignant melanoma may be seen on the back of the legs, particularly in susceptible females. Most lesions start as an irregular pigmented lesion with the characteristics

A   (Asymmetry)

B   (Irregular border)

C   (Color—black, red, white, and blue)

D   (Diameter > 0.6 cm)

Ulceration occurs only in late lesions or nodular melanomas. Excisional biopsy for diagnosis is the treatment of choice.

6. CONCLUSION

The astute clinician should recognize the signs and symptoms of venous disease in order to initiate treatment early in the course of the disease. The clinician must have a rudimentary understanding of the pathogenesis of leg ulcers in order to choose the appropriate therapy and take precautions to avoid ulcer recurrence. Should there be an awareness of the many conditions that can mimic venous leg ulceration to avoid unnecessary or ineffective treatment. The recognition of underlying pathology will improve the overall quality of care of these patients.

Case Study: The patient had an arterial Doppler performed with an ABI of 0.9. Venous reflux was demonstrated with a Duplex Doppler in the vascular lab. The ulcer was treated with a hydrocolloid and high compression therapy (four-layer bandage) with healing in 16 weeks. Our patient lost 40 lb and has worn knee high compression stockings with 20–30 mmHg compression with no ulcer recurrence in the last 5 years.

REFERENCES

1. London NJ, Donnelly R. ABC of arterial and venous disease. Ulceration lower limb. Br Med J 2000; 320(7249):1589–1591.
2. Nelzen O, Bergqvist D, Lindhagen A. Venous and non-venous leg ulcers: clinical history and appearance in a population study. Br J Surg 1994; 81(2):182–187.
3. Valencia IC, Falabella A, Kirsner RS, Eaglstein WH. Continuing medical education: chronic venous insufficiency and venous leg ulceration. J Am Acad Dermatol 2001; 44(3):401–421.
4. Scott TE, LaMorte WW, Gorin DR, Mesoian JO. Risk factors for chronic venous insufficiency: a dual case-control study. J Vasc Surg 1995; 22:622–628.
5. Browaw NL, Brunand KG. The cause of venous ulceration. Lancet 1982; 2:243–245.
6. Falanga V. Venous ulceration. J Dermatol Surg Oncol 1993; 19:764–771.

7. Brunand KG, Whimster I, Naidoo A, Browaw NL. Precapillary fibrin in the ulcer-bearing skin of the lower leg: the cause of lipodermatosclerosis and venous ulceration. Br Med J (Clin Res Ed) 1982; 285:1071–1072.

8. Padres JD, Tonneson MG, Falanga V, Eaglstein WH, Clark RA. Skin capillaries surrounding chronic venous ulcers demonstrate smooth muscle hyperplasia and increased laminin type IV collagen. J Invest Dermatol 1991; 9(suppl 1):A127.

9. Mani R, White JE, Barret DF, Weaver PW. Tissue oxygenation, venous ulcers, and fibrin cuffs. J R Soc Med 1989; 82:345–346.

10. Scott HJ, Coleridge Smith PD, Scurr JH. Histological study of white blood cells and their association with lipodermosclerosis and venous ulceration. Br J Surg 1991; 78:210–211.

11. Goudin FW, Smith JG. Etiology of venous ulceration. Southern Med J 1993; 86: 1142–1146.

12. Falanga V, Eaglstein WH. The trap hypothesis of venous ulceration. Lancet 1993; 341:1006–1008.

13. Higley HR, Ksander GA, Gerhardt CO, Falanga V. Extravasation of macromolecules and possible trapping of transforming growth factor beta in venous ulceration. Br J Dermatol 1996; 192:79–85.

14. Orsted HL, Radke L, Gorst R. The impact of musculoskeletal changes on the dynamics of the calf muscle pump. Ostomy Wound Manage 2001; 47(10):18–24.

15. Phillips JAAD 1994.

16. Venous Ulcer Guidelines.

17. Sibbald RG, Williamson D, Falanga V, Cherry GW. Venous leg ulcers. In: Krasner DL, Rodeheaver GT, Sibbald RG, eds. Chronic Wound Care: A Clinical Source Book for Healthcare Professionals, 3rd ed. Wayne, PA: HMP Communications, 2001:483–494.

18. Sibbald RG. Ostomy Wound Manag 1998; 44(9):52–64.

19. Sibbald RG, Cameron J. Dermatological aspects of would care. In: Krasner DL, Rodeheaver GT, Sibbald RG, eds. Chronic Wound Care: A Clinical Source Book for Healthcare Professionals, 3rd ed. Wayne, PA: HMP Communications, 2001:273–285.

20. Ryan S, Eager C, Sibbald RG. Venous leg ulcer pain. Ostomy Wound Manage 2003; 49(suppl A):16–23.

21. Margolis DJ, Berlin JA, Strom BL. Risk factors associated with the failure of a venous leg ulcer to heal. Arch Dermatol 1991; 135:950–956.

22. Tallman P, Muscoare E, Carson P, et al. Initial rate of healing predicts complete healing of venous ulcers. Arch Dermatol 1997; 133:1231–1234.

23. Sibbald RG. An approach to leg and foot ulcers: a brief overview. Ostomy Wound Manage 1998; 44(9):28–35.

24. Von der Driesh. Pyoderma gangrenosum: a report of 44 cases with follow up. Br J Dermatol 1997; 137:1000–1005.

25. Sibbald RG, Orsted H, Schultz GS, Coutts P, Keast D. Ostomy Wound Management 2003; 49(11):24–51.

26. Grayson ML, Gibbons GW, Balogh K, Levin E, Karchmer AW. Probing to bone in infected pedal ulcers. A clinical sign of underlying osteomyelitis in diabetic patients. JAMA 1995; 273:721–723.

27. Hoffman F, Cameron J. Malignancy and pre-malignancy in leg ulceration. Abstract. 10th Conference of European Wound Management Association, May 18–20, 2000, Stockholm, Sweden.

11

Peripheral Vascular Disease

Daniel G. Federman, Chris B. Ruser, and Jeffrey D. Kravetz
Department of Medicine, Yale University School of Medicine,
West Haven, Connecticut, U.S.A.

1. INTRODUCTION

Health-care professionals frequently encounter patients with lower extremity wounds, many of which may be recalcitrant and refractory to therapy. Venous disease, arterial insufficiency, neuropathy, and a broad category of miscellaneous causes, such as pyoderma gangrenosum, vasculitis, and malignancy, should be considered. In this chapter, we will focus on arterial disease and describe how the health-care provider is in a unique situation to diagnose and treat not only an entity that may be causing or delaying healing in lower extremity wounds, but also an entity that is a part of a systemic process that has serious implications to those affected.

2. EPIDEMIOLOGY

Peripheral vascular disease (PVD) is a common manifestation of the atherosclerotic process and is defined as abnormal arterial flow to the lower extremities. The age-adjusted prevalence of PVD is ~12%, and as many as 20–30% of those over 75 years of age may be affected (1–3). The all-cause mortality rate is similar for men and women with PVD, although males are two to five times more likely to develop symptomatic disease during their lifetime (4). However, even asymptomatic patients with PVD have an increased mortality when compared with those without PVD.

Atherosclerosis is a common link between peripheral vascular, cardiovascular, and cerebrovascular disease, and it is therefore not surprising that patients with PVD experience frequent complications from these two other processes. Even in the absence of a previous history of myocardial infarction, patients with PVD have a similar risk of cardiovascular death than patients with known coronary artery or cerebrovascular disease (5). The 10-year mortality rate for cardiovascular events is three to six times greater for patients with PVD than for those without manifestations of this disease (6), and among the patients with abnormal ankle–brachial indices (ABIs), the lower the index, the higher the rate of cardiovascular events (7). The annual mortality rate for patients with critical leg ischemia, those with the lowest ABI values, approaches 25%, a figure much higher than that for many malignancies (8).

2.1. Clinical Manifestations

Although the majority of patients with PVD are asymptomatic (9), those with symptoms often complain of intermittent claudication, which is typically described as cramping pain in the calf or buttocks that occurs with exercise and is relieved very quickly with cessation of exercise and rest. Patients with aorto-iliac disease may present with Leriche's syndrome, with claudication of the buttocks and thighs, along with impotence, due to decreased flow through the pudendal artery.

The disease progresses slowly in the lower extremities in symptomatic patients. When claudicants were followed for 5 years, 25% experienced worsening claudication and 5% underwent amputation (10).

2.2. Diagnosis

Although the prevalence of this disease is high, physician awareness is relatively low. Furthermore, the underdiagnosis of PVD appears to be a barrier to the use of effective secondary preventive measures, such as aggressive treatment of hypertension and lipid disorders, as well as the use of antiplatelet therapy, in order to reduce the high cardiovascular risk in these patients (11). It therefore behooves clinicians to be facile with various methods of diagnosis.

Various modalities, other than patient history, can be used to establish a diagnosis of PVD. A survey composed of eight questions, the Rose questionnaire was aimed at standardizing and further categorizing claudication (12). However, it became apparent that the Rose questionnaire was imperfect and was later modified by Leng and Fowkes (13) to a six-question survey, with a reported sensitivity of 91% and specificity of 99%.

The physical examination often can be extremely helpful in supporting a diagnosis of PVD. On the basis of published studies, investigators found that abnormal pedal pulses, a unilaterally cool extremity, prolonged venous filling time, or the presence of a femoral bruit was helpful in establishing the diagnosis. An abnormal femoral pulse, lower extremity bruits, and warm knees were helpful in determining the extent and distribution of vascular disease. However, the capillary refill test, foot discoloration, atrophic skin, and hairless extremities are not helpful in making diagnostic decisions (14).

The ABI is a simple, noninvasive tool used in diagnosis of PVD and to assess the effects of intervention. Abnormally low values identify patients with angiographically proven occlusions with a sensitivity of 96% and a specificity of 94–100% (15,16). In order to perform an ABI properly, the patient should be in the supine position and appropriately sized arm and ankle blood pressure cuffs should be used. Using a 5–10 mHz hand-held Doppler, systolic-pressure measurements are obtained in both brachial arteries and posterior tibial and dorsalis pedis arteries. The ABI for each lower extremity is calculated by dividing the higher of the two lower extremity pressures on each leg by the higher of the two brachial pressure measurements. Whereas a normal ABI is > 0.9, an ABI of 0.71–0.90 is consistent with mild obstruction, an ABI of 0.41–0.70 is consistent with moderate obstruction, and an ABI of < 0.40 is considered severe obstructive disease.

The ABI confers not only diagnostic utility, but also prognostic and other useful information as well. Those with ABIs < 0.4 may develop rest pain, and this value or less bodes poorly for the healing of ischemic wounds. Among patients with abnormally low ABIs, the lower the ABI, the worse the long-term prognosis is. Those with an ABI ≤ 0.3 had a relative risk of death nearly double those whose ABIs were between 0.5 and 0.91 when followed for 52 months (17). The ABI has been shown to be more closely associated with leg function in patients with PVD than claudication or other leg symptoms (18).

Exercise testing, which can be performed by walking on a treadmill at 1.5–2 miles per hour at 10–15% incline for up to 5 min, increases the sensitivity of the ABI (19). Exercise testing should not be performed in those with unstable coronary syndromes, those with critical ischemia, or in symptomatic patients with rest pain. Stiff, calcified, noncompressible vessels may cause an ABI >1.30, especially in diabetics and the elderly, and in this situation, other diagnostic modalities should be used. In patients with diabetes mellitus, the digital arteries of the toes tend to be relatively spared of the medial calcinosis, and therefore, a toe/brachial index may be helpful.

Alternative accepted noninvasive diagnostic modalities, which can be useful in those with noncompressible vessels, include segmental leg pressures, pulse volume recordings, Doppler waveform analysis, color duplex and color Doppler imaging (19), and magnetic resonance angiography (MRA) (20).

2.3. Segmental Leg Pressures

Although a single ABI measurement can be useful for diagnosing PVD, it does not provide anatomic localization of the obstruction. However, if multiple blood pressure recordings are obtained along the lower extremity and indexes calculated with respect to the brachial blood pressure, one can identify the site of obstruction. Most vascular laboratories use appropriately sized pneumatic cuffs placed on (1) the proximal thigh, just below the perineum, (2) the distal thigh, just superior to the patella, (3) the proximal calf, just inferior to the knee, (4) the lower calf, just superior to the ankle, and (5) the first toe (21). A drop of ≥ 20–30 mmHg between a more proximal and an adjacent distal segment implies obstruction in the arterial segment between the two pneumatic cuffs.

This modality may help the clinician ascertain whether a patient's symptoms are attributable to vascular disease. For example, it would be unlikely for infrapopliteal disease to be responsible for a patient's complaint of thigh pain with exercise, whereas it could be responsible for a patient's ischemic foot. Similarly, if a patient with a low ABI developed a traumatic wound in the thigh or proximal calf, one could help localize the site of obstruction and determine whether the wound would likely heal without more aggressive intervention.

2.4. Doppler Waveform Analysis, Color Duplex Imaging

Analysis of the Doppler arterial waveform can also help in diagnosis. The finding of a lower-resistance waveform, as one records waveforms distally down the lower extremity, implies an obstructing lesion in the arterial segment where the normal arterial waveform and the abnormal waveforms were obtained. This information can be additive to that obtained with segmental leg pressures in which specific vessels can often be identified as responsible culprit arteries (21).

Color duplex imaging combines real-time B-mode imaging with pulsed and color Doppler imaging. Whereas B-mode imaging provides anatomic detail of the vessel, color Doppler provides not only easier identification of the vessel, but also the information about the direction of flow and the presence of turbulence. This modality allows for both anatomic and physiologic evaluation but, when compared with segmental leg pressures or arterial waveform analysis, requires longer examination time, a more skilled technologist, and more expensive equipment.

Other means of diagnosis requiring technology not readily available in most clinicians' offices include the use of transcutaneous oxygen tension measurements (22) and photoplethysmography, which can be used to determine ABIs (23). Enthusiasm for pulse oximetry as a means of detecting PVD was tempered when it was found to be insensitive for the detection of early PVD (24).

2.5. Magnetic Resonance Angiography

Magnetic resonance angiography has emerged as a noninvasive imaging modality that avoids risks associated with the current "gold standard," conventional angiography (e.g., arterial puncture, plaque embolization, and contrast-induced nephropathy) and provides adequate preoperative evaluation of inflow and runoff vessels (25). A meta-analysis demonstrated that MRA is highly accurate for assessing the entire lower extremity for arterial disease. The three-dimensional gadolinium-enhanced MRA is superior when compared with a two-dimensional MRA (20).

2.6. Wound Healing and Tissue Loss

The noninvasive assessment can provide information beyond diagnosis alone. Although a variety of other variables impact on the success or rate of wound healing (nutritional status, presence of infection or coexistent venous disease, patient adherence, and aggressiveness of health-care provider), a great deal of useful information with respect to wound healing and tissue loss can be learned by the noninvasive assessment. Such information includes the likelihood that a conservative approach will result in satisfactory healing, whether revascularization attempts should be employed to promote healing, and where an amputation should be performed to ensure adequate healing if it is considered. Patients with an ABI < 0.4 are unlikely to have ischemic lesions heal without attempts at revascularization. Studies have also demonstrated that $\sim$80% of distal ischemic lesions will heal if the ankle pressure is at least 80 mmHg (21,26). Conversely, if the ankle pressure is < 50–55 mmHg, healing rates of 0–11% can be expected (21,27,28).

Toe pressures can also be useful in predicting the likelihood of healing in patients with ischemic tissue loss of the toes or forefoot or for those with minor forefoot amputations. If a toe is gangrenous, the measurement should be obtained from an adjacent digit. Healing rates of 86–90% for ischemic foot lesions have been demonstrated if the toe pressure is found to be at least 30 mmHg (21,27,28), 14–50% if toe pressures are in the 20–30 mmHg range, and 0–29% if toe pressures are < 20 mmHg (29).

Transcutaneous oxygen tension (tcPO_2) measurements, which can be obtained using a sensor composed of a centrally located platinum cathode surrounded by a circular silver–silver chloride anion and a heating element to cause vasodilation, can also be helpful in predicting whether an amputation at that site will heal. A tcPO_2 value of >10 mmHg is associated with healing in 75–94% of patients, whereas lower values were associated with failure of healing in 51–100% (30,31). However, others have found that higher tcPO_2 levels, ranging from 20 to 50 mmHg, were predictors of whether ulcers or amputations would heal (32–35).

2.7. Therapy

As PVD is associated with the atherosclerotic process, therapy is aimed not only at the affected extremity, but also at the entire disease process. A variety of pharmacological and nonpharmacological measures should be employed to target atherosclerotic risk factors, improve the functional status of the patient with claudication, and decrease the rates of amputation, myocardial infarction, and stroke.

2.7.1. Risk-Factor Modification

Traditional atherosclerotic risk factors should be treated aggressively. Emphasis should be placed on smoking cessation, as it may be one of the most important risk factors. Over 90% of hospitalized vascular patients with PVD in one study were the current or recent smokers (36). There is ample evidence supporting the beneficial effects of smoking cessation, for those without or with PVD (37). In the Framingham study, men who stopped smoking had lower rates of coronary heart disease and stroke than subjects who continued to smoke (38). In another study, smokers with claudication that continued to smoke developed rest pain 16% of the time, whereas none of those who stopped smoking developed rest pain at 7 years (39). The antidepressant bupropion or nicotine replacement, in the form of transdermal patches, spray, gum, or inhaler, combined with behavioral modification therapy enhances the rate of smoking cessation (40).

Dyslipidemia is a major independent risk for atherosclerosis. Several large, well-done clinical trials have demonstrated the beneficial effects of lipid lowering in patients with coronary artery disease (41). Furthermore, treatment of dyslipidemia in patients with PVD reduces disease progression and claudication (42–44). Therapy with statins is preferred, though niacin can be used if contraindications to statins preclude their use.

Diabetes mellitus is a common disorder associated with significant morbidity and mortality. Although intensive control of blood glucose has been shown to reduce microvascular complications (nephropathy, retinopathy, and neuropathy), it has not been shown to reduce the risk of PVD (45) or the risk of amputation due to PVD (46). Although these findings do not support aggressive glucose control for control of PVD, it should be attempted in order to reduce other complications.

Hypertension is a known risk factor for atherosclerosis; however, it is not presently known whether treatment of hypertension alters the natural progression of PVD. The Joint National Committee on Prevention, Detection, Evaluation, and Treatment of High Blood Pressure has recommended that beta-blockers and diuretics be chosen as initial drug therapy, unless there are specific indications for another medication (47), but more recently, the use of angiotensin-converting-enzyme inhibitors has been shown to confer cardiovascular protection beyond what would be expected from their blood pressure lowering effects alone (48).

2.7.2. Exercise and Specific Medical Therapy

The role of exercise therapy has been studied in several small trials. A review of the literature demonstrated that exercise increases maximal walking distance, with an overall improvement of 150% (range, 74–230%) (49). Additional studies are needed to ascertain the long-term benefits of exercise for PVD patients, as well as the cost-effectiveness of different exercise regimens.

Pentoxifylline, a xanthine derivative, increases walking distances in claudicants when used for up to 6 months (50), though its exact mechanism of action is not clearly understood and its effects often are not dramatic (51).

Cilostazol, a phosphodiesterase III inhibitor, is generally well tolerated and has been found to be superior to pentoxifylline (52), though it is more expensive. It is contraindicated for patients with congestive heart failure, as chemically related agents have been found to increase mortality in these patients (53).

Antiplatelet therapy has a role in the treatment of patients with PVD. Aspirin, at doses of 81–325 mg/day, has been recommended for those afflicted (54). Ticlopidine, which inhibits adenosine 5′-diphosphate-stimulated fibrinogen binding to its platelet receptor, has been shown superior to placebo in its ability to increase walking distances (55). However, due to the risk of neutropenia and thrombotic thrombocytopenic purpura, it has been supplanted by a newer, chemically related drug, clopidogrel. This agent has been shown to reduce cardiovascular risk when compared with aspirin in patients with atherosclerosis (56).

Other agents that may prove useful include naftidrofuryl, levocarnitine, propionyl levocarnitine, and prostaglandins (57), though further evidence to support their use is warranted.

REFERENCES

1. Criqui MH, Fronek A, Barrett-Connor E, et al. The prevalence of peripheral arterial disease in a defined population. Circulation 1985; 71:510–515.
2. Hiatt WR, Marshall JA, Baxter J, et al. Diagnostic methods for peripheral arterial disease in the San Luis Valley Diabetes Study. J Clin Epidemiol 1990; 43:597–606.
3. Fowkes FG. Epidemiology of peripheral vascular disease. Atherosclerosis 1997; 131 (suppl):S29–S31.
4. Fowkes FG. Epidemiology of atherosclerotic disease in the lower limbs. Eur J Vasc Surg 1988; 2:283–291.
5. Newman AB, Shemanski L, Manolio TA, et al. Ankle–arm index as a predictor of cardiovascular disease and mortality in the Cardiovascular Health Study. Arterioscler Thromb Vasc Biol 1999; 19:538–545.
6. Criqui MH, Langer RD, Fronek A, et al. Mortality over a period of 10 years in patients with peripheral arterial disease. N Engl J Med 1992; 326:381–386.
7. McKenna M, Wolfson S, Kuller L. The ratio of ankle and arm arterial pressure as an independent predictor of mortality. Atherosclerosis 1991; 87:119–128.
8. Dormandy JA, Heeck L, Vig S. The fate of patients with critical leg ischemia. Sem Vasc Surg 1999; 12:142–147.
9. Stoffers HE, Rinkens PE, Kester AD, et al. The prevalence of asymptomatic and unrecognized peripheral arterial occlusive disease. Int J Epidemiol 1996; 25:282–290.
10. Imperato AM, Kim GE, Davidson T, Crowley JG. Intermittent claudication: its natural course. Surgery 1975; 78:795–799.
11. Hirsch AT, Criqui MH, Treat-Jacobson D, Regensteiner JG, Creager MA, Olin JW, Krook SH, Hunninghake DB, Comerota AJ, Walsh MMME, McDermott MM, Hiatt WR. Peripheral arterial disease detection, awareness, and treatment in primary care. JAMA 2001; 286:1317–1324.
12. Rose GA. The diagnosis of ischemic heart pain and intermittent claudication in field surveys. Bull Org Mond Sante 1962; 27:645–658.
13. Leng GC, Fowkes FGR. The Edinburgh claudication questionnaire: an improved version of the WHO/Rose questionnaire for use in epidemiological surveys. J Clin Epidemiol 1992; 45:1101–1109.

14. McGee SR, Boyko EJ. Physical examination and chronic lower-extremity ischemia. Arch Intern Med 1998; 158:1357–1364.
15. Carter SA. Indirect systolic pressures and pulse waves in arterial occlusive disease of the lower extremities. Circulation 1968; 37:624–637.
16. Ouriel K, McDonnell AE, Metz CE, Zarins CK. A critical evaluation of stress testing in the diagnosis of peripheral vascular disease. Surgery 1982; 91:686–693.
17. McGrae McDermott M, Feinglass J, Slavensky R, Pearce WH. The ankle–brachial index as a predictor of survival in patients with peripheral vascular disease. J Gen Intern Med 1994; 49:445–449.
18. McDermott MM, Greenland P, Liu K, Guralnik JM, Celic L, Criqui MH, et al. The ankle-brachial index is associated with leg function and physical activity: the walking and leg circulation study. Ann Intern Med 2002; 136:873–883.
19. Gathan V. The noninvasive vascular laboratory. Surg Clin N Am 1998; 78:507–518.
20. Koelemay MJ, Lijmer JG, Stoker J, Legemate DA, Bossuyt P. Magnetic resonance angiography for the evaluation of lower extremity arterial disease: a meta-analysis. JAMA 2001; 285:1338–1345.
21. Rose SC. Noninvasive vascular laboratory for evaluation of peripheral arterial occlusive disease: part II—clinical applications: chronic usually atherosclerotic, lower extremity ischemia. J Vasc Intervent Radiol 2000; 11:1257–1275.
22. Byrne P, Provan JL, Ameli FM, Jones DP. The use of transcutaneous oxygen tension measurements in the diagnosis of peripheral vascular insufficiency. Ann Surg 1984; 200:159–165.
23. Whitely MS, Horrocks M, Fox AD. Photoplethysmography can replace hand-held Doppler in the measurement of ankle/brachial indices. Am R Coll Surg Engl 1998; 80:96–98.
24. Joyce WP, Walsh K, Gough DB, Gorey TF, Fitzpatrick JM. Pulse oximetry: a new non-invasive assessment of peripheral arterial occlusive disease. Br J Surg 1990; 77:1115–1117.
25. Velazquez OC, Baum RA, Carpenter JP. Magnetic resonance angiography of lower-extremity arterial disease. Surg Clin N Am 1998; 78:519–537.
26. Nicholas GG, Myers JL, DeMuth WE Jr. The role of vascular laboratory criteria in the selection of patients for lower extremity amputation. Ann Surg 1982; 195:469–473.
27. Carter SA. The relationship of distal systolic pressures to healing of skin lesions in limbs with arterial occlusive disease, with special reference to diabetes mellitus. Scand J Clin Lab Invest 1973; 31(suppl):239–243.
28. Baker WH, Barnes RW. Minor forefoot amputations in patients with low ankle pressure. Am J Surg 1977; 133:331–332.
29. Holstein P, Noer I, Tonnesen KH, Sager P, Lassen NA. Distal blood pressure in severe arterial insufficiency: strain-gauge, radioisotopes, and other methods. In: Bergan JJ, Yao ST, eds. Gangrene and Severe Ischemia of the Lower Extremities. New York: Grunes & Straton, 1978:95–114.
30. Harward TRS, Volny J, Golbranson F, Bernstein EF, Fronek A. Oxygen inhalation-induced transcutaneous PO_2 changes as a predictor of amputation level. J Vasc Surg 1985; 2:220–227.
31. Karanfilian RG, Lynch TG, Zirul VT, Padberg FT, Jamil Z, Hobson RW II. The value of laser Doppler velocimetry and transcutaenous oxygen tension determination in predicting healing of ischemic forefoot ulcerations and amputations in diabetic and nondiabetic patients. J Vasc Surg 1986; 4:511–516.
32. Cina C, Katsamouris A, Megerman J, et al. Utility of transcutaneous oxygen tension measurements in peripheral arterial occlusive disease. J Vasc Surg 1984; 1:362–371.
33. Katsamouris A, Brewster DC, Megerman J, Cina C, Darling RC, Abbott WM. Transcutaneous oxygen tension in selection of amputation level. Am J Surg 1984; 147:510–517.
34. Ratliff DA, Clyne CAC, Chant ADB, Webster JHH. Prediction of amputation wound healing: the role of transcutaneous PO_2 assessment. Br J Surg 1984; 71:219–222.
35. Ballard JL, Eke CC, Bunt TJ, Killeen JD. A prospective evaluation of transcutaneous oxygen measurements in the management of diabetic foot problems. J Vasc Surg 1995; 22:485–492.

36. Celermajer DS, Sorenson KE, Georgakopoulos D, et al. Cigarette smoking is associated with dose-related and potentially reversible impairment of endothelium-dependent dilation in healthy young adults. Circulation 1993; 88:2149–2155.
37. Quick CRG, Cotton LT. The measured effect of stopping smoking on intermittent clausication. Br J Surg 1982; 69(suppl):S24–S26.
38. Gordon T, Kannel WB, McGee D, Dawber TR. Death and coronary attacks in men after giving up cigarette smoking: a report from the Framingham study. Lancet 1974; 2:1345–1348.
39. Jonasson T, Bergstrom R. Cessation of smoking in patients with intermittent claudication. Effects on the risk of peripheral vascular complications, myocardial infarction, and mortality. Acta Med Scand 1987; 221:253–260.
40. Hughes JR, Goldstein MG, Hurt RD, Shiffman S. Recent advances in the pharmacotherapy of smoking. JAMA 1999; 281:72–76.
41. LaRosa JC, He J, Vupputurri S. Effect of statins on risk of coronary disease: a meta-analysis of randomized controlled trials. JAMA 1999; 282:2340–2346.
42. Leng GC, Price JF, Jepson RG. Lipid-lowering for lower limb atherosclerosis Cochrane Database of Systematic Reviews. 2000; 2:CD000123.
43. Blankenhorn DH, Azen SP, Crawford DW, et al. Effects of colestipol–niacin therapy on human femoral atherosclerosis. Circulation 1991; 83:438–447.
44. Lewis B. Randomised controlled trial of the treatment of hyperlipidemia on progression 1f atherosclerosis. Acta Med Scand Suppl 1985; 701:53–57.
45. The Diabetes Control and Complications Trail (DCCT) Research Group. Effect of intensive diabetes management on macrovascular events and risk factors in the diabetes control and complications trial. Am J Cardiol 1995; 75:894–903.
46. UK Prospective Diabetes Study (UKPDS) Group. Intensive blood-glucose control with sulphonylureas or insulin compared with conventions treatment and risk of complications in patients with type 2 diabetes (UKPDS 33). Lancet 1998; 352:837–853.
47. The Joint National Committee on Prevention, Detection, Evaluation and Treatment of High blood Pressure. The sixth report of the Joint National Committee on Prevention, Detection, Evaluation, and Treatment of High Blood Pressure. Arch Intern Med 1997; 157:2413–2446.
48. The Heart Outcomes Prevention Evaluation Study Investigators. Effects of an angiotensin-converting-enzyme inhibitor, ramipril, on cardiovascular events in high-risk patients. N Engl J Med 2000; 342:145–153.
49. Leng GC, Fowler B, Ernst E. Exercise for intermittent claudication. Cochrane Database of Systematic Reviews. 2000; 2:CD000990.
50. Gillings D, Koch G, Reich T, et al. Another look at the pentoxifylline efficacy data for intermittent claudication. J Clin Pharmacol 1987; 27:601–609.
51. Green RM, McNamara JA. The effects of pentoxifylline on patients with intermittent claudication. J Vasc Surg 1988; 7:356–362.
52. Dawson DL, Cutler BS, Hiatt WR, et al. A comparison of cilostazol and pentoxifylline for treating intermittent claudication. Am J Med 2000; 109:523–530.
53. Packer M, Carver JR, Rodenheffer RJ, et al. Effect of oral milrinone on mortality in severe chronic heart failure. The PROMISE Study Research Group. N Engl J Med 1991; 325:1468–1475.
54. Sachdev GP, Ohlrogge KD, Johnson CL. Review of the fifth American college of chest physicians consensus conference on antithrombotic therapy: outpatient management for adults. Am J Health Syst Pharm 1999; 56:1505–1514.
55. Arcan JC, Blanchard J, Boissel JP, et al. Multicenter double-blind study of ticlopidine in the treatment of intermittent claudication and the prevention of its complications. Angiology 1988; 39:802–811.
56. CAPRIE Steering Committee. A randomized, blinded, trial of clopidogrel vs. aspirin in patients at risk of ischemic events (CAPRIE). Lancet 1996; 348:1329–1339.
57. Hiatt WR. Medical treatment of peripheral arterial disease and claudication. N Engl J Med 2001; 344:1608–1621.

12
Ulceration Due to Arterial Occlusion

Morris D. Kerstein
*Department of Surgery, Jefferson Medical College, Philadelphia, Pennsylvania and
VA Medical and Regional Office Center, Wilmington, Delaware, U.S.A.*

Occlusive vascular disease may involve the common femoral artery, as well as distal branches, above-the-knee (AK) and below-the-knee (BK) popliteal, and anterior tibial and posterior tibial, peroneal vessels or their branches. The involvement can begin at any time in one's adult life and move forward, produce flow-reducing narrowing, and finally, occlusion. The atherosclerotic involvement, one identifies in the lower extremity, is also manifest in other parts of the body; atherosclerosis is a multivessel process. This diffuse involvement may modify or mitigate the surgeon's attempts at maintaining function. The focus is often an isolated extremity, but an assessment of the risk–benefit analysis of any intervention must be undertaken. Active intervention is based on disability, threat to limb loss, or interference of normal daily function. Therefore, the indication for surgical intervention may be claudication if it interferes with the patient's lifestyle. A wound, unresponsive to conservative management, with rest pain or tissue breakdown, more likely than not, will require reconstructive vascular surgery (1,2).

Stenosis or narrowing, or occlusion may be impacted upon due to collateral pathways. Therefore, the symptoms are a reflection of the narrowing or stenosis, as well as occlusion and the lack of collaterals. Thus, the patient who has a nonhealing ulcer or tissue necrosis, more likely than not, also has multiple sequential occlusions or the combined segment disease of hemodynamically significant lesions at the tibial level and superficial femoral–popliteal level.

Lesions with significant nonhealing ulceration and stenosis, or occlusion as the precipitating factor may be present in one of the four categories: no signs or symptoms, or intermittent claudication less than one block; with significant claudication (the patient frequently has dependent rubor and decreased temperature; rest pain associated with atrophy, cyanosis, or dependent rubor); and nonhealing ischemic ulcer or gangrene. Invasive diagnostic and therapeutic intervention is sometimes indicated with claudication if it interferes with one's lifestyle. Invasive diagnostic and therapeutic intervention is usually indicated for the patient with rest pain and tissue breakdown. Rest pain alone may sometimes be difficult to evaluate, in particular, when the patient's disease is combined or compounded by diabetes mellitus. One would have to ensure no evidence exists of arthritis, neuritis, or neuropathy. Obviously, such pain will not be relieved by reconstructive vascular surgery. With a confusing or complex etiology, it may be necessary to perform noninvasive laboratory studies. Angiographic evaluation is withheld until operative intervention is planned. Whether conservative management of the nonhealing arterial ulcer will progress is a judgment call. Should it progress, one must consider intervention. If it remains the same or improves, particularly in the patient more than 75 or 80 years of age, one must proceed more slowly because of cardiopulmonary, renal, or cerebrovascular disease (3). If pain becomes intolerable and the ulcer is progressive, the patient should be assessed to determine the risk–benefit analysis of local ulcer control, vascular intervention, or amputation. The relative ease and simplicity of percutaneous balloon angioplasty, alone or in combination with other endovascular reconstructive treatments, have decreased the risk and risk–benefit analysis for many patients with nonhealing ulcers and vascular disease. The combined efforts of surgeons, radiologists, and cardiologists in the field of peripheral vascular occlusive disease have decreased the risk and, more importantly, the patient is then a better candidate for varying degrees of intervention. These less-invasive processes can initiate the healing process and further delay or prevent aggressive open high-risk arterial reconstructive surgery (2).

Intermittent claudication is the pain brought on by exertion and relieved by rest. It is a distinct symptom and manifestation of arterial vascular occlusive disease (4). The patient describes a sense of heaviness, weakness, or fatigue in the limb without pain. One must differentiate neuromuscular disorders from vascular occlusive disease. On occasion, leg symptoms also can be produced by spinal cord or chorda equina compression. This form of neurogenic pseudoclaudication is most often produced by spinal stenosis and is to be expected when peripheral pulses are apparently normal. A thorough assessment is required because on rare occasions, both neurologic and vascular occlusive problems can coexist. Finally, the patient may require both invasive angiography and invasive myelography (Table 1), or preferably magnetic resonance imaging.

A typical arterial or ischemic ulcer is more painful than a venous ulcer or other manifestations of ischemia. The arterial ulcer usually has a necrotic base and is located in an area of pressure or trauma. The arterial ulcer is seen in the distal areas of vascular supply; for example, the end of the digit over the metatarsal head or over the malleolus. One must address the local phenomenon of the "blue toe" and assess whether it represents progression of chronic atherosclerotic vascular disease with occlusion or another etiology. The "blue toe syndrome," for example, is related to atheromatous emboli, originating higher up in the aorta or femoral region. Local infection often seen in diabetic patients may appear in the same fashion. Noninvasive arterial tests must be included in the evaluation, and therefore, one can determine

Table 1   Evaluation of Peripheral Vascular Arterial Disease

History and physical examination
   Decreased to absent pulse
   Pallor
   Paresthesias/claudication
   Rest pain
   Tissue loss
Noninvasive vascular laboratory tests (Doppler)
   Segmental pressures
Angiography or magnetic resonance angiography

Table 2 Peripheral Artery Disease

Risk factors
  Hypertension
  Diabetes
  Elevated cholesterol, especially low-density lipoprotein
  Poor healing of cuts, injuries
  History of smoking
  Pain in the calf on walking (claudication) and relieved at rest
  Pain in the foot/leg at rest
  Decreased activity or exercise
  History of heart disease

Source: From Refs. 21, 27.

whether it is a systemic or local process. Radical local excision and drainage with a good proximal blood supply may result in a healed foot if one is dealing with a diabetic distal digital occlusion. Diagnosis may be more complex when the infection coexists with more proximal vascular occlusive disease. An embolic process must be considered for the "blue toes" and vascular occlusion with the associated nonhealing lesion. Such emboli may result from the heart or aorta. The five etiologies of cardiac emboli include atrial fibrillation, mural thrombus, myocardial infarction with an akinetic segment of the wall, vegetations on the valve, paradoxical embolus, and atrial myxoma. Often, an acute thrombosis cannot be differentiated easily from embolus. Therefore, cardiac and peripheral arterial evaluation is a requirement (Table 2).

    A physical examination may disclose discoloration and swelling, but a thorough assessment will include pulses, sensation, and temperature. The extent of infection or necrosis deep to the skin may be an assessment of pulses, temperature, touch, pressure, greater than one expects from initial examination. Further identification or assessment of the foot may be carried out without anesthesia if the patient has diminished sensation from diabetic neuropathy. If this is not the case, exploration and subsequent debridement should be performed in the operating room with anesthesia.

    The assessment focuses on previous operative scars, a reflection of vascular construction and possible sympathectomy. Scars provide evidence as to the extent of the vascular disease to some degree. Particular attention must be directed to the heel and between the toes. Vascular disease is usually symmetrical; the opposite limb must be inspected as well. Palpable pulses are graded 0 to 4; a thorough assessment includes the noninvasive vascular laboratory with Doppler ultrasound—particularly in the absent or diminished pulse. The presence or absence of a dorsalis pedis and posterior tibial pulse and the ankle–brachial ratio (ABR) may further confirm

Table 3 Doppler Ankle–Brachial Ratio

0.85–1.2	Normal
0.5–0.85	Claudication (mild-to-moderate disease)
	A wound can heal
0.5–0.25	Threat of tissue and limb loss
> 1.2	May be due to DM, MS, RD

Note: DM, diabetes mellitus; MS, Mönckeberg's sclerosis; and RD, renal disease.
Source: From Ref. 5.

small-vessel disease (Tables 1 and 3) (5). In the patient with associated proximal disease (e.g., a femoral bruit), arterial reconstruction or angioplasty above the inguinal ligament may be indicated.

Systemic factors are important in evaluation of the patient with a nonhealing ulcer of the lower extremity in the presence of arterial disease. The presence of heart disease, diabetes, kidney disease, hypertension and chronic pulmonary disease must be assessed. A cardiac assessment would include a thorough history, physical examination, and electrocardiogram, often combined with a thallium-persantine stress test. The presence of cardiac failure may require a Swan-Ganz catheter for further assessment. Renal function is measured by blood chemistry, including creatinine clearance, and sometimes by ultrasound of the kidneys (6–8).

The noninvasive vascular laboratory not only assesses the degree of vascular occlusive disease, but also represents a baseline that one can use for further assessment for testing. One can localize the level of disease, in addition using not only pressure and ABR, but also decreased waveforms, which suggest the inflexible artery. The noninvasive testing can help predict when amputation has little chance of healing. For example, an ankle pressure below 30 mmHg may indicate a toe amputation, or other local foot procedure for an ischemic lesion will not heal without major revascularization. Toe pressures in the range of 30 mmHg represent the cut-off zone where they will heal. One can be falsely directed with diabetes and Mönckeberg's sclerosis; both have rigid pipestem vessels in the disease configuration and yield falsely elevated pressures. The waveform is usually flat (9,10).

One may require angiography not to necessarily detect the presence of vascular occlusive disease but to determine whether it is reconstructable. The arterial tree from groin-to-forefoot should be visualized in continuity by a transfemoral route. Multiple exposures of large boluses of contrast media are often necessary. The oblique views are important when performing optimal bypass surgery and often require augmentation with further digital studies. Currently, expanded use of magnetic resonance imaging/magnetic resonance angiography has safely and more effectively improved the diagnostic ability in peripheral vascular occlusive disease.

One must undertake vascular reconstructive disease for the limb with a nonhealing ulcer (11). If the extensive gangrene proceeds into the deeper tissues, amputation will be/is necessary. More than 60% of these patients have diabetes mellitus, and their mean age is 65–70 years. The general medical management should include assessment of cardiopulmonary, renal disease, as well as a diabetic status, before proceeding with arteriography, surgical reconstruction, or both. With the threat to limb loss because of nonhealing ulcers, the patient should undergo arterial assessment and, if appropriate, femoral–popliteal bypass. It may be necessary to bypass into an isolated vascular segment, although this is not the procedural choice (12). The sequential bypass or bypass from femoral-to-distal vessel may be necessary and performed in one or two stages (13). Small-vessel bypasses to the posterior-tibial or anterior-tibial vessels, or to the peroneal arteries, are necessary when proximal obliteration of the vessel is present. The absence of a plantar arch and vascular calcification is not an absolute contraindication to reconstruction; < 5% of patients are now considered unreconstructable or inoperable (14–16). Surgical interventions, including axillo-popliteal bypass, profundoplasty with endarterectomy, and saphenous vein patch, are further surgical considerations (13). Until 1976, the reversed autogenous saphenous vein graft was the material of choice (17). Since then, a variety of Dacron grafts and polytetrafluoroethylene grafts have become available and are used (18). Good results are noted in the femoral–popliteal region; however, one should consider using autogenous tissue in the distal–popliteal position (19,20). Currently, multiple variations and additions are available in terms of prosthetic material, including rings that support the Dacron fabric. If one considers use of arm veins, nearly ≥60% of all patients may be operated on with autogenous tissue to reconstruct their vessels. The issue of in situ grafts vs. reversed has generated a significant amount of research and controversy; however, no clear answer exists as to which type of vein graft is best or in which type of position the vein graft is most effective in situ, reversed, or not reversed (17).

Nearly 75% of all patients have gangrenous, necrotic foot lesions, or nonhealing ulcers. These patients need an assessment of their vascular status initially and then debridement with excision of one or more toes. Attempts should be considered to excise enough bone so sufficient skin and soft tissue are available to cover the wound. Particularly in diabetic patients, one may use multiple secondary operative procedures, often to achieve a healed foot.

The graft may fail due to intimal hyperplasia, progression of proximal or distal disease, or lesions within the graft itself, which produce signs and symptoms of hemodynamic deterioration in the patient with arterial reconstruction (18–20). Importance of the failing-graft concept implies frequent follow up in a noninvasive vascular laboratory. The reoperation at an early stage may protect the graft, and more importantly, heal the foot or distal foot ulcer.

The 30-day mortality rate for all patients who undergo infrainguinal arterial reconstruction is 5%. Operative mortality rate is somewhat higher for the infrapopliteal and axillopopliteal bypass than for patients who require femoral–popliteal bypass. The most common cause of death is myocardial infarction and the second most common cause of death is stroke. The cause of death is a reflection of the advanced stage of tissue atherosclerotic vascular change present in this patient population. Salvage rates are better for femoral–popliteal bypass than for distal or axillofemoral bypass. The success of various reconstructive procedures is a reflection of the total systemic assessment of the patient, patient selection, and variations in the methods of reporting or analyzing results.

The issue of cost–benefit analysis regarding limb salvage remains unresolved. The question is reflected by one's philosophy and perspective on the subject of quality of life and ability to live and function independently. One may consider a primary BK amputation for the nonhealing distal lesion in some or all of these patients to achieve a more rapid rehabilitation. Experience has shown that older, poor-risk patients do not ambulate easily or quickly with an AK prosthesis. Many patients may never walk or require 2–3 months of institutional training. One could also argue that repeated attempts at reconstruction often result in loss of the knee and, therefore, increased cardiopulmonary demands with the use of a prosthesis.

The cost of an aggressive approach to salvage of limbs has a mean cost of $20,000 for a femoral–popliteal bypass and $30,000 for a small-vessel bypass. These figures include all physician, hospital, and rehabilitation costs, as well as those of reoperation. The mean total cost of a BK amputation, in which 26% of patients result in failed rehabilitation, is $27,000. Therefore, limb salvage and surgery are expensive but more so than the less-attractive alternate of amputation. Arterial ulcers are less common than ulcers of venous origin, but are more difficult to treat because of an underlying disease process. The ischemic ulcer represents a potential limb loss, often refractory to healing unless tissue perfusion can be improved. Arterial ulcers are more prone to invasive infection, gangrene, or both, which may necessitate amputation. Management of the ischemic limb may require significant changes

Table 4 Tests of Vascular Supply

Doppler ultrasound
Pulse volume recording
Color-flow duplex imaging
Transcutaneous oxygen assessment
Segmental pressure

Source: From Refs. 22, 28.

in the patient's lifestyle. Treatment of this group of patients is, therefore, multifaceted with the need to improve perfusion and circulation, decrease the risk of infection, local management of the wound proper, interventions to reduce pain, and finally, the need for patient education regarding lifestyle changes. Severe ischemia appears in < 25% of patients with leg ulcers and symptomatic arterial disease; 3–5% of the symptomatic population require amputation. Ischemia portends a poor outcome if less-aggressive intervention and reconstruction are undertaken. This group of patients has an annual mortality rate of nearly 20%; the most common cause of death is coronary artery disease. Reducing those risk factors for the nonhealing ulcer is necessary. They include hypertension, tobacco use, elevated cholesterol (low-density lipoprotein), diabetes mellitus, and abnormal metabolism of homocysteine (Table 2) (21). Vascular studies are often warranted to determine further adequacy or assessment of perfusion and include noninvasive, as well as invasive, studies. Noninvasive studies include pulse-volume recording, segmental-pressure analysis, transcutaneous oxygen, and color-flow duplex imaging (Table 4) (22).

Management of the patient with arterial ulceration should include methods to improve circulation. Options include bypass grafting, angioplasty, and placement of stents. Further methods of improving oxygenation of the tissue include hyperbaric oxygen therapy to increase the amount of oxygen dissolved in the plasma and pharmacologic options including anticoagulants and anticoagulant agents (3,23–25).

Topical therapy for ischemic ulcers includes the consideration of occlusive vs. nonocclusive dressings. This subject is discussed further in other chapters. Appropriate management of the patient with ischemic ulcer is based on an accurate assessment of the circulatory status, as well as the presence or absence of infection.

Ulcerations of the lower extremities may represent the arterial, diabetic, or both, as etiology (26). The wound-care specialist must be aware of the various diagnostic tests to confirm the ulcer etiology and concurrent management approaches for the various conditions. One must address the systemic need, as well as the local/regional requirements. A multidisciplinary approach is necessary for successful management of the peripheral vascular arterial ulcer.

ACKNOWLEDGMENT

The author thanks Gae O. Decker-Garrad for editorial assistance.

REFERENCES

1. Boyd AM. The natural course of arteriosclerosis of the lower extremities. Proc R Soc Med 1962; 55:591–593.
2. Ouriel K. Peripheral arterial disease. Lancet 2001; 358(9289):1257–1264.

3. Goodfield M. Optimal management of chronic leg ulcers in the elderly. Drugs Aging 1997; 10(5):341–348.

4. Donnely R. Assessment and management of intermittent claudication: importance of secondary prevention. Int J Clin Pract Suppl 2001; 119:2–9.

5. Ray SA, Buckenham TM, Belli AM, Taylor RS, Dormandy JA. The nature and importance of changes in toe-brachial pressure indices following percutaneous transluminal angioplasty for leg ischaemia. Eur J Vasc Endovasc Surg 1997; 14(2):125–133.

6. Altemose GT, Wiener DH. Control of risk factors in peripheral vascular disease: management of hypertension. Surg Clin North Am 1998; 78(3):369–384.

7. Rockson SG, Cooke JP. Peripheral arterial insufficiency: mechanisms, natural history, and therapeutic options. Adv Intern Med 1998; 43:253–277.

8. Terry MB, Berkowitz HD, Kerstein MD. Tobacco: its impact on vascular disease. Surg Clin North Am 1998; 78(3):409–429.

9. Stubbing NJ, Bailey P, Poole M. Protocol for accurate assessment of ABPI in patients with leg ulcers. J Wound Care 1997; 6(9):417–418.

10. Smith FB, Lowe GD, Lee AJ, Rumley A, Leng GC, Fowkes FG. Smoking, hemorheologic factors, and progression of peripheral arterial disease in patients with claudication. 1998; 28(1):129–135.

11. Treiman GS, Oderich GS, Ashrafi A, Schneider PA. Management of ischemic heel ulceration and gangrene: an evaluation of factors associated with successful healing. J Vasc Surg 2000; 31(6):1110–1118.

12. Mannick JA, Jackson BT, Coffman JD. Success of bypass vein grafts in patients with isolated popliteal artery segments. Surgery 1967; 61:17–35.

13. Galland RB, Whiteley MS, Gibson M, Simmons MJ, Torrie EP, Magee TR. Remote superficial femoral artery endarterectomy: medium-term results. Eur J Vasc Endovasc Surg 2000; 19(3):278–282.

14. Ascer E, Veith FJ, Morin L, Lesser ML, Gupta SK, Samson RH, White-Flores SA. Components of outflow resistance and their correlation with graft patency in lower extremity arterial reconstructions. J Vasc Surg 1984; 1(6):817–828.

15. Ascer E, Veith FJ, Gupta SK. Bypasses to plantar arteries and other tibial branches: an extended approach to limb salvage. J Vasc Surg 1988; 8(4):434–441.

16. Towne JB, Bernhard VM, Rollins DL, Baum PL. Profundaplasty in perspective: limitations in the long-term management of limb ischemia. Surgery 1981; 90:1037–1046.

17. Schulman ML, Badley MR. Late results and angiographic evaluation of arm veins as long bypass grafts. Surgery 1982; 92:1032–1041.

18. Quinones-Baldrich WJ, Busuttil RW, Baker JD, Vescera CL, Ahn SS. Is the preferential use of polytetrafluoroethylene grafts for femoropopliteal bypass justified? J Vasc Surg 1988; 8(3):219–228.

19. Bergan JJ, Veith FJ, Bernhard VM, Yao JS, Flinn WR, Gupta SK, Scher LA, Samson RH, Towne JB. Randomization of autogenous vein and polytetrafluoroethylene grafts in femoral–distal reconstruction. 1982; 92(6):921–930.

20. Szilagyi DE, Hageman JH, Smith RF, Elliott JP, Brown F, Dietz P. Autogenous vein grafting in femoropopliteal atherosclerosis: the limits of its effectiveness. Surgery 1979; 86(6):836–851.

21. O'Brien SP, Mureebe L, Lossing A, Kerstein MD. Epidemiology, risk factors, and management of peripheral vascular disease. Ostomy Wound Manage 1998; 44(9):68–75; quiz 85–86.

22. Bianchi J, Douglas WS, Dawe RS, Lucke TW, Loney M, McEvoy M, Urcelay M. Pulse oximetry: a new tool to assess patients with leg ulcers. J Wound Care 2000; 9(3):109–112.

23. Cooke JP, Ma AO. Medical therapy of peripheral arterial occlusive disease. Surg Clin North Am 1995; 75(4):569–579.

24. McNamara DB, Champion HC, Kadowitz PJ. Pharmacologic management of peripheral vascular disease. Surg Clin North Am 1998; 78(3):447–464.

25. Moon RE. Use of hyperbaric oxygen in the management of selected wounds. Adv Wound Care 1998; 11(7):332–334.
26. Hampton S. Identifying and managing arterial ulceration. Community Nurse 2000; 6(7):49–52.
27. O'Hare A, Johansen K. Lower-extremity peripheral arterial disease among patients with end-stage renal disease. J Am Soc Nephrol 2001; 12(12):2838–2847.
28. Jorneskog G, Djavani K, Brismar K. Day-to-day variability of transcutaneous oxygen tension in patients with diabetes mellitus and peripheral arterial occlusive disease. J Vasc Surg 2001; 34(2):277–282.

13

Pressure Ulcers: Epidemiology and Pathophysiology

Carlos A. Charles and Anna F. Falabella
Department of Dermatology and Cutaneous Surgery, University of Miami School of Medicine, Miami, Florida, U.S.A.

1. INTRODUCTION

Pressure ulcers are a common, serious, and expensive medical problem, imposing a significant burden on the health care system. Of historical significance, pressure ulcers have been reported since the time of Egyptian mummies (1). In the early 1800s Brown-Sequard (2) suggested that skin pressure and prolonged moisture were the most essential etiologic components in the development of pressure ulcers, this idea stemmed from experiments in which animal spinal cords were transected and ulcers were not produced as long as the animal skin was maintained dry. Subsequently, in 1873, researchers suggested that pressure ulcers were caused by the sloughing and mortification or death of tissue produced by continual pressure (3). While Charcot introduced the pessimistic belief that pressure sores occurred in all paraplegic patients, and that they are inevitable in anesthetic skin, therapeutic interventions during World War I demonstrated that pressure ulcers could be prevented and successfully treated (4). These modalities were further explored over time, and World War II provided the impetus for the beginnings of modern reconstructive surgical approaches to wound healing (5). As research has evolved, investigators have further pursued both surgical and noninvasive approaches to better understand the pathophysiology and successful therapeutic interventions for pressure ulcers. Most importantly, researches and clinicians alike have begun to recognize the role and biomechanics of pressure as a direct cause of ulcer formation and this has led to a concerted effort towards prevention, which remains the foundation for successful clinical outcomes.

1.1. Definition

Pressure ulcers are wounds that present as restricted areas of tissue necrosis . They develop in the setting of prolonged compression of soft tissue between bony prominences and external surfaces (6). Many synonyms are commonly employed for pressure ulcers, including but not limited to, decubitus ulcers, bedsores, ischemic ulcers, and pressure sores. The moniker, decubitus ulcer, is derived from Latin and is translated "to lie down" (7), as it has been thought that pressure ulcers are simply the result of prolonged recumbency. It is now well known that the prolonged application of pressure to the soft tissues in any position can lead to ulceration, therefore, "pressure ulcer" seems to be the most appropriate terminology.

The most common anatomic sites for the development of pressure ulcers appear to be cutaneous sites overlying bony prominences, such as the sacrum, greater trochanters, heels, lateral malleoli, and the ischial tuberosities (Fig. 1). Both intrinsic and extrinsic risk factors have been identified for the development of pressure ulcers. The strongest intrinsic predictors of pressure ulcer development include limited mobility and poor nutrition (8). Increased age, incontinence, diabetes mellitus, stroke, skin abnormalities, white race, and male sex have also been associated with pressure ulcer formation by multivariate analysis by some studies (9). Extrinsic factors include pressure, shear stress, friction, and moisture; of these, prolonged pressure appears to be the most critical. Ninety-five percent of all pressure ulcers develop on the caudal aspect of the body, with 65% involving the pelvic area and 30% arising on the lower limbs.

2. EPIDEMIOLOGY

The available epidemiologic data for describing pressure ulcers are variable. Primarily because various definitions have been used to describe pressure ulcers, additionally, distinct populations have been studied. While some studies have focused on pressure ulcers limited to hospitalized patients, others have focused on particular patient groups such as maternity, pediatric or ambulatory surgical patients (10,11). The following discussion will outline the epidemiology of pressure ulcers in the US population in various clinical settings and describe the economic burden imposed by this condition. Data available describing overall prevalence and incidence figures will be discussed. Due to the difficulties with making an accurate clinical assessment of Stage I pressure ulcers, the following discussion will describe prevalence and incidence data from studies that examined the occurrence of Stage II and greatecr ulcers separately from those that focused on Stage I ulcer data.

2.1. Prevalence

The prevalence of Stage II and greater pressure ulcers is variable among divergent populations of patients. Among hospitalized patients, studies have found the prevalence to range from 3.0% to 11.0% (12–14), 1.2% to 11.2% among nursing home patients (15–17) 15.0% to 30.0% for spinal cord injury patients and patients of physical rehabilitation units (14), and approximately 7% among patients in home care settings (18), with higher estimates when Stage I ulcers are included (Table 1). Prevalence estimates of pressure ulcers appear to be higher among spinal cord injury and physical rehabilitation center patients, while the frequency of ulcers is similar in patients of nursing homes, acute care hospitals, and home care settings.

The age and sex distribution of a sample of patients with pressure ulcers identified by a Danish community-based survey demonstrated that the prevalence of pressure ulcers is bimodal (13). This survey found that there was a small peak in prevalence between the ages of 20 and 30 and a much greater peak between the ages 70 and 80. Within this survey, greater than 50% of the patients with pressure ulcers were

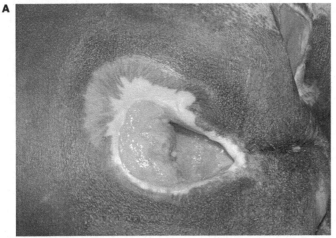

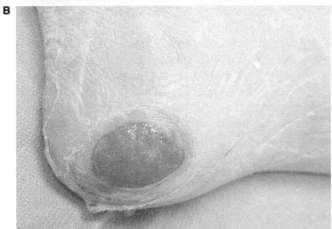

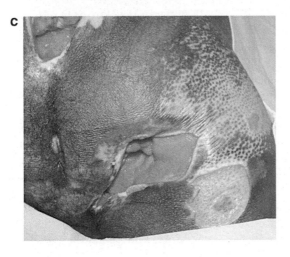

Figure 1 (A) Stage 3 sacral pressure ulcer. (B) Stage 2 pressure ulcer overlying the heel bony prominence. (C) Multiple sacral pressure ulcers in various stages.

Table 1 Pressure Ulcer Prevalence Data by Setting and Ulcer Stage

Pressure ulcer stage	Hospitals	Nursing homes	Spinal cord injury/ rehabilitation centers	Hospice/ home care	Community
Stage II and greater	3.0–11.0%	1.2–11.2%	20.0–30.0%	8.7%	—
Stage I and greater	4.0–29.7%	17.4–28.0%	25.0–60.0%	13.8–19.0%	0.04–0.08%

Source: Adapted from Ref. 9.

aged 70 years or older, and the majority of the younger patients were male. This male predominance in the younger patient population reflected the greater number of male patients who had suffered spinal cord injuries. On the contrary, the older population of pressure ulcer patients was more likely to be female, reflecting the greater proportion of women in the geriatric population.

In sum, the prevalence data suggest that pressure ulcers are primarily a problem of older persons, but do not establish that increased age directly affects the incidence of pressure ulcers. The prevalence data do suggest that particular groups of patients, such those with hip fractures, bed- or chair-bound patients, those with spinal cord injuries, and the elderly, are at particularly high risk for developing pressure ulcers. Additionally, age specific cutaneous alterations may in fact predispose patients to pressure ulcer development (19). Physiologic changes associated with age such as a decrease in epidermal turnover, with a decrease in the cutaneous vascular supply, and flattening of the dermal–epidermal junction, all may lead to a propensity for pressure ulcer development.

2.2. Incidence

Previous reports demonstrate that 1.2–2.7% of all patients develop Stage II or greater pressure ulcers while hospitalized (20,21). Assessing patients who developed Stage I pressure ulcers during hospitalization increased these estimates to 5.4% (20). Furthermore, an additional study suggests that when a Stage I ulcer develops, the risk of a higher stage ulcer occurring increases by up to 10-fold (22). The majority of the hospital-based studies of pressure ulcer incidence have focused on high-risk groups, such as patients whose activity is limited to a bed or chair, or those with hip fractures. Amongst newly admitted patients aged 55 or older, as many as 10.6% may be confined to a bed or chair (23). The incidence of the development of a Stage II or greater pressure ulcer in these patients has been reported to range from approximately 7.7% to 29.5% (24). Additionally, in one study, estimating the incidence of hospital-acquired pressure ulcers among elderly patients hospitalized for hip fracture surgery the incidence of hospital-acquired pressure ulcers was 8.8% (25). In this study, after adjusting for confounding variables, longer wait before surgery, intensive care unit stay, longer surgical procedure, and general anesthesia were all significantly associated with higher pressure ulcer risk.

A number of hospital-based studies have observed other patient populations of significant concern. The incidence of Stage I and greater ulcers among elective surgery patients has been demonstrated to range from 12.0% to 17.0% after follow-up periods of 10 days to 3 weeks (26,27). The incidence of Stage I and greater pressure ulcers among patients with mechanical restraints has been found to be approximately 22% (28). Additionally, studies have reported that 33% of patients admitted to an adult medical and surgical intensive care unit developed a Stage I or greater pressure ulcer at a period of 2 weeks follow-up (29).

Numerous studies suggest that the majority of pressure ulcers occur during acute care hospitalizations. One study demonstrated that 57% of ulcers amongst community-based individuals had occurred during recent hospitalizations, while 18% occurred at home and 18% occurred in a nursing home (30). Furthermore, in randomized, controlled clinical trial of 65 hospitalized patients with pressure ulcers, 54% of the patients had developed the ulcer while in the hospital (31).

2.3. Long-Term Care Settings

Several studies investigating the incidence of pressure ulcers from long-term care settings or nursing home databases currently exist (16,32,33). The bulk of these data was obtained by evaluating all residents at 3- to 6-month intervals. The calculated incidence from these studies of 0.20 to 0.56/1000 patient days (Table 2) may be lower than expected since Stage 1 ulcers were not included because of their potential difficulty of reliable identification for research purposes. In a 2-week prospective cohort study of patients at risk for developing pressure ulcers, defined by a Braden score of less than 17, the incidence pressure ulcers, including Stage 1, was 14/1000 patient days (34). As a comparison, the incidence among all admissions to an adult intensive care unit was 28/1000 patient days (29). While high-risk patients, defined by patients with an APACHE II score more than 15, admitted to an intensive care unit was 28/1000 patient days (35). In the assessment of patients that went on to develop

Table 2 Epidemiologic Data on Pressure Ulcers in the Nursing Home

Variable	Observation
Patients admitted with ulcers	17–35%
Prevalence among residents	7–23%
Of patients with ulcers, prevalence by ulcer stage	
Stage 1	24%
Stage 2	41%
Stage 3	22%
Stage 4	13%
Common Ulcer sited	
Sacrum or coccyx	36%
Hips (over trochanter)	17%
Buttocks (over ischium)	15%
Heels	12%
Ankles (over malleolus)	7%
Other	13%
Range of ulcers per resident	1.6–2.5
Range of incidence computed from databases, n/1000 patient days	0.20–0.56
Incidence in high-risk patients, n/1000 patient days	14
Proportion of initial ulcers developing in high-risk patients	
By 7 days	53%
By 14 days	82%

Source: Adapted from Smith DM. Pressure ulcers in the nursing home. Ann Intern Med 1995; 123: 433–442.

pressure ulcers after nursing home admission, most ulcers occurred within the first 7–14 days of admission (34). This phenomenon may be due to the fact that the patients were still recovering from an acute event. Therefore, it is imperative that patients at risk are identified when admitted to the nursing home and that preventive measures are initiated as soon as possible.

2.4. Mortality

Pressure ulcers have been linked to increased mortality rates in both acute and long-term health care settings. Previous reports indicate that deaths occur during acute hospitalization in 67% of patients who develop a pressure ulcer compared with 15% of at-risk patients without pressure ulcers (12). Additionally, patients who develop a new pressure ulcer within 6 weeks of hospitalization are three times more likely to die compared to patients who do not develop a pressure ulcer (36). In long-term healthcare environments, the development of a pressure ulcer within 3 months upon admission was associated with a 92% mortality rate, compared with a mortality rate of 4% among residents who did not develop a pressure ulcer (34). In a skilled nursing facility, residents who had pressure ulcers experienced a 6-month mortality rate of 77.3%, whereas patients without pressure ulcers had a mortality rate of 18.3% (37). Additionally, patients whose pressure ulcers healed within 6 months had a significantly lower mortality rate than those whose ulcers did not heal, 11% vs. 64%, respectively (38).

Although pressure ulcers clearly have some association with death rates, it is not completely clear how they contribute to increased mortality. Despite numerous reports citing up to a threefold increase in mortality with the development of a new pressure ulcer, a correlation has not been described between the severity of the pressure ulcer and the magnitude of increased risk. Patients with Stage II pressure ulcers are equally as likely to die as patients with Stage IV pressure ulcers (38), suggesting that pressure ulcers may not directly cause death, but their association with increased mortality may be due to their occurrence in a debilitated, sick patient population. This was further exemplified in a prospective study of residents of 51 nursing homes, in which pressure ulcers were associated with an increased rate of mortality but not with the rate of acute hospitalization (36). Furthermore, the association between pressure ulcers and increased mortality is nearly eliminated when correcting for the presence and severity of comorbid conditions (39).

2.5. Costs

Pressure ulcers have imposed a significant economic burden on both patients and the healthcare system. In the acute-care setting the average variable costs, defined as the additional costs sustained to treat the pressure ulcers, have been estimated to be $1300 per patient or $80 per day (40). In cases in which the patient was admitted specifically for treatment of pressure ulcers, the average variable costs then increased to $3746 per patient. In the long-term care or nursing home setting, the average variable costs were estimated to be $751 per patient and $5.35 per day (range $0 to $128 per day) (41). For some individual nursing home residents, the costs may range from $4255 to 23,300 per patient (42). These costs were procured from the perspective of the care-taking institution and are a conservative measure from the patient perspective. The costs of the primary physician are not included in these figures. Additionally, the costs before or after admission to the health-care facility are not included, nor are the costs related to the hospital admission being prolonged because of the ulcer. Also, the costs not directly associated to pressure ulcer treatment, such as expenditures for physical therapy to improve mobility, were not assessed. Lastly, the reports from the nursing home did not account for the costs of pressure-relieving devices nor hospitalizations for pressure ulcers. Therefore, from the patient perspective, treatment costs for pressure ulcers can be significantly higher.

3. PATHOPHYSIOLOGY

The four most important features implicated in the development of pressure ulcers are prolonged pressure, friction, shearing forces, and moisture. The following will describe the role of each of these features in detail.

3.1. Pressure

Pressure is defined as force per unit area, and it is the single most important causative factor for pressure ulcer formation. External pressures are generally greatest overlying bony prominences (43). These localized increases in pressure lead to compromised capillary circulation. Normal capillary pressures usually fall in the range of 12–32 mmHg (44). Prolonged pressures of greater than 32 mm Hg lead to increased interstitial pressures resulting in compromised tissue perfusion and oxygenation. Additionally, as local pressures increase, the potential for pressure ulcer formation also increases (45). The duration of localized pressure also plays an integral role in pressure ulcer formation. Studies have demonstrated that a constant pressure of 70 mmHg for 2 hr may result in localized tissue death and ulceration, while intermittent pressure relief can prevent tissue damage and result in minimal changes (46). Damage to the deep tissues can occur with relatively minimal superficial injury, as interstitial pressures tend to be highest at the bone/muscle interface (Fig. 2). As a result, caregivers may not be immediately aware of the initial signs of tissue damage.

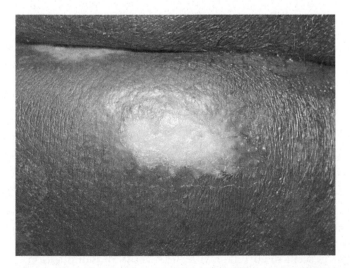

Figure 2   Early sacral pressure ulcer in a bed bound patient. Damage to the deep tissues can occur with relatively minimal superficial injury and caregivers must be aware of the initial signs of tissue damage.

3.2. Friction

Friction leads to superficial damage of the protective stratum corneum; consequently the amount of pressure necessary for ulcer formation is reduced (46). Friction is specifically defined as the amount force that resists relative motion between two surfaces that are in direct contact. By injuring the innate protection of the stratum corneum, the function of the skin as a barrier is diminished and the propensity for ulceration is enhanced. This is a common phenomenon in the clinical setting in which chronically bedridden patients slide or are dragged across moistened bed sheets (47).

3.3. Shearing Forces

Shearing forces are an integral factor in the development of pressure ulcers. Specifically, they play a principal role in influencing the size and grade of the resultant ulcer. Shearing forces are produced from the sliding and relative displacement of two apposing surfaces (48). In the clinical environment, movement of the recumbanct patient produces shearing forces. Specifically, in a supine patient with the head raised at an angle of greater than 30°, shearing forces are produced at the sacral and coccygeal areas. With patient movement, pressure is transmitted to the deep fascia and sacrum, as the outer sacral skin remains fixed due to friction with the stationary bed. These physical forces create thromboses and undermining of the dermis, as well as angulation of the vessels within the superficial fascia, all of which predispose the tissue to ulceration (49).

3.4. Moisture

A chronic moist environment secondary to perspiration, fecal or urinary incontinence, can lead to tissue maceration and an increased risk of pressure ulcer formation (50). The combination of prolonged moisture, along with pressure, shearing forces, and friction create an environment in which ulceration is nearly unavoidable without the implementation of appropriate preventive measures.

4. RISK FACTORS

Unrelieved pressure, friction, shearing forces, and moisture cannot account for the entire pathogenesis of pressure ulcers. Endogenous factors predisposing patients to pressure ulcers such as old age, chronic illness, sepsis, neurological and vascular disease, have all been implicated in the formation of pressure ulcers. The following discussion will focus on the role of some of these critical risk factors in the development of pressure ulcers.

4.1. Poor Nutrition

Many studies have identified an association between malnutrition and pressure ulcer formation (51,52). Malnutrition results in a reduction of subcutaneous fat and can predispose to prolonged wound healing. The likelihood of pressure ulcer development and the extent of pressure ulcers seem to correlate with the severity of malnutrition. Total lymphocyte count and serum albumin levels are readily accessible tests that can be performed on patients to assess their level of nutrition (53). Clinically significant malnutrition is often defined as a serum albumin level of less than 3.5 mg/dL, a total lymphocyte count of less than $1800/mm^3$, or a decrease in body weight of more than 15% (54). From a practical standpoint, it is important to determine the patient's nutritional status, and to implement appropriate measures to optimize healing.

4.2. Prolonged Immobilization

There are many factors predisposing patients to prolonged immobilization, including severe debilitating diseases such as arthritis, extended stays in intensive care units, or neurological compromise from spinal cord injury. Studies have measured the number of spontaneous nocturnal movements in geriatric patients and have found that the incidence of pressure ulcers was inversely correlated to this number (55). Additionally, prospective studies have found that being in bed or chair-bound is associated with a significantly increased risk of presenting with a pressure ulcer or with the development of a new ulcer during a long-term care facility admission (53).

4.3. Sensory Deficit

The existence of a sensory deficit mitigates the patient's ability to detect painful stimuli resulting from prolonged pressure. Additionally, patients with spinal cord deficits leading to sensory loss may have concomitant motor deficits with spasticity, further limiting motion and predisposing to ulcer formation (50).

4.4. Circulatory Compromise

Circulatory compromise resulting in poor oxygen perfusion may augment skin ulcerations and delay wound healing. This phenomenon is common in this patient population in which factors such as cardiovascular compromise, blood dyscrasias, anemia, and/or interstitial edema are widespread.

5. COMPLICATIONS

When addressed promptly, pressure ulcers can be managed expeditiously. However, complications that may even be life threatening are common and should be managed accordingly. The following section will address the source of these complications and briefly describe their initial steps in their management.

5.1. Infection

The topic of wound infection is one of controversy. As is the case for the majority chronic wounds, swab cultures taken from pressure ulcers commonly reveal polymicrobial growth. A myriad of aerobic organisms are often recovered such as *Staphylococcus aureus, Staphylococcus epidermidis, Escherichia coli*, and *Pseudomonas aeruginosa*; additionally, anaerobic organisms may also be present. However, the clinical distinction between bacterial colonization and bacterial infection is important. Colonization refers to the harmless existence of microorganisms within wounds. While most wounds are colonized, the presence of microorganisms in this capacity is not thought to impede wound healing (56). In this scenario, the clinical signs of infection, such as tenderness, redness, and heat, may not be present.

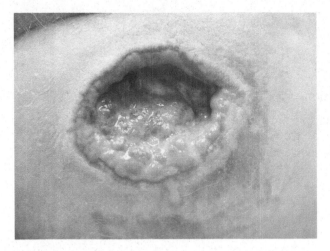

Figure 3 Clinically infected pressure ulcer with associated redness, tenderness, purulent discharge, and malodor.

Additionally, histological features reveal a lack of heavy polymorphonuclear leukocyte infiltration or bacteria within the tissue (57).

Alternatively, infected chronic wounds demonstrate tissue invasion by microorganisms. Earlier studies have stated that the presence of more than 10^6 microorganisms per gram of tissue could mitigate wound healing and regeneration (58,59); however, the validity of this numerical value as a determinant for active wound infection has come into question since clinical experience has shown that wounds with this level of microbial contamination, and without clinical signs of infection, will often not require antimicrobial treatment. Wound infections have also been subdivided into clinically apparent and unapparent infections (60). Apparent infections are easily identified by the presence of associated redness, warmth, and tenderness, along with occasional purulent discharge, malodor, and systemic signs of infection (Fig. 3). While unapparent infection is manifested by the attenuation of the common signs of infection. In the pressure ulcer population of patients comorbid medical problems can often lead to a mitigated host response to infection and decreased sensation, leading to the absence or attenuation of leukocytosis, pain, and/or fever, consequently it may be difficult to distinguish between colonization and unapparent infection in the setting of a positive microbial culture. Unapparent infections should be considered in wounds that fail to heal despite optimization of other factors important for pressure ulcer treatment, such as pressure relief and nutritional supplementation, and the administration of antibiotics may be beneficial.

5.2. Osteomyelitis

It has been reported that approximately one-third of all nonhealing pressure ulcers may be associated with an underlying bone infection that can occur through direct microbial extension or by hematogenous spread (61). Diagnosing osteomyelitis may be difficult. Findings from radiographic nuclear imaging as well as soft-tissue culture may be falsely negative adjacent to the pressure ulcer. The indium 111-labeled leukocyte scanning is the most accurate nuclear study for diagnosing osteomyelitis; however, the test is expensive and often difficult to interpret in the setting of overlying soft-tissue inflammation. Gram-negative bacilli and anaerobes are the usual causative pathogens of osteomyelitis.

5.3. Sinus Tracts

Sinus tracts frequently appear in pressure ulcers. They may extend deep within the affected area causing osteomyelitis and communicating with deep viscera such as the bowel or bladder. A sonogram or fistulogram may be helpful to determine the extent of sinus tract penetration, and thereby for appropriate planning for surgical intervention if necessary. Additionally, case reports have demonstrated success in treating recalcitrant sinus tracts within pressure ulcers with tissue-engineered therapies, including the use of a dermal matrix substitute to stimulate healing (63).

5.4. Squamous Cell Carcinoma

The term Marjolin's ulcer is used to describe a cancer arising from any chronic wound. Malignant degeneration of nonhealing pressure ulcers has been reported with an estimated incidence of 0.5% (63). Histologically, they most commonly present as a well-differentiated squamous cell carcinoma that behave aggressively have a high potential for metastasis. Pressure ulcer carcinomas behave differently than other Marjolin's ulcers.

They are most commonly aggressive well-differentiated squamous cell carcinomas. Previous studies have reported an 80% 2-year mortality rate in patients presenting with local disease who were treated only with surgical excision (64). Additionally, a 66% 2-year mortality rate from local or metastatic disease in pressure ulcer carcinoma patients has been reported (63). An aggressive surgical approach with wide excision of the cancer is recommended. Prophylactic node dissection may also be considered. However, cure may not be possible even in the most aggressive resection.

6. SUMMARY

Pressure ulcer is a serious and costly medical problem, imposing a considerable burden on the health care system. This brief review of the literature illustrating the epidemiology and pathophysiology of pressure ulcers provides some background information on the extent, natural history, and predisposing factors of the problem. Additionally, the review also demonstrates some of the common problems inherent to the reliability of data collected and misinterpretation of results.

The prevalence studies presented herein provide a general guide to the extent of the problem. Between 5% and 10% of patients may be affected at any one point of time. Additionally, factors that seem to predispose patients to pressure ulcer formation such as increasing age, reduced mobility, malnutrition, and incontinence have been identified. However, the results suggest that no single cause exists. The incidence studies seem to support the prevalence data and reinforce the evidence regarding the predisposing factors.

In sum, while the exact pathophysiology for pressure ulcer development is multifactorial and not completely understood, the data concerning their epidemiology do provide clinicians with valuable information about how many and which patients are at high risk for their development. This information is of great value and provides some insight for pressure ulcer treatment and prevention.

REFERENCES

1. Thompson RJ. Pathological changes in mummies. Proc R Soc Med 1961; 54:409–415.
2. Brown-Sequard E. Experimental Researches Applied to Physiology and Pathology. New York: H. Bailliere, 1852.
3. Paget J. Clinical lecture on bedores. Students J Hosp Gaz 1873; 1:144–146.
4. Marie P, Roussy G. Sur la possibilite de prevenir la formation des escarres dans les traumatismes de guerre. Bull Acad Med Paris 1915; 73:602.
5. Scoville WB. Cited by B.N. Bailey. In: Bedores. London: Edward Arnold, 1976.
6. Margolis DJ. Definition of a pressure ulcer. Adv Wound Care 1995; 8:8–10.
7. Stedman's Online Medical Dictionary. Baltimore: Lippincott Williams & Wilkins, 2003.
8. Livesley NJ, Chow AW. Infected pressure ulcers in elderly individuals. Clin Infect Dis 2002; 35:1390–1396.
9. Allman RM. Pressure ulcer prevalence, incidence, risk factors, and impact. Clin Geriatr Med 1997; 13:421–437.
10. The National Pressure Ulcer Advisory Panel. Pressure ulcers prevalence, cost, and risk assessment: consensus development conference statement. Decubitus 1989; 2:24–28.
11. Phillips TJ. Chronic cutaneous ulcers: etiology and epidemiology. J Invest Dermatol 1994; 102(suppl):38S–41S.
12. Allman RM, Laprade CA, Noel LB, et al. Pressure ulcers among hospitalized patients. Ann Intern Med 1986; 105:337–342.
13. Peterson MC, Bittman S. The epidemiology of pressure sores. Scand J Plast Reconstr Surg. 1971; 5:62–66.
14. Shannon ML, Skorga P. Pressure ulcer prevalence in two general hospitals. Decubitus 1989; 2:38–43.
15. Brandeis GH, Berlowitz DR, Hossain M, et al. Pressure ulcers: the minimum data set and the resident assessment protocol. Adv Wound Care 1995; 8:18–25.
16. Brandeis GH, Morris JN, Nash DJ, et al. The epidemiology and natural history of pressure ulcers in elderly nursing home residents. JAMA 1990; 264:2905–2909.
17. Kennedy KL. The prevalence of pressure ulcers in an intermediate care facility. Decubitus 1989; 2:44–45.
18. Meehan M, O'Hara L, Morrison YM. Report on the prevalence of skin ulcers in a home health agency population. Adv Wound Care 1999; 12:459–467.
19. Allman RM. Pressure ulcers among the elderly. N Engl J Med 1989; 320(30):850–853.
20. Gosnell DJ, Johannsen J, Ayres M. Pressure ulcer incidence and severity in a community hospital. Decubitus 1992; 5:56–58.
21. Anderson KE, Kvorning SA. Medical aspects of the decubitus ulcer. Int J Dermatol 1982; 21:265.
22. Allman RM, Goode PS, Patrick MM, et al. Pressure ulcer risk factors among hospitalized patients with activity limitation. JAMA 1995; 273: 865–870.
23. Allman RM, Damiano AM, Strauss MJ. Pressure ulcer status and post-discharge health care resource utilization among older adults with activity limitations. Adv Wound Care. 1996; 9:38–44.
24. Clarke M, Kadhom HM. The nursing prevention of pressure sores in hospital and community patients. J Adv Nurs 1988; 13:365–373.
25. Baumgarten M, Margolis D, Berlin JA, et al. Risk factors for pressure ulcers among elderly hip fracture patients. Wound Repair Regen 2003; 11:96–103.
26. Kemp MG, Keithley JK, Smith DW et al. Factors that contribute to pressure sores in surgical patients. Res Nurs Health 1990; 13:293–301.
27. Stotts NA. Predicting pressure ulcer development in surgical patients. Heart Lung 1988; 17(6 Pt 1):641–647.
28. Lofgren RP, MacPherson DS, Granieri R. Mechanical restraints on the medical wards: are protective devices safe? Am J Public Health 1989; 79:735–738.

29. Bergstrom N, Demuth PJ, Braden BJ. A clinical trial of the Braden Scale for Predicting Pressure Sore Risk. Nurs Clin North Am 1987; 22:417–428.

30. Guralnik JM, Harris TB, White LR, et al. Occurrence and predictors of pressure sores in the National Health and Nutrition Examination Survey follow-up. J Am Geriatr Soc 1998; 36:807.

31. Allman RM, Walkr JM, Hart MK, et al. Air-fluidized beds or conventional therapy for pressure sores: a randomized trial. Ann Intern Med 1987; 107:641.

32. Brandeis GH, Ooi WL, Hossain M, Morris, et al. A longitudinal study of the risk factors associated with the formation of pressure ulcers in nursing homes. J Am Geriatr Soc 1994; 42:388–393.

33. Rudman D, Mattson DE, Alverno L, et al. Comparison of clinical indicators in two nursing homes. J Am Geriatr Soc 1993; 41:1317–1325.

34. Bergstrom N, Braden B. A prospective study of pressure sore risk among institutionalized elderly. J Am Geriatr Soc 1992; 40:747–758.

35. Inman KJ, Sibbald WJ, Rutledge FS. Clinical utility and cost-effectiveness of an air suspension bed in the prevention of pressure ulcers. JAMA 1993; 269:1139–1143.

36. Berlowitz DR, Wilking SVB. The short-term outcome of pressure sores. J Am Geriatr Soc 1990; 38:748–752.

37. Michoki RJ, Lamy PP. The problem of pressure sores in a nursing home population: statistical data. J Am Geriatr Soc 1976; 24:323–328.

38. Reed JW. Pressure ulcers in the elderly: prevention and treatment utilizing the team approach. Maryland State Med J 1981; 30:45–50.

39. Thomas DR, Goode PS, Tarquin PH, et al. Pressure ulcers and risk of death. J Am Geriatr Soc 1996; 44:1435–1440.

40. Alterescu V. The financial costs of inpatient pressure ulcers to an acute care facility. Decubitus 1989; 2:14–23.

41. Frantz RA, Gardner S, Harvey P. The cost of treating pressure ulcers to an acute care facility. Decubitus 1989; 2:14–23.

42. Frantz RA. Pressure ulcer costs in long-term care. Decubitus 1989; 2:56–57.

43. Reuler JB, CooneyTG. The pressure sore: pathophysiology and principles of management. Ann Intern Med 1981; 94:661–666.

44. Kosiak M, Kubicek WG, Olson M, et al. Evaluation of pressure as a factor in the production of ischial ulcers. Arch Phys Med Rehabil 1959; 40:60–69.

45. Falanga V. Chronic wounds. Pathophysiologic and experimental considerations. Prog Dermatol 1992; 26:1–8.

46. Dinsdale SM. Decubitus ulcers: role of pressure and friction in causation. Arch Phys Med Rehab 1974; 55:147–152.

47. Jastremski CA. Pressure relief bedding to prevent pressure ulcer development in critical care. J Crit Care 2002; 17:122–125.

48. Tepperman PS, De Zwirek CS, Chiarcossi AL, et al. Pressure sores: prevention and set-up management. Postgrad Med 1997; 60:309–314.

49. Reichel SM. Shearing force as a factor in decubitus ulcers in paraplegics. JAMA 1958; 166:762–763.

50. Herman LE, Rothman KF. Prevention, care and treatment of pressure (decubitus) ulcers in intensive care unit patients. J Intensive Care Med 1989; 4:117–133.

51. Breslow RA, Halfrisch J, Goldberg AP. Malnutrition in tube fed nursing home patients with pressure sores. J Parenteral Enteral Nutr 1991; 15:663–668.

52. Berlitz DR, Van B, Wilking S. Risk factors for pressure sores: a comparison of cross sectional and cohort derived data. J Am Geriatr Soc 1989; 37:1043–1050.

53. Pinchcofsky-Devin GD, Kaminski MV. Correlation of pressure sores and nutritional status. J Am Geriatr Soc 1986; 34:435–440.

54. Bergstrom N, Bennett MA, Carlson CE, et al. Treatment of pressure ulcers. Clinical Practice Guideline No. 15. (AHCPR Publication No. 95–0652). Rockville, MD: U.S.

Department of Health and Human Services, Public Health Service, Agency for Health Care Policy and Research, December 1994.

55. Exton-Smith AN, Sherwin RW. The prevention of pressure sores: significance of spontaneous bodily movements. Lancet 1961; 2:1124–1126.

56. Mertz PM, Eaglstein WH. The effect of semiocclusive dressing on the microbial population in superficial wounds. Arch Surg 1984; 119:287–289.

57. Hutchinson JJ. Prevalence of wound infection under occlusive dressings: a collective survey of reported research. Wounds 1989; 1:287–289.

58. Sapico FL, Ginunas VJ, Thornhill-Joynes M, et al. Quantitative microbiology of pressure sores in different stages of healing. Diagn Microbiol Infect Dis 1986; 5:31–38.

59. Bendy RH, Nuccio PA, Wolfe E, et al. Relationship of a quantitative wound bacterial count to healing of decubiti: effect of topical gentamicin. Antimicrob Agents Chemother 1964; 4:147–155.

60. Parish LC, Witkowski JA. The infected decubitus ulcer. Int J Dermatol 1989; 28:643–647.

61. Surgarmann B M, Hawes S, Mucher DM, et al. Osteomyelitis and pressure sores. Arch Intern Med 1983; 143:638–648.

62. Banta MN, Eaglstein WH, Kirsner RS. Healing of refractory sinus tracts by dermal matrix injection with Cymetra. Dermatol Surg 2003; Aug; 29:863–866.

63. Mustoe T, Upton J, Marcellino V, et al. Carcinoma in chronic pressure ulcers: a fulminant disease process. Plast Reconstr Surg 1986; 77:116–121.

64. Grotting JC, Bunkis J, Vasconez LO. Pressure sore carcinoma. Ann Plast Surg 1987; 18:527–532.

14

Treatment and Prevention of Pressure Ulcers

Lia van Rijswijk
*La Salle University School of Nursing, La Salle Neighborhood Nursing Center,
Newtown and Philadelphia, Pennsylvania, U.S.A.*

Janice M. Beitz
La Salle University School of Nursing, Philadelphia, Pennsylvania, U.S.A.

1. INTRODUCTION

Three themes pervade the current pressure ulcer literature: (1) pressure ulcers are multifactorial, expensive, and painful complications of immobility, increasing morbidity and the risk of mortality; (2) pressure ulcer prevention strategies and treatment effectiveness are a reflection of the quality of care delivered; and (3) prevention is always better than treatment. Given the overwhelming consensus on these three perspectives, the critical focus on maintaining skin integrity is intensifying as the number of frail and vulnerable elderly is increasing in the United States and other developed nations. The spotlight on pressure ulcers has become so intense that treatment and prevention strategies are now scrutinized and used as "quality indicators." While important gaps in the understanding of effective pressure ulcer prevention and treatment strategies remain (1), pressure ulcer prevention and treatment strategies should, as much as possible, be evidence-based, timely, and effective (2).

2. THE ELEMENTS OF PREVENTION

Pressure ulcer prevention targets several areas of concern. The literature suggests that interventions aimed at reducing predisposing risk factors can help prevent many ulcers and minimize the severity of those that do occur. Pressure ulcer prevention begins with a comprehensive risk assessment followed by a plan of care with its associated interventions (3). Optimal pressure ulcer prevention strategies include: (1) identification and assessment of risk level based on predisposing factors; (2) regular risk reassessment, skin inspection, and the provision of good basic skin care and early treatment if needed; (3) evaluation and implementation of appropriate pressure reducing support surfaces; and (4) most especially, education of patients and all caregivers.

3. RISK FACTORS, RISK ASSESSMENT, AND PREVENTION STRATEGIES

The positive effect of risk assessment and targeted prevention strategies to reduce the incidence and prevalence of pressure ulcers has been extensively documented (3–7).

3.1. Risk Factors

Even though the primary cause of pressure ulcers is pressure, questions about the relationships among the amount of external force, time, and various extrinsic and intrinsic variables remain. Time and pressure interact. High pressures can cause damage during a short-time frame, while low external force can cause damage over a longer time period of time. During partial or full capillary occlusion, anoxia and the build up of metabolites occur. Reactive hyperemia is observed when the pressure is released and blood starts flowing through the deprived tissue (8). Tissue damage can occur during both the occlusion and reperfusion phase, and the often-cited 32 mm Hg cutoff for capillary closing and pressure ulcer development is exceedingly viewed with caution. Indeed, the necessary pressure to cause ischemia or reperfusion injury may be much less in vulnerable persons (9) and relative, rather than absolute, blood flow deficits may increase the risk of pressure ulcer formation (10).

The ability of the skin and underlying tissues to withstand pressure may be referred to as "tissue tolerance" (11).

Extrinsic risk factors that affect a person's tissue tolerance include the presence of skin irritants (moisture) and the effects of friction and shearing on the skin. Friction (from sliding) and shear (caused by, among other things, sliding down in bed) reduce the requisite pressure needed to produce vessel occlusion with resultant tissue ischemia (12). Moisture (e.g., fecal and/or urinary incontinence) weakens the skin cell wall and alters skin pH, increasing its vulnerability to the effects of friction and shearing.

In addition to the above, there are many known, and possibly more unknown, intrinsic "tissue tolerance" factors unique to individuals that may determine whose skin breaks down or not (13,14). Known intrinsic risk factors include: reduced or impaired mobility, nutritional deficiencies, extremes of age, chronic illnesses (e.g., diabetes mellitus), selected medication use (e.g., steroids, antineoplastic agents, sedatives), vascular disease, and a history of pressure ulcers. For example, in 13 of 15 recent prevalence and incidence studies conducted in a variety of health and home care settings, reduced mobility was found to be a risk factor for the development of pressure ulcers (15).

The second most commonly identified risk factor was nutritional deficiencies (10 of 15 studies). Thus, prototypical at-risk persons are the very young or, more commonly, the elderly, who have limited mobility, a less-than-optimal nutritional status, and suffer from chronic illnesses. The combination of decreased mobility and sensation, as seen in persons who are paralyzed (spinal cord injury), also warrants vigilance: all persons with spinal cord injuries are at high risk for developing pressure ulcers (7).

Nutritional risk factors for the development of pressure ulcers (e.g., impaired nutritional intake, low dietary protein intake, and recent weight loss) continue to be identified across populations (16). Low albumin levels are associated with pressure ulcer development as well as delayed wound healing (17). Extremes of body weight (morbid obesity or cachexia) can increase risk to bony prominences, and a history of smoking is considered a risk factor because of its vasoconstrictive effects (18).

A risk factor that is receiving greater attention in the literature is the need for a long operative procedure; that is, the operating room intervention as an etiologic factor (19–21). Surgical patients identified as the highest risk for skin breakdown include hip fracture repair, cardiac and vascular surgery patients, and persons positioned on the OR table for longer than 4 hr. While research on the incidence of OR acquired pressure ulcers remains limited both in number and methodological rigor (7), the risk is real and these patients need to be included in comprehensive prevention and assessment initiatives.

Finally, recent studies suggest that not all risk factors are patient related. After controlling for all known pressure ulcer risk factors, several studies have found significant differences in pressure ulcer rates between different facilities (15). Indeed, compliance with processes of care to prevent pressure ulcers has been found to vary significantly (22), and an inverse relationship between the number of hours of care delivered by registered nurses and the incidence of pressure ulcers has also been observed (23). According to Olshansky, there are ample data to suggest that a focus on patient-specific risk factors is incomplete and that the "main determining factor affecting pressure ulcer incidence is not patients' high-risk potential—it is the staff taking care of those patients" (24).

At this time, risk assessment remains an inexact and incomplete science. Meehan submits that the contemporary pressure ulcer "blame game" is exacerbated because "we do not know enough about the dynamic process of skin breakdown that occurs in conjunction with a series of medically complex events or exacerbation of long-standing chronic diseases to reliably and consistently prevent pressure damage" (25).

3.2. Risk Assessment

Given these limitations, why is risk assessment crucial? Recognizing high-risk patients is crucial to implementing appropriate and timely prevention strategies. Several risk assessment instruments are in use including the Gosnell scale, the Norton scale and the Braden scale. The latter is the most commonly used pressure ulcer risk assessment tool in the United States. It is valid and reliable, but there are some problems with specificity and sensitivity (26,27).

Though an in-depth description of all risk assessment instruments is beyond the scope of this chapter, a common theme exists—all are designed to alert users to patient skin breakdown risk and all include some of the risk factors described earlier. For example, the lower the score on the Braden scale (potential range 23–6), the higher a patient's risk for altered skin integrity. While research continues to compare risk assessment instruments and tests their reliability across settings, the absolute value of risk scores may be less vital than identification of major patient risk factors and the institution of appropriate care interventions (28,29). Of course, knowing the score is half of what is needed; the risk assessment must be linked to prevention protocols and interventions (30).

3.3. Prevention Strategies

Once a patient has been found to be at risk, critical steps in prevention should ensue, including: daily skin inspection, documentation of overall health, hydration, nutrition, and continence status. Risk assessments should be repeated weekly or when a patient's condition changes significantly. Use of harsh soaps should be avoided and skin should be kept clean and moisturized (31). To protect the skin of incontinent patients, basic nursing interventions should include the use of protective skin cleansers and appropriate moisture barrier products.

Shearing and friction can be controlled by using positioning and repositioning aids like trapeze bars, draw, or lift sheets. Patients should not be placed in high Fowlers position unless absolutely necessary. Skin may be protected from friction by use of transparent film dressings, as well as heel and elbow protectors. Sheepskins also help decrease friction but are not effective in pressure reduction/relief (32).

A major component of pressure ulcer prevention is reducing the effect of pressure through repositioning and use of appropriate pressure support surfaces. All attempts at preventing or healing these wounds will be futile, if pressure is not reduced. Pressure support surfaces work mainly by redistributing pressure, but some are also designed to reduce friction, shear, or manage moisture. The choice of surface differs when the purpose is prevention of skin damage. Generally speaking, more costly surfaces such as air fluidized or low air loss beds and kinetic turning surfaces are not utilized, and not reimbursed, for prevention. However, there is some evidence to suggest that low air loss beds may reduce the incidence of pressure ulcers compared to standard intensive care beds (33). For prophylaxis, "low tech" alternatives to the standard hospital mattress, such as foam overlays (at least 4 inches thick), gel pads, static air or water filled mattresses, can reduce the incidence of ulcers in high risk patients (33). For persons with more risk factors, or those who already have an ulcer, alternating pressure support mattress overlays or replacement systems can be used (33). Advantages of the latter "higher tech" interventions include their ability to help keep patients' skin drier which is especially helpful for incontinent clients, but well-controlled clinical studies comparing their effectiveness are lacking (33). Because support surface performance characteristics have not yet been standardized and variations between surfaces (including those in the same category) exist, clinicians need to evaluate whether the clinical effectiveness of pressure reduction/relief relief surfaces lives up to their advertising (34,35).

Three noteworthy issues are associated with the use of support and redistribution surfaces. First, regular hospital mattresses do not meet the need for optimal pressure reduction in high-risk patients unless they are specifically manufactured for that purpose and are within warranty (usually less than 3–5 years of use) (26). Second, patients on pressure support surfaces still need to be frequently repositioned to off-load pressure from bony prominences. A 30° tilt is better than full side lying position, and cushions should be placed to pad bony prominences. This intervention is crucial for heels because currently marketed support surfaces do not prevent heel breakdown (36). Heels should be positioned on devices (e.g., pillows, etc.) that allow them to hang free from the bed surface. If a heel protective device is used, the selection process must be individualized (12).

Finally, dated procedures affecting pressure reduction should be discarded. Donut-shaped products, ring cushions or the practice of massaging reddened areas should be avoided since these interventions may actually cause tissue damage (37). Adherence to these "ritualistic" practices may result from a lack of knowledge and skills that creates fear of change (38).

Because pressure ulcer prevention in general, and risk assessment and pressure reduction/relief measures to prevent pressure ulcers in particular have been classified as "quality indicators" and "quality of care issues," implementation of these strategies is crucial in all health care settings (2,39,40).

3.4. Nutrition

A nutritional status assessment and timely implementation of dietary interventions are major components of pressure ulcer prevention and healing protocols of care. Across different populations, strong associations between nutritional deficiencies and the development as well as healing status of pressure ulcers have been found (16). Nutritional assessment should be conducted in light of the patient's medical status and the nutritional goal should be to maintain or improve the dietary intake. No single assessment variable provides a complete reflection of nutritional status. The client's medical and surgical history, background of the current health problem, as well as physical signs and symptoms should be evaluated. For example, nutritional factors that may contribute to skin breakdown include: reduced calorie intake, protein deficiency, anemia, dehydration, and increased blood glucose levels (16,41). Anthropometric markers of nutritional deficiencies, e.g., height and weight, % weight loss, and body mass index, should be obtained. Biochemical markers of protein and calorie malnutrition as well as metabolic disorders include: serum albumin, prealbumin, transferrin, lymphocyte current, hemoglobin, hematocrit, and blood glucose levels. If deficits exist (albumin less than 3.5 g/dL, a total lymphocyte count less than $1800/mm^3$, and weight loss greater than 15%), fluid, vitamin, minerals, protein, and calorie supplementation should be initiated. If oral intake will not suffice or if swallowing is damaged, enteral tube feedings or parenteral nutrition may be required (42). Appetite stimulants such as megestrol acetate or anabolic agents like oxandrolone may help increase weight, specifically, lean body mass (43).

If a pressure ulcer develops, protein loss from the wound may cause or exacerbate existing protein deficiency. The potential positive effects of enteral feeding on pressure ulcer prevention and healing must be considered in light of the high rate of complications associated with long-term tube feeding (44). Even though research evidence to support the use of nutritional supplements for pressure ulcer prevention and healing is limited, preclinical and acute wound healing studies have shown that nutrition, including levels of Vitamin C and A, does play a very important role (16). Nutritional deficiencies are an important risk factor for patient morbidity and, while awaiting the results of much-needed pressure ulcer research, clinicians should address the nutritional needs of all persons who are at risk for, or who have, a pressure ulcer. This common-sense approach may not only prevent pressure ulcers, it may also prevent costly litigation. A recent study in hospitals and long-term care facilities found that monetary recovery for patients whose pressure ulcers were caused by poor nutrition alone was nearly five times higher than for patients whose pressure ulcers were caused by poor pressure management (45).

3.5. Education and System Concerns

Education of patients and caregivers is vital to the success of pressure ulcer prevention strategies. Many examples of constituents and components to include in a quality educational program are available, providing helpful guidelines for patient and staff education (29,46–48). Whatever the delivery method, education must be immediate, intense, relevant, and motivational (49). Dlugacz, Stier, and Greenwood (50) suggest that the larger picture must also be considered. They submit that improving care for pressure ulcer prevention requires that caregivers at all levels embrace a "common clinical culture." Using care maps and performance measures, the authors described a process in which caregivers learned to change the way in which they thought about the problem of pressure ulcer prevention. Research suggests that organizational culture (a culture of quality care) is a major determinant of whether barriers to quality skin care and integration of evidence-based protocols can be overcome (51).

Pressure ulcer prevention is also a "team sport" and optimal skin care practices may be easiest to achieve using a multidisciplinary approach (46). Prevention efforts must also include education about the need for documentation to promote continuity of care as well as to obtain adequate reimbursement (52,53).

4. THE ELEMENTS OF TREATMENT

Discussions of pressure ulcer treatment strategies often, erroneously, focus on the wound itself. Though the observation "You can put anything on a pressure ulcer except the patient" is oversimplified, it helps remind clinicians that pressure ulcer treatment strategies include: (1) removing or reducing the effects of pressure, shear and friction, (2) addressing underlying conditions that may delay healing (e.g., nutritional deficiencies), and (3) using wound management strategies that foster repair. Of course, these strategies should always be placed in the context of a patient's overall goal of care. Especially, in the frail elderly or terminally ill patient, the risk or discomfort associated with some interventions needs to be weighed against their potential to facilitate healing. Indeed, while optimal wound treatment strategies are always indicated, their purpose may be to facilitate healing, to reduce discomfort, or to prevent deterioration and complications (54).

4.1. Removing the Cause

To facilitate healing and prevent the development of additional ulcers, prevention strategies discussed earlier need to be implemented for all patients with pressure ulcers. If at all possible, patients should not be placed directly on their ulcer and, when a patient is incontinent, measures to prevent contamination of the wound with feces and/or urine are crucial. As discussed, robust evidence of support surface effectiveness for the prevention of pressure ulcers is limited. Evidence of a causal relationship between these surfaces and pressure ulcer healing is similarly sparse. With the exception of two prospective-controlled clinical studies comparing air-fluidized beds to a range of standard beds and special mattresses, most studies are too small, not controlled, or poorly designed (33,55). Until research findings suggest otherwise, common sense and indirect evidence indicate that all persons with pressure ulcers must be placed on a surface that redistributes pressure and/or reduces shear and friction (56,57). At this time, the type of support surface to use can only be based on product characteristics and the patient's clinical condition (55).

In addition to using positioning/repositioning techniques and support surfaces (see prevention strategies), efforts to maximize patient mobility will not only release pressure and improve patient sense of well-being, but also they may improve respiratory function, cardiac output, venous return, and maintenance of muscle mass (11). When able to transfer to a chair, patients must be placed on pressure-reducing chair cushions. If at all possible, attempts to address the most important cause of these wounds, immobility, will go a long way toward healing and preventing the development of new ulcers.

4.2. Supporting the Patient

To help wounds heal, general nutritional assessment and intervention strategies (see Sec. 3.4. Nutrition) need to be implemented and the proposed treatment plan reviewed and discussed with patients and/or their caregivers (56). Pressure ulcers are a source of procedural and chronic pain, although sometimes difficult to measure in the frail and elderly, they have a negative effect on patient quality of life (58,59). Because improving patient quality of life should always be a goal of care and because stress has been shown to delay healing in acute wounds, clinicians should be mindful of the stress associated with these chronic wounds and consider measures to reduce its potential negative effects on patient well-being and healing (60,61).

4.3. Wound Care

4.3.1. Assessment

For many years, pressure ulcer staging has been used to describe ulcer depth. Indeed, in many health care settings in the United States, pressure ulcer staging is mandatory. The most commonly used system, the national pressure ulcer advisory panel (NPUAP) staging system (56) has recently been modified to help assess Stage I ulcers in patients with darkly pigmented skin. See Table 1. This new definition remains to be tested but there is evidence to suggest that visual and nonvisual indicators should be used in the assessment of Stage I ulcers (62). While useful as an initial diagnosis, staging has inappropriately been adapted to monitor healing. During the past 10 years, much has been learned about wound assessment rationale and techniques (See also: Part 4: Noninvasive wound measurement techniques). Wound assessments are crucial to guide treatment and help monitor treatment

Table 1 NPUAP Staging System[a]

Stage	Definition
Stage I	A Stage I pressure ulcer is an observable pressure related alteration of intact skin whose indicators as compared to the adjacent or opposite area on the body may include changes in one or more of the following: skin temperature (warmth or coolness), tissue consistency (firm or boggy feel), and/or sensation (pain, itching). The ulcer appears as a defined area of persistent redness in lightly pigmented skin, whereas in darker skin tones, the ulcer may appear with persistent red, blue, or purple hues.
Stage II	Partial thickness skin loss involving epidermis, dermis, or both. The ulcer is superficial and presents clinically as an abrasion, blister, or shallow crater.
Stage III	Full thickness skin loss involving damage to, or necrosis of, subcutaneous tissue that may extend down to, but not through, underlying fascia. The ulcer presents clinically as a deep crater with or without undermining of adjacent tissue.
Stage IV	Full thickness skin loss with extensive destruction, tissue necrosis, or damage to muscle, bone, or supporting structures (e.g., tendon, joint capsule). Undermining and sinus tracts also may be associated with Stage IV pressure ulcers.

[a] Available at: http://www.npuap.org

Table 2 Clinical Pressure Ulcer Assessment

Pressure ulcer characteristic	Technique (instrument)	Rationale/comment
Location	Clinical assessment	Facilitates continuity of care.
Stage/depth	Clinical assessment Probing instrument and measuring tape (PSST©)[a]	Staging is useful for diagnostic purposes, should not be used to monitor healing. Ulcer depth guides treatment.
Size	Measuring tape (length/width) Tracing and manual or computerized Planimetry (PSST© & PUSH© tool [b])	Change in size is predictor of healing. Validity/ reliability of manual measurement technique sufficient for clinical practice.
Tissue type	Clinical assessment (predominant tissue type or as % of wound bed) (PSST© and PUSH© tool)	Guides treatment and monitors effectiveness.
Exudate amount	Clinical assessment/rating scale (PSST© and PUSH© tool)	Helps guide treatment. Subjective. Affected by treatment used.
Surrounding skin condition/ wound edges	Clinical assessment (PSST©+)	Helps guide treatment, diagnosis of infection, and adverse reactions to treatments used.

[a] PSST = Pressure Sore Status Tool.
[b] PUSH tool = Pressure Ulcer Scale for Healing.

effectiveness (2). For example, change in wound size after 2–4 weeks of care has been found to predict healing in pressure ulcers and other chronic wounds (63–65). Two standardized instruments for the assessment and documentation of pressure ulcers are available: The Pressure Sore Status Tool© (PSST) and the Pressure Ulcer Scale for Healing (PUSH)©. While the content validity and reliability of both instruments has been established, their prospective validity remains to be studied (1,2,66). The instruments are also not designed to guide treatment choices. Clinicians may, or may not, decide to use the PSST or PUSH instrument to monitor healing. However, the wound characteristics included in these instruments (Table 2) need to be assessed on a regular basis, usually once a week, to guide treatment and monitor changes in the wound.

4.3.2. Treatment

All wound treatment decisions are based on: (1) ulcer status, (2) product safety and effectiveness, and (3) wound pain and caregiver concerns. While treatment costs are an important consideration, they are primarily a function of treatment appropriateness (ulcer status), safety, and effectiveness. When comparing treatment costs in chronic wound care, direct costs (e.g., product purchase price, provider time) are often less important than treatment outcome (67).

Because the actual wound healing process of pressure ulcers is essentially similar to the process of healing other wounds, general principles of pressure ulcer care are based on the principles of acute and surgical wound care. For example, because there is no reason to believe that wounds caused by pressure respond differently to the presence of necrotic tissue than wounds caused by trauma, results of acute and surgical preclinical and clinical wound healing studies are used to support recommendations for the removal of necrotic tissue and cleansing of pressure ulcers with nontoxic cleansing agents (56,57,68).

Because wound care decisions are based on wound status, specifically, levels of exudate, predominant tissue type (e.g., necrotic vs. granulation tissue), wound depth, surrounding skin condition, and condition of wound edges (69), wound treatments often change during the course of healing.

4.3.2.1. Cleansing and Debridement. One wound treatment requirement that generally remains the same during the entire healing process is the need to cleanse the wound between dressing changes. Use of a nontoxic wound cleanser (e.g., normal saline) and enough irrigation pressure to dislodge and remove yellow slough (if present) is recommended (56). The use of tap water as a cleansing agent remains a topic of discussion, particularly in home care. A recent review of available evidence suggests that, providing the quality of the water is good, tap water may be considered acceptable (70). Whirlpool treatments may also help cleanse pressure ulcers but their use in clinical practice is limited by practical (e.g., access, mobility) and infection control concerns.

Necrotic tissue may support the growth of pathological organisms and its presence in pressure ulcers is associated with slower healing (56,71). There are no studies comparing the effectiveness of the four commonly used debridement methods: surgical or sharp, mechanical, enzymatic, and autolytic. Sharp debridement is usually recommended for patients whose wounds contain large amounts of dry, adherent, necrotic tissue, who are at high risk for infection, and who are able to tolerate the procedure. It is essential when cellulitis or sepsis is present. Because sharp debridement requires the availability of a skilled professional who is able to perform the procedure and manage potential problems (e.g., bleeding), many pressure ulcers are debrided using less-invasive methods.

Knowledge about the effectiveness of mechanical debridement, which is usually accomplished using wet-to-dry dressings, is limited to a few small studies (72). Their results varied greatly and because this debridement method is not selective, potentially painful, and labor-intensive, it is not considered a treatment of choice.

Enzymes, once activated in the presence of moisture, will break down and/or digest necrotic tissue. The effectiveness of applying enzymes to debride wounds has been established in burn wounds (72). Results in pressure ulcer research are less unambiguous and this method is generally slow and costly (1). For example, in one 4-week pressure ulcer study, only 46% of collagenase and 36% of fibrinolysin/ deoxyribonuclease-treated wounds exhibited a $\geq 50\%$ decrease in necrotic tissue (73). The difference between these two agents was not statistically significant.

Autolytic debridement, another selective and noninvasive method, involves the retention of moisture at the wound site, liquefying devitalized tissue. In addition, the natural enzymes that degrade fibrin and necrotic tissue are retained when wounds are covered with moisture retentive dressings (1,72). Research evaluating autolytic debridement is limited but appears to suggest that a 50% reduction in eschar should be observed after 10–5 days of treatment (72). While different debridement methods are usually described separately, in clinical practice, a combination of treatments will expedite the process. For example, sharp debridement to remove dry eschar is commonly followed by the application of a moisture retentive dressing to dissolve the fibrinous slough that cannot be surgically removed without traumatizing the wound bed.

4.3.2.2. Dressings. Another constant in topical pressure ulcer care is maintenance of a moist environment (1,2,57). While excess exudate needs to be absorbed
and contained so as to prevent maceration of the surrounding skin, wounds should
never be allowed to dry out. If the wound is dry, moisture should be added (for
example, by applying an amorphous gel dressing) prior to applying a dressing that
will retain it (69). Indeed, clinicians using gauze-based dressings on pressure ulcers,
whether moistened or dry, will be hard pressed to find any evidence to support their
practice. Moisture-retentive dressings facilitate pressure ulcer healing, reduce the
number of dressing changes required, and, as a result, are cost-effective
(2,56,57,67,71). See Table 3. Even though there is ample research to substantiate
the use of moisture retentive dressings in the management of wounds in general
and pressure ulcers in particular, it is important to note that a recent review of
the literature yielded only 3 topical treatment modalities with enough data ($\geq$100
ulcers) to be included in a meta-analysis (67). Hence, the second principle upon
which to base treatment decisions is product safety and effectiveness. Because most
wound treatment (and prevention) products are devices that are exempt from pre-
marketing studies, many have not been subjected to the rigors of prospective, controlled clinical studies. As a result, clinicians need to critically review the safety
and effectiveness profile of these products.

4.3.2.3. Infection. Chronic wounds frequently contain a variety of bacteria.
Whether or not their presence will lead to invasion and subsequent infection depends
on many factors, including bacterial virulence and the ability of the host to mount an
adequate response. For example, the significantly reduced infection rates observed
when using moisture retentive instead of gauze-type dressings is believed to be the
result of their ability to protect against contamination while retaining viable macrophages at the wound site (74,75). In everyday practice, determining whether or not a
pressure ulcer is infected remains problematic. Because all wounds are colonized,
nonquantitative swab cultures will not facilitate the diagnosis of an infection (29).
Also, the classic symptoms of wound infection (redness, swelling, warmth, odor)
may, or may not, be present when an ulcer is infected. A clinician's most important
diagnostic tool is monitoring the ulcer's response to care. If the ulcer fails to exhibit
signs of healing after 2–4 weeks of providing appropriate systemic and local care
(63), the wound may be infected. In these instances, results of a quantitative swab

Table 3 Outcomes and Costs of Pressure Ulcer Protocols of Care

Dressing type (number of studies/ulcers[a])	Average (range) proportion of ulcers healed		Average (range) number of dressing changes per week	Cost per patient healed[a]
	After 6 weeks	After 12 weeks		
Saline gauze (6/102)	28% (0–83)	51% (0–100)	14.41 (7–21)	$ 2,179
Hydrocolloid C (3/136)	28% (15–56)	48% (29–80)	2.47 (1.8–7)	$ 1,267
Hydrocolloid D (9/281)	32% (17–89)	61% (33–100)	2.19 (1.0–3.4)	$ 910

[a] Costs include direct wound care costs (labor and materials) only.
Source: Adapted from Ref. 67.

or tissue biopsy culture (if available) are useful to help guide antibiotic therapy. Research ascertaining the effectiveness of topical antibiotic therapy is limited but an antibiotic that is effective against Gram-negative, Gram-positive, and anaerobic organisms is usually recommended (29,56). If the wound still fails to improve, imaging studies (e.g., computed tomography, MRI) or a bone biopsy and histopathological evaluation should be considered since the latter is still the gold standard for detecting osteomyelitis (76). While awaiting the results of much-needed research in this area, an optimal treatment approach to prevent life-threatening infections includes: (a) timely removal of necrotic tissue, (b) protecting the wound against contamination by using a dressing that has been shown to be impermeable to bacteria, (c) providing a wound environment that optimizes the body's own defense mechanisms, (d) aggressive monitoring of the ulcer's response to treatment and timely changes in the plan of care when the wound fails to heal.

   4.3.2.4. Surgery and Other Treatment Modalities.   Surgical repair of pressure ulcers may be the treatment of choice for patients who are otherwise in good health and able to tolerate the procedure and postoperative follow-up. As a result, surgical repair of extensive, e.g., Stage III and IV pressure ulcers using muscle and musculo-cutaneous flap closure is most often performed in persons with spinal cord injuries (56,57). Postoperative care requirements are extensive and complications, including recurrence, are common. Careful patient selection and education are crucial to reducing recurrence rates.

   Because pressure ulcers can present a formidable clinical challenge, many different treatment modalities have, at one time or another, been applied to these wounds. The most extensively evaluated adjunctive therapy for use if conventional treatments fail is the application of electrical current to stimulate healing (1,29,56). Unfortunately, questions about the optimal electrical charge needed to stimulate pressure ulcer healing and concerns about the methodological limitations of the studies remain (77). Even though some studies have been conducted, the efficacy of potentially promising therapies such as therapeutic ultrasound, radiant heat, topical negative pressure, topical or systemic hyperbaric oxygen has not been established, in part because of study limitations such as small sample size, lack of appropriate control treatments (e.g., moisture retentive dressings), or faulty study design (inclusion of patients with multiple wounds) (1,78–80). The ability of ultraviolet light C to inhibit bacterial growth including the growth of antibiotic-resistant bacteria is intriguing because patients with pressure ulcers are a frequent source of MRSA and VRSA (81). Research to establish its role in the management of pressure ulcers is needed.

   Research suggests that topically applied growth factors could play an important role in the treatment of pressure ulcers who fail to respond to conventional, moisture-retentive dressing therapy (1,57). However, a variety of growth factors are involved in the wound healing process. At this time, it is not known which growth factor, or combination of growth factors, is more effective than conventional pressure ulcer therapy. At this time, the magic bullet to heal pressure ulcers remains elusive.

5. SUMMARY

Throughout history, pressure ulcers have challenged providers and frustrated patients. Their presence has been blamed on everything and everyone and they have been treated with every imaginable ointment and treatment modality. Most have disappointed. Fortunately, the majority of ulcers heal within a reasonable period of time when the cause of the ulcer is removed, systemic measures to support healing are implemented, and the wound is free of necrotic tissue, protected against contamination, and kept moist. Healing the recalcitrant ulcer, however, will remain a challenge until understanding of the etiology and pathophysiology of these wounds improves.

Similarly, despite many years of research, much remains unknown about pressure ulcer prevention. Though quality pressure ulcer treatment and prevention are dependent upon a number of factors, the current and upcoming nursing shortage will likely adversely affect the pressure ulcer-related goals of health care and public policy initiatives that strive to reduce the financial and human factor burden of chronic conditions (53). Ironically, in the best of times for pressure ulcer technological innovations and developments, the worst of times may be emerging for the quality and availability of persons needed to use them. Given this trend and current knowledge base, improved patient outcomes cannot occur without much-needed research to improve the evidence-base of prevention and treatment strategies and without increasing emphasis on patient and caregiver education.

REFERENCES

1. Lyder CH. Pressure ulcer prevention and treatment. In: Fitzpatrick JJ, Archbold PG, Stewart BJ, Lyons KS, eds. Annual Review of Nursing Research. New York: Springer Publishing Company, 2002:35–61.
2. Bates-Jensen BB. Quality indicators for prevention and management of pressure ulcers in vulnerable elders. Ann Inter Med 2001; 135(8):744–751.
3. Nelson M. Pressure ulcer assessment and documentation: the beginning of a plan of care. J Legal Nurse Consulting 2001; 12(4):22–25.
4. Andrychuk MA. Pressure ulcers: causes, risk factors, assessment, and intervention. Orthopedic Nurs 1998; 17(4):65–83.
5. Bryant RA, Rolstad BS. Utilizing a systems approach to implement pressure ulcer prediction and prevention. Ostomy/Wound Manage 2001; 47(9):26–36.
6. Gould D, James T, Tarpey A, Kelly D, Pattison D, Fox C. Prevention studies to reduce the incidence of pressure sores: a literature review. J Clin Nurs 2000; 9:163–177.
7. National pressure ulcer advisory panel. In: Cuddigan J, Ayello EA, Sussman C, eds. Pressure Ulcers in America: Prevalence, Incidence and Implications for the Future. Reston, VA: NPUAP, 2001.
8. Nixon J. The pathophysiology and aetiolgy of pressure ulcers. In: Morrison MJ, ed. The Prevention and Treatment of Pressure Ulcers. London: Harcourt Publ. Limited, 2001: 17–36.
9. DeFloor T. The risk of pressure sores: a conceptual scheme. J Clin Nurs 1999; 8:206–216.
10. Mayrovitz HN, Sims N, Taylor MC. Sacral skin blood perfusion: a factor in pressure ulcers? Ostomy/Wound Manage 2002; 48(6):34–42.
11. Braden B, Bergstrom N. A conceptual schema for the study of the etiology of pressure sores. Rehabil Nurs 1987; 12(1):8–16.
12. Graff MK, Bryant J, Beinlich N. Preventing heel breakdown. Orthopedic Nurs 2000; 19(5):63–69.
13. DeFloor T, De Schuijmer. Preventing pressure ulcers: an evaluation of four operating-table mattresses. Appl Nurs Res 2000; 13(3):134–141.
14. Tomaselli N. Clinical decision making for pressure ulcers. Care Manage 2001; 5(3): 10–13.

15. van Rijswijk L. Epidemiology. In: Morrison MJ, ed. The Prevention and Treatment of Pressure Ulcers. London: Harcourt Publ. Limited, 2001:7–13.

16. Thomas DR. Improving outcome of pressure ulcers with nutritional interventions: a review of the evidence. Nutrition 2001; 17:121–125.

17. Anthony D, Reynolds T, Russell L. An investigation into the use of serum albumin in pressure sore prediction. J Adv Nurs 2000; 32(2):359–365.

18. Banks V. Pressure sores: topical treatment and the healing process. J Wound Care 1998; 7(5):265–266.

19. Armstrong D, Bortz P. An integrative review of pressure relief in surgical patients. AORN J 2001; 73(3):645–674.

20. Byers PH, Carta SG, Mayrovitz HN. Pressure ulcer research issues in surgical patients. Adv Skin Wound Care 2000; 13:115–121.

21. Schultz A, Bien M, Dumond K, Brown K, Myers A. Etiology and incidence of pressure ulcers in surgical patients. AORN J 1999; 70(3):434–449.

22. Lyder CH, Preston J, Grady JN, Scinto J, Allman R, Bergstrom N, Rodeheaver G. Quality of care for hospitalized medicare patients at risk for pressure ulcers. Arch Intern Med 2001; 161:1549–1554.

23. Blegen MA, Goode CJ, Reed L. Nurse staffing and patient outcomes. Nurs Res 1998; 47(1):43–50.

24. Olshansky K. Rethinking our approach to pressure ulcers. Ostomy/Wound Manage 2001; 47(5):6.

25. Meehan M. Beyond the pressure ulcer blame game: reflections for the future. Ostomy/Wound Manage 2000; 46(5):46–52.

26. Day D, Hayes K, Kennedy AM, Diercksen D. Pressure ulcer prevention: review of the literature. J N Y State Nurses Assoc 1997; 28(2):12–17.

27. Halfens R. Risk assessment scales for pressure ulcers: a theoretical methodological, and clinical perspective. Ostomy/Wound Manage 2000; 46(8):36–44.

28. Bergquist S. Subscales, subscores or summative score. Evaluating the contribution of Braden scale items for predicting pressure ulcer risk in older adults receiving home health care. J WOCN 2001; 28:279–289.

29. Dolynchuk K, Keast D, Campbell K, Houghton P, Orstead H, Sibbald G, Atkinson A. Best practices for the prevention and treatment of pressure ulcers. Ostomy/Wound Manage 2000; 46(11):38–52.

30. Ayello E, Braden B. Why is pressure ulcer risk assessment so important? Nursing 2001; 31:74–80.

31. Nesselroth S, Gahtan V. Management of pressure ulcers in the home care setting. Home Health Care Consultant 2000; 7(4):34–42.

32. Sharp C, Burr G, Broadbent M, Casey R, Merriman M. Pressure ulcer prevention and care: a survey of current practice. J Qual Clin Pract 2000; 20(4):150–157.

33. Cullum N. Pressure ulcer prevention and treatment: a synopsis of the current evidence from research. Crit Care Nurs Clin North America 2001; 13(4):547–554.

34. Krouskop T, van Rijswijk L. Standardizing performance-based criteria for support surfaces. Ostomy/Wound Manage 1995; 4(1):34–45.

35. Whittemore R. Pressure-reduction support surfaces: a review of the literature. J WOCN 1998; 25(1):6–25.

36. Ratliff CR, Rodeheaver G. Pressure ulcer assessment and management. Lippincott's Primary Care Pract 1999; 3(2):242–258.

37. Maklebust J. Pressure ulcers: decreasing the risk for older adults. Geriatric Nurs 1997; 18:250–254.

38. Moore Z. Improving pressure ulcer prevention through education. Nurs Stand 2001; 16(6):64–70.

39. Panel for the Prediction and Prevention of Pressure Ulcers in Adults. Pressure ulcers in adults: prediction and prevention. Clinical Practice Guideline #3. Rockville, MD:

Agency for Health Care Policy and Research, Public Health Service, US Department of Health & Human Services, May, 1992.

40. U.S. Department of Health and Human Services. Healthy People 2010. Conference Edition (in Two Volumes), Washington, DC, January, 2000.

41. Gibbons RB. Nutritional aspects of wound management. Home Healthcare Consultant 2000; 7(4):19–22.

42. Ferguson M, Cook A, Rimmasch H, Benders, Voss A. Pressure ulcer management: the importance of nutrition. MEDSURG Nurs 2000; 9(4):163–177.

43. Ferguson M, Cook A, Bender S, Rimmasch H, Voss A. Diagnosing and treating involuntary weight loss. MEDSURG Nurs 2001; 10(4):165–175.

44. Mathus-Vliegen E. Nutritional status, nutrition, and pressure ulcers. Nutr Clin Pract 2001; 16:286–291.

45. Sheridan SG, Hahn PW, Malkoff TL. Report and Results of Research on Nursing Home Liability for Pressure Ulcers. Columbus, OH: Buckingham, Doolittle & Burrough, 1999.

46. Flynn MB, Fink R. Committing to evidence-based skin care practice. Crit Care Nurs Clini North America 2001; 13(4):555–568.

47. Hall P, Schumann L. Wound care: meeting the challenge. J Amer Acad Nurse Pract 2001; 13(6):258–268.

48. Junkin J. Promoting healthy skin in various settings. Nurs Clin North America 2000; 35(2):339–348.

49. Pieper B. General considerations for the management of wounds in home care. Home Health care Consultant 2000; 7(12):25–32.

50. Dlugacz Y, Stier L, Greenwood A. Changing the system: a quality management approach to pressure injuries. J Healthcare Qual 2001; 23(5):15–21.

51. Frantz R, Gardner S, Specht J, McIntire G. Integration of pressure ulcer treatment protocol into practice: clinical outcomes and care environment attributes. Outcomes Manage Nurs Pract 2001; 5(3):112–120.

52. Gunningberg L, Lindholm C, Carlsson M, Sjoden P. The development of pressure ulcers in patients with hip fractures: inadequate nursing documentation is still a problem. J Adv Nurs 2000; 31(5):1155–1164.

53. Gallagher S. Pressure ulcers, outcomes, and the nursing shortage. Ostomy/Wound Manage 2001; 47(8):49–51.

54. Ennis WJ. Healing: can we? Must we? Should we? Ostomy/Wound Manage 2001; 47(9):6, 8.

55. Maklebust J. An update on horizontal support surfaces. Ostomy/Wound Manage 1999; 45(suppl 1A):70S–77S.

56. Bergstrom N, Bennett MA, Carlson CE, et al. Treatment of pressure ulcers. Clinical Practice Guideline No. 15. Rockville, MD: US Department of Health and Human Services, Public Health Service, Agency for Health Care Policy and Research, December, 1994.

57. Consortium for Spinal Cord Medicine. Pressure Ulcer prevention and Treatment Following Spinal Cord Injury: A Clinical Practice Guideline for Healthcare Professionals. Paralyzed Veterans of America, 2000. Available at: www.pva.org. Date accessed: September 30, 2002.

58. Clark M. Pressure ulcers and quality of life. Nurs Stand Tissue Viability Suppl 2002; 16(22):74–78, 80.

59. van Rijswijk L, Gottlieb D. Like a terrorist. Ostomy/Wound Manage 2000; 46(5):25–26.

60. Marucha PT, Kiecolt-Glaser JK, Favagehi M. Mucosal wound healing is impaired by examination stress. Psychosom Med 1998; 60:362–365.

61. Cole-King A, Harding KG. Psychological factors and delayed healing in chronic wounds. Psychosom Med 2001; 63:216–220.

62. Sprigle S, Linden M, Riordan B. Analysis of localized erythema using clinical indicators and spectroscopy. Ostomy/Wound Manage. 2003; 49(3):42–52.

63. van Rijswijk L, Polansky M. Predictors of time to healing deep pressure ulcers. Ostomy/Wound Manage 1994; 40:40–42, 44, 46–48 passim.

64. van Rijswijk L, The Multi-Center Leg Ulcer Study Group. Full thickness leg ulcers: patient demographics and predictors of healing. J Fam Pract 1993; 36:625–632.

65. Tallman P, Muscare E, Eglstein WH, Falanga V. Initial rate of healing predicts complete healing of venous ulcers. Arch Dermatol 1997; 133:1231–1234.

66. Stotts NA, Rodeheaver GT, Thomas DR, Frantz R, et al. An instrument to measure healing in pressure ulcers: development and validation of the pressure ulcer scale for healing (PUSH). J Gerontol 2001; 56A(12):M795–M799.

67. Kerstein MD, Gemmen E, van Rijswijk L, Lyder CH, Phillips T, et al. Cost and cost effectiveness of venous and pressure ulcer protocols of care. Dis Manage Health Outcomes 2001; 9(11):651–663.

68. Blunt J. Wound cleansing: ritualistic or research-based practice? Nurs Stand 2001; 16(1):33–36.

69. Beitz JM, van Rijswijk L. Using wound care algorithms: a content validation study. JWOCN 1999; 26:238–249.

70. Fernandez R, Griffiths R, Ussia C. Water for wound cleansing. *The Cochrane Database of Systematic Reviews* 2002, Issue 1. Art. No.: CD003861. DOI: 10.1002/14651858. CD003861.

71. Xakellis GC, Chrischilles EA. Hydrocolloid versus saline-gauze dressings in treating pressure ulcers: a cost-effectiveness analysis. Arch Phys Med Rehabil 1992; 73:463–469.

72. Fowler E, van Rijswijk L. Using wound debridement to help achieve the goals of care. Ostomy Wound manage 1995; 41(7A):23S–35S.

73. Püllen R, Popp R, Volkers P, Füsgen I. Prospective randomized double-blind study of the wound-debriding effects of collagenase and fibrinolysin/deoxyribonuclease in pressure ulcers. Age Age 2002; 31:126–130.

74. Hutchinson J, McGuckin M. Occlusive dressings: a microbiologic and clinical review. Am J Infect Control 1990; 18:257–268.

75. Bowler PG. The 10^5 bacterial growth guideline: Reassessing its clinical relevance in wound healing. *Ostomy Wound Manage* 2003; 49(1):44–53.

76. Livesley NJ, Chow AW. Infected pressure ulcers in elderly individuals. Clin Infect Dis 2002; 35(11):1390–1396.

77. Flemming K, Cullum N. Electromagnetic therapy for treating pressure sores. *The Cochrane Database of Systematic Reviews* 2001, Issue 1. Art. No.: CD002930. DOI: 10.1002/14651858.CD002930.

78. Flemming K, Cullum N. Therapeutic ultrasound for pressure sores. *The Cochrane Database of Systematic Reviews* 2000, Issue 4. Art. No.: CD001275. DOI: 10.1002/14651858.CD001275.

79. Evans D, Land L. Topical negative pressure for treating chronic wounds. *The Cochrane Database of Systematic Reviews* 2001, Issue 1. Art. No.: CD001898. DOI: 10.1002/14651858.CD001898.

80. Ford CN, Reinhard E, Yeh D, Syrek D, et al. Interim analysis of a prospective, randomized trial of vacuum-assisted closure versus the healthpoint system in the management of pressure ulcers. Ann Plast Surg 2002; 49:55–61.

81. Thai TP, Houghton PE, Keast DH, Campbell KE, Woodbury MG. Ultraviolet light C in the treatment of chronic wounds with MRSA: a case study. Ostomy/Wound Manage 2002; 48(11):52–60.

ADDITIONAL READINGS

Bogie K, Regers, Levine S, Sahgal V. Electrical stimulation for pressure sore prevention and wound healing. Assistive Technol 2000; 12(1):50–66.

Brandeis GH, Berlowitz DR, Katz P. Are pressure ulcers preventable? A survey of experts. Adv Skin Wound Care. 2001; 14:244–248.

Brasseur K, Liske T. Critical care formula improves outcomes for a patient with chronic pressure ulcers. Nutr Clin Pract 2001; 25:218–222.

Brienza DM, Geyer MJ. Understanding support surface technologies. Adv Skin Wound Care 2000; 13(5):237–244.

Buss IC, Halfens RG, Abu-Saad H. The most effective time interval for repositioning subjects at risk of pressure sore development: a literature review. Rehabil Nurs 2002; 27(2):59–77.

Cervo F, Cruz A, Posillico J. Pressure ulcers analysis of guidelines for treatment and management. Geriatrics 2000; 55(3):55–60.

Cuddigan J, Berlowitz DR, Ayello E. Pressure ulcers in America: prevalence, incidence, and implications for the future. Adv Skin Wound Care 2001; 14(4):208–215.

Davis C. Prevalence and incidence studies of pressure ulcers in two long-term facilities in Canada. Ostomy/Wound Manage 2001; 47(11):28–34.

DeFloor T, Grypdonck M. Do pressure relief cushions really relieve pressure? West J Nurs Res 2000; 3:335–350.

Dukich J, O'Connor D. Impact of practice guidelines on support surface selection, incidence of pressure ulcers and fiscal dollars. Ostomy/Wound Manage 2001; 47(3):44–53.

Fletcher J, Kopp P. Framework guidelines for wound care. Professional Nurse 2000; 16(2):917–921.

Fontaine R. Investigating the efficacy of a non-powered pressure-reducing therapeutic mattress: a retrospective multi-site study. Ostomy/Wound Manage 2000; 46(9):34–43.

Fontaine R, Risley S, Castellino R. A quantitative analysis of pressure and shear in the effectiveness of support surfaces. J WOCN 1998; 25(5):233–239.

Garber S, Krouskop T. Technical advances in wheelchair and seating systems. Phys Med Rehabil 1997; 11(1):93–106.

Geyer MJ, Brienza DM, Karg P, Trefler E, Kelsey S. A randomized control trial to evaluate pressure-reducing seat cushions for elderly wheelchair users. Adv Skin Wound Care 2001; 14(3):120–129.

Gould D, Kelly D, Goldstone L, Gammon J. Examining the validity of pressure ulcer risk assessment scales: developing and using illustrated patient simulations to collect the data. J Clin Nurs 2001; 10(5):697–705.

Guenter P, Malyszek R, Bliss D, Steffe T, O'Hara D, La Van F, Montiero D. Survey of nutritional status in newly hospitalized patients with stage III or stage IV pressure ulcers. Adv Skin Wound Care 2000; 13(4):164–168.

Halfens R, Haalboom J. A historical overview of pressure ulcer literature of the past 35 years. Ostomy/Wound Manag 2001; 47(11):36–43.

Harker J. Role of the nurse consultant in tissue ability. Nurs Stand 2001; 15(49):39–42.

Hart BD, Birkas J, Lachmann M, Saunders L. Promoting positive outcomes for elderly persons in the hospital: prevention and risk factor modification. AACN Clin Issues 2002; 13(1):22–33.

Hendrix T, Foreman S. Optimal long-term care nurse-staffing levels. Nurs Econ 2001; 19(4):164–175.

Jones I, Tweed C, Marron M. Pressure area care in infants and children: nimbus. Pediatric system. Br J Nurs 2001; 10(12):789–795.

Jordan R. Supporting healing. Adv Directors Rehabil 2001; 10(10):23–24, 38.

Kramer JD, Kearney M. Patient, wound, and treatment characteristics associated with healing in pressure ulcers. Adv Skin Wound Care 2000; 13:17–24.

Krause JS, Vines C, Farley T, Sniezek J, Coker J. An exploratory study of pressure ulcers after spinal cord injury: relationship to protective behaviors and risk factors. Arch Phys Med Rehabil 2001; 82:107–113.

Langemo D, Melland H, Hanson D, Olson B, Hunter S. The lived experience of having a pressure ulcer: a qualitative analysis. Adv Skin Wound Care 2000; 13:225–235.

Lyne P, Papanikolaou P, Lycett E. An empirical investigation of pressure ulcer risk factors. Nurs Stand 2000; 14:46–53.

Margolis D, Knauss J, Bilker W. Hormone replacement therapy and prevention of pressure ulcers and venous leg ulcers. Lancet 2002; 359(23):672–675.

Olson K, Trachuk L, Hanson J. Preventing pressure sores in oncology patients. Clin Nurs Res 1998; 7(2):207–224.

Parsons L, Kraus SD, Ward K. Orthopedic trauma-managing secondary medical problems. Crit Care Nurs Clin North America 2001; 13(3):433–442.

Pieper B, Templin T, Dobal M, Jacox A. Home care nurses' rating of appropriateness of wound treatment and wound healing. J WOCN 2002; 29:20–28.

Richardson J, Prentice D, Rivers S. Developing an interdisciplinary evidence-based skin care pathway for long-term care. Adv Skin Wound Care 2001; 14:197–205.

Russell L. Malnutrition and pressure ulcers: nutritional assessment tools. Br J Nurs 2000; 9(4):194–198.

Russell L. The importance of patients' nutritional status in wound healing. Br J Nurs 2001; 10(6):S42–S49.

Scott EM, Leaper DJ, Clark M, Kelly PJ. Effects of warming therapy on pressure ulcers—a randomized trial. AORN J 2001; 73(5):921–938.

Sibbald G, Williamson D, Orstead H, Campbell K, Keast D, Krasner D, Sibbald D. Preparing the wound bed-debridement, bacterial balance, and moisture balance. Ostomy/Wound Manage 2000; 46(4):14–35.

Singhal A, Reis ED, Kerstein MD. Options for non-surgical debridement of necrotic wounds. Adv Skin Wound Care 2001; 14:96–103.

Spoelhof GD. Management of pressure ulcers in the nursing home. Ann Long-Term Care 2000; 8(8):69–72.

Spoelhof GD. Treatment of pressure ulcers. Home Health Care Consultant 2001; 8(3):10–16.

Stanton J. A nurse's aid to clinical selection of pressure-reducing equipment. Br J Nurs 2001; 10(5):S16–S24.

Warren JB, Yoder LH, Young-McCaughan S. Development of a decision tree for support surfaces: a tool for nursing. MEDSURG Nurs 1999; 8(4):239–248.

Weaver V, McCausland D. Revised medicare policies for support surfaces: a review. J WOCN 1998; 25(1):26–35.

Xakellis GC, Frantz R, Lewis A, Harvey P. Translating pressure ulcer guidelines into practice: it's harder than it sounds. Adv Skin Wound Care 2001; 14:249–256, 258.

Zevola DR, Raffa M, Brown K. Using clinical pathways in patients undergoing cardiac valve surgery. Crit Care Nurse 2002; 22(1):31–50.

Zulkowski KM, Tellez R, Van Rijswijk L. Documentation with MDS section M: skin condition. Adv Skin Wound Care 2001; 14:81–89.

15

Diabetic Foot and Ulceration: Epidemiology and Pathophysiology

Andrew J. M. Boulton
Department of Medicine, Division of Endocrinology, Diabetes and Metabolism, University of Miami School of Medicine, Miami, Florida, U.S.A. and Department of Medicine, University of Manchester, Manchester, U.K.

David G. Armstrong
Department of Surgery, Doctor William M. Scholl College of Podiatric Medicine, Rosalind Franklin University of Medicine and Science, Chicago, Illinois, U.S.A.

1. INTRODUCTION

Coming events cast their shadows before.

—Thomas Campbell

Although not referring to diabetic foot problems when writing these lines, the Scottish poet's words can usefully be applied to the breakdown of the diabetic foot. Ulceration does not occur spontaneously, rather it is a combination of causative factors that result in the development of a lesion. There are many warning signs or "shadows" that can identify those at risk. The famous Boston diabetes physician, Elliott Joslin, realized this almost 70 years ago when, after observing many clinical cases of diabetic foot disease he remarked "Diabetic gangrene is not heaven-sent, but earth-born" (1). Thus, it is not an inevitable consequence of having diabetes that foot ulceration will occur: ulcers invariably occur in certain individuals as a consequence of an interaction between specific pathologies of the lower limb and environmental hazards.

One might ask–why does the diabetic foot warrant two chapters in a text on advanced wound care? Similarly, why are there no articles on the osteoarthritic or rheumatoid foot? The answer to these questions lies in one word—neuropathy (2). Until the middle of the 20th Century, patients with Leprosy (Hansen's disease) were frequently removed from society as it was believed that the disfiguring lesions of the extremities occurred as a consequence of infection. In biblical times, leprosy colonies are described; early last century patients in the United States were sent to the National Hansen's Disease Center in Louisiana. It was Dr. Paul Brand, working in south India, who later realized that the foot ulcers did not result directly from infection, but from loss of sensation caused by the leprosy infection. It was Brand who described pain as "God's greatest gift to man" (3). Thus, in diabetes, the loss of pain sensation as a consequence of distal sensory neuropathy, results in the many problems collectively described or referred to as "the diabetic foot."

The traditional medical model of disease suggests that a patient goes to the doctor because of symptoms, treatment is prescribed and then the patient recovers. Because this cannot apply in the case of insensitive feet, health care professionals have difficulty in comprehending the diabetic foot syndrome: they find it difficult to take the initiative and look for early lesions or warning signs of imminent breakdown. Many doctors regard these patients as stupid—how can a sensible person walk on a swollen, red foot with an active infected foot ulcer? What we must realize is that an insensitive foot is not only painless, but also does not feel as if it belongs to the individual (3). Our task is to identify diabetic patients at risk of ulceration and help them to cope with this health state by avoiding exposure to environmental hazards that may result in ulceration.

In this chapter, the epidemiology and economics of diabetic foot lesions will first be described. The many "shadows" or risk factors that might predict the coming event of foot ulceration will then be discussed. Throughout the chapter, the term "diabetic foot" will be used to refer to the foot at risk of breakdown as a consequence of one or more pathologies.

2. EPIDEMIOLOGY OF THE DIABETIC FOOT

One day everything will be well—that is our hope.
Everything is fine today—that is our illusion.

—Voltaire

The words of Voltaire summarize the depressing statistics that follow regarding the incidence and prevalence of foot ulceration and amputation in diabetes. Foot ulceration is much more common in diabetic patients with neuropathy and vascular disease: the annual incidence rises from <1% in those without neuropathy, for example, to more than 7% in those with established neuropathy (4–6). A selection of epidemiological data for ulceration and amputation, originating from several countries, as provided in Table 1. Globally, the diabetic foot remains a major medical, social, and economic problem that is seen in every continent (7). However, the reported frequencies of ulceration and amputation do vary considerably on the basics of the diagnostic criteria used as well as regional differences. It is likely that up to 10% of patients with diabetes have past or present ulceration and approximately 1% have already undergone amputations. Diabetes remains the major cause of nontraumatic amputation in most Western countries: rates are as much as 15 times higher than in the nondiabetic population. However, the study of the epidemiology of diabetic foot disease and amputation has been beset by numerous problems relating to both diagnostic tests and population selection. Until proper registers of people with diabetes that are population based are fully available, reliable data relating to accurate estimates of prevalence and incidence of these late complications will remain limited.

The effects of racial influences on the epidemiology of foot ulceration and amputation have recently been assessed. Resnick et al. (8) reported that amputation was more common amongst black subjects with diabetes than in white Americans with diabetes, although the effect of race diminished after adjustment for smoking,

Table 1 Epidemiology of Foot Ulceration and Amputation

Author (Ref.)	Country	Year	N	Prevalence		Incidence		Risk factors for foot ulcers (%)
				Ulcers (%)	Amputations (%)	Ulcers (%)	Amputation (%)	
Abbott et al. (6)	U.K.	2002	9710	1.7	1.3	2.2	–	>50
Manes et al. (12)	GR	2002	821	4.75	–	–	–	>50
Muller et al. (13)	NL	2002	665	–	–	2.1	0.6	–
Ramsey et al. (14)	U.S.A.	1997	8965	–	–	5.8[a]	0.9[a]	–
Vozar et al. (15)	SL	1997	1205	2.5	0.9	0.6	0.6	–
Moss et al. (16)	U.S.A.	1992	2900	–	–	10.1[b]	2.1[b]	–

Key: GR, Greece; NL, Netherlands; SL, Slovakia.
[a] Incidence figures over 3 years.
[b] Incidence figures over 4 years

education, and diabetes. However, no such ethnic differences were observed in a recent study of potential ethnic disparities in an insured population (9). The situation appears to be different in the United Kingdom, where Leggetter et al. (10) recently reported no ethnic differences in diabetes-related amputation in women, whereas in males the amputation rates are lower in Afro-Caribbeans than Europeans. Similarly, Asians of Indian subcontinent origin have a lower incidence of amputation and foot ulceration than their European counterparts (11).

Studies from Germany have attempted to measure trends in the incidence of amputations in recent years. Unfortunately, no change in amputation rates was observed during a 9-year follow-up period (17). The strong association between risk of amputation and diabetes therefore persists, and seems to be strongest in younger age groups (18).

In summary, the study of the epidemiology of foot ulceration and amputation in diabetes have been clouded by a lack of agreement over diagnostic criteria and by variation in subject selection methods. However, there can be little doubt that both amputation and foot ulceration remain all too common in diabetic populations. It must be assumed that at least 50% of older Type 2 diabetic subjects have identifiable risk factors for foot ulceration.

3. ECONOMIC ASPECTS OF DIABETIC FOOT PROBLEMS

One of several reasons that resulted in the American Diabetes Association holding a consensus conference on diabetic wound care in 1999 (19) was the vast cost of diabetic foot disease in the United States, and the real need to develop cost-effective measures to treat and prevent ulcers. The 1997 average inpatient hospital costs were: foot ulcers, $16,580; toe or transmetatarsal amputation, $25,241; and transtibial amputation, $31,436 (20). Subsequently, Holzer et al. (21) estimated that the total expenditure for diabetic foot ulcers amongst a population of 7 million U.S. patients was $16 million over a 2-year period. Harrington et al. (22) studied costs in the Medicare system and found that expenditure for a diabetic foot ulcer was on average three times higher than those for Medicare patients in general. Diabetic foot ulcers cost the Medicare system $1.5 billion in 1995. More recently, data from 8905 diabetic patients in an HMO estimated the cost for a middle-aged patient with a new foot ulcer to be $28,000 over a 2-year period (14).

Turning now to potential savings by preventing ulcers and amputations, a report from Sweden analyzed the cost effectiveness of an intensive prevention program (23). They showed that an intensified prevention strategy which included education, foot care, and footwear would be cost effective and ever cost saving if applied to those patients with risk factors for foot ulcers. However, there is no benefit is providing patients with healthy feet and no risk factors, with this level of education and care.

The next section discuses the major risk factors for foot ulceration and amputation.

4. PATHOGENESIS OF DIABETIC FOOT ULCERATION

An understanding of the contributory factors that ultimately result in foot ulceration is likely to help in the planning of effective preventative strategies. There is no doubt that foot ulcers rarely result from a single pathology. The neuropathic foot, for example, does not spontaneously ulcerate. It is a combination of insensitivity with some other factors that results in ulceration. Such factors may be extrinsic (e.g., walking barefoot and treading on a sharp object, or simply wearing ill-fitting shoes) or intrinsic (such as the patient with insensitivity and high foot pressures who develops callus that results in ulceration) (24).

The breakdown of the diabetic foot has traditionally been considered to result from a combination of neuropathy, vascular disease, and infection. There is, however, no compelling evidence to implicate infection. Infection is normally a consequence rather than a cause of skin breakdown. As noted above, neuropathy is the most important contributory cause in the pathway to ulceration (25). This will be discussed in some detail in addition to peripheral vascular disease (PVD) and other risk factors.

4.1. Diabetic Neuropathy

The diabetic neuropathies comprise a heterogeneous group of conditions that may, on clinical grounds, be divided in various polyneuropathies and mononeuropathies (26). It is the distal sensorimotor and peripheral autonomic (sympathetic) neuropathies that play important roles in the pathogenesis of foot ulceration.

Distal sensorimotor neuropathy is by far the commonest of all the neuropathies. Some recent studies reporting on the prevalence are summarized in Table 2. It can be assumed safely that at least half of older Type 2 diabetic patients have significant sensory loss. The onset of this type of neuropathy tends to be insidious and, in some cases, patients never experience any symptoms simply developing insensitive feet. Those who get symptoms may experience burning, shooting or electrical pain, paresthesiae, stabbing or lancinating pain, all of which are prone to nocturnal exacerbation. Contact hyperesthesiae and allodynia are also common. Clinical examination reveals a distal sensory loss to large and small fiber functions: small muscle wasting and absent ankle reflexes are also usually found.

It must be realized that there is a spectrum of symptomatic severity in sensory neuropathy. At one extreme, severe symptoms may be experienced, at the other, symptoms may be absent. Thus, a diagnosis of neuropathy *cannot be made on history alone: assessment of foot ulcer risk cannot be made without a careful exam with shoes and socks removed.*

Autonomic neuropathy involves the sympathetic nervous system in the lower limb resulting in anhidrosis, and dry skin which cracks and is liable to callus formation. In addition, in the absence of large vessel PVD, sympathetic dysfunction results in increased skin blood and a warm foot. Hence, the warm, dry insensate foot is truly the high-risk foot.

Peripheral neuropathy can easily be diagnosed by a simple clinical assessment of large fiber function (e.g., loss of perception of vibration using a 128-Hz turning fork), small fiber function (e.g., pin-prick sensation) in the feet together with an assessment of ankle reflexes (30,31). Simple tests of sensory function may also be useful, such as pressure perception using a log monofilament (31,32). Neuropathic feet usually have a typical appearance on clinical observation: clawed toes, prominent metatarsal heads, small muscle wasting, and dry, flaky skin.

4.2. Neuropathy—The Major Contributory Factor in Ulceration

Several longitudinal studies confirm the key role of neuropathy in the pathway to ulceration. Loss of small and large fiber function have been shown to predict

Table 2 Epidemiologic Data on Diabetic Sensorimotor Neuropathy

	Author (Ref.)	Country	Year	Number of subjects	Prevalence (%)
1. Population-based studies	Abbott et al. (6)	UK	2002	9710	23
	Manes et al. (12)	Greece	2002	821	34
	Partanen et al. (27)	Finland	1995	133	8[a]
					42[b]
2. Clinic-based studies	Tesfaye et al. (28)	Europe	1996	3250	28
	Cahezas-Cerrato (29)	Spain	1998	2644	23

[a] At diagnosis of Type 2 diabetes.
[b] After 10 years of diagnosed Type 2 diabetes.

ulceration (5,33,34). Abbott et al. (6), in a large prospective study of almost 10,000 patients, demonstrated that a simple neuropathy disability of some was a powerful predictor of ulceration. Most recently, a 6-year prospective study confirmed that the most reproducible measure of nerve function, motor nerve conduction velocity assessed by electrophysiological means, is a robust surrogate endpoint for foot ulceration (35).

Considering all the above data, there can be little doubt that neuropathy can lead to foot ulceration with or without ischemia. Other risk factors that are associated with foot ulceration will now be considered.

4.3. Peripheral Vascular Disease

A number of large epidemiological studies have confirmed the frequency of all forms of ischemic PVD in diabetes (24,36). The Framingham Study (36), for example, reported a 50% excess of absent foot pulses in diabetic females, with similar results in males. Reports from Europe and the United States have confirmed that PVD is a major contributory factor in the pathogenesis of foot ulceration and subsequent amputation in diabetes (37,38). Major factors in the etiology of PVD are hyperglycemia, smoking, dyslipidemia, and hypertension (39). In the clinical assessment of PVD, Doppler pressure measures at the ankle may overestimate the true pressure reading due to stiff or calcified arteries, giving a false sense of security. Recently, a new pulse oximetric toe pressure method has been shown to be more reliable (40).

In the pathogenesis of ulceration, PVD is rarely the sole cause: a combination of risk factors in common. Thus, PVD together with minor trauma might permit infection, and the increase in blood supply cannot be met, resulting in a painful, infected ischemic ulcer. Perhaps more dangerous is the neuroischemic ulcer which is becoming more common in diabetic foot clinics. The neuropathic patient might not experience the pain of claudication, and, unless examined for, early PVD might be missed in such a patient. Similarly, ulcer development might go unnoticed in such a patient.

4.4. Foot Pressure Abnormalities in Diabetic Patients

As noted above, the insensate diabetic neuropathic does not spontaneously ulcerate. Traumatic ulcers result as a consequence of trauma to the insensate foot, as in the patient who purchases shoes of insufficient size and fails to experience any discomfort whilst wearing them. Pressure ulcers on the plantar surface of the foot result as a consequence of pressure that would not normally cause ulceration, but which because of intrinsic abnormalities of the neuropathic foot, leads to plantar ulceration when repetitively applied. Abnormalities of pressures and loads under the diabetic foot are very common as confirmed in cross-sectional studies (41). Thus, the combination of insensitivity, abnormally high foot pressures and repetitive stress from, for example, walking, may lead to break down under high-pressure areas such as the metatarsal head. In a prospective study, Veves et al. (42) observed a 28% incidence of ulceration in neuropathic feet with high plantar pressures during a 2.5-year follow-up period. In contrast, no ulcers developed in patients with normal pressure. Thus, biomechanics, the branch of science concerned with the consequences of forces applied to living tissues, is clearly relevant to diabetic foot disease since the majority of neuropathic foot ulcers result from repetitive stress which is not perceived by patients.

A number of methodologies are available to assess plantar pressures and may be useful in research studies (24). More recently, a semiquantitative estimation of pressure distribution based upon the Harris mat technique has been developed and is known as "Podotrack" or "Pressurestat." This is a portable and expensive device with disposable methodology that has been confirmed as a useful screening tool to identify areas under the neuropathic foot at risk of ulceration (43).

4.4.1. Callus

The presence of plantar callus, especially in the neuropathic foot, is associated with an increased risk of ulceration. In one study, the risk was 77-fold increased in the cross-sectional part, whereas in the prospective follow-up, ulceration only occurred at sites of callus, representing an infinite increase in risk (44).

4.4.2. Edema

The presence of peripheral edema impairs local blood supply and has been associated with an increased risk of ulceration (25,37).

4.4.3. Postural Instability

Poor balance and instability are increasingly being recognized as troublesome symptoms of diabetic neuropathies, presumably secondary to loss of proprioception. The relationship between body sway, postural instability, and foot ulceration has been confirmed (45).

4.4.4. Deformity

Any deformity occurring in a diabetic foot, such as prominence of the metatarsal heads, clawed toes, Charcot prominences, or hallux valgus, increases ulcer risk (30,31).

4.4.5. Previous Foot Ulceration

Several studies have confirmed that foot ulceration is most common in those patients with a past history of ulceration or amputation, and also in those from a poor social background. Indeed, annual occurrence rates of up to 50% have been reported (24).

5. THE PATHWAY TO ULCERATION

For one mistake made for not knowing, ten mistakes are made for not looking.

—*J.A. Lindsay*

It is a combination of factors that results in ulceration of the diabetic foot. Reiber et al. (25) assessed the component causes that when combined, completed the causal chain that resulted in ulceration. Of all the individual component causes, neuropathy was the most important being present in 78% of new foot ulcer cases. The commonest combination of risk factors occurring together was neuropathy, deformity, and trauma. Deformity was frequent prominence of the metatarsal heads and clawing of the toes, and the trauma was most frequency inappropriate footwear. As Lindsay pointed out, the essential factor in the identification of the patient at risk of foot ulceration is the careful clinical examination of the foot after shoes and socks have been removed. A simple assessment of the presence of neuropathy, vascular disease, abnormal shape, skin texture, circulation and so on will help in the identification of the patient at increased risk of what should be a preventable problem.

6. CHARCOT NEUROARTHROPATHY

Charcot neuropathy is a rare and disabling condition affecting the bones and joints of the feet. It particularly affects patients with long-standing diabetes who have both somatic and autonomic peripheral neuropathy, but in whom the peripheral circulation is intact (24,46). Diabetes is now the commonest cause of Charcot neuroarthropathy in the Western world and should be suspected in any diabetic patient with no neuropathy who presents with a warm and swollen foot. Although traditionally, texts state that the Charcot foot is painless, up to 50% of patients may experience nonspecific pain and discomfort in the affected foot. Although the pathogenesis of the Charcot foot is poorly understood, it is generally believed to occur in patients with moderate-to-severe sensorimotor neuropathy whose feet are subjected to repetitive minor trauma which often goes unnoticed. Less commonly, there is a clear history of a significant injury. The acute condition may be mistaken for osteomyelitis or inflammatory arthropathy. The foot is warm and one useful diagnostic test is to compare the skin temperature with the contralateral foot. The Charcot foot is usually at least 2°C warmer than the unaffected foot.

Treatment goals in Charcot neuropathy are firstly to have a high index of suspicion and to aim for early diagnosis. In the very early stages, there may not be specific abnormalities on x-ray examination but later typical changes include bone and joint destruction, fragmentation, and remodeling in advanced cases. The joints most frequently affected are those of the mid-foot, especially the cuneiform-metatarsal area, but up to 10% may occur at the ankle level. Bone scans initially demonstrate increased blood flow and bone uptake and to exclude incidental osteomyelitis, and indium-labeled white cell scan or MRI examination may be required. Once diagnosed, the treatment goals are to reduce disease activity, to achieve stable joint and to reduce deformity. Initial treatment involving mobilization usually using a cast and very recent evidence suggests that bisphosphonates such as Pamidronate may be useful in reducing disease activity in the early stage (47). In the later stages, when the foot has achieved a stable shape, surgery may be necessary to remove bony lumps and more extensively constructive surgery has in some centers led to excellent clinical results (24).

REFERENCES

1. Joslin EP. The menace of diabetic gangrene. N Engl J Med 1934; 211:16–20.
2. Boulton AJM. The diabetic foot—from art to science. Diabetologia 2004; 47:1343–1353.
3. Brand PW. The diabetic foot. In: Ellenberg M, Rifkin H, eds. Diabetes Mellitus. Theory and Practice. 3rd ed. New York: Medical Examining Company, 1983:829–849.
4. Young MJ, Veves A, Breddy JL, Boulton AJM. The use of vibration perception thresholds to predict diabetic neuropathic foot ulceration: a prospective study. Diabetes Care 1994; 17:557–561.
5. Abbott CA, Vileikyte L, Williamson S, Carrington AL, Boulton AJM. Multicenter study of the incidence of and predictive risk factors for diabetic neuropathic foot ulceration. Diabetes Care 1998; 21:1071–1075.
6. Abbott CA, Carrington AL, Ashe H, Every L, Whalley A, Van Ross ERE, Boulton AJM. The North West diabetes foot care study: incidence of and risk factors for new diabetic foot ulceration in a community-based cohort. Diabetic Medicine 2002; 19:377–384.

7. Boulton AJM, Vileikyte L. Diabetic foot problems and their management around the world. In: Bowker JH, Pfeifer MA, eds. Levin and O'Neal's The Diabetic Foot. 6th ed. Mosby: St. Louis, 2001:261–271.

8. Resnick HE, Valsania P, Phillips CL. Diabetes mellitus and nontraumatic lower extremity amputation in black and white Americans: the national health and nutrition examination survey epidemiologic follow-up study 1971–1992. Arch Intern Med 1999; 159:2470–2475.

9. Karter AJ, Ferrara A, Liiu JY, Moffet HH, Ackerson LM, Selby JV. Ethnic disparities in diabetic complications in an insured population. JAMA 2002; 287:2519–2527.

10. Leggetter SY, Chaturvedi N, Fuller JH, Edmonds ME. Ethnicity and risk of diabetes-related lower-extremity amputation: a population-based, case-control study of African Caribbeans and Europeans in the United Kingdom. Arch Intern Med 2002; 162:73–78.

11. Chaturvedi N, Abbott CA, Whalley A, Widdows P, Leggetter SY, Boulton AJM. Risk of diabetic-related amputation in Sough Asians vs. Europeans in the UK. Diabetic Med 2002; 19:99–104.

12. Manes C, Papazoglou N, Sassidou E, Soulisk K, Milarakis D, Satsoglou A, Sakallerou A. Prevalence of diabetic neuropathy and foot ulceration: identification of potential risk factors—a population-based study. Wounds 2002; 14:11–15.

13. Muller IS, de Grauw WJ, van Gerwen WH, Bartelink ML, Rutton GE. Foot ulceration and lower-limb amputation in type 2 diabetic patients in Dutch primary health care. Diabetes Care 2002; 25:570–574.

14. Ramsey SD, Newton K, Blough D, McCulloch DK, Sandhu N, Reiber GE, et al. Incidence, outcomes and cost of foot ulcers in patients with diabetes. Diabetes Care 1999; 22:382–387.

15. Vozar J, Adamka J, Holeczy P, Seilingerova R. Diabetics with foot lesions and amputations in the region of Horny Zitny Ostrov 1993–1995. Diabetologia 1997; 40(suppl 1): A465.

16. Moss S, Klein R, Klein B. The prevalence and incidence of lower extremity amputation in a diabetic population. Am Intern Med 1992; 152:610–616.

17. Trautner C, Haastert B, Spraul M, Giani G, Berger M. Unchanged incidence of lower-limb amputations in a German city, 1990–1998. Diabetes Care 2001; 24:855–859.

18. Trautner C, Haastert B, Giani G, Berger M. Amputations and diabetes: a case control study. Diabetic Med 2002; 19:35–40.

19. Consensus development conference on diabetic wound care. Diabetes Care 1999; 22:1354–1360.

20. Assal JP, Mehnert H, Tritschler HJ, Sidorenko A, Keen H. 'On your feet' workshop on the diabetic foot. J Diabet Comp 2002; 16:183–194.

21. Holzer SES, Camerota A, Martens L, Cuerdon T, Crystal-Peters J, Zagari M. Costs and duration of care for lower extremity ulcers in patients with diabetes. Clin Ther 1998; 20:518–524.

22. Harrington C, Zagari MJ, Corea J, Klitenic J. A cost analysis of diabetic lower-extremity ulcers. Diabetes Care 2000; 23:1333–1338.

23. Tennvall GR, Apelqvist J. Prevention of diabetes-related foot ulcers and amputations: a cost–utility analysis based on Markov model simulations. Diabetologia 2001; 44: 2077–2087.

24. Boulton AJM, Kirsner RS, Vileikyte L. Neuropathic diabetic foot ulcers. N Engl J Med 2004; 351:48–55.

25. Reiber GE, Vileikyte L, Boyko EJ, Del Aguila M, Smith DG, Lavery LA, Boulton AJM. Casual pathways for incident lower-extremity ulcers in patients with diabetes from two settings. Diabetes Care 1999; 22:157–162.

26. Boulton AJM, Malik RA. Diabetic neuropathy. Med Clin N Am 1998; 82:909–929.

27. Partanen J, Niskanen L, Lehtinen J, Siitonen OI. Natural history of peripheral neuropathy in patients with non-insulin dependent diabetes mellitus. N Eng J Med 1995; 333: 89–96.

28. Tesfaye S, Stavers L, Stephenson J, Fuller JH, Pozza G, Ward JD. Prevalence of diabetic peripheral neuropathy and its relation to glycaemic control and potential risk factors: the Eurodiab IDDM Complication Study. Diabetologia 1996; 39:1377–1384.

29. Cahezas-Cerrato J. The prevalence of clinical diabetic polyneuropathy in Spain. Diabetologia 1998; 41:1263–1969.

30. Lavery LA, Gazewood JD. Assessing the feet of people with diabetes. J Fam Pract 2000; 49(suppl):S9–S16.

31. Lavery LA, Armstrong DG, Vela SA, Quebedeaux TL, Fleischli JG. Practical criteria for screening patients at high risk for diabetic foot ulceration. Arch Intern Med 1998; 158:157–162.

32. Mayfield JA, Sugarman JR. The use of the Semmes–Weinstein monofilament and other threshold tests for preventing foot ulceration and amputation in persons with diabetes. J Fam Pract 2000; 49(suppl):S17–S29.

33. Boyko EJ, Ahroni JH, Stengel V, Forsberg RC, Davignon DR, Smith DG. A prospective study of risk factors for diabetic foot ulcers: the Seattle Diabetic Foot Study. Diabetes Care 1999; 22:1036–1042.

34. Litzelman DK, Marriott DJ, Vinicor F. Independent physiological predictors of foot lesions in patients with NIDDM. Diabetes Care 1997; 20:1273–1278.

35. Carrington AL, Shaw JE, Van Schie CHM, Abbott CA, Vileikyte L, Boulton AJM. Can motor nerve conduction velocity predict foot problems in diabetes over a six-year outcome period? Diabetes Care 2002; 25:2010–2015.

36. Abbott RD, Brand FN, Kannel WB. Epidemiology of some peripheral arterial findings in diabetic men and women: experiences from the Framingham Study. Am J Med 1990; 88:376–381.

37. Pecoraro R, Reiber GE, Burgess EM. Pathways to diabetic limb amputation. Diabetes Care 1990; 13:513–521.

38. Siitonen OI, Niskanen LK, Laakso M, Siitonen JF, Pyorala K. Lower extremity amputation in diabetic and non-diabetic patients: a population-based study in Eastern Finland. Diabetes Care 1993; 16:16–20.

39. Adler AJ, Steens RJ, Neil A, Stratton IM, Boulton AJM, Holman RR. UKPDS 59: hyperglycemia and other potentially modifiable risk factors for peripheral vascular disease in type 2 diabetes. Diabetes Care 2002; 25:894–899.

40. Johansson KEA, Marklund BRG, Fowelin JHR. Evaluation of a new screening method for detecting peripheral arterial disease is a primary health care population of patients with diabetes. Diabetic Med 2002; 19:307–310.

41. Frykberg RG, Lavery LA, Pham H, Harvey C, Armstrong DG, Harkless LB, Veves A. Role of neuropathy and high foot pressures in diabetic foot ulceration. Diabetes Care 1998; 21:1714–1719.

42. Veves A, Murray HJ, Young MJ, Boulton AJM. The risk of foot ulceration in diabetic patients with high foot pressure: a prospective study. Diabetologia 1992; 35:660–663.

43. Van Schie CMH, Abbott CA, Vileikyte L, Shaw JE, Hollis S, Boulton AJM. A comparative study of the Podotrack, a simple semiquantitative plantar pressure measuring device, and the optical pedobarograph in the assessment of pressures under the diabetic foot. Diabetic Med 1999; 16:154–159.

44. Murray HJ, Young MJ, Hollis S, Boulton AJM. The association between callus formation, high pressures and neuropathy in diabetic foot ulceration. Diabetic Med 1996; 13:979–983.

45. Katoulis EC, Ebdon-Parry M, Hollis S, Vileikyte L, Van Ross ERE, Boulton AJM. Postural instability in diabetic neuropathic patients at risk of foot ulceration. Diabetic Med 1997; 14:296–300.

46. Shaw JE, Boulton AJM. The Charcot foot. Foot 1995; 5:65–70.

47. Jude EB, Selby PL, Burgess J, Lilleystone P, Mawer EB, Page SR, Foster AV, Edmonds ME, Boulton AJM. Bisphosphonates in the treatment of Charcot neuroarthropathy: a double-blind randomised controlled trial. Diabetologia 2001; 44:2032–2037.

16

Practical Local Treatment of the Diabetic Foot Wound

David G. Armstrong
*Department of Surgery, Doctor William M. Scholl College of Podiatric Medicine,
Rosalind Franklin University of Medicine and Science, Chicago, Illinois, U.S.A.*

Lawrence A. Lavery
*Department of Surgery, Scott & White Memorial Hospital,
Texas A&M University College of Medicine, Temple, Texas, U.S.A.*

Andrew J. M. Boulton
*Division of Endocrinology, Diabetes and Metabolism, University of Miami School of
Medicine, Miami, Florida, U.S.A. and Department of Medicine, University of
Manchester, Manchester, U.K.*

1. INTRODUCTION

For the short life of "modern" medical history, treatment of wounds in general and diabetic foot wounds specifically has been identified as a branch of therapeutics that is decidedly unappealing and lacking in merit. This has changed in recent years, as is clearly illustrated by works such as this text. The purpose of this chapter is to discuss and identify specific treatments for active wounds and potential therapies for prevention. To do this, we will revisit the pathogenesis of wounds of the diabetic foot and then specifically identify intervention strategies to treat and prevent wounds.

2. PATHWAYS TO ULCERATION: CURRENT CONCEPTS

The fundamental pathway leading to foot ulceration in persons with diabetes involves a number of factors. Understanding the causal pathway and risk factors is an essential part of evaluating treatment strategies.

Neuropathy is a major component of most diabetic ulcerations, being present in over 82% of diabetic patients with foot wounds (1,1a). It is this lack of sensation when combined with unaccommodated structural deformity, that exposes the patient to undue sudden or repetitive stress, eventual tissue breakdown, subsequent infection, and possible amputation (2). Neuropathy alone, however, is generally not enough to cause ulceration. In most cases, foot deformity and repetitive stress on that deformity must also be present. Regions of high planter pressure are directly associated with foot deformity. When this abnormal focus of pressure is coupled with lack of painful feedback (neuropathy) and varying degrees of stress, the result can be a foot ulcer. There are two main mechanisms by which refers to prolonged low pressure over a small radius of curvature (i.e., bunion or hammertoe deformity). This usually results in wounds over the medial, lateral, and dorsal prominence of the forefoot. The second and most common mechanism involves prolonged repetitive moderate stress. This normally occurs on the planter aspect of the foot, secondary to prominent metatarsal heads with an atrophied or anteriorly displaced fat pad. The other mechanism of skin breakdown in the insensate diabetic foot (puncture wounds and thermal injuries) are not related to foot deformity. The deformities listed above are believed to be more common in the diabetic due to atrophy of the intrinsic musculature responsible for stabilizing the digits as well as increased prevalence of limited joint mobility (3,4).

2.1. Debridement and Offloading

Wound debridement is a critical element of wound care. Debridement should reduce or eliminate factors that can impede healing and stimulate the normal wound-healing cascade. The objective of debriding a wound is to remove nonviable tissue and chronic inflammatory byproducts (5–7). Surgical debridement can help "convert" a chronic wound to an acute one. There are a variety of techniques to debride a wound with little specific documentation addressed in the medial literature to compare chemical, mechanical, insect, or surgical methods (8). In patients with adequate blood flow, surgical debridement and excision of devitalized tissue is preferable. Steed et al. (9), in an important post hoc analysis of patients enrolled in a randomized controlled trial of topical growth factors, reported that significantly more patients healed in centers that had more frequent wound debridement regardless of the treatment group.

2.1.1. Maggot Debridement Therapy

In patients for whom surgical debridement is not appropriate, such as those with marginal vascular perfusion to the extremity, we have found maggot debridement therapy (MDT) to be a useful adjunct. Maggots have been shown to be safe and effective to treat difficult wounds (10). This technique is relatively inexpensive and not technically demanding. It is surprisingly well tolerated by patients.

3. OFFLOADING: CURRENT CONCEPTS

Reducing pressure and shear forces on the foot is a pivotal part of ulcer healing. Unfortunately, it may be the most neglected aspect of ulcer care. We observe in many centers that persons with diabetic foot ulcers walk out with the same shoes that contributed to the development of the ulceration in the first place.

Total contact casting (TCC) has been called the gold standard modality in offloading the diabetic foot (8). Total contact casting is perhaps one of the most extensively studied methods to facilitate wound healing in persons with diabetes and leprosy. Without question, it is as effective at offloading the foot as any other existing therapeutic modality Table 1 (11).

Table 1   A Review of Healing Times by Offloading Modality

Modality	Author	Type of ulcer	Mean healing time	Percentage healed
Total contact cast	Myerson	Wagner grades I and II	Forefoot ulcers: 30.0 days Midfoot/hindfoot ulcers: 63.0 Days	90%
Total contact cast	Helm	Wagner grades I, II, and III	38.3 days	73%
Total contact cast	Mueller	Wagner grades I and II	42.0 days	90%
Total contact cast	Sinacore	Not reported	43.6 days	82%
Total contact cast	Walker	Wagner grade I, II, and III	Forefoot ulcers: 30.6 days Nonforefoot ulcers: 42.1 days	Not reported
Total contact cast	Armstrong	Meggitt–Wagner grade I	38.8 days	100%
Total contact cast	Lavery	Meggitt–Wagner grade I	Midfoot ulcers: 28.4 days	100%
Half-shoe	Chantelau	Apelqvist grades I, II, III, and IV	70 days	96%
Insoles	Holstein	Not reported	108 days	97%
Custom splint	Boninger	Not reported	300 days	Not reported
TCC, Aircast boot, half-shoe	Armstrong	Wagner grade I	TCC=Aircast= half-shoe=	TCC=Aircast= half shoe=
Scotch cast boot	Knowles	Wagner grades I, II, and III	130.5 ± 106.7 days	80%

Our group published results of a randomized clinical trial comparing the proportion of healing of ulcers treated with the TCC compared with two other readily available and popular devices: removable cast walkers and half shoes. We found that a significantly higher proportion of patients healed in the TCC compared with either of the other devices (12). One additional interesting aspect of the study above was the evaluation of activity in the three groups. Interestingly, we found that approximately the same activity level between patients wearing a TCC compared to those wearing a removable cast walker. Previous studies have suggested that certain removable cast walkers (including the one reviewed in the above study) reduce pressure in the laboratory approximately as well as the TCC (13,11). One may therefore rightly question why a higher proportion of patients healed in the TCC than in the removable cast walker. Logical arguments would be either that pressure reduction is unimportant (and that some other characteristic of the cast promotes healing better than other modalities) or that patients remove their removable cast walker and walk without protective footwear. Certainly, there have been numerous studies that have suggested that plantar pressure is an important aspect in the pathogenesis and healing of diabetic foot wounds (14–19). There have been two descriptive reports in the literature evaluating compliance with offloading modalities in persons at high risk for lower extremity amputation (both of them evaluating shoes).

Knowles and coworkers identified that of patients at high risk for ulceration, only 22% of the 50-patient population regularly wore their protective shoes.(20) Armstrong et al. (21) evaluated a similar patient population using a novel computerized, Internet based continuous activity monitor. In this study, only 15% of patients indicated that they wore their shoes at home, a place where they took over 50% of their daily activity. Based on these results and our clinical experience in patients with profound neuropathy, we would suggest that the easier a device is to remove, the more difficult it may be for the patient to reapply.

The removable cast walker is a very attractive offloading device. It is probably less expensive than the repetitive application of total contact casts in terms of time and material costs. It requires very little training to apply. It is reusable and is in our experience better tolerated than a total contact cast by many patients and clinicians. We would argue that the least attractive attribute of the removable cast walker is its ease of removal. Over the past several years, we have used a technique that incorporates the ease of use of a ready-made removable cast boot and the "forced compliance" (22) that is available with a total contact cast. One may use the removable cast walker of their choice for this technique. We generally prefer either the Aircast removable cast walker (Aircast, Summit, NJ, U.S.A.) or the DH Pressure Relief Walker (Centec Orthopaedics, Camarillo, CA, U.S.A.). The devices can be applied in the recommended manner. As is warranted, one may also consider applying cast padding to the leg of these patients. We will then apply two layers of 4-in. cohesive bandage or plaster of Paris around the removable cast walker (Figs. 1–3). If utilizingz the plaster of Paris, the device should be covered with 14-in. cohesive bandage or stockinette prior to application of plaster of Paris to prevent soiling of the removable cast walker from the plaster and to facilitate its repeated use. Care should be taken not to extend proximal to the foam padding of the walker to avoid any skin irritation or impingement of the common peroneal nerve as it courses near the fibular head. If one wants to cover the toes to protect from foreign objects entering the cast walker, then one should consider padding the digits well using self adhesive foam (Reston foam, 3M, St. Paul, MN, U.S.A.) as is used on the same area in a TCC. The clinician may then consider dispensing a cast protector to allow the patient to shower more easily. Alternatively, the patient may use a large, thick trash bag to protect the cast walker. This simple technique provides quick and effect mechanism to protect the foot from repetitive injury by converting a removable cast walker into a device that cannot be easily removed by the patient.

4. ACTIVITY MONITORING

Activity level is one of the key factors determining the success or failure of treatment regimes instituted in foot care, in particular, or in medicine, in general. I believe that objectively monitoring this level and using this information to modulate our patients' course may certainly improve our ability to assist in caring for our patients and helping them care for themselves.

Over the past few years, a number of research groups have embarked on projects that use pedometers (step counters) to monitor and document activity levels (23,12,24–26). These devices range in complexity from the very simple (Sportline, Campbell, CA, U.S.A., US$17.95) to the sophisticated device used in the present study (Sportbrain, Sunnyvale, CA, U.S.A., US$99.00). The most simple of these

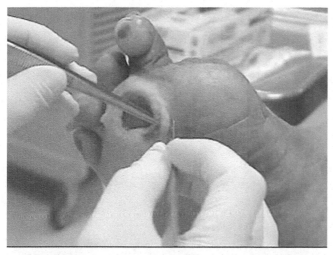

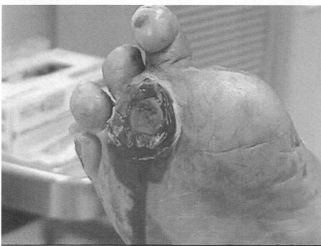

Figure 1 Appropriate debridement of a plantar forefoot ulcer. Note all undermining and non-viable tissue has been removed from the periphery. This is commonly performed with a scalpel or a tissue nipper.

devices merely count steps and rely on the patient to record them judiciously in a logbook which is provided them. The more sophisticated devices upload their information to a webpage, which can then be monitored graphically continuously by the clinician and patient.

In using these devices clinically, my group has previously anecdotally observed that many high-risk patients take nearly as many steps at home as they do while working. It appears as though this anecdotal observation was supported by the data collected in this study. This observation is true despite the fact that most of our offloading modalities are designed to be removable and are, in many instances, removed immediately by the patients when he or she arrives at home. Additionally, by using activity monitors that time-stamp steps have taken, it has been possible to identify hidden pockets of activity which can be modified at home or at the workplace to better suit the status of the patient. For example, a patient

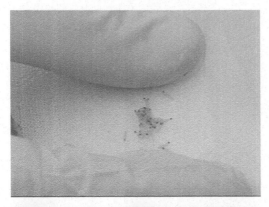

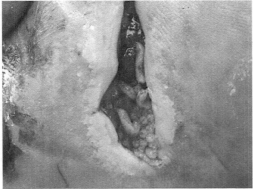

Figure 2   Therapeutic larvae (maggots) are a potentially effective means of adjunctive debridement for necrotic diabetic foot wounds.

with a history of diabetic foot ulceration might be able to use this technology coupled with dermal thermometry (27) to monitor and dose their activity with the clinician as guide much in the way they monitor their blood glucose and dose their insulin. A patient with ill-defined heel pain may be able to log the points during the day when he/she notices onset of pain and then compare this to his/her activity level (as measured by the pedometer) at or before the onset of symptoms. A competitive

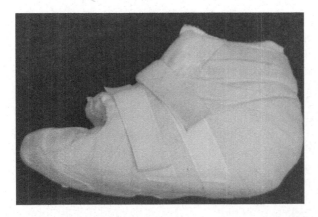

Figure 3   The Scotchcast boot.

athlete having undergone reconstructive foot surgery may be able to begin rehabilitation using objective goals of activity rather than merely allowing pain to be his/her guide. I see a time when formulas may be instituted for medical and surgical intervention that take not only the patients' age, sex, and medical history into account, but also their specific objectively measured level of activity.

To date, there have been numerous studies which have used activity monitors to evaluate groups of patients. Research in the area of claudication (28), prosthesis wear (25), chronic obstructive pulmonary disease (24), diabetes control (26), diabetic foot ulcer recurrence (23), and offloading wounds (12) have all suggested that activity level plays a significant role in outcomes of many disparate maladies. I believe that more robust work in these different areas of medicine will potentially yield even more information about the care of patients.

4.1. Therapeutic Shoes and Insoles

One of the mainstays of programs designed to reduce ulcer occurrence or recurrence involves the use of therapeutic shoes with accommodative insoles to accommodate high-pressure areas on the sole of the foot. Unfortunately, at the present time, there is little scientific information to help clinicians make decisions about shoe and insole design or material selection.

However, therapeutic shoes and insoles represent a relatively inexpensive intervention strategy that can make a substantial impact on the prevalence of pathology (29–33). In the United States, congressional legislation has provided funding for Medicare recipients with diabetes to receive one pair of therapeutic shoes and three pairs of insoles each year (34,35).

Therapeutic shoes and viscoelastic inserts are commonly used as an artificial shock absorber in high-risk diabetics to prevent the development of neuropathic foot ulcerations by decreasing pressure on the sole of the foot. By providing an extrinsic mechanism (viscoelastic insoles) to reduce pressure on the sole of the foot, the risk of developing an ulceration can be substantially reduced (Uccioli). Clinical studies by Uccioli and Chantelau suggest that the development of new ulcerations in high-risk diabetics can be significantly decreased with therapeutic footwear and insoles. However, even in treatment groups that received therapeutic footwear and insoles, the rate of ulceration was still very high, 28% and 50%.

Chantelau found that patients who were compliant with wearing therapeutic footwear were significantly less likely to ulcerate than subjects who did not (36). The results of the present project indicate that therapeutic shoes are worn primarily during periods outside the home, with little attention being given to the period while the patient is in the home—a period amounting to at least one-half of the daily activity of these high risk patients. It would stand to reason that more attention paid to accommodation of these patients during nonworking hours through use of modalities such as accommodative slippers or sandals might be an effective means of improving compliance with this potentially effective prophylactic regime.

5. CONCLUSION

In this brief chapter, we have revisited the etiology and effective local treatment of the diabetic foot including debridement, offloading, and activity modulation. We believe that consistently addressing these local factors, coupled with the critical factors of infection, control and vascular intervention can and will, with dissemination, reduce the unnecessarily high incidence of lower extremity ulceration and amputation which exists today.

REFERENCES

1. Pecoraro RE, Reiber GE, Burgess EM. Pathways to diabetic limb amputation: basis for prevention. Diabetes Care 1990; 13:513–521.
1a. Singh N, Armstrong DG, Lipsky BA. Preventing foot ulcers in patients with diabetes. JAMA 2005; 293(2): 217–228.
2. Brand PW. The insensitive foot (including leprosy). In: Jahss M, ed. Disorders of the Foot and Ankle. Philadelphia: Saunders, 1991:2170–2175.
3. Fernando DJ, Masson EA, Veves A, Boulton AJ. Relationship of limited joint mobility to abnormal foot pressures and diabetic foot ulceration. Diabetes Care 1991; 14(1):8–11.
4. Rosenbloom AL. Skeletal and joint manifestations of childhood diabetes. Pediatr Clin North Am 1984; 31:569–589.
5. Armstrong DG, Jude EB. The role of matrix metalloproteinases in wound healing. J Am Podiatr Med Assoc 2002; 92(1):12–18.
6. Jude EB, Rogers AA, Oyibo SO, Armstrong DG, Boulton AJM. Matrix metalloproteinase and tissue inhibitor of metalloproteinase expression in diabetic and venous ulcers. Diabetologia 2001; 44(suppl 1):A3.
7. Nwomeh BC, Liang HX, Cohen IK, Yager DR. MMP-8 is the predominant collagenase in healing wounds and nonhealing ulcers. J Surg Res 1999; 81(2):189–195.
8. American Diabetes Association. Consensus Development Conference on diabetic foot wound care. Diabetes Care 1999; 22(8):1354.
9. Steed DL, Donohoe D, Webster MW, Lindsley L. Effect of extensive debridement and treatment on the healing of diabetic foot ulcers. Diabetic Ulcer Study Group. J Am Coll Surg 1996; 183(1):61–64.
10. Armstrong DG, Mossel J, Nixon BP, Knowles EA, Boulton AJM. Maggot debridement therapy: a primer. J Am Podiatr Med Assoc 2002a; 92:398–401.
11. Lavery LA, Vela SA, Lavery DC, Quebedeaux TL. Reducing dynamic foot pressures in high-risk diabetic subjects with foot ulcerations. A comparison of treatments. Diabetes Care 1996; 19(8):818–821.
12. Armstrong DG, Nguyen HC, Lavery LA, van Schie CH, Boulton AJM, Harkless LB. Offloading the diabetic foot wound: a randomized clinical trial. Diabetes Care 2001b; 24:1019–1022.
13. Baumhauer JF, Wervey R, McWilliams J, Harris GF, Shereff MJ. A comparison study of plantar foot pressure in a standardized shoe, total contact cast, and prefabricated pneumatic walking brace. Foot Ankle Int 1997; 18:26–33.
14. Boulton AJ, Betts RP, Franks CI, Newrick PG, Ward JD, Duckworth T. Abnormalities of foot pressure in early diabetic neuropathy. Diabet Med 1987a; 4(3):225–228.
15. Boulton AJ, Betts RP, Franks CI, Ward JD, Duckworth T. The natural history of foot pressure abnormalities in neuropathic diabetic subjects. Diab Res 1987b; 5:73.
16. Boulton AJ, Betts RP, Newrick PG, Ward JD. Foot pressure abnormalities—a sensitive marker of early sensory neuropathy. Diabetes 1986; 12A(suppl 1):35.
17. Boulton AJ, Hardisty CA, Betts RP, Franks CI, Worth RC, Ward JD, Duckworth T. Dynamic foot pressure and other studies as diagnostic and management aids in diabetic neuropathy. Diabetes Care 1983; 6(1):26–33.
18. Boulton AJM. The importance of abnormal foot pressure and gait in causation of foot ulcers. In: Connor H, Boulton AJM, Ward JD, eds. The Foot in Diabetes. Chichester: John Wiley and Sons, 1987:11–26.

19. Frykberg RG, Lavery LA, Pham H, Harvey C, Harkless L, Veves A. Role of neuropathy and high foot pressures in diabetic foot ulceration (In Process Citation). Diabetes Care 1998; 21(10):1714–1719.

20. Knowles EA, Boulton AJ. Do people with diabetes wear their prescribed footwear? Diabet Med 1996; 13(12):1064–1068.

21. Armstrong DG, Abu Rumman PL, Nixon BP, Boulton AJM. Continuous activity monitoring in persons at high risk for diabetes-related lower extremity amputation. J Am Podiatr Med Assoc 2001a; 91:451–455.

22. Armstrong DG, Short B, Nixon BP, Boulton AJM. Technique for fabrication of an "instant" total contact cast for treatment of neuropathic diabetic foot ulcers. J Am Podiatr Med Assn 2002b; 92:405–408.

23. Ahrweiler F, Chantelau E. Recurrent vs. non-recurrent diabetic foot ulcer disease: impact of physical activity. Diabetologia 1997; 40(suppl 1):A486.

24. Barchfeld T, Schonhofer B, Jones P, Kohler D. Evaluation of daily activity in patients with COPD. Med Klin 1999; 94(1 Spec No):93–95.

25. Schmalzried TP, Szuszczewicz ES, Northfield MR, Akizuki KH, Frankel RE, Belcher G, Amstutz HC. Quantitative assessment of walking activity after total hip or knee replacement. J Bone Joint Surg Am 1998; 80(1):54–59.

26. Yamanouchi K, Shinozaki T, Chikada K, Nishikawa T, Ito K, Shimizu S, Ozawa N, Suzuki Y, Maeno H, Kato K, et al. Daily walking combined with diet therapy is a useful means for obese NIDDM patients not only to reduce body weight but also to improve insulin sensitivity. Diabetes Care 1995; 18(6):775–778.

27. Armstrong DG, Lavery LA. Predicting neuropathic ulceration with infrared dermal thermometry. J Amer Podiatr Med Assoc 1997; 87(7):336–337.

28. Sieminski DJ, Gardner AW. The relationship between free-living daily physical activity and the severity of peripheral arterial occlusive disease. Vasc Med 1997; 2(4):286–291.

29. Chantelau E, Kushner T, Spraul M. How effective is cushioned therapeutic footwear in protecting diabetic feet? A clinical study. Diabet Med 1990; 7(4):335–339.

30. Edmonds ME, Blundell MP, Morns ME, Thomas EM, Cotton LT, Watkins PJ. Improved survival of the diabetic foot: the role of a specialized foot clinic. Q J Med 1986; 60:763–771.

31. Lippman HI, Perrotto A, Farrar R. The neuropathic foot of the diabetic. Bull NY Acad Med 1976; 52:1159.

32. Litzelman DK, Marriott DJ, Vinicor F. The role of footwear in the prevention of foot lesions in patients with NIDDM. Conventional wisdom or evidence-based practice? Diabetes Care 1997; 20(2):156–162.

33. Uccioli L, Faglia E, Monticone G, Favales F, Durola L, Aldeghi A, Quarantiello A, Calia P, Menzinger G. Manufactured shoes in the prevention of diabetic foot ulcers. Diabetes Care 1995; 18(10):1376–1378.

34. Sugarman JR, Reiber GE, Baumgardner G, Prela CM, Lowery J. Use of the therapeutic footwear benefit among diabetic Medicare beneficiaries in three states, 1995. Diabetes Care 1998; 21(5):777–781.

35. Wooldridge J, Bergeron J, Thornton C. Preventing diabetic foot disease: lessons from the Medicare therapeutic shoe demonstration. Am J Public Health 1996; 86(7):935–938.

36. Chantelau E, Haage P. An audit of cushioned diabetic footwear: relation to patient compliance. Diabet Med 1994; 11(1):114–116.

17

Skin Changes and Wound Care After Radiation Injury

Stefanie J. Schluender
Department of Surgery, The Mount Sinai Medical Center, New York, New York, U S A

Felicia A. Mendelsohn
Department of Internal Medicine, Yale University School of Medicine, New Haven, Connecticut, U.S.A.

Celia M. Divino
Division of General Surgery, The Mount Sinai School of Medicine, New York, New York, U.S.A.

1. INTRODUCTION

Radiotherapy has proved an effective modality for cancer treatment with more than 50% of all cancer patients undergoing some form of radiation treatment. It has been reported as curative in several malignancies including, Hodgkin's lymphoma, seminoma, basal cell, and squamous carcinomas of the head and neck (1). Radiotherapy has demonstrated efficacy in reducing local recurrence and producing downstaging as adjuvant therapy and has been used as palliation for unresectable malignancies. Radiation-induced skin and subcutaneous tissue damage is the most common side effect of radiotherapy with up to 95% of the patients experiencing some degree of reaction (2–4). As the efficacy and application of radiotherapy has increased and the life expectancy of cancer patients has risen, there has been a corresponding rise in the number of patients suffering from radiation-induced injury despite improvements in radiation techniques. Ionizing radiation produces functional and morphological changes in noncancerous tissue. These complications can range from mild skin reactions to nonhealing ulcers that are susceptible to life-threatening infections (5). Energy transference from ionizing radiation generates highly reactive chemical products with a burst of free radicals that react with proteins, lipids, and carbohydrates to ultimately cause damage to cellular and nuclear membranes and deoxyribonucleic acid (DNA). Morbidity of radiation is dependent on the individual cell sensitivity, rate dose accumulation, volume of tissue irradiated, quality or type of radiation, chemotherapy, and surgical trauma (6).

2. RADIATION THERAPY

The unit of radiation dose is the Gray (Gy) which equals 1 J of energy absorbed per 1 kg of tissue or 100 rad. Radiation used in cancer treatments can be delivered by beam sources or brachytherapy. For external beam radiotherapy, megavoltage photon irradiation is given by cobalt-60 sources (gamma rays) or high-energy linear accelerators (x-rays). Brachytherapy, however, uses radioactive sources adjacent to or within tumors, allowing high dosages to be delivered to the area immediately adjacent to the source.

With low-dose radiation exposure, such as one dose of 100 mGy, single-strand DNA breaks may be produced, but are rapidly repaired using the intact DNA strand as a guide. With higher doses of radiation, between 0.5 and 5 Gy, cellular death usually occurs after one or more reproductive divisions and is usually the result of irreparable double-strand DNA breaks. After doses of radiotherapy above 5 Gy, as used in cancer therapy, direct cell death occurs before reproductive division. This is known as "interphase death" and is a result of direct interaction of free radicals upon essential cellular enzymes and mechanisms (6).

Fractionation of doses can be used to minimize the injury to normal tissues during radiotherapy. The total dose of radiation is protracted over a period of time, reducing the adverse effects and allowing time for repair of sub-lethal injury and proliferation of healthy surviving cells. Similarly, a given dose of radiation administered at a high-dose rate produces more skin injury than the same total dose given at a low-dose rate. Larger doses of radiation may be tolerated if focused on highly specific regions, rather than distributed over larger areas (7).

3. EFFECTS OF RADIATION THERAPY

After low doses of radiation, immediate morphological changes occur in the nucleus with clumping of nuclear chromatin and swelling of the nucleus. With higher doses of radiation, the cell nucleus becomes dense and disfigured with loss of the nuclear membrane. The cytoplasm may demonstrate swelling, the mitochondria may be distorted, and the endoplasmic reticulum may degenerate (6). Low-dose cellular changes are due to an apoptotic mechanism, whereas high-dose changes are probably due to direct cellular necrosis.

Acute effects result from necrosis of the rapidly proliferative stem cell lines, including epithelial, endothelial, and mesenchymal cells. Radiation inhibits mitotic activity in the germinal cells of the epidermis, hair follicles, and sebaceous glands with resulting epilation and dryness. Acute vascular changes include degenerative changes of the basement membrane, increased vascular permeability and thrombosis with loss of capillary segments. A transient, faint erythema may appear during the first week of treatment due to dilatation of capillaries and is associated with an increase in vascular permeability. By the third or fourth week, erythema is localized to the radiation field accompanied by edema, warmth, and tenderness. Larger vessels such as arterioles are obstructed by fibrin thrombi with prominent edema and small foci of hemorrhage. If the total radiation dose does not exceed 3000 rad, the erythema phase is followed during the fourth or fifth week by the "dry desquamation" phase. This phase is characterized by pruritus, scaling, and an increase in melanin deposition in the basal layer. By two months, the inflammatory exudate and edema have subsided, leaving the skin healed, but hyperpigmented.

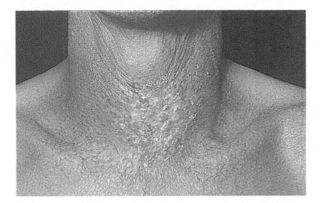

Figure 1 Deep, nonhealing radiation ulcer following bullous formation and necrosis.

If the total radiation dose is 4000 rad or greater, the erythema phase is followed by "moist desquamation." This stage begins in the fourth week and is accompanied by considerable discomfort. Suprabasal and subepidermal bullous formation occurs with eventual unroofing and possible loss of the entire irradiated epidermis. The edema and fibrinous exudate persist and re-epithelization of the denuded skin usually begins within 10 days (Fig. 1). Following high-dose radiation, melanocytes are often destroyed resulting in areas of hypopigmentation. Ulcers may appear at any time beginning two weeks after radiation exposure. Ulcers formed in the early stage are a result of direct necrosis of the epidermis and usually heal, but tend to recur (6,7).

Chronic effects of radiation are progressive and irreversible, caused by cellular dysfunction and involution with epithelial atrophy, fibroblast depletion and fibrosis,

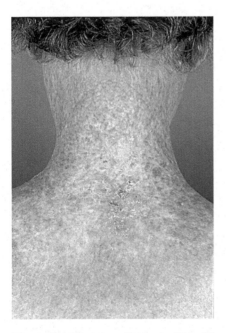

Figure 2 Chronic radiodermatitis with erythema, atrophy, keratosis, hypopigmentation, and hyperpigmentation.

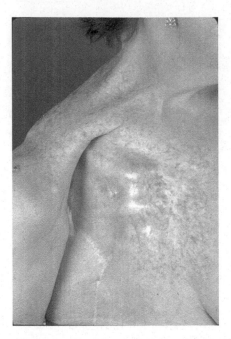

Figure 3 Telangectasias with reticular pattern and atrophic skin.

and endothelial necrosis (Fig. 2). One year after radiation treatment, the epidermis is thin, dry, and semi-translucent with telangiectasias (Fig. 3). Hair follicles, sebaceous glands, and sweat glands are absent. Collagen and subcutaneous adipose tissue become progressively replaced by dense fibrous tissue which leads to thickened, indurated skin with limitation of motion. A characteristic feature of radiation injury in soft tissues is the accumulation of fibrinous exudate under the epidermis. Delayed radiation lesions are also characterized by eccentric myointimal proliferation of the small arteries and arterioles (Fig. 4). These changes are progressive with thrombosis or complete obstruction and are compounded by the lack of angiogenesis secondary to endothelial stem cell loss and increasing fibrosis resulting in decreased tissue partial pressures of oxygen. Delayed ulcers are more common than acute ulcers and heal slowly, persisting for years (Fig. 5). The skin in the chronic stage

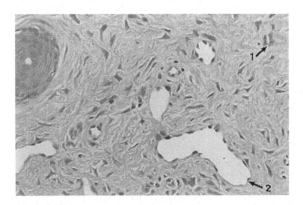

Figure 4 Histopathology of chronic radiation dermatitis (hematoxylin and eosin). Atypical fibroblasts (1) and telangiectasia (2) following radiation with dermal fibrosis.

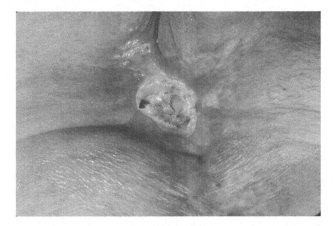

Figure 5 Chronic radiation dermatitis with evidence of atrophy and fibrosis of dermis and vessels.

is thin, hypovascular, painful, and injured by slight trauma or infection (6,7). Chronic radiation changes have the potential for tumorigenesis.

Individual patient factors have been defined to predict the severity of radiation reactions. These include radiosensitizers, anatomic site, genetics, age, comorbidity, and nutritional status (1). Combined modality treatment with chemotherapy enhances the effect of radiation on both malignant cells and normal cells. Adriamycin, actinomycin D, bleomycin sulfate, hydroxyurea, 5-fluorouracil, and methotraxate have the highest likelihood of creating an additive effect (8). In addition to chemotherapy, any drug that impairs the healing process can be associated with radiosensitizing, including steroids and NSAIDS. The anatomic site can also affect the increased sensitivity to radiotherapy. Areas of the body with appositional skin, such as the axilla, inframammary fold, groin, and perineum, are at increased risk secondary to moisture, warmth, and friction (9). Genetic syndromes associated with radiotherapy hypersensitivity include ataxia telangectasia, Bloom's syndrome, Fanconi's anemia, retinoblastoma, Down's syndrome, basal cell nevus syndrome, progeria, and cancer prone families (10,11). Personal characteristic also plays a role in the response to radiation. Increasing age is associated with poor healing overall due to decreased cell turnover with thinning of the epidermis, loss of collagen, and a decreased capillary network. Diabetes, autoimmune disorders, and collagen vascular diseases have all been associated with poor healing and increased infection rates for radiated skin. Nutritional status obviously plays an important role in healing and can be responsible for additional delay in healing. Studies concerning UV light exposure and cigarette use have yielded conflicting results.

4. TREATMENT OF RADIATION-INDUCED WOUNDS

Acute skin changes present primarily with erythema, appearing in the irradiated area approximately three weeks into treatment (12). Recommendations for care include gentle washing with water, saline, or a soap solution rinsed thoroughly to avoid excessive irritation. Powders, deodorant, lotions, perfumes, and cosmetics should be avoided and friction should be minimized by wearing loose cotton clothing and avoiding rubbing or shaving (9). Numerous skin-care products are available that can be used to reduce discomfort (Table 1). Eucerin® (Beiersdorf, Norwalk, CT) and Lubriderm® (Warner-Lambert, Morris Plains, NJ) are hydrophilic preparations that absorb water and act as mild lubricants. Protective ointments, such as A and D Ointment® (Schering, Kenilworth, NJ) or gels, are effective for protecting dry lesions. Any products that contain alcohol or menthol should be avoided due to loss of natural lipids.

Dry desquamation also may appear during this same time period; the treated area can appear red or tanned, dry, itchy, and peeling. All the products used for the erythematous reaction also can be applied in this situation. Eucerin® and Lubriderm® both protect and lubricate the scaly or flaking skin produced as a result of loss of sweat and sebaceous gland function (13). To decrease itching, products such as Aveeno Bath® (Rydelle Laboratories, Edison, NJ), cornstarch, and mild steroids (i.e., hydrocortisone cream 1%; Topicort®, Medicis, Scottsdale, AZ) can be used. Bathing daily, however, is not recommended due to the drying effect, unless a low-pH, moisturizing cleanser is used. Cornstarch should be avoided on moist skin, such as the axilla, breast, or groin, as it may promote a fungal infection. Corticosteroids should be used with caution to reduce itching, secondary to delayed healing by inhibiting inflammation and reducing blood flow. Steroids can also cause atrophy of dermal collagen, resulting in thinning of the skin and increased susceptibility to infection.

By the fourth week of treatment, moist desquamation may occur, especially with radiation treatment to the chest wall, supraclavicular region, axilla, groin, or intact breast. Care involves the use of astringent soaks, cleansers, antibiotics, and irrigations. Hydrogen peroxide has an antibacterial effect and is effective in cleansing wounds of purulent debris. Full-strength hydrogen peroxide is harmful to granulation tissue and should be avoided. Dressings that provide a barrier are used to protect from external contamination and infection, promote wound healing, prevent soiling of clothing, and prevent further irritation, friction, or shearing. Moistened dressings or soaks with an astringent precipitate protein and cleanse, dry, and seal exudative surfaces, preventing evaporative heat loss and decreasing inflammation and tissue dessication (Table 1). The dressing should be changed from 1 to 3 times daily depending on the drainage, except for hydrocolloids such as DuoDERM® CGF® (ConvaTec, A Bristol-Myes Squibb Company, Princeton, NJ) that may be left in place for 5–7 days. Tegaderm® (3M Health Care, St. Paul, MN) and Op-site® (Smith & Nephew, Largo, FL) do not adhere to areas with skin folds such as the axilla, but have advantages in comparison to hydrocolloids and hydrogels. The ability to irradiate through these thicker dressings without creating a bolus effect remains to be explored. All dressings discussed are beneficial due to the preservation of moisture enhancing re-epithelialization, enzymatic lysis of necrotic tissue, and inflammatory cell phagocytosis of necrotic debris and bacteria (14). If infection is proven by wound culture, topical antibiotics such as Neosporin® (Warner-Lambert, Morris Plains, NJ) or Bacitracin® (Warner-Lambert, Morris Plains, NJ) should be used, and a systemic antibiotic as indicated. Silver sulfadiazine 1% cream® (Watson Laboratories, Corona, CA) is recommended as an effective preparation against gram-positive and gram-negative organisms and Candida albicans.

In the long term, irradiated skin often results in chronic localized xerosis. Mild soaps and bath oils may be used during bathing. Lowila Cake® (Westwood-Squibb, Buffalo, NY) and Dove® (Lever Brothers, New York, NY) are neutral soap preparations made with synthetic detergents with a pH of < 7.5. Basis® (Beiersdorf, Norwalk, CT) contains higher amounts of fat, which leave a film of protective oil on the skin. Some skin cleansers, such as Aloe Veste 2-n-1 Body Wash and

Table 1 Skin Care Products Used for Different Radiation Skin Reactions

Erythema	Dry desquamation	Moist desquamation	Long-term treatments
Natural Care Gel®	All products used for erythema	Normal saline	Mild soaps (Lowila Cake®, Basis®, Dove®)
Special Care Cream®	Aloe Veste 2-n-1 Body Wash and Shampoo®	Sterile water	Bath oils (Alpha Keri®, Lubrex®)
Carrington Wound Gel®	Aveeno Bath®	Half- or third-strength hydrogen peroxide and water	Lubricants (petrolatum, mineral and baby oils, Eucerin®)
Eucerin®	Cornstarch (not in moist skin areas)	Domeboro Soaks®	Dry skin lotions (Alpha Keri®, Lubrex®, Lubriderm®, U-Lactin®)
Lubriderm®	Mild steroids (hydrocortisone cream 1%, Topicort®)	Biolex Wound Cleanser®	Creams (Alpha Keri®, Nivea®)
A and D Ointment®		Carra Klenz Wound Cleanser®	Thick preparations (Eucerin®, Aquaphor®)
Aloe Veste 2-n-1 Protective Ointment®		Film Dressings: Tegaderm®, Opsite®	
Avoid products containing alcohol or menthol		Hydrocolloid dressings: DuoDERM® CGF® Gel dressing: Vigilon®	

Natural Care Gel®, Special Care Cream®, Biolex Wound Cleanser® (Bard, Murray Hill, NJ); Carrington Wound Gel®, Cara Cleanse® (Carrington, Irving, TX); Eucerin®, Basis®, Nivea®, Aquaphor® (Beiersdorf, Norwalk, CT); Lubriderm® (Warner-Lambert, Morris Plains, NJ); A and D Ointment® (Schering, Kenilworth, NJ); Aveeno Bath® (Rydelle Laboratories, Edison, NJ); Topicort® (Medicis, Scottsdale, AZ); Domeboro Soaks® (Miles, West Haven, CT); Tegaderm® (3M Health Care, St. Paul, MN); Op-site® (Smith & Nephew, Largo, FL); DuoDERM® CGF® Extra Thin, DuoDERM® Hydroactive® Aloe Veste 2-n-1 Body Wash and Shampoo®, and Aloe Veste 2-n-1 Protective Ointment® (ConvaTec, A Bristol-Myers Squibb Company Princeton, NJ; Lowila Cake®, Alpha-Keri® (Westwood-Squibb, Buffalo, NY); Dove® (Lever Brothers, New York, NY); Lubrex®, U-Lactin® (T/I Pharmaceuticals, Irvine, CA); Vigilon® (Bard Medical Division, Covington, GA).

Table 2 Dressings and Skin and Substitutes Used for Severe Radiation Wounds That May Require Skin Grafting

Type of dressing	Applications
Biosynthetic and synthetic (Biobrane®, OpSite®, and Tegaderm®)	Biobrane: Protects clean, superficial, partial thickness burns; can be used to protect a wound between widely meshed autograft; also used for intermediate closure of an excised wound until autograft becomes available; Covers donor graft sites
	OpSite or Tegaderm: covers clean partial thickness wounds and donor sites; reduces pain from wounds; provides moist environment for re-epithelization
Artificial skin (Integra®)	Dermal substitute used for closure of excised full-thickness burns
Bioengineered skin (Apligraf®)	Indicated for chronic venous and diabetic foot ulcers; can serve many functions of human skin, including providing a barrier for the wound against mechanical damage and infection, producing structural and regulatory substances (e.g., growth factors or cytokines), and interacting with underlying tissue to promote more effective wound care; low antigenicity, greater likelihood of graft acceptance, and greater proliferative potential

Biobrane: Bertek, Morgantown, WV; OpSite: Smith & Nephew, Largo FL; Tegaderm: 3M Health Care, St Paul, MN; Integra: Integra Life Science, Plainsboro, NJ; Apligraf: Organogenesis, Canton, MA and Novartis Pharmaceuticals Corporation, East Hanover, NJ.

Shampoo® (ConvaTec, A Bristol-Meyers Squibb Company, Princeton, NJ), are formulated to cleanse and moisturize the skin while preserving naturally low pH. Lubricants such as petrolatum, mineral and baby oils, and Eucerin® are more effective, but tend to be less aesthetically pleasing. Dry skin lotions, creams, or thicker preparations may be used to lubricate the skin and prevent fissures.

Irradiated skin may appear normal after completion of radiotherapy, but changes may become evident, adversely affecting quality of life. With higher doses of radiation, more delayed changes such as fibrosis of tissues and small blood vessels should be expected. Patients should be instructed to protect treated skin from excessive sun exposure and trauma, due to the irradiated skin's inability to respond to trauma and delayed healing. In some rare cases, radiation wounds may be so severe that skin grafting is necessary and dressings used for thermal burns may be applied to the radiation wounds and donor graft sites (15–27) (Table 2).

5. EXPERIMENTAL TREATMENT STRATEGIES

Investigation into possible treatments for radiation-induced skin injury has included growth factors, cytokines, antioxidants, topical steroids, and nonsteroidal anti-inflammatory preparations, aloe vera, and lasers.

After tissue injury, transforming growth factor-Beta-1 (TGF-beta 1) is released from platelets to modulate chemotaxis of macrophages and fibroblasts, stimulate production of extracellular matrix, collagen, and fibronectin and increase angiogenesis. Studies demonstrate that TGF-beta 1 improved tensile strength, increased mature collagen, and improved flap survival (28) with increases in wound bursting strength (29). TGF-beta 1 is also considered to act as a master switch for tissue fibrosis in late radiation damage, causing remodeling of the extracellular matrix, decreased matrix-degrading proteases, and increased inhibitors of proteases (30–32). TGF-beta 1's ability to induce apoptosis can favor parenchymal damage and replacement by fibrotic tissue. Research has also been conducted to determine effectiveness of granulocyte-macrophage colony-stimulating factor (GM-CSF) in managing acute radiation dermatitis, based on its therapeutic effect in burn patients. Application of GM-CSF stimulates wound healing by promoting the migration and maturation of monocytes, increasing fibroplasia and keratinization, inducing the growth of new blood vessels, and promoting the chemotaxis of inflammatory cells. The most important role of GM-CSF is its stimulation of proliferation and differentiation of basal epithelial stem cells. The use of the GM-CSF impregnated gauze with steroid cream was shown with statistical significance to reduce the duration of symptoms, the healing period of radiation dermatitis, the pain, and the severity of radiation dermatitis when compared to steroid cream alone (33).

A growing body of evidence supports a causative role of oxidative stress in fibrogenesis. Super oxide dismutase (SOD) is a scavenging enzyme that catalyzes destruction of the superoxide anion radicals formed by irradiation. Results have been conflicting (34,35). Vitamin C has also been studied as an antioxidant and scavenger of peroxyl radicals for prevention of radiation dermatitis and improved collagen synthesis (36,37). Systemic ascorbic acid before whole-body radiation increased the dose of radiation required for skin desquamation (6). Topical ascorbic acid has been found to lack significant radioprotective effect due to poor absorption (37).

Topical corticosteroids are commonly prescribed for anti-inflammatory effects in radiation dermatitis. Acute and chronic effects of radiation are accompanied by production of prostaglandin, prostacyclin, thromboxane, and leukotriene responsible for vasodilatation, increased vascular permeability, thrombosis, and chemotaxis. Administration of glucocorticoid or NSAIDs attenuates the effects of radiation in humans (38). Hydrocortisone cream has demonstrated reduction in the erythematous skin reactions following radiotherapy, but requires further studies (39,40). Aloe vera gel has been studied as a prophylactic agent for radiation-induced skin toxicity (41,42). The three active compounds that may serve to decrease inflammation are carboxypeptidase (hydrolyzes bradykinin and angiotensin I), salicylic acid (inhibits prostaglandin synthesis), and magnesium lactate (antihistamine). Human studies demonstrate conflicting results when compared to placebo and soap (43,44).

Low-intensity helium-neon laser irradiation was demonstrated to have a beneficial effect on wound healing of recalcitrant skin ulcers after radiotherapy, enhancing metabolic pathways through ATPase, induction of reactive oxygen species, stimulation of calcium (Ca^{2+}) influx and mitosis rate, and formation of mRNA and protein secretion. Laser treatment also enhances cell proliferation and motility of fibroblasts and keratinocytes with improvement of skin circulation and induction of neoangiogenesis.

As the indications for radiotherapy increase along with cancer survival rates, the number of patients suffering from radiodermatitis will exponentially rise. The diagnosis and appropriate management of radiation-induced skin changes will prove an important clinical skill and there are promising developments for new treatment options.

ACKNOWLEDGMENTS

The authors thank Robert G. Phelps, MD, Associate Professor, Department of Pathology, Division of Dermatopathology, The Mount Sinai Medical Center, New York, NY for providing the histopathological sections and the NYU Department of Dermatology, New York, NY for providing the radiation dermatitis photographs.

REFERENCES

1. Porock D. Factors influencing the severity of radiation skin and oral mucosal reactions: development of a conceptual framework. Eur J Cancer Care 2002; 11:33–43.
2. King KB, Nail LM, Kreamer K, et al. Patients' descriptions of the experience of receiving radiation therapy. Oncol Nurs Forum 1985; 12:55–61.
3. De Conno F, Ventafridda V, Saita L. Skin problems in advanced and terminal cancer patients. J Pain Symptom Manage 1991; 6:247–255.
4. Porock D, Kristjanson L. Skin reactions during radiotherapy: the use and impact of topical agents and dressing. Eur J Cancer Care 1999; 8:143–153.
5. Vuilleumier HA, Reis ED. Radiation injury. In: Marti MC, Givel JC, eds. Surgical Management of Anorectal and Colonic Disease. Heidelberg: Springer-Verlag, 1998:423–435.
6. Mettle FA Jr, Moseley RD Jr. Medical Effects of Ionizing Radiation. Orlando: Grune & Stratton, 1985.
7. McLean AS. Early adverse effects of radiation. Br Med Bull 1973; 29:69–73.
8. McDonald A. Altered protective mechanisms. In: Dow, KH Hindered LJ, eds. Nursing Care Radiation Oncology. Philadelphia: W.B. Saunders, 1992:96–126.
9. Sitton E. Early and late radiation-induced skin alterations. Part II: nursing care of irradiated skin. Oncol Nurs Forum 1992; 19:907–912.
10. Mahon SM, Casperson DS. Hereditary cancer syndrome: Part 1–clinical and educational issues. Oncol Nurs Forum 1995; 22:763–771.
11. Peters LJ. The ESTRO Regaud Lecture. Inherent radiosensitivity of tumor and normal tissue cells as a predictor of human tumour response. Radiotherapy Oncol 1990; 17: 177–190.
12. Dunne-Daly CF. Skin and wound care in radiation oncology. Cancer Nurs 1995; 18: 144–160.
13. Ratliff C. Impaired skin integrity related to radiation therapy. J Enterostomal Ther 1990; 17:193–198.
14. Varghese M, Balin AD, Carter DM, Caldwell D. Local environment of chronic wounds under synthetic dressings. Arch Dermatol 1986; 122:52–57.
15. Bayley EW. Wound healing in the patient with burns. Nurs Clin North Am 1990; 25:205–222.
16. Hansbrough JF. Use of Biobrane for extensive posterior donor site wounds. J Burn Care Rehabil 1995; 16(3 Pt 1):335–336.
17. Smith DJ Jr. Use of Biobrane in wound management. J Burn Care Rehabil 1995; 16(3 Pt 1): 317–320.
18. Housinger TA, Wondrely L, Warden GD. The use of Biobrane for coverage of the pediatric donor site. J Burn Care Rehabil 1993; 14:26–28.

19. Winfrey ME, Cochran M, Hegarty MT. A new technology in burn therapy: INTEGRA artificial skin. Dimens Crit Care Nurs 1999; 18:14–20.

20. Boyce ST, Kagan RJ, Meyer NA, Yahkuboff KP, Warden GD. The 1999 clinical research award. Cultured skin substitutes combined with Integra Artificial Skin to replace native skin autograft and allograft for the closure of excised full-thickness burns. J Burn Care Rehabil 1999; 20:453–461.

21. Pandya AN, Woodward B, Parkhouse N. The use of cultured autologous keratinocytes with integra in the resurfacing of acute burns. Plast Reconstr Surg 1998; 102:825–828.

22. Clayton MC, Bishop JF. Perioperative and postoperative dressing techniques for Integra Artificial Skin: views from two medical centers. J Burn Care Rehabil 1998; 19:358–363.

23. Falanga V, Sabolinski M. A bilayered living skin construct (APLIGRAF®) accelerates complete closure of hard-to-heal venous ulcers. Wound Repair Regen 1999; 7:201–207.

24. Eaglstein WH, Falanga V. Tissue engineering and the development of Apligraf a human skin equivalent. Adv Wound Care 1998; 11(suppl 4):1–8.

25. Falanga V. Apligraf treatment of venous ulcers and other chronic wounds. J Dermatol 1998; 25:812–820.

26. Kirsner RS. The use of Apligraf in acute wounds. J Dermatol 1998; 25:805–811.

27. Trent JF, Kirsner RS. Tissue engineered skin: Apligraf, a bi-layered living skin equivalent. Int J Clin Pract 1998; 52:408–413.

28. Nall AV, Brownlee RE, Colvin CP, et al. Transforming growth factor-1 improves wound healing and random flap survival in normal and irradiated rats. Arch Otolaryngol Head Neck Surg 1996; 122:171–177.

29. Bernstein EF, Harisiadis L, Salomon G, et al. Transforming growth factor-improves healing of radiation-impaired wounds. J Invest Dermatol 1991; 97:430–434.

30. Martin M, Vozenin MC, Gault N, et al. Coactivation of AP-1 activity and TGF-1 gene expression in the stress response of normal skin cells to ionizing radiation. Oncogene 1997; 15:981–989.

31. Randall K, Coggle J. Expression of TGF-1 in mouse skin during the acute phase of radiation damage. Int J Radiat Biol 1995; 68:301–309.

32. Martin M, Lefaix J, Delanian S. TGF-1 and radiation fibrosis: a master switch and a specific therapeutic target? Int J Radiat Oncol Biol Phys 2000; 47:277–290.

33. Kouvaris JR, Kouloulias VE, Plataniotis GA, Balafouta EJ, Vlahos LJ. Dermatitis during radiation for vulvar carcinoma: prevention and treatment with granulocyte-macrophage colony-stimulating factor impregnated gauze. Wound Repair Regen 2001; 9: 187–193.

34. Sanchiz F, Milla A, Artola N, et al. Prevention of radioinduced cystitis by orgotein: a randomized study. Anticancer Res 1996; 16(4A):2025–2028.

35. Cividalli A, Adami M, De Tomasi F, et al. Orgotein as a radioprotector in normal tissues: experiments on mouse skin and a murine adenocarcinoma. Acta Radiol Oncol 1985; 24:273–277.

36. Okunieff P. Interactions between ascorbic acid and the radiation of bone marrow, skin, and tumor. Am J Clin Nutr 1991; 54(suppl 6):1281S–1283S.

37. Halperin EC, Gaspar L, George S, Darr D, Pinnell S. A double-blind, randomized, prospective trial to evaluate topical vitamin C solution for the prevention of radiation dermatitis. Int J Rad Oncol Biol Phys 1993; 26:413–416.

38. Michalowski AS. On radiation damage to normal tissues and its treatment. II. Anti-inflammatory drugs. Acta Oncol 1994; 33:139–157.

39. Glees JP, Mameghan-Zadeh H, Sparkes CG. Effectiveness of topical steroids in the control of radiation dermatitis: a randomized trial using 1% hydrocortisone cream and 0.05% clobetasone butyrate (Eumovate). Clin Radiol 1979; 30:397–403.

40. Simonen P, Hamilton C, Ferguson S, et al. Do inflammatory processes contribute to radiation induced erythema observed in the skin of humans? Radiother Oncol 1998; 46:73–82.

41. Vogler BK, Ernst E. Aloe vera: a systematic review of its clinical effectiveness. Br J Gen Pract 1999; 49:823–828.

42. Williams MS, Burk M, Loprinzi CL, et al. Phase III double-blind evaluation of an aloe vera gel as a prophylactic agent for radiation-induced skin toxicity. Int J Radiat Oncol Biol Phys 1996; 36:345–349.

43. Olsen DL, Raub W Jr, Bradley C, Johnson M, Macias JL, Love V, Markoe A. The effect of aloe vera gel/mild soap versus mild soap alone in preventing skin reactions in patients undergoing radiation therapy. Oncol Nurs Forum 2001; 28:543–547.

44. Schindl A, Schindl M, Pernerstorfer-Schon H, Mossbacher U, Schindl L. Low intensity laser irradiation in the treatment of recalcitrant radiation ulcers in patients with breast cancer: long-term results of 3 cases. Photodermatol Photoimmunol Photomed 2000; 16:34–37.

18
Factitial Ulcers

Georgette Rodriguez
Department of Dermatology and Cutaneous Surgery,
University of Miami School of Medicine, Miami, Florida, U.S.A.

Factitious disorders in dermatology are varied and complex. These self-inflicted diseases span diagnostic categories and vary in clinical presentations. Among the spectrum of these disorders are dermatitis artefacta and malingering, both of which can manifest as ulcers. The difference between dermatitis artefacta and malingering lies in the intent of the patient. In dermatitis artefacta, however, lesions are produced either consciously or unconsciously for purposes of satisfying a psychological need of which he or she is not aware (1–3). This is in contrast to the malingerer, who consciously produces self-inflicted lesions for an external secondary gain such as money, getting out of work, obtaining privileges, or narcotics (1). Although the differential diagnosis for ulcers is extensive, the patient history of the ulcers and the clinical features of the lesions can provide clues in the diagnosis of factitial ulcers.

1. EPIDEMIOLOGY

Factitious disorders, specifically dermatitis artefacta, can be seen in all races and occur at any age (2). The highest incidence occurs in adolescence and young adulthood, with a female to male ratio reported from 3:1 to 20:1 (2–5). Many of these women are single, immature, or divorced (1,6). In contrast, malingering is more common in men (1,5). There is a high incidence of patients with self-inflicted lesions that are employed or are closely related to someone in the medical field (1,5,7). These patients also represent a wide range of educational backgrounds (2).

2. CLINICAL FEATURES

Factitial dermatoses should be suspected in cases of chronic, non-healing lesions (1,6,9). As mentioned, the lesions can vary; however, there are some clinical features that can help in diagnosing factitial disease. The morphology of lesions is described as having a "bizarre" appearance (1). The lesions are usually sharply angulated or linear; some form sharply demarcated geometric shapes (Fig. 1). Different patterns of presentation may be present secondary to the mechanism of injury production (1,10). The locations of lesions are variable but usually involve accessible sites to

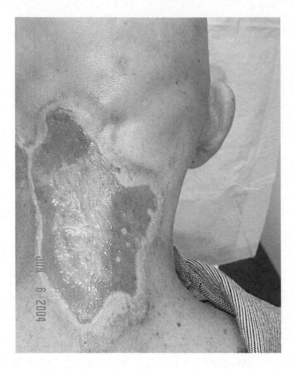

Figure 1   Well-demarcated ulcer on the neck, with linear borders in a rectangular shape.

the dominant hand of the patient (1,6,10). The lack of descriptive details to learn the evolution and development of lesions is also characteristic, and lesions appearing overnight on previously normal skin are not unusual (2,4). Another common feature is the presence of lesions in different stages of healing. As the patient starts to heal, new lesions are produced resulting in lesions of varying age, for example, ulcers, blisters, and hyperpigmented plaques or patches in the same patient (1). There are also laboratory data that can raise a suspicion. For example, wound cultures demonstrating fecal or unusual bacteria may be suggestive of manipulation of wounds.

3. "HOLLOW HISTORY"

Gandy describes the patient's inability and unwillingness to discuss the evolution of the lesions and the tendency to deviate in tangents as a "hollow history" (8). Redirection to the patient's history of current lesions is usually met with hostility and frustration by the patient. There may also be a history of previous unusual illnesses in the past. He or she has also seen numerous physicians in a variety of fields and has tried a number of medicaments without success (1,2,4). If malingering is suspected, the patient may have legal problems or potential for financial reward.

4. DIAGNOSIS

Diagnosis of factitial disease is challenging to the practitioner. Neither the malingerer nor the patient with dermatitis artefacta has any desire to be discovered or cured since it provides some secondary gain or psychological satisfaction (5). The diagnosis should be based not only on the appearance of lesions and the history, but on the patient's personality as well (6). Lyell (1) describes the importance of the nature of the lesion as well as the personality of the patient. He describes the type of patient as being emotionally immature, under stress and possessing "hysterical traits." These hysterical manifestations include paralyses, anesthesia, blindness, deafness, aphonia, or abdominal pain (1,2). These traits lead to exhaustive negative work-ups by numerous physicians before making a diagnosis. Biopsies are usually performed to exclude other diagnoses. Controversy exists as to whether the biopsy is helpful in making a diagnosis of dermatitis artefacta. Two reviews discuss that the histopathology is not characteristic (1,7). On the other hand, Joe et al. (6) describe the histopathology as characteristic. They describe injury to the epidermis with necrolytic changes without an immunogenic response. If the injury extends to the dermis, there is a minimal inflammatory response (6). Other studies describe polarized light microscopy and electron probe microanalysis to evaluate for exogenous material used to induce the lesions (6,8,9). Protective dressings such as Unna boots may lead to the healing of lesions which may help in clarifying the diagnosis as well (1,3). Other authors mention the use of cameras or surveillance to catch patients manipulating or creating wound in an in-patient setting (1,2). Despite these efforts, often the diagnosis of dermatitis artefacta or malingering is one of exclusion. One recent retrospective study of dermatitis artefacta reported the mean time of onset of disease to time of diagnosis as 10 months and in some cases as long as 4 years (7). This is due to frequent misdiagnoses and/or numerous physicians involved in the care (1,7).

5. TREATMENT

Recommendations in the literature for treatment of factitial ulcers secondary to dermatitis artefacta or malingering are few. Universal to these disorders is the difficulty in treatment. Very little is known of the prognosis of these patients since follow-up is poor (1,7). One long-term follow-up of 43 patients with self-inflicted injury showed that 30% continue to produce lesions 12 years after onset of lesions (11). In one-third of dermatology patients, the management of skin conditions involves consideration of psychiatric and psychosocial factors (12). Many patients with dermatitis artefacta suffer from depression or personality disorders (1,7,12). In children posttraumatic stress disorder (PTSD) with dissociative symptoms that occur in child abuse or sexual abuse should be ruled out (12). Antidepressants, especially selective serotonin reuptake inhibitors (SSRI), are effective in the treatment of PTSD and depression (12). Olanzapine, an antipsychotic medication, has also been used in the treatment of self-inflicted dermatoses when other modalities have failed. One study showed an excellent clinical response in patients treated (13). Pimozide, a neuroleptic and a selective blocker of dopamine D_2 receptors, has also been reported in the treatment of dermatitis artefacta at low doses (2). In some cases, behavior therapy, hypnosis, and other psychotherapeutic interventions may be effective as well (4,12). No studies exist comparing different treatment options. In the case of malingering, treatment may involve uncovering the secondary gain.

In either case, a multidisciplinary approach needs to be taken in the treatment of factitial disorders. The physician needs to establish rapport and confidence in the patient–doctor relationship. Some suggestions include frequent short visits and supervision of treatment (1,6,7). For example, if the patient has an ulcer, protective dressings can be placed that are only changed by the physician or his/her team (1,2,14). Once a rapport is established and the patient trusts the doctor, an opportunity to discuss possible psychiatric care or referral may arise (4).

6. CONCLUSION

Factitial ulcers are one of the many presentations of dermatitis artefacta and malingering. The care of these patients falls into the hands of numerous physicians including family practitioners, internists, dermatologists, to mention a few. A general awareness of clinical and historical clues in making this diagnosis can lead to a more rapid and cost-effective diagnosis and treatment of this disease. There are many reports in the dermatological and psychiatric literatures that discuss confronting the patients about the nature of their self-inflicted wounds. Many authors believe that it is counterproductive to confront the patient (1–3,8). This may lead to an angry patient that will seek medical care elsewhere. Providing support for the patient and establishing a relationship will create trust and lead to further discussions for treatment options mentioned above.

REFERENCES

1. Lyell A. Cutaneous artifactual disease. J Am Acad Dermatol 1979; 1:391–407.
2. Koblenzer C. Cutaneous manifestations of psychiatric disease that commonly present to the dermatologist—diagnosis and treatment. Int J Psychiatry Med 1992; 22:47–63.
3. Koenig TW, Garnis-Jones S, Rencic A, Tausk FA. Psychological aspects of skin diseases. In: Freedberg IM, Eisen AZ, Wolff K, Austen KF, Goldsmith LA, Katz SI, eds. Fitzpatrick's Dermatology in General Medicine. New York: McGraw-Hill, 2003:389–398.
4. Koblenzer C. Psychodermatology of women. Clin in Dermatol 1997; 15:127–141.
5. Halprin KM. The art of self-mutilation. JAMA 1967; 199(2):155.
6. Joe EK, Li VW, Magro CM, Arndt KA, Bowers KE. Diagnostic clues to dermatitis artefacta. Cutis 1999; 63:209–214.
7. Saez-de-Ocariz M, Orozco-Covarrubias L, Mora-Magana I, Duran-McKinster C, Tamayo-Sanchez L, Gutierrez-Castrellon P, Ruiz-Maldonado R. Dermatitis artefacta in pediatric patients: experience at the national institute of pediatrics. Ped Dermatol 2004; 21:205–211.
8. Antony SJ, Mannion SM. Dermatitis artefacta revisited. Cutis 1995; 55:362–364.
9. Jackson RM, Tucker SB, Abraham JL, Millins JL. Factitial cutaneous ulcers and nodules: the use of electron probe microanalysis in diagnosis. J Am Acad Dermatol 1984; 11:1065–1069.
10. Gandy DT. The concept and clinical aspects of factitial dermatitis. South Med J 1953; 46:551–555.
11. Sneddon I, Sneddon J. Self-inflicted injury: a follow up study of 43 patients. Br Med J 1975; 3:527–530.
12. Gupta MA, Gupta AK. The use of antidepressant drugs in dermatology. JEADV 2001; 15:512–518.
13. Garnis-Jones S, Collins S, Rosenthal D. Treatment of self mutilation with olanzapine. J Cutan Med Surg 2000:161–163.
14. Falabella A, Falanga V. Uncommon causes of ulcers. Clin Plas Surg 1998; 25:467–478.

19
Calciphylaxis

Paolo Romanelli and Shasa Hu
Department of Dermatology and Cutaneous Surgery, University of Miami School of Medicine, Miami, Florida, U.S.A.

1. INTRODUCTION

Calcific uremic arteriolopathy (CUA), also known as calciphylaxis, is a syndrome of cutaneous microvascular calcification of unknown etiology causing painful violaceous skin lesions. These then progress to nonhealing ulcers and gangrene. It is a serious complication of end-stage renal disease (ESRD) associated with high mortality. The pathogenesis and risks for CUA remain poorly understood. At the present time, there are no standard treatments.

1.1. Historical Background

The term calciphylaxis is based on a syndrome described by Hans Selye in experimental rats in 1962 (1). He hypothesized that two steps are required to produce ectopic systemic calcifications in nonuremic experimental animals. Firstly, the animals were sensitized by agents such as parathyroid hormone (PTH), vitamin D, or a diet high in calcium (Ca) and phosphorus (P). Secondly, after a "critical period" of sensitization, the animals were given subcutaneous or intraperitoneal injection of challenging agents. The challenging agents included local trauma, injection of iron salt, egg albumin, polymycin, or glucocorticoids. These agents induced an "anaphylactic" inflammatory reaction that days later resulted in macroscopically visible deposits of calcium salts (hydroxyapatite) systemically and at the site of injection. Selye coined the term calciphylaxis for this condition of "systemic hypersensitivity in which tissues respond to appropriate challenging agents with rapid deposition of calcium." A few years later, a syndrome characterized by peripheral tissue necrosis, ulcerations, and vascular calcifications was reported in uremic patients on dialysis or after renal transplantation. Because of its resemblance to Selye's animal model, it was also named calciphylaxis (2–5). However, Selye's animal model lacked vascular calcification that was the hallmark of calciphylaxis in humans. Ischemia was not a usual outcome of his experiments. The term "calciphylaxis" implied a hypersensitivity reaction, which is also inappropriate, as IgE plays no role in the human condition. Subsequently, a variety of nomenclatures were proposed in the literature, including calcifying panniculitis, uremic gangrene syndrome, necrotizing panniculitis, and calcinosis cutis. Recently, the term "calcific uremic arteriolopathy" was proposed, and it is considered a more appropriate term than calciphylaxis as it describes the characteristic histology of the disease (6,7). In this chapter, the terms "calcific uremic arteriolopathy" and "calciphylaxis" will be used interchangeably.

2. CLINICAL FEATURES

2.1. Clinical Presentation

Calcific uremic arteriolopathy, historically considered rare, has been reported with increasing frequency in the last decade (6–9). The syndrome primarily affects patients with ESRD, commonly secondary to diabetes mellitus, and cardiovascular disease. These patients often have concomitant secondary hyperparathyroidism from their renal failure, and are either on dialysis or postrenal transplantation. The range of ages reported is 6 months to 83 years with a mean age of 48 years (8). The prevalence of the syndrome is estimated to be between 1% and 4% of the dialysis population (10,11). Occasionally, patients with predialysis renal insufficiency can also manifest calciphylaxis (12–16). A small number of cases occurred in patients with cancer [breast carcinoma (17–19) and leukemia (20)], alcoholic cirrhosis (15), inflammatory bowel disease (21), and primary hyperparathyroidism without renal insufficiency (22).

In addition to having ESRD, patients with calciphylaxis are more likely to be white, female, and obese (7,9,10,12,23–25). Patients with diabetes may also be at greater risk for calciphylaxis (26). The implication of such demographic features of CUA on its pathogenesis will be discussed in "Pathogenesis" section. Table 1 lists the main medical conditions associated with calciphylaxis.

Calcific uremic arteriolopathy can be a localized cutaneous or systemic form. Cutaneous manifestation of calciphylaxis is characterized by intensely painful plaques or indurated subcutaneous nodules and ulcers, usually with eschar. The nodules and plaques may represent the earlier stage of CUA; they often appear violaceous and mottled, resembling livedo reticularis. The eruptions can rapidly become bullous, necrotic, and progressing into hemorrhagic, nonhealing ulcers with gangrene. The skin lesions are pruritic and intensely painful, often necessitating strong analgesics. Ulcerations usually have irregular borders and can become circumferential with eschar formation (Fig. 1). Both distal and proximal sites can be affected, although regions with greater adipose tissue, such as the breast, abdomen, and thighs, are more frequently involved. Gangrene of the digits is a common presentation. Ulceration of the penis from calciphylaxis has also been reported (27–30). Other characteristic findings are bilaterality, superficial nature of skin lesions, and persistence of palpable pulses distal to the necrotic ulcers (6,26,31,32). Secondary infection leading into a sepsis is a common and often fatal sequela. In the systemic form of CUA, kidneys,

Table 1 Risk Factors for Calciphylaxis

Female	Hyperparathyroidism, secondary or primary
Caucasian race	Warfarin therapy
Obesity	Protein C or S abnormality
Diabetes mellitus	Excess calcium salts intake
End-stage renal disease	Immunosuppression

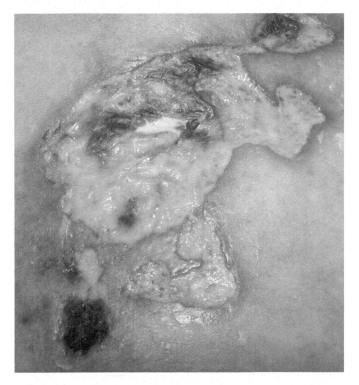

Figure 1 Irregularly bordered ulcers with black eschar and necrosis located on the anterior thigh of a patient with calciphylaxis.

skeletal muscles, and less frequently the lungs, heart, and gastrointestinal tract can have the characteristic vascular calcification in addition to the skin (33–37). While visceral organ ischemia from CUA is not a common consequence of systemic CUA, mesenteric ischemia despite patency of mesenteric arteries has been reported (7,38–41).

2.2. Laboratory Findings

Calciphylaxis has been associated with severe derangement of calcium phosphate metabolism. Commonly reported abnormalities include elevated serum phosphorus levels, elevated calcium × phosphorus (Ca × P) product, and elevated intact PTH (42,43). Serum calcium level can be either normal or mildly elevated. However, these abnormalities are common in patients with ESRD, and none of them are consistently associated with CUA. The absence of these abnormalities also does not exclude the diagnosis (17,24,44). Table 2 summarizes the common laboratory findings in calciphylaxis.

Table 2 Common Laboratory Findings in Calciphylaxis

Normo- or hypercalcemia	Hyperphosphotemia
Elevated calcium X phosphate products	Elevated parathyroid hormone

The diagnosis of calciphylaxis usually is made clinically. In clinically equivocal cases, x-ray and bone scan can aid in the diagnosis. On plain radiographic films of the affected area, vessel calcification is a prominent finding. Diffuse reticular pattern or gross confluent patches of calcification can also be present (9). This finding, however, is not specific as vascular calcification is a frequent finding in patients on dialysis (45). Subcutaneous calcium deposition can be better detected by bone scan (9,46). Bone scan shows increased uptake in the subcutaneous, clinically apparent diseased areas. In area of deep ulceration, however, bone scan can be negative as the amount of calcium-containing tissue can be significantly decreased through necrosis and denudation of subcutaneous tissue (9).

2.3. Histology

When a patient with fitting medical profile presents with the characteristic skin lesions, biopsy is usually not needed to diagnose calciphylaxis, and can lead to ulceration or poor healing at the biopsy site. Furthermore, biopsy result is not always positive in clinically evident areas. Histologic examination characteristically shows calcium deposits within the walls of small subcutaneous arteries/arterioles with diameters from 300 to 600 μm, averaging 100 μm (32,47). Von Kossa stain can be applied to confirm the calcium deposition. The vascular calcification may be in the intima or media, although the medial location is more distinctively seen in calciphylaxis (23,24,43,48). The arteriolar calcification is often superimposed by intimal fibroblastic hyperplasia causing marked luminal narrowing (Figs. 2–4). Calcification precedes the endovascular fibrosis (32,48). A complete spectrum of histological changes can be observed: from vessels with fine calcifications without fibrosis, to vessels with calcification and proliferating endothelial fibroblasts, to vessels with both calcification and well-developed endovascular fibrosis and stenosis (32). Giant cells may be present in the earliest stages of endovascular fibrosis. Such a distinctive vasculopathy appears to be the primary cause of the ischemia in CUA. Microvascular thromboses, calcific panniculitis, extravascular calcification with an infiltrate of neutrophils, and macrophages can be present as well. Vasculitic features are not present. Electron microscopic spectral analysis of the mineral content of the calcific lesions in the subcutaneous tissue showed only calcium and phosphorus (7).

The vascular calcification in calciphylaxis has been compared to that in Monckeberg's medial calcific stenosis and atherosclerotic vascular disease. Both calciphylaxis and medial calcific stenosis share the medial location of calcium deposits. However, the calcification in medial calcific stenosis is not accompanied by fibroplasia and inflammation, as in calciphylaxis. In comparison to atherosclerotic peripheral vascular disease, calciphylaxis lacks smooth muscle proliferation, lipid-laden macrophages, or connective tissue extracellular lipid deposits.

2.4. Differential Diagnosis

Diseases that may present with similar associated similar ulcerations as CUA include peripheral vascular disease, cholesterol embolization, vasculitis, marantic endocarditis, coumadin necrosis, cellulitis, systemic lupus erythematosus, protein C deficiency, cryoglobulinemia, scleroderma, CREST syndrome, metastatic calcification, pancreatic panniculitis, disseminated intravascular coagulation, Henoch–Schonlein purpura, Weber–Christian syndrome, and homocysteinemia (32,35,40,49,50). The distinguishing features of CUA are the lack of associated immunoglobulin deposition

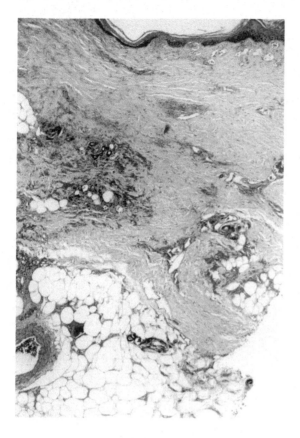

Figure 2 Calcific metaplasia with a subcutaneous artery imbedded in adipose tissue.

or vasculitic features on histology and negative serology (32,40). Acral lesions of CUA differ from gangrene from peripheral vascular disease in that peripheral pulses are often preserved in CUA. Pancreatic panniculitis is often more widespread with involvement of the pretibial region, and accompanied by amylase abnormality. The histology of CUA further distinguishes it from the other clinical entities.

Calciphylaxis should be differentiated from other forms of cutaneous calcification. There are four major categories of calcinosis cutis: dystrophic, metastatic, idiopathic, and iatrogenic (51). Dystrophic calcification is the most common type of calcinosis cutis. It occurs in the setting of local tissue injury or abnormalities. The local tissue abnormalities precipitate calcification while serum calcium and phosphate levels and calcium metabolism remain normal. Causes of dystrophic calcification include collagen vascular disease (such as calcinosis cutis in CREST syndrome), panniculitis, porphyria cutanea tarda, Ehlers–Danlos syndrome, Werner syndrome, cutaneous neoplasms, infections, and trauma. The internal organs usually are spared in dystrophic calcification. In contrast to dystrophic calcification, metastatic calcification results from abnormal calcium and/or phosphate metabolism. Subsequently, calcification of cutaneous, subcutaneous, and deep tissue may occur. The internal organs may be affected as well. Calciphylaxis is considered a type of metastatic calcification. Other causes of metastatic calcification include Albright hereditary osteodystrophy, sarcoidosis, hypervitaminosis D, pseudohyperparathyroidism,

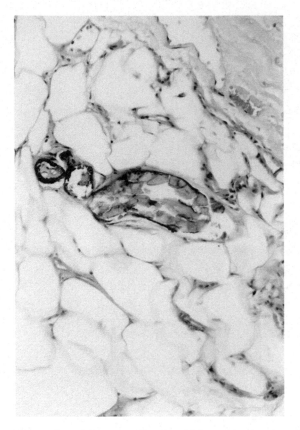

Figure 3 Higher magnification of the same vessel reveals both intimal and medial calcification leading to vessel lumen stenosis.

pseudoxanthoma elasticum, lymphoma, leukemia, and metastatic carcinoma; all of which are associated with abnormal calcium metabolism. Idiopathic calcification develops without identifiable underlying tissue abnormalities or abnormal calcium metabolism. Examples include subepidermal-calcified nodules, idiopathic calcification of the scrotum, and tumoral calcinosis. These lesions are usually chronic and rarely associated with ulceration of the overlying skin. Calciphylaxis can also be readily differentiated from iatrogenic calcification, as the latter is often a complication of intravenous calcium chloride and calcium gluconate therapy.

3. PATHOGENESIS

The pathogenesis of CUA has not been fully elucidated. The syndrome appears to result from a multitude of predisposing and/or sensitizing events that are commonly present in the uremic milieu. The key pathology of CUA is microvascular calcification, especially that of arterioles, accompanied by cutaneous tissue ischemia and necrosis. A variety of theories behind the vessel calcification in CUA have been evaluated. None of them have been consistently demonstrated by clinical studies. However, the inconsistency of these studies may be the result of their small sample size and limited statistical power. The following section focuses on the role of

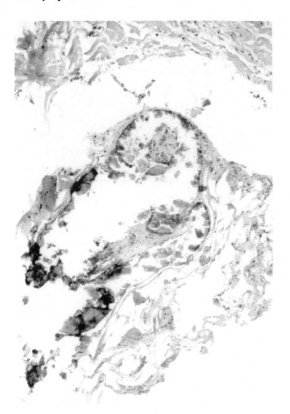

Figure 4 A medium-sized subcutaneous artery with intramual calcification, intimal hyperplasia, and vessel wall necrosis.

adipose tissue, serum divalent ions (calcium, phosphorus, and Ca × P products) and PTH, and presents recent advances in the research on pathophysiology of calciphylaxis.

As mentioned previously, in patients with renal failure, risk factors for the development of CUA include female gender, obesity, and diabetes mellitus (9,12,24,52). The increased adipose tissue is a common feature shared by obese, female (as opposed to males), and diabetic population. The role of adipose tissue may be of that it predispose to relative hypoperfusion of the skin and subcutaneous tissue (53). The increased susceptibility to small vessel damages of adipose tissue may then promote calcifications before cutaneous lesions and tissue necrosis becomes clinically apparent (6). The predominant occurrence of calciphylaxis in locations with more adipose tissue also supports this hypothesis (24).

Because of the characteristic calcification of small vessels, much attention has focused on the role of calcium toxicity, or disregulation of calcium and phosphate metabolism in the pathogenesis of CUA. Elevated serum markers of calcium metabolism, such as calcium, phosphate, and Ca × P products, were thought to promote the extraskeletal calcification via passive precipitation, thereby, increase the risk of calciphylaxis. Hypercalcemia was found to be a risk factor by some case-control studies (10). The role of elevated serum calcium level has also been evaluated through oral $CaCO_3$ intake in dialysis patients. Studies have demonstrated a greater risk of calciphylaxis from increased calcium salts intake (9,12,14,54). The rise in incidence of CUA in the past 15 years has been postulated to be related to cessation of aluminum-containing P binders and the wide usage of Ca-containing phosphate binders (6). However, subsequent studies did not find significant association between serum calcium level, calcium salt intake, and CUA (12,23). Moreover, while all dialysis patients suffer from disordered calcium metabolism, relatively few dialysis patients develop calciphylaxis (24).

The association of calciphylaxis with serum phosphorus and $Ca \times P$ product levels is inconsistent as well. Majority of clinical studies implicated elevated serum phosphorus and $Ca \times P$ levels as risk factors (9,10,12,23,55), while a small number of studies did not (14,24). Calcific uremic arteriolopathy has also occurred after renal transplant when the $Ca \times P$ product is normalized (3,48).

The importance of PTH remains speculative. Based on the animal model by Selye, it is postulated that elevated PTH may sensitize tissue to calciphylaxis through disregulated calcium metabolism (1,8,10,26,43). Occurrence of CUA in the absence of hyperparathyroidism (56), after parathyroidectomy (4,36,57), or even in patients with biopsy-proven low-turnover bone disease with low levels of PTH challenges the importance of PTH (42). Furthermore, recent case-control studies have failed to demonstrate a role for PTH, instead finding elevated serum P to be more important (9,12,23,58).

Recent evidence suggests that smooth muscle cells play an active role in vascular calcification. Studies indicate that vascular calcification in calciphylaxis is also a cell-mediated process resembling osteogenesis in bone, rather than passive precipitation of calcium and phosphorus in the setting of disregulated mineral metabolism (59). In in vitro experiments, both uremic and hyperphosphatemic sera induced phenotypic transformation of vascular smooth muscle cells to osteoblast-like cells with subsequent calcification and expression of osteopontin (60). Osteopontin is a bone matrix protein produced by osteoblasts. Although initially isolated from bone, it is localized in many tissues and appears that have increased expression in tissues at risk or known to calcify (61). Immunostaining of calcified vessels in CUA patients on dialysis demonstrated the presence of osteopontin and several other bone-related proteins including bone sialoprotein, alkaline phosphatase, and type I collagen, while noncalcified vessels stained negative for osteopontin (23). It is suggested that these bone-forming proteins mineralize in the presence of elevated $Ca \times P$ product and/or calcium load (59). Electron microscopic examination of calcified vessels further revealed that calcium deposits were in the form of large masses and in small 50–150 nm round particles. The patterns of small round calcium deposits were similar to those seen in in vitro calcification of smooth muscle cells, and in normal calcification in osteoblasts and chondrocytes, as the small calcium deposits were intertwined among collagen fibrils (23). In the light of these findings, the role of hyperphosphatemia in the pathogenesis of CUA may be its inductive effect on dedifferentiation of vascular smooth muscle cells into osteoblast-like cells with subsequent mineralization. However, CUA appears to be mediated only partially by hyperphosphatemia, because the addition of inorganic phosphorus to vascular smooth muscle cells in vitro failed to augment the osteopontin expression induced by uremic serum (60). This suggests that additional factors present in uremic milieu participate in the pathogenesis of CUA in patients with ESRD. In calciphylaxis occurring in the absence of renal failure or hyperphosphatemia (17,18), it is not known which biochemical agents take on the role of phosphorus if a similar process of cell-mediated calcification occurs.

Table 3 Reported Precipitants of Calciphylaxis

Local trauma	Albumin infusion
Iron dextran injection	Chemotherapy
Protein malnutrition	Corticosteriods

Coagulopathy from warfarin administration and abnormal protein C or S function have been implicated in the development of CUA. Warfarin can lead to a reduction of plasma protein C levels. The use of warfarin prior to the onset of calciphylaxis was a significant risk factor in some studies (7,38), while not in others (9). Calciphylaxis has reported to occur in patients with functional protein C or S deficiency or antiphospholipid antibodies (12,62,63). The hypercoagulable or prothrombotic state from warfarin therapy, protein C or S deficiency, or antiphospholipid may contribute to skin necrosis via small vessel thrombosis in CUA (62). However, most patients on dialysis are successfully anticoagulated with heparin or warfarin without developing CUA (64), and normal functional protein C activity has been recorded in the majority of cases (25,26). Local trauma, such as subcutaneous injections of insulin (24), and iron dextran (65) are other possible precipitants of calciphylaxis (66). Additional triggering factors, listed in Table 3, such as protein malnutrition (12,24), albumin infusion (15), corticosteroids (67), chemotherapy, and immunosuppressants (16,18,36), have also been suggested. Despite their inconsistent and unclear association with CUA, all the above factors may act as the challenging agents used by Selye in his animal models; they cause cellular injury in an environment that has already been "sensitized" to calcification.

In summary, it appears that CUA is associated a host of predisposing factors with varying degree of significance in individuals. The vascular calcification in CUA may be a subacute to chronic process that precedes clinically evident disease. In patients with ESRD, hyperphosphatemia together with other unidentified toxins in the uremic milieu may create an inductive environment in which vascular smooth muscles of subcutaneous vessels, in response to cellular injuries, dedifferentiate into osteoblast-like cells and lead to calcification. It is not known whether the same cell-mediated process occurs in patients with calciphylaxis but without renal insufficiency or hyperparathyroidism. Also, in these patients, other conditions such as coagulopathy and immunosuppression may play more important roles in inducing vascular calcification. The tissue ischemia from vascular calcification and fibrosis becomes clinically evident with inciting events, such as acute changes in serum electrolyte levels, systemic illness, and local trauma. However, the fact that calciphylaxis only affects a very small subpopulation of ESRD patients and others without apparent risk factors, suggests that there may be a yet defined genetic predisposition for vascular mineralization in individuals.

4. CLINICAL COURSE/PROGNOSIS

The clinical course of CUA is characterized by rapid progression of cutaneous lesions with often fatal outcome, and high morbidity with slow healing of the ulcers if the patient survives. Mortality from CUA ranges between 60% and 80%, mainly from overwhelming sepsis from wound infection (9,26,44). Patients with ulceration and proximal lesions have even worse prognosis (8,9,44,48), with mortality as high as 89% (9). In addition to sepsis, other causes of death from calciphylaxis include myocardial infarction, refractory hypotension, and cerebrovascular accidents (9,36). It is not uncommon for a patient to have overwhelming sepsis within weeks of the diagnosis of calciphylaxis, and ensuing death within months of diagnosis. Debilitating pain, high risk of limb amputation, complicated hospital course with prolonged rehabilitation further adds to the disease burden of calciphylaxis. Many of the survivors are severely disabled as a consequence of limb amputations and reconstructive surgeries.

The high mortality rate in CUA patients is partly explained by their comorbid conditions, such as diabetes, cardiovascular disease, peripheral arterial occlusive disease, and chronic protein malnutrition. Additionally, the vasculopathy seen in CUA appears to be irreversible even after aggressive therapies (3,32,43). All of these factors contribute to delayed healing of ulcers in these patients, and consequently, increased risk for wound infection and sepsis. Coexistent peripheral arterial disease in patients with ESRD also decreases the success rate of limb salvage in calciphylaxis (39).

5. MANAGEMENT

5.1. Medical Management

With the lack of understanding of its pathophysiology and the lack of clinical trials, there are no standardized treatments of CUA. None of the current treatments appear satisfactory in a majority of cases (available management options are listed in Table 4). The difficulty in managing calciphylaxis partly arises from the irreversible nature of the vasculopathy at the diagnosis of clinical lesions. Because of its rapidly progressive course and often fatal outcome, the main principles of managing calciphylaxis are early recognition of the disease, prevention of sepsis, and aggressive supportive therapy and wound care with a multidisciplinary approach. Supportive therapy should target fluid-electrolyte balance, PTH level, coagulopathy, nutritional status, and pain control. At the present time, lowering of elevated serum phosphorus, calcium, and $Ca \times P$ product, together with aggressive wound care may contribute to the successful outcome of patients with CUA (68).

Since most of patients with CUA are on dialysis, serum phosphorus, calcium, and $Ca \times P$ product should be managed by dietary compliance, increased dialysis

Table 4 Management Options for Patients with Calciphylaxis

Medical	Surgical
Adjust dialysis dose/frequency	Subtotal parathyroidectomy
Low calcium dialysate	Cervical or lumbar sympathectomy
Discontinue calcium salts	Wound debridement
Substitute with non-calcium phosphate binders	Amputation or excision of affected region
Dietary restriction of phosphorus	Skin graft
Appropriate systemic or topical antibiotics	
Steroid and cimetidine	
Etidronate disodium	
Analgesics	
Nutritional support	
Minimize local trauma	
Eliminate known inciting factors	
Hyperbaric oxygen therapy	
Wound dressing	

dose/frequency, and use of appropriate phosphate binders. In patients with hyper-phosphatemia, strict control of serum P level has been shown to reverse CUA (69,70). Ca-containing phosphate binders should be discontinued. Sevelamer hydrochloride (Renagel)—a calcium-free phosphate binder—can be used instead (6,9,68,71). Another possible consideration is to switch calcitriol to paricalcitol, a less calcemic form of vitamin D replacement therapy. A low dialysate Ca has been advocated in some centers as the dialysis-induced hypocalcemia may favor a shift of Ca from soft tissue to intravascular space (6,72,73).

Calciphylaxis with only nonulcerating plaques may respond to oral steroid therapy, although steroids have been reported as an inciting factor in some cases (9). In a case-controlled series of 36 patients, steroid administration resulted improvement and reduced risk of ulceration when given to patients with plaques only. However, in the presence of any ulcer or high risk of infection, steroid treatment should be cautioned.

Pain should be controlled with appropriate and adequate amount of analgesics. Low molecular weight heparin may be of some benefits as it may limit further thrombosis and tissue ischemia (7). Known predisposing factors of CUA should be avoided or minimized. For instance, local injections and physical trauma to affected site should be limited if possible.

5.2. Other Approaches

The role of parathyroidectomy in CUA remains controversial. The procedure has resulted in an improved outcome in some studies (8,26,32,35,43,67), while others have not found this effective (26,36,44). In the first case series describing 11 patients with calciphylaxis in 1976, most patients had chronic, severe hyperparathyroidism. Seven of them benefited from parathyroidectomy (43). However, a later review study did not find significant increase in survival from parathyroidectomy (48). Calcific uremic arteriolopathy also developed in patients after parathyroidectomy. Because of its invasive nature, with added metabolic stress to the patient, and debatable benefit, parathyroidectomy should be performed only in patients with proven elevated plasma PTH level.

Hyperbaric oxygen therapy (HOT) is a noninvasive procedure that may benefit some patients with calciphylaxis. It consists of patient breathing 100% O_2 inside a sealed chamber with pressure at least 1.4 times of ambient pressure. Each treatment session lasts between 60 and 90 min. Hyperbaric oxygen therapy has been used with some success in the treatment of selected problem wounds. It is hypothesized that hyperbaric oxygen restores and improves tissue PO_2 thus enhancing fibroblast proliferation and collagen production as well as angiogenesis in hypoxic wounds (74). In support of the use of HOT in calciphylaxis, low skin oxygen tensions have been found in limbs of patients with calciphylaxis (52,75). Hyperbaric oxygen therapy has demonstrated successful outcomes, albeit mixed, in some calciphylaxis wounds (75–79). It is worth noting that the cases of positive outcomes required a minimum average of 23 sessions, or about 4–5 weeks of therapy (76). No direct adverse effects of HOT on wounds were reported. Therefore, HOT deserves a trial as an adjuvant therapy in patients who are committed and without contraindication to hyperbaric oxygen. Other therapeutic modalities that have been anecdotally reported include cervical or lumbar sympathectomy (31,43), etidronate disodium (17,80), and gluco-corticoids with subsequent cimetidine (81). Anticoagulation has been beneficial in patients with protein C and protein S deficiencies (18).

6. WOUND CARE

Aggressive wound care is an integral part of managing calciphylaxis. One of the primary goals should be the prevention of fulminant sepsis, which is the cause of death in the majority of patients with calciphylaxis. It is important to obtain regular wound cultures followed by judicious use of systemic antibiotic. Local wound care is complicated by the predilection for eschar formation and tissue ischemia in calciphylaxis ulcers. Selection of the topical dressing should be based the character of the wound bed and marginal skin, ulcer depth, and the amount of exudate. Moist wound dressings would be preferable in relieving pain, assisting debridement of necrotic tissue, and encouraging formation of granulation tissue (49). Debridement of necrotic tissue is advocated by some authors (18,31). Whirlpool may be utilized to facilitate debridement. Surgical debridement can be complicated by nonhealing wound or spread of necrotic tissue base, given the poor wound healing baseline of patients who develop calciphylaxis. Subsequent to debridement, grafting with autologous skin and tissue-engineered skin has been used to promote wound closure (82).

Host nutrition status is another important aspect of wound healing. Patients with CUA require special attention to their nutritional status. Low albumin is associated with poor wound healing and an increased susceptibility to infection (83,84). In case-controlled studies of patients of CUA, it was demonstrated CUA patients had lower serum albumin than control population on dialysis (12,24). Nutritional supplements can be given to patients in accordance with their other medical conditions. Prevention of ulcer development during the nodule/plaque stage is important as well since ulceration dramatically increase the mortality in these patients (9).

Amputation of the affected limb is a last resort. It should be performed above the level of involvement by calciphylaxis. Punch biopsies can be utilized to assess dermal involvement at the planned level of amputation. However, more proximal disease may occur subsequently.

6.1. Preventive Measure

It is equally important to focus medical care on the prevention of future episodes of calciphylaxis. Attention is especially warranted in known at-risk population, i.e., female sex, Caucasian race, obesity, and diabetes. Their serum calcium, phosphate, PTH levels, and nutritional status should be monitored and managed accordingly (53). If possible, oral calcium salts may be substituted by noncalcium phosphate binders. These patients may also benefit from weight reduction, since obesity is associated with increased risk of CUA in dialysis patients.

7. CONCLUSION

Calcific uremic arteriolopathy, or calciphylaxis, remains to be a poorly understood, life-threatening syndrome characterized by calcification and intimal fibroplasia of small-to-medium vessels. It is often a serious complication of ESRD. Patients present with rapidly progressive cutaneous ulcers and gangrene, often leading to secondary infection and sepsis. Proximal involvement results in a worse prognosis than involvement limited to distal areas. Many endogenous and exogenous factors are proposed pathogenic agents, but none of them have been consistently proven. With limited understanding of its pathogenesis, there are no universally effective treatment of CUA. Wound care of calciphylaxis ulcers is challenging. Sepsis from wound infection is the main cause of high mortality of this disease. Calciphylaxis is an important diagnosis to consider in patients with renal failure, because early recognition followed by aggressive treatment may decrease the mortality and morbidity of the disease. Recent studies suggest that the vascular calcification in calciphylaxis in ESRD patients is an active cell-mediated process. This raises hope that directed intervention may arrest vascular calcification and improve survival.

REFERENCES

1. Selye H. Calciphylaxis. Chicago, IL: University of Chicago Press, 1962.
2. Anderson DC, Stewart WK, Piercy DM. Calcifying panniculitis with fat and skin necrosis in a case of uraemia with autonomous hyperparathyroidism. Lancet 1968; 2:323 325.
3. Massry SG, Gordon A, Coburn JW, Kaplan L, Franklin SS, Maxwell MH, Kleeman CR. Vascular calcification and peripheral necrosis in a renal transplant recipient. Reversal of lesions following subtotal parathyroidectomy. Am J Med 1970; 49:416–422.
4. Conn J Jr, Krumlovsky FA, Del Greco F, Simon NM. Calciphylaxis: etiology of progressive vascular calcification and gangrene? Ann Surg 1973; 177:206–210.
5. Cobb JJ, Krumlowshy PA, Delgrasso F et al. Calciphylaxis etiology of progressive vascular calcification and gangrene. Ann Surg 1973; 177:206–210.
6. Llach F. Calcific uremic arteriolopathy (calciphylaxis): an evolving entity? Am J Kidney Dis 1998; 32:514–518.
7. Coates T, Kirkland GS, Dymock RB, Murphy BF, Brealey JK, Mathew TH, Disney AP. Cutaneous necrosis from calcific uremic arteriolopathy. Am J Kidney Dis 1998; 32:384–391.
8. Hafner J, Keusch G, Wahl C, Sauter B, Hurlimann A, von Weizsacker F, Krayenbuhl M, Biedermann K, Brunner U, Helfenstein U. Uremic small-artery disease with medial calcification and intimal hyperplasia (so-called calciphylaxis): a complication of chronic renal failure and benefit from parathyroidectomy. J Am Acad Dermatol 1995; 33: 954–962.
9. Fine A, Zacharias J. Calciphylaxis is usually non-ulcerating: risk factors, outcome and therapy. Kidney Int 2002; 61:2210–2217.
10. Angelis M, Wong LL, Myers SA, Wong LM. Calciphylaxis in patients on hemodialysis: a prevalence study. Surgery 1997; 122:1083–1089; discussion 1089–1090.
11. Levin A, Mehta RL, Goldstein MB. Mathematical formulation to help identify the patient at risk of ischemic tissue necrosis—a potentially lethal complication of chronic renal failure. Am J Nephrol 1993; 13:448–453.
12. Mazhar AR, Johnson RJ, Gillen D, Stivelman JC, Ryan MJ, Davis CL, Stehman-Breen CO. Risk factors and mortality associated with calciphylaxis in end-stage renal disease. Kidney Int 2001; 60:324–332.
13. Smiley CM, Hanlon SU, Michel DM. Calciphylaxis in moderate renal insufficiency: changing disease concepts. Am J Nephrol 2000; 20:324–328.
14. Zacharias JM, Fontaine B, Fine A. Calcium use increases risk of calciphylaxis: a case-control study. Perit Dial Int 1999; 19:248–252.
15. Fader DJ, Kang S. Calciphylaxis without renal failure. Arch Dermatol 1996; 132: 837–838.
16. Kent RB III, Lyerly RT. Systemic calciphylaxis. South Med J 1994; 87:278–281.
17. Banky JP, Dowling JP, Miles C. Idiopathic calciphylaxis. Australas J Dermatol 2002; 43:190–193.
18. Goyal S, Huhn KM, Provost TT. Calciphylaxis in a patient without renal failure or elevated parathyroid hormone: possible aetiological role of chemotherapy. Br J Dermatol 2000; 143:1087–1090.
19. Mastruserio DN, Nguyen EQ, Nielsen T, Hessel A, Pellegrini AE. Calciphylaxis associated with metastatic breast carcinoma. J Am Acad Dermatol 1999; 41:295–298.

20. Lestringant GG, Masouye I, El-Hayek M, Girardet C, Revesz T, Frossard PM. Diffuse calcinosis cutis in a patient with congenital leukemia and leukemia cutis. Dermatology 2000; 200:147–150.

21. Barri YM, Graves GS, Knochel JP. Calciphylaxis in a patient with Crohn's disease in the absence of end-stage renal disease. Am J Kidney Dis 1997; 29:773–776.

22. Pollock B, Cunliffe WJ, Merchant WJ. Calciphylaxis in the absence of renal failure. Clin Exp Dermatol 2000; 25:389–392.

23. Ahmed S, O'Neill KD, Hood AF, Evan AP, Moe SM. Calciphylaxis is associated with hyperphosphatemia and increased osteopontin expression by vascular smooth muscle cells. Am J Kidney Dis 2001; 37:1267–1276.

24. Bleyer AJ, Choi M, Igwemezie B, de la Torre E, White WL. A case control study of proximal calciphylaxis. Am J Kidney Dis 1998; 32:376–383.

25. Walsh JS, Fairley JA. Calciphylaxis. J Am Acad Dermatol 1996; 35:786–787.

26. Hafner J, Keusch G, Wahl C, Burg G. Calciphylaxis: a syndrome of skin necrosis and acral gangrene in chronic renal failure. Vasa 1998; 27:137–143.

27. Handa SP, Strzelczak D. Uremic small artery disease: calciphylaxis with penis involvement. Clin Nephrol 1998; 50:258–261.

28. Jhaveri FM, Woosley JT, Fried FA. Penile calciphylaxis: rare necrotic lesions in chronic renal failure patients. J Urol 1998; 160:764–767.

29. Wood JC, Monga M, Hellstrom WJ. Penile calciphylaxis. Urology 1997; 50:622–624.

30. Ivker RA, Woosley J, Briggaman RA. Calciphylaxis in three patients with end-stage renal disease. Arch Dermatol 1995; 131:63–68.

31. Duh QY, Lim RC, Clark OH. Calciphylaxis in secondary hyperparathyroidism. Diagnosis and parathyroidectomy. Arch Surg 1991; 126:1213–1218; discussion 1218–1219.

32. Fischer AH, Morris DJ. Pathogenesis of calciphylaxis: study of three cases with literature review. Hum Pathol 1995; 26:1055–1064.

33. Asirvatham S, Sebastian C, Sivaram CA, Kaufman C, Chandrasekaran K. Aortic valve involvement in calciphylaxis: uremic small artery disease with medial calcification and intimal hyperplasia. Am J Kidney Dis 1998; 32:499–502.

34. Edelstein CL, Wickham MK, Kirby PA. Systemic calciphylaxis presenting as a painful, proximal myopathy. Postgrad Med J 1992; 68:209–211.

35. Khafif RA, DeLima C, Silverberg A, Frankel R. Calciphylaxis and systemic calcinosis. Collective review. Arch Intern Med 1990; 150:956–959.

36. Adrogue HJ, Frazier MR, Zeluff B, Suki WN. Systemic calciphylaxis revisited. Am J Nephrol 1981; 1:177–183.

37. Richardson JA, Herron G, Reitz R, Layzer R. Ischemic ulcerations of skin and necrosis of muscle in azotemic hyperparathyroidism. Ann Intern Med 1969; 71:129–138.

38. Igaki N, Moriguchi R, Hirota Y, Sakai M, Akiyama H, Tamada F, Oimomi M, Goto T. Calciphylaxis in a patient with end-stage renal disease secondary to systemic lupus erythematosus associated with acral gangrene and mesenteric ischemia. Intern Med 2001; 40:1232–1237.

39. Mureebe L, Moy M, Balfour E, Blume P, Gahtan V. Calciphylaxis: a poor prognostic indicator for limb salvage. J Vasc Surg 2001; 33:1275–1279.

40. Gilson RT, Milum E. Calciphylaxis: case report and treatment review. Cutis 1999; 63:149–153.

41. Tamura M, Hiroshige K, Osajima A, Soejima M, Takasugi M, Kuroiwa A. A dialysis patient with systemic calciphylaxis exhibiting rapidly progressive visceral ischemia and acral gangrene. Intern Med 1995; 34:908–912.

42. Mawad HW, Sawaya BP, Sarin R, Malluche HH. Calcific uremic arteriolopathy in association with low turnover uremic bone disease. Clin Nephrol 1999; 52:160–166.

43. Gipstein RM, Coburn JW, Adams DA, Lee DB, Parsa KP, Sellers A, Suki WN, Massry SG. Calciphylaxis in man. A syndrome of tissue necrosis and vascular calcification in 11 patients with chronic renal failure. Arch Intern Med 1976; 136:1273–1280.

44. Budisavljevic MN, Cheek D, Ploth DW. Calciphylaxis in chronic renal failure. J Am Soc Nephrol 1996; 7:978–982.

45. Mathur RV, Shortland JR, el-Nahas AM. Calciphylaxis. Postgrad Med J 2001; 77: 557–561.

46. Fine A, Fleming S, Leslie W. Calciphylaxis presenting with calf pain and plaques in four continuous ambulatory peritoneal dialysis patients and in one predialysis patient. Am J Kidney Dis 1995; 25:498–502.

47. Essary LR, Wick MR. Cutaneous calciphylaxis. An underrecognized clinicopathologic entity. Am J Clin Pathol 2000; 113:280–287.

48. Chan YL, Mahony JF, Turner JJ, Posen S. The vascular lesions associated with skin necrosis in renal disease. Br J Dermatol 1983; 109:85–95.

49. Burkhart C, Burkhart CN, Milan A. Calciphylaxis: a case report and review of literature. Wounds 1999; 11:58–61.

50. Sankarasubbaiyan S, Scott G, Holley JL. Cryofibrinogenemia: an addition to the differential diagnosis of calciphylaxis in end-stage renal disease. Am J Kidney Dis 1998; 32:494–498.

51. Walsh JS, Fairley JA. Calcifying disorders of the skin. J Am Acad Dermatol 1995; 33:693–706; quiz 707–610.

52. Wilmer WA, Voroshilova O, Singh I, Middendorf DF, Cosio FG. Transcutaneous oxygen tension in patients with calciphylaxis. Am J Kidney Dis 2001; 37:797–806.

53. Wilmer WA, Magro CM. Calciphylaxis: emerging concepts in prevention, diagnosis, and treatment. Semin Dial 2002; 15:172–186.

54. Campistol JM, Almirall J, Martin E, Torras A, Revert L. Calcium-carbonate-induced calciphylaxis. Nephron 1989; 51:549–550.

55. Torok L, Kozepessy L. Cutaneous gangrene due to hyperparathyroidism secondary to chronic renal failure (uraemic gangrene syndrome). Clin Exp Dermatol 1996; 21:75–77.

56. Fernandez E, Amoedo ML, Borras M, Pais B, Montoliu J. Tumoral calcinosis in haemodialysis patients without severe hyperparathyroidism. Nephrol Dial Transplant 1993; 8:1270–1273.

57. Wilkinson SP, Stewart WK, Parham DM, Guthrie W. Symmetric gangrene of the extremities in late renal failure: a case report and review of the literature. Q J Med 1988; 67:319–341.

58. Bleyer AJ, White WL, Choi MJ. Calcific small vessel ischemic disease (calciphylaxis) in dialysis patients. Int J Artif Organs 2000; 23:351–355.

59. Reslerova M, Moe SM. Vascular calcification in dialysis patients: pathogenesis and consequences. Am J Kidney Dis 2003; 41:S96–S99.

60. Chen NX, O'Neill KD, Duan D, Moe SM. Phosphorus and uremic serum up-regulate osteopontin expression in vascular smooth muscle cells. Kidney Int 2002; 62:1724–1731.

61. Rittling SR, Denhardt DT. Osteopontin function in pathology: lessons from osteopontin-deficient mice. Exp Nephrol 1999; 7:103–113.

62. Mehta RL, Scott G, Sloand JA, Francis CW. Skin necrosis associated with acquired protein C deficiency in patients with renal failure and calciphylaxis. Am J Med 1990; 88:252–257.

63. Perez-Mijares R, Guzman-Zamudio JL, Payan-Lopez J, Rodriguez-Fernandez A, Gomez-Fernandez P, Almaraz-Jimenez M. Calciphylaxis in a haemodialysis patient: functional protein S deficiency? Nephrol Dial Transplant 1996; 11:1856–1859.

64. Goldsmith DJ. Calciphylaxis, thrombotic diathesis and defects in coagulation regulation. Nephrol Dial Transplant 1997; 12:1082–1083.

65. Rees JK, Coles GA. Calciphylaxis in man. Br Med J 1969; 2:670–672.

66. Handa SP, Sohi PS. Proximal calciphylaxis in four insulin-requiring diabetic hemodialysis patients. Am J Kidney Dis 1997; 29:812.

67. Fox R, Banowsky LH, Cruz AB Jr. Post-renal transplant calciphylaxis: successful treatment with parathyroidectomy. J Urol 1983; 129:362–363.

68. Russell R, Brookshire MA, Zekonis M, Moe SM. Distal calcific uremic arteriolopathy in a hemodialysis patient responds to lowering of Ca × P product and aggressive wound care. Clin Nephrol 2002; 58:238–243.

69. McAuley K, Devereux F, Walker R. Calciphylaxis in two non-compliant patients with end-stage renal failure. Nephrol Dial Transplant 1997; 12:1061–1063.

70. Richens G, Piepkorn MW, Krueger GG. Calcifying panniculitis associated with renal failure. A case of Selye's calciphylaxis in man. J Am Acad Dermatol 1982; 6:537–539.

71. Kleinpeter MA. Spectrum of complications related to secondary hyperparathyroidism in a peritoneal dialysis patient. Adv Perit Dial 2000; 16:286–290.

72. Lipsker D, Chosidow O, Martinez F, Challier E, Frances C. Low-calcium dialysis in calciphylaxis. Arch Dermatol 1997; 133:798–799.

73. Fernandez E, Montoliu J. Successful treatment of massive uraemic tumoral calcinosis with daily haemodialysis and very low calcium dialysate. Nephrol Dial Transplant 1994; 9:1207–1209.

74. Zamboni WA, Browder LK, Martinez J. Hyperbaric oxygen and wound healing. Clin Plast Surg 2003; 30:67–75.

75. Vassa N, Twardowski ZJ, Campbell J. Hyperbaric oxygen therapy in calciphylaxis-induced skin necrosis in a peritoneal dialysis patient. Am J Kidney Dis 1994; 23:878–881.

76. Basile C, Montanaro A, Masi M, Pati G, De Maio P, Gismondi A. Hyperbaric oxygen therapy for calcific uremic arteriolopathy: a case series. J Nephrol 2002; 15:676–680.

77. Podymow T, Wherrett C, Burns KD. Hyperbaric oxygen in the treatment of calciphylaxis: a case series. Nephrol Dial Transplant 2001; 16:2176–2180.

78. Benedetto BJ, Emhoff TA. The use of hyperbaric oxygen for the management of calciphylaxis. Curr Surg 2000; 57:507.

79. Dean SM, Werman H. Calciphylaxis: a favorable outcome with hyperbaric oxygen. Vasc Med 1998; 3:115–120.

80. Whittam LR, McGibbon DH, MacDonald DM. Proximal cutaneous necrosis in association with chronic renal failure. Br J Dermatol 1996; 135:778–781.

81. Elamin EM, McDonald AB. Calcifying panniculitis with renal failure: a new management approach. Dermatology 1996; 192:156–159.

82. Trent JT, Kirsner RS. Calciphylaxis: diagnosis and treatment. Adv Skin Wound Care 2001; 14:309–312.

83. Jaar BG, Hermann JA, Furth SL, Briggs W, Powe NR. Septicemia in diabetic hemodialysis patients: comparison of incidence, risk factors, and mortality with nondiabetic hemodialysis patients. Am J Kidney Dis 2000; 35:282–292.

84. Doweiko JP, Nompleggi DJ. The role of albumin in human physiology and pathophysiology, Part III: albumin and disease states. J Parenter Enteral Nutr 1991; 15:476–483.

20
Burn Wounds: Pathophysiology and Treatment

Nicholas Namias

Division of Burns and Department of Surgical Infectious Diseases, University of Miami/Jackson Memorial Medical Center, Miami, Florida, U.S.A.

1. TYPES OF BURN WOUNDS

Burn wounds encompass a wide variety of insults to the integument. An overview of several types is given here. While this chapter provides an overview of burn care, it is not intended to prepare every wound care practitioner for comprehensive burn care. The American Burn Association has established guidelines for who should be referred to a burn center (Table 1).

1.1. Thermal

Thermal burns are most commonly caused by scalding liquids, ranging from cooking grease, which can be several hundred degrees Fahrenheit, to simple tap water, which at 140°F can cause serious burns in infants, the elderly, or those with sensory deficits. Other causes of thermal burns include flame burns, flash burns, and contact burns. Flame burns are generally deep burns and usually can be expected to require excision and grafting (Figs. 1–4). Flash burns can be variable. These occur when there is a source of great heat but no direct contact with the heat. Examples are electrical flash burns (heat given off by an arc) and propane explosion flash burns from cooking supplies for grills, boats, or mobile homes. The depth of these is highly variable but even the lightest layer of clothing can prevent them; it is not unusual to see a v-distribution burn where a collar button was left open, while the rest of the chest is spared. Contact burns that come to medical attention are generally deep. These are the result of direct contact with a hot solid, and an inability to free oneself from the heat source or a source so hot that even momentary contact causes a deep burn. Examples include contact with motor vehicle mufflers and industrial machinery. These can be expected to require excision and grafting or, when possible, primary closure.

1.2. Electrical

Electrical injuries are deceptive. Major electrical injuries can be associated with cardiac dysrrhytmias, muscle necrosis, myoglobinuria, and renal failure (Fig. 5). It

Table 1 American Burn Association Criteria for Patients to Be Referred to a Burn Center

1. Partial thickness burns greater than 10% total body surface area (TBSA)
2. Burns that involve the face, hands, feet, genitalia, perineum, or major joints
3. Third-degree burns in any age group
4. Electrical burns, including lightning injury
5. Chemical burns
6. Inhalation injury
7. Burn injury in patients with pre-existing medical disorders that could complicate management, prolong recovery, or affect mortality
8. Any patients with burns and concomitant trauma (such as fractures) in which the burn injury poses the greatest risk of morbidity or mortality. In such cases, if the trauma poses the greater immediate risk, the patient may be initially stabilized in a trauma center before being transferred to a burn unit. Physician judgment will be necessary in such situations and should be in concert with the regional medical control plan and triage protocols
9. Burned children in hospitals without qualified personnel or equipment for the care of children
10. Burn injury in patients who will require special social, emotional, or long-term rehabilitative intervention

is beyond the scope of this chapter to discuss the management of these issues. Consultation with a surgeon and/or a critical care physician is mandatory for major electrical injuries. Although technically the severity of injury is dependent upon amperage, it is the voltage that is commonly discussed clinically. Household current of 120 or 220 V generally cause small wounds without significant systemic physiologic sequelae. An EKG should be done to rule out dysrrhytmias but generally the muscular problems are not present at this voltage. Industrial electricity, in the thousands of volts, can cause the problems described above. As the current passes through the body, various tissues resist the current based on their composition. Bone, as a relatively dry tissue, acts as a resistor and generates heat, causing thermal injury to

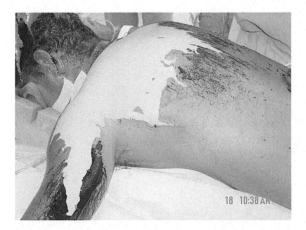

Figure 1 Full thickness (third-degree) burns to the back from molten tar. Note the white color.

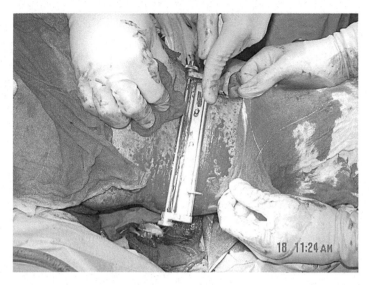

Figure 2 Tangential excision of the burn wound. The Watson knife is a protected straight edge razor used to remove thin successive layers until bleeding viable tissue is reached.

adjacent deep muscles and thrombosis of adjacent vessels. The injured patient may present only with small external injuries where the current entered and exited, but the degree of underlying injury may be far greater than expected by the untrained observer.

1.3. Chemical

Chemical injuries can be caused by acids or alkalis. Acids tend to cause coagulation of proteins that they come in contact with, essentially "tanning" the skin and creating a protective layer for the underlying tissues. Alkalis, however, continue the burning process by saponification until the alkali is removed. Whether acid or alkali,

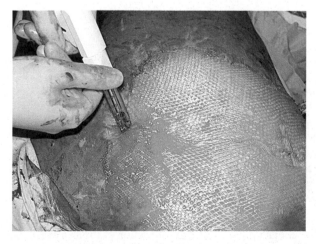

Figure 3 A meshed split thickness skin graft is applied to the excised wound.

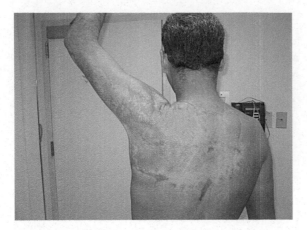

Figure 4 The result of early excision and grafting several weeks postoperatively.

the treatment is irrigation with water or any physiologic crystalloid, e.g., saline solution. This should be continued until symptoms abate or it is clear that the offending agent has been removed. It is not unusual to continue irrigation for an hour. One common unique exception to the rule of not neutralizing the offending agent is hydrofluoric acid. It is used in glass etching, circuit board manufacture, and as a cleaning agent for boats. It injures by binding calcium from the tissues (Fig. 6). The treatment is to administer exogenous calcium, either as a calcium gluconate topical slurry, intravenous calcium gluconate or chloride, or intra-arterial calcium gluconate or chloride. Calcium should be administered until symptoms abate or systemic calcium levels are unacceptable.

1.4. Radiation

Fortunately, most burns due to radiation are sunburns. These burns are superficial and generally require no treatment. Occasionally a patient will develop a second-degree

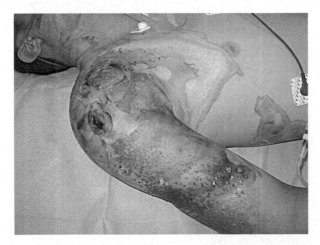

Figure 5 Injury from a 7000 V source. Notice the gray discoloration of the full thickness burn, the tissue destruction at electrical contact points, and the constriction of the arm causing underlying muscle necrosis. This patient did develop myoglobinuria.

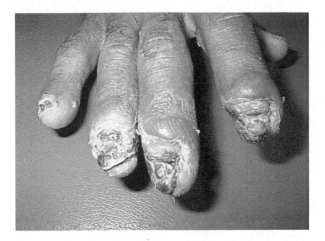

Figure 6 Tissue loss from hydrofluoric acid burns. There was at least a 12-hr delay from exposure to presentation.

burn with blistering, and these can be treated as any other second-degree burn. Radiation burns due to laboratory accident, medical overexposure, or acts of war are varied in their presentation. At total doses less than 5 Gy, there can be an immediate erythema which resolves in several days, followed by a second erythema and desquamation of keratinocytes and possible loss of hair at 2–3 weeks after exposure. At doses of 12–20 Gy, a "moist desquamation" occurs, with blistering, and is treated as any other second-degree burn. At doses of radiation in excess of 25 Gy, skin necrosis and ulceration may present several weeks to months after exposure due to occlusion of the microvascular supply. These patients are at risk for skin cancers, which may present months or years later (1). The wounds are treated as other burns are treated. The unique set of complications of these injuries are due to associated physiologic effects of radiation or associated injuries in the case of war, and are beyond the scope of this text.

2. PATHOPHYSIOLOGY

2.1. Partial vs. Full Thickness

Burn depth is characterized either by "degree" or by qualitative description of the thickness of the burn. Laypersons are most familiar with the terms "first degree" (epidermis only, e.g., sunburn), "second degree" (epidermis and partial thickness of the dermis, e.g., scalding injuries), and "third degree" (full thickness of the dermis, e.g., long exposure to flames). Physicians caring for burns generally discuss burns in terms of "partial" or "full" thickness. "First-degree" burns require no specific care. Second-degree or partial thickness burns generally are recognized by either blistering or denudation of the dermis. Depending on the depth, they may be of variable moistness, color, and pain (Fig. 7). Third-degree or full thickness burns are recognized by the fact that they are dry, leathery, and insensate. Some burns are a combination of the above and defy categorization; these are termed "indeterminate." Burns that are initially partial thickness can convert to full thickness either by infection or hypoperfusion of the wounds.

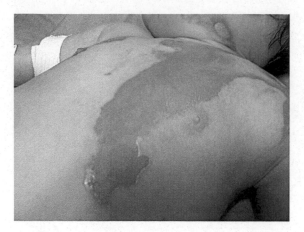

Figure 7 Typical scald burn. Notice moist pink appearance.

2.2. Nature of Thermal Contact vs. Depth of Wound

The depth of burn is dependent on the temperature of the burning agent and the duration of contact. Work from 1947 (2) first demonstrated quantitatively the contributions of temperature and time in the depth of burning. Tap water at 120 °F will provide a satisfactorily hot shower for an adult but will spare an infant from second-degree burns for 8 minutes. Water at 140 ° F will scald an infant in 3 sec! The principle of specific heat applies to scalding liquids. Water or aqueous-based liquids cool relatively rapidly, and run off of the wound rapidly. Oil-based liquids (cooking oil, grease, fat-based soups) adhere to the wound, reach temperatures much higher than boiling water, are slow to cool, and subsequently tend to cause deeper burns. Molten tar is an extreme example, while grease burns from cooking are common in burn centers.

2.3. Nature of the Burn Wound

It is obvious to the casual observer that the partial thickness burn will have associated insensible water losses. What is not so obvious is that the full thickness burn, which appears dry and leathery, also has associated insensible losses. If full thickness burn eschar is used to cover a container of water, evaporative loss from the container is unimpeded. The moist partial thickness burn wound is exquisitely painful, triggered by even the slightest air currents passing over it. To the contrary, the full thickness burn wound has no viable nerve endings, and is insensate

The burn wound is the nidus for a local inflammatory response, or, in burns approaching 15% TBSA, a systemic inflammatory response, the most obvious clinical manifestation being edema. The edema is both interstitial, from an increase in microvascular permeability, and intracellular, from an influx of sodium caused by a change in the resting membrane potential of cells after a significant burn injury. Aside from the inflammatory response caused by the presence of ischemic or necrotic tissue, and the inflammatory response derived from reperfusion injury once resuscitation has begun, the undebrided burn wound can serve as a focus for infection. In partial thickness burns, the protective epidermis is lost, creating a portal of entry for microorganisms. Colonization of burn wounds is common, and does not necessarily mandate systemic antibiotic therapy. Swab culture of wounds will universally yield organisms; therapeutic decisions cannot be made on the results of these cultures. In superficial partial thickness burns (e.g., hot water scald), the most likely evidence of infection is cellulitis surrounding the wound. A small rim of erythema around a burn wound can normally be expected. When this spreads from the immediate area of the perimeter of the wound, cellulitis is suspected, and systemic antibiotics are begun. The author's preference is oxacillin. In full thickness burns, when the organism burden exceeds 10×5 organisms per cubic centimeter of tissue, as measured by quantitative culture of a wound biopsy, the risk for invasion of unburned subjacent tissue increases. It is this invasion and the systemic response to it that is termed burn wound sepsis. Definitive diagnosis requires quantitative culture and histologic evidence of invasion of normal tissues. Unfortunately, this technique is limited to very few specialized centers. In the absence of this technique, one must rely on gross observation of new dark discoloration in a burn wound accompanied with systemic illness. This mandates excision of the suspect wounds, topical and systemic antimicrobials, and appropriate physiologic support in the intensive care unit.

2.4. Natural History

The natural history of burn wounds is well known. Until the 1970s, effective topical antimicrobials were not available, and early operative intervention had not yet been introduced. Superficial second-degree burns can be expected to heal spontaneously in 2–3 weeks, with minimal hypertrophic scarring. Deeper second-degree burns will take longer to heal. This will be accompanied by significant hypertrophic scarring, contraction, and potential for functional deficit due to contractures. Third-degree burns, in which, by definition, all of the dermal elements needed for regeneration of the skin are destroyed, cannot heal spontaneously except by contraction. This contraction does not occur until the burn eschar separates from the underlying wound. Untreated, the burn wound becomes colonized, and bacteria invade the space between the eschar and the normal underlying tissue. The eschar undergoes digestion by bacterial collagenases. Additionally, pus form under the eschar, and the eschar lifts from the underlying granulating wound bed; this process is known as suppuration. If the patient survives this without developing systemic sepsis, the wound then must heal by contraction. This contraction can render limbs useless, impair the ability to close the eyes or mouth, and even double over entire bodies across the waist (Fig. 8).

2.5. Hypertrophic Scarring

Hypertrophic scarring arises when the wound takes longer than 2–3 weeks to heal spontaneously, at the borders and seams of skin grafts, and in the interstices of meshed split thickness skin grafts. The entity is on a continuum that includes keloids, and histopathologically they are both disorders of collagen alignment. In normal burn wound scarring, the collagen fibers align parallel to the surface of the skin. In hypertrophic scarring, they take on a whorled pattern. Clinically, these scars are raised from the surface of the wound after maturation has otherwise completed (Fig. 9). Common practice to prevent or to treat hypertrophic scarring is to apply elastic pressure garments to the affected areas. This is supported by years of experience and by nonrandomized trials. A prospective, randomized trial

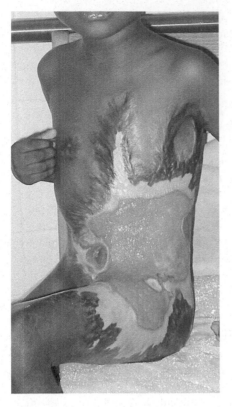

Figure 8 Child from Third World country with full thickness burns closing by contraction. The hip cannot be extended.

concluded that pressure garments did not affect the frequency of hypertrophic scarring after burns (3). It is unclear why the practice of using pressure garments persists, but some possible reasons include the perceived effects on pain, itching, and edema reported by patients, and the need of both patients and caregivers to "do something."

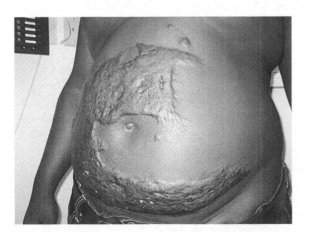

Figure 9 Hypertrophic scar in a healed burn wound.

3. NONOPERATIVE AND PREOPERATIVE WOUND MANAGEMENT

Although it is common practice to use antimicrobial topical therapy on all burn wounds, this practice, in fact, has only been shown to reduce burn wound sepsis in large (20–40%) but not extremely large (>40%) burn wounds, and has not been shown to be of benefit in small wounds. Despite this, topical antimicrobial use is near universal and the available agents will briefly be discussed here. For all of the modalities discussed below, near aseptic technique should be used. It is not possible to maintain operating room levels of sterility for daily wound care; in fact, tap water is used to clean the wounds. However, the author prefers to start with sterile gloves, a clean disposable apron so as not to transfer contamination between patients, a cap to prevent hair from falling into the wound, and a surgical mask. Gloves worn to remove old dressings are changed before applying new dressings. Attention is paid to adequate analgesia and anxiolysis as needed. Intravenous morphine and midazolam are preferred for large wounds, with doses titrated to effect. Oral acetaminophen/hydrocodone combinations or hydromorphone are used for smaller wounds. Prescriptions are given for home use for outpatients. Slow release oxycodone is commonly given for durable pain relief between dressing changes. No burn care should ever be rendered without adequate analgesia.

3.1. Silver Sulfadiazene

Silver sulfadiazene cream 1% was introduced in the 1970s. It is the most commonly used topical antimicrobial in American burn centers. It has broad-spectrum antimicrobial fsactivity including Gram-positive and negative organisms, methicillin-resistant *Staphylococcus aureus*, and *Candida* spp. It is ideally changed twice daily, being washed off with soap and water at each dressing change. When not removed, it combines with proteinaceous exudates from the wounds to create a pseudo-eschar that make evaluation of the wound difficult. It is soothing on application. It does not penetrate eschar well, and is not suitable for reducing bacterial burden once organisms have invaded the wound. Its predominant adverse effect is a transient leukopenia that resolves spontaneously without withdrawal of the drug. Uncommonly, patients will develop a maculopapular rash in response to the drug. Despite its ability to delay wound colonization and prevent burn wound sepsis, silver sulfadiazene is known to slow epithelialization.

3.2. Mafenide Acetate

Mafenide acetate is available as an 11% cream or a 5% solution. Mafenide acetate has activity against most Gram-negative organisms, but poor activity against *Staphylococci* and *Candida*. In the cream form, it is painful on application. It is a carbonic anhydrase inhibitor, and when used on large areas can cause a metabolic acidosis. Despite these serious shortcomings, it remains useful in the patient with invasive infection being prepared for the operating room.

3.3. AgNO$_3$

Silver nitrate solution 0.5% is the silver-based predecessor to silver sulfadiazene. Its spectrum of activity is similar to silver sulfadiazene but is in an aqueous solution that has several advantages and disadvantages. The main advantages are that: (1) it does not leave a pseudoeschar, maintaining an easily evaluable wound, and (2) it does not have to be wiped off of the wound, which provides a pain control advantage. Its main disadvantage is that it stains everything it comes into contact with brown or black, including linens, beds, floors, and unburned skin. It is a hypotonic solution with the described complication of causing loss of electrolytes from the wound, but this has not been a problem in the authors' experience. Wet solution needs to be added every 2–4 hr, and the gauze needs to be replaced twice a day to avoid accumulation of crystalline silver nitrate, which can be histotoxic.

3.4. Collagenase and Papain-Urea

Collagenase and papain-urea debriding ointments are commercially available. Collagenase has been compared to silver sulfadiazene as a topical therapy for burns, and led to faster re-epithelialization (4). However, it provides no antimicrobial effect, and is not appropriate for large wounds at risk for burn wound sepsis. There are no comparative studies of the two debriding agents against each other. Their value is in speeding the removal of eschar in situations where there is eschar to be removed but the wound is too small to merit a trip to the operating room, or if other reasons preclude a trip to the operating room. Collagenase is pain free on application. Papain-urea is painful on application, and is probably best used on insensate full thickness eschar.

3.5. Acticoat/Arglaes/Silverlon

These dressings represent a new method of delivering silver to the wound. All are essentially silver containing dressings that release silver to the wound directly, without a carrier cream or solution. The need for frequent dressing changes is eliminated. Once the dressing is applied, it remains in place for several days. Conceptually they are promising, and have rapidly been embraced by burn care practitioners to replace silver sulfadiazene. Each has a proprietary method of delivering the silver, and each bandage has different physical properties. There are no good comparative studies of these dressings. The market will decide which prevails.

3.6. Biobrane/Transcyte

These are synthetic dressings combined with biologic agents that provide for protection of superficial wounds while they re-epithelialize. Biobrane has porcine collagen-coated nylon fibers on the surface that comes in contact with the wound. It has been shown in small studies to reduce the time to wound closure and cause less pain when compared to silver sulfadiazene (5,6). Transcyte has human dermal proteins, glycosaminoglycans, and growth factors. There are several small studies to suggest that it can shorten the time to wound closure and with one study claiming a reduction in the need for surgical grafting (7–9). The acquisition cost of Transcyte is significant. Large controlled trials are needed before it will be universally adopted.

4. OPERATIVE MANAGEMENT

Operative excision is undertaken when it appears that the wound will not close spontaneously in 2–3 weeks. Early excision, within several days of injury, has become the standard of care. This includes some indeterminate wounds, deep second-degree wounds, and all third-degree wounds.

4.1. Tangential Excision

Tangential excision involves slicing off thin layers of the burn successively until punctate bleeding from viable tissue is obtained. This is done with specialized instruments (e.g., Watson knife, Goulian knife) that are essentially razor blades with a guard to help guide the depth of excision. The guards provide a minimum margin of safety; these instruments are dangerous in untrained hands. Blood loss can be prodigious in these operations

4.2. Full Thickness Excision

Full thickness excision is performed when it is clear that there is no viable dermis remaining. Blood loss can be minimized in this way by operating in an avascular surgical plane, as opposed to slicing through tissue in tangential excision. The excision can be taken down to subcutaneous fat or to fascia. Excision to fat had been thought to yield a poor graft take but less cosmetic deformity, although recent data refute the resulting poor graft take (10). Excision to fascia yields a good graft take but greater cosmetic deformity.

4.3. Temporary Coverage for the Excised Wound

When the size of the excision outstrips the availability of donor skin with which to close the wound, the open wounds must either be treated with topical antimicrobials or have a temporary covering. Various options for temporary coverage are described below.

4.3.1. Allograft

Allograft (also known as homograft) is human cadaver skin. It is processed and screened from donors in much the same way as other organ donations, thus minimizing the risk of disease transmission from donor to recipient. Allograft will temporarily "take" (vascularize) for several weeks before being rejected by the host immune system. It is available in a cryopreserved state from tissue banks. Aside from providing heat and moisture retention, the interface between the allograft and the wound provides a milieu in which host phagocytes can engulf invading bacteria. The allograft is left in place until harvested donor sites have healed and can be reharvested for further grafting.

4.3.2. Xenograft

Xenograft (graft from another species) provides a biologic cover but does not vascularize in the way that allograft does. Porcine xenograft is commonly used in the United States. It is commercially available in several forms; some forms require no refrigeration and have a long shelf life. In Brazil, frog skin, which is readily available, has been used with great success. Xenografts provide the heat and moisture retention of allografts, but do not vascularize as do allografts. Porcine xenograft is the authors' treatment of choice for superficial scald burns. It is wrapped for 24 hr in gauze soaked in 0.5% $AgNO_3$ aqueous solution, and then exposed to air (11).

4.3.3. Biobrane/Transcyte

Biobrane and Transcyte are described above. These can also be used for temporary coverage of excised wounds. There are no good data to support the superiority of these over any of the other temporary coverings.

4.3.4. Apligraf

Apligraf is a bioengineered wound dressing containing cells cultured from a neonatal foreskin cell line. It is indicated for use in diabetic foot ulcers. There is only anecdotal evidence for its use in burns. The author has had mixed results. It universal acceptance in burn care awaits further research.

4.4. Permanent Coverage

Excised wounds will eventually require permanent coverage. Donor skin from the patient is required in some amount for all forms of permanent coverage.

4.4.1. STSG

Split thickness skin graft (STSG) is the gold standard for permanent coverage. The surgical technique for skin grafting is described in Chapter 46. Only some salient points will be discussed here. Meshing of skin grafts allows for greater surface area to be covered, as meshed grafts can be expanded. Meshing also allows serum and blood to escape from under the graft, avoiding the graft failure that results from the accumulation of such fluid under unmeshed grafts. Additionally, hypertrophic scarring can develop in the interstices of meshed grafts. Despite these drawbacks, mesh grafts are often used in burn care because of the need to cover the maximal area with the minimal donor, and the perceived greater likelihood for graft take with a meshed graft in the frequently contaminated, inflamed burn wound. Full thickness grafts are infrequently used in burn 2 wounds but remain an option for small wounds.

4.4.2. Alloderm

Alloderm® is human cadaver skin processed to be completely acellular. All that remains is the connective tissue scaffolding. The concept is that the Alloderm is applied to the excised wound, and ingrowth from the excised bed creates a neodermis. Autografting with a very thin split thickness skin graft can be done at the first operation or in a delayed fashion. The intuitive benefit is that in large burns, immediate coverage can be obtained with Alloderm, and application of autograft superthin split thickness skin grafts can proceed as donor sites heal and become available for repeated harvest. Another claimed benefit is superior function and cosmesis. Evidence for these claims at this time is largely anecdotal.

4.4.3. Integra

Integra® is a synthetic skin substitute synthesized from bovine collagen and shark glycosaminoglycans. It is paired with a thin silastic membrane that acts as a temporary epidermis. Integra is applied to a freshly excised burn wound, and ingrowth from the underlying wound creates a neodermis. When that is completely vascularized (approximately 2 weeks), a superthin split thickness skin graft must be applied to replace the silastic membrane. Similar to Alloderm, it allows for immediate coverage of large wounds, and has claimed benefits of superior cosmesis and function.

Although there is large experience supporting that it is safe and effective (12), pro-spective, randomized evidence for its superiority to other methods of wound closure is lacking at this time.

4.4.4. Cultured Epidermal Autograft

Epicel® cultured epidermal autograft is cultured from the patients' own cells. A small biopsy is taken from the patient and sent to a central processing laboratory. The cells from this skin are then cultured into large sheets, which are ready in several weeks. These epidermal sheets can then be applied to either an open excised burn wound, or as the epidermal component of a wound that has already been grafted with Alloderm or Integra. The cultured epidermal autograft is only several cells thick, and is chal-lenging to handle and apply. Graft take is not as good as with split thickness skin grafting. Prospective evidence of the superiority of this product to autografting in small burns is not available, but in cases of very large burns where donor sites are very limited, this may be the only technique to salvage the patient.

REFERENCES

1. Milner SM, Herndon DN. Radiation injuries, vesicant burns, and mass casualties. In: Herndon DN, ed. Total Burn Care. 2nd ed. Ch 38. WB Saunders: New York, 2002:481–491.
2. Moritz AR, Henriques FC Jr. The relative importance of time and surface temperature in the causation of cutaneous burns. Am J Pathal 1947; 23:695–719.
3. Chang P, Laubenthal KN, Lewis RW II, Rosenquist MD, Lindley-Smith P, Kealey GP. Prospective, randomized study of the efficacy of pressure garment therapy in patients with burns. J Burn Care Rehabil 1995; 16(5):473–475.
4. Hansbrough JF, Achauer B, Dawson J, Himel H, Luterman A, Slater H, Levenson S, Salzberg CA, Hansbrough WB, Dore C. Wound healing in partial-thickness burn wounds treated with collagenase ointment versus silver sulfadiazine cream. J Burn Care Rehabil 1995; 16(3 Pt 1):241–247.
5. Gerding RL, Emerman CL, Effron D, Lukens T, Imbembo AL, Fratianne RB. Outpa-tient management of partial-thickness burns: Biobrane versus 1% silver sulfadiazine. Ann Emerg Med 1990; 19(2):121–124.
6. Barret JP, Dziewulski P, Ramzy PI, Wolf SE, Desai MH, Herndon DN. Biobrane versus 1% silver sulfadiazine in second-degree pediatric burns. Plast Reconstr Surg 2000; 105(1):62–65.
7. Lukish JR, Eichelberger MR, Newman KD, Pao M, Nobuhara K, Keating M, Golonka N, Pratsch G, Misra V, Valladares E, Johnson P, Gilbert JC, Powell DM, Hartman GE. The use of a bioactive skin substitute decreases length of stay for pediatric burn patients. J Pediatr Surg 2001; 36(8):1118–1121.
8. Noordenbos J, Dore C, Hansbrough JF. Safety and efficacy of TransCyte for the treat-ment of partial-thickness burns. J Burn Care Rehabil 1999; 20(4):275–281.
9. Demling RH, DeSanti L. Management of partial thickness facial burns (comparison of topical antibiotics and bio-engineered skin substitutes). Burns 1999; 25(3):256–261.
10. Thourani VH, Ingram WL, Feliciano DV. Factors affecting success of split-thickness skin grafts in the modern burn unit. J Trauma 2003; 54(3):562–568.
11. Still JM Jr, Law EJ. Primary excision of the burn wound. Clin Plast Surg 2000; 27(1):23–47.
12. Heimbach DM, Warden GD, Luterman A, Jordan MH, Ozobia N, Ryan CM, Voigt DW, Hickerson WL, Saffle JR, DeClement FA, Sheridan RL, Dimick AR. Multicenter postapproval clinical trial of integra(r) dermal regeneration template for burn treatment. J Burn Care Rehabil 2003; 24(1):42–48.

21
Pyoderma Gangrenosum

Mark D. Hoffman

Department of Dermatology, Rush-Presbyterian-St. Luke's Medical Center, Chicago, Illinois, U.S.A.

1. INTRODUCTION

Pyoderma gangrenosum (PG) is an inflammatory ulcerative condition of unclear etiology. Originally described by Brunsting et al. in 1930 and felt to represent a bacterial infection (1), their designation for these lesions is in fact a misnomer. PG is neither an infectious disease nor result in devitalized tissue requiring debridement. Rather, it is a reactive disorder that typically responds favorably to anti-inflammatory agents. Surgical debridement rarely serves to contain the process, and may in fact aggravate and extend it. Because of the peculiar tendency of PG to be expressed in tissues that have been injured, traumatized, or surgical manipulated—a phenomenon known as "pathergy"—it is important for clinicians to be able to recognize PG and distinguish it from its simulators.

Pyoderma gangrenosum frequently occurs in connection with an extra-cutaneous disease process. Inflammatory bowel disease, arthritis, and hematologic disorders including malignancy are most common, and may precede or follow the development of skin ulceration. Knowledge of these disease associations both assists in the diagnosis of PG, and prompts farther evaluation for attendant co-morbidity.

2. EPIDEMIOLOGY

Pyoderma gangrenosum typically affects middle-aged adults (average age = 50 years (2)), but may occur in infancy (3) or childhood (4). The reported female/male ratio has varied from 1:1 (5) to 3:1 (6). Although pyoderma gangrenosum is uncommon, it is not rare. The incidence of the disease has been estimated to be 2 cases per million population per year (2); academic dermatologic referral centers may encounter as many as 10 cases annually (7).

Pyoderma gangrenosum is nearly always sporadic. However, 7 kindred have been reported with familial clustering of the disease (8,9). In addition, PG is a component of the so-called "PAPA syndrome" (pyogenic arthritis, pyoderma gangrenosum, and acne), an autosomal-dominant condition whose disease-locus has been mapped to chromosome 15q (10).

3. CUTANEOUS LESIONS OF PYODERMA GANGRENOSUM

The skin ulcerations of PG are unique both in their manner of evolution, and in their appearance when fully mature. When the characteristic features of PG are present in a case under consideration, a presumptive diagnosis can often be made.

Pyoderma gangrenosum has been divided into a number of clinical subtypes. It is surprising for some to discover that these subtypes are based largely on *pre-ulcerative* or "primary" features in the skin lesions–not on the characteristics of the ensuing "secondary" ulcerations themselves. Pyoderma gangrenosum ordinarily first arises either as pustules or as bullae (primary lesions). These early, incipient lesions may be relatively inconspicuous and few in number. However, it is important that clinicians search for them, since their presence allow for the more specific assignment into a PG-subtype. Since each of the various subtypes of PG has been correlated with specific systemic diseases, subclassification may be of considerable value to the practitioner. Regrettably, different classification schemes for PG do exist in the literature (5,11), and not all of the variants that have been proposed enjoy universal acceptance (7).

The most common expression of PG is in its "classical" (a.k.a. "typical" or "ulcerative") form. This subtype is often associated with arthritis or inflammatory bowel disease. Lesions begin as single or grouped sterile inflammatory pustules (Figure 1) or sometimes as deep red nodules, which subsequently devolve into hemorrhagic ulcerations. Occasionally a patient with PG will develop inflammatory pustules that do not ulcerate. This "pustular" form of PG is also associated with inflammatory bowel disease, and may represent a *forme fruste* of classical PG.

Another well-recognized variant of PG is the "bullous" (a.k.a. "atypical") form (12). In this pattern lesions begin as grey, occasionally hemorrhagic vesicles

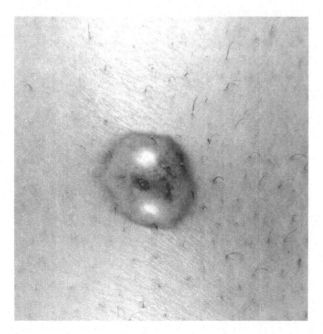

Figure 1   The initial blush of PG—an inflammatory pustule destined to ulcerate in a patient with ulcerative colitis.

and bullae, and the ulcerations tend to be more superficial than those found in the classical variant. This subtype of PG may accompany myeloproliferative disease.

Peristomal pyoderma gangrenosum is an unusual subtype that may follow the creation of an enterostomy or colostomy outlet (by months to decades). The ulcers or fistulous tracts that develop may be confused with a wound infection, a contact dermatitis, or a stitch abscess. Peristomal PG occurs in patients having inflammatory bowel disease or abdominal malignancy (13).

Regardless of their initial form of presentation, the resultant ulcerations of pyoderma gangrenosum display features highly suggestive of this diagnosis (Figure 2). Especially notable are the ulcer margins—they are elevated, boggy and violaceous, and often overhang the ulcer base by several millimeters (Figure 3). Just beyond the ulcer margin is a peripheral zone of erythema. Newly formed ulcerations display a hemorrhagic crust at their bases; later, a fibrinoid, mucopurulent exudate is observed.

Ulcer expansion can occur rapidly, with lesions sometimes enlarging by one to two centimeters in a single day. As ulcers widen, the inflammatory process may proceed at different rates at different fronts, so that their borders become serpiginous. In PG, the inflammatory response to noxious stimuli is abnormal and exaggerated, and lesions may be initiated by even minor trauma. Patients often volunteer or can be prompted to recall an inciting injury during the initial history taking. This phenomenon, known as pathergy, is another diagnostically helpful feature and is seen in approximately 25% of patients (14). The ulcerations of PG are nearly always painful—sometimes exceedingly so. A lack of pain without explanation (e.g., neuropathy) should cast doubt on the diagnosis of PG.

PG has a proclivity for the legs, which are affected in about 80% of cases. Other areas may also be targeted, albeit less frequently—the trunk is involved about 10% of the time; the head, groin, or upper extremities in fewer than 5% of patients (14). Multiple ulcers are usually present simultaneously. Lesion size in PG is highly

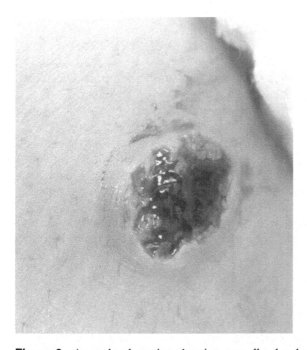

Figure 2 An early ulceration showing a swollen border and hemorrhagic base.

(a)   (b)

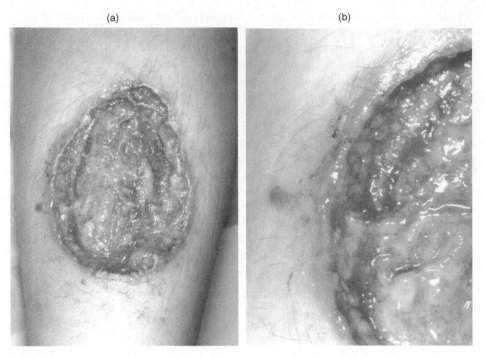

Figure 3   (a) A large mature lesion of pyoderma gangrenosum. (b) The characteristic active
and undermined ulcer margin.

variable, ranging from under one centimeter to over 30 centimeters. Although most
ulcers are less than 3 cm, 80% of patients have at least one ulcer > 3 cm (15). Healing, when it occurs, results in atrophic and sometimes cribriform scarring.

4. EXTRACUTANEOUS LESIONS OF PYODERMA GANGRENOSUM

Extracutaneous involvement by the pyoderma gangrenosum disease process is unusual but does occur; patients with inflammatory colitis may be at higher risk (16).
Sterile neutrophilic infiltrates may develop in one or several organ systems: lungs,
eyes, heart (13), CNS (17), muscle (18), bone, liver, or spleen (19). The lung is most
commonly affected; in one series of 21 cases, 2 patients had fatal pulmonary involvement (20). Pulmonary symptoms include cough, dyspnea, or chest pain (16). Chest
radiography may show a consolidated, cavitary pneumonia (21), a unilateral opacity
(22), or multiple and bilateral nodules (23). Eye disease expressed as peripheral
ulcerative keratitis may lead to blindness if it goes unrecognized and untreated.
Patients complain of decreased visual acuity, eye pain, redness, and/or irritation
(24). Extracutaneous PG may precede but usually appears simultaneously with or
following the onset of skin lesions.

5. DISEASE ASSOCIATIONS

It has been estimated that 50% of patients with PG have a concomitant disease or
systemic abnormality (5). As previously discussed, the manner in which PG develops
may help to predict potential disease associations.

Inflammatory bowel disease (both ulcerative colitis and Crohn's disease) occurs in approximately one third of patients with PG (14). Some have observed that cutaneous disease activity seems to parallel that of the intestinal tract, and there exist reports describing the healing of skin ulcerations following intestinal resection (25,26). However, PG has also first appeared many years after total proctocolectomy (27).

Arthritis complicates nearly 40% of cases. Both a symmetrical polyarthritis (7) and an asymmetrical monoarticular inflammation affecting large joints (5) have been cited as the most common form. The arthritis may be seropositive or seronegative.

Hematologic abnormalities may also occur, especially in the context of bullous PG. Myelogenous leukemia, lymphoblastic leukemia, and myeloid metaplasia have all been described (28). A monoclonal gammopathy, usually IgA and usually benign, may be detected in up to 20% of patients (15).

A number of reports have linked PG with Takayasu arteritis, particularly in Japan (29).

6. HISTOPATHOLOGY

The histopathologic findings in PG are not specific but are supportive. The microscopic findings are governed in part by the site of the biopsy (pre-ulcerative lesion; erythematous margin of ulcer; ulcer edge; or ulcer base), which in turn will reflect the stage and maturity of the inflammatory process.

Disagreement exists as to the nature of the changes in the earliest phases of PG. Some propose that PG arises initially as a neutrophilic, suppurative, and necrotizing folliculitis (30,31). Others report that the earliest and most characteristic histologic feature is a lymphoeytic vasculitis–seen most reliably at the erythematous margin of an ulcer (described as the preferred biopsy site) (32). In this schema, the mixed infiltrate of neutrophils and lymphocytes seen at the ulcer edge, and the dermal necrosis and abscess formation contained within the ulcer floor are deemed secondary changes.

Although a secondary leukocytoclastic vasculitis may be observed in areas of pronounced tissue damage, it should not otherwise be conspicuous. Direct immunofluorescence is positive in 55% of cases, typically showing IgM, C3, and fibrin in the papillary and reticular dermal vessels (32); these deposits likely reflect non-specific tissue injury (33).

One study has suggested that the finding of histiocytic giant cells within the inflammatory infiltrate may signal the presence of inflammatory bowel disease, particularly Crohn's disease (34). In PG associated with leukemia, the cellular infiltrate may be clonal (35–37).

7. ETIOLOGY/PATHOGENESIS

Pyoderma gangrenosum is one of a group of so-called "neutrophilic dermatoses" (38)—which includes Sweet's syndrome and others—characterized by an infiltrate rich in polymorphonuclear leukocytes. However, the fundamental cause of this abnormal assembly of neutrophils into lesional tissue remains speculative. Some reports suggest that the underlying defect inheres within the neutrophil itself (39,40), and recent studies have found unique aberrations in integrin expression and behavior on the neutrophils of patients with PG (41,42). Moreover, PG has occurred in patients with leukocyte adhesion1 deficiency type (43), a heritable condition whose mutation results in the depletion or absence of β2 integrins on neutrophils.

Other evidence, however, points to a primary and pivotal role for T-cells in the pathogenesis of this disease. PG often responds favorably to medications (e.g. cyclosporine) which specifically target T-cells and alter their cytokine production, but whose affect on neutrophils is only indirect.

Cytokine abnormalities may be important in the pathogenesis of PG. IL-8 is a potent activator and chemoattractant for neutrophils, and is over-expressed in lesional tissue from patients with PG (44). The source of this IL-8 is unclear. A number of cell types may generate IL-8 including T-cells, B-cells, NK cells, basophils, eosinophils, monocytes, fibroblasts, endothelial cells, keratinocytes, and even neutrophils themselves. IL-1 may be germane in the subset of PG patients with the PAPA syndrome. These individuals have mutations in CD2-binding protein 1, which result in excessive production of IL-1 (45). This cytokine would be expected to activate a number of pathways which might lead to the recruitment of inflammatory cells, including neutrophils, into the skin.

TNF-α may play a key role in some cases of PG, particularly those associated with inflammatory bowel disease. TNF-α is a "primary" cytokine (along with IL-1) which mediates innate immunity and has a broad range of effects, including activation of granulocytes, induction of other cytokines (IL-8 and others), and up-regulation of adhesion molecules. Serum TNF-α has been reported to be elevated in a patient with PG–its levels correlating with ulcer activity (46). Serum TNF-α concentrations are also noted to be increased during inflammatory bowel disease relapses (47), and inhibition of TNF-α has led to improvement of skin lesions in patients with both inflammatory bowel disease and PG.

One potential model for the pathogenesis of PG that may explain the links between skin ulcerations, inflammatory bowels disease, TNF-α, and pathergy is the Schwartzman reaction. This is a form of cytokine-primed, neutrophil-dependent skin destruction occurring at a site(s) of previous infection or inflammation. Its histology is characterized by neutrophil aggregation, endothelial damage, hemorrhage, and microthrombi, but a significant T-cell component and immune-complexes are both absent. In its classic form the Schwartzman reaction proceeds through 3 stages: first the skin is "prepared" by injecting it with endotoxin (LPS); next LPS is given systemically; and finally necrosis is observed within the prepared site(s) (48). The Schwartzman reaction was initially proposed as a paradigm for PG by Rostenberg in 1953 when ulcerative colitis was thought to represent a septic process (49), but this model was essentially abandoned as the understanding of inflammatory bowel disease pathogenesis shifted away from infectious etiologies towards an immune disturbance. However, more recent observations relating to the Schwartzman reaction might suggest that this phenomenon be revived as a model for PG: for instance, it is now know that a variety of organisms (streptococci, corynebacterium viruses) are capable of "preparing" the skin in place of LPS, and moreover, that TNF-α can substitute for LPS in the second step (48). One might conjecture, therefore, that during relapses-of IBD elevated serum THF-α levels act upon skin tissue(s) previously prepared by infection (or skin injury secondary to trauma (50)), leading to the development of ulcerations.

In a handful of cases medications have triggered outbreaks of PG. Reports have implicated isotretinoin (51,52), sulpiride (53) (a form of respiridone), and GM-CSF(54). Drug-induced folliculitis/furunculosis may be mechanistic in cases linked to isotretinoin and respiridone, while cases precipitated by GM-CSF might be driven by its direct effect on neutrophil numbers, function, and/or differentiation. Discontinuation of the offending medication in these instances has led to improvement or clearing of the ulcers.

Speculation has also focused on roles for *Chlamydia pneumoniae* (55), as well as on putative cross-reactive skin/intestinal antibodies (targeting tropomyosin-5 (56) or cytokeratin 18 (57)), but these hypotheses remain unproven.

It is difficult to reconcile all of these disparate clinical and laboratory findings into a completely unified framework for pathogenesis. PG may ultimately represent the end phenotype of a variety of abnormalities that result in inappropriate neutrophil trafficking, leading to tissue neutrophilia within the skin and potentially elsewhere.

8. DIAGNOSIS AND EVALUATION

The diagnosis of pyoderma gangrenosum is made clinically. The appearance of painful, rapidly evolving ulcerations with shaggy, violaceous, and undermined borders is highly suggestive. If moreover such lesions occur on the legs and are multiple, a provisional diagnosis of PG can often be made. The skin should be inspected for any primary lesions (pustules or bullae), since their presence might lend support to this diagnosis and give additional direction to the investigation for associated diseases.

Many disease processes can resemble PG and share one or more of its key features (Table 1). The diagnosis of PG is thus assured only when these conditions have been reasonably excluded from consideration (58). A skin biopsy should be obtained and tissue cultures submitted–even if this may result in pathergic ulcer enlargement—to exclude vasculitic, vaso-occlusive, infectious, and neoplastic etiologies. Laboratory analyses are performed to help rule out alternative diagnostic possibilities and to search for associated conditions.

Additional procedures may be warranted based on the findings of a complete history and physical examination (Table 2).

Perhaps due to a lack of familiarity, physicians commonly fail to recognize PG when they are confronted with it. A recent study evaluated clinicians' diagnostic

Table 1 Differential diagnosis of pyoderma gangrenosum

Infection
  Bacterial
  Atypical mycobacterial
  Deep fungal
  Viral
Vascular disease
  Systemic vasculitis
  Antiphospholipid antibody syndrome
  Venous or arterial insufficiency
Factitial ulceration
Cutaneous malignancy
Brown recluse spider bite
Drug reaction
  Halogenoderma
  Hydroxyurea

Table 2 Evaluation of a patient with suspected pyoderma gangrenosum

---

To assure diagnosis:
  History and physical examination
  Skin biopsy
    Histology
    Cultures (bacterial, fungal, viral)
  Laboratory
    ANCA
    Antinuclear antibodies
    Antiphospholipid antibodies
    Cryoglobulins
To investigate for associated conditions:
  History and physical examination
  Laboratory
    CBC with examination of peripheral smear
    Serum protein electrophoresis and immunoelectophoresis
    Rheumatoid factor
  Studies of gastrointestinal tract
  Bone marrow aspirate/biopsy (if indicated)
  Radiographs (if indicated)
    CXR
    Joints

---

accuracy when presented with images of skin ulcers, and found that PG lesions were especially likely to be misdiagnosed (59). Pyoderma gangrenosum ulcerations were incorrectly diagnosed as venous ulcerations (32% of the time), neuropathic ulcers and arterial ulcers (20% of the time for each), and vasculitic lesions and neoplastic wounds (6% of the time for each). The diagnosis of ulcerative PG was correctly made in only 10% of the cases. Depending on the presentation, any of the causes mentioned above may reasonably enter into the differential diagnosis of pyoderma gangrenosum. However, venous ulcers generally lack the pain and rapid evolution of PG, while displaying the chronic inflammatory changes of hyperpigmentation and fibrosis at their periphery. Clinical features, the histology, and an evaluation giving close attention to the neurologic and arterial systems can usually exclude the remaining alternatives.

9. MANAGEMENT

Unfortunately, no treatment for PG has been subjected to a controlled trial. Although general guidelines for the management of PG can be offered, the physician needs to be flexible and sensitive to the particularities of the case at hand. Therapy for PG is either local, or local and systemic, as dictated by the number and severity of the skin lesions. The presence of non-cutaneous disease may at times circumscribe the therapeutic options. Local therapy alone may be sufficient for small and stable lesions. Attention to wound hygiene is important in order to optimize the milieu for healing. Saline compresses are often utilized for PG, but the application of an occlusive dressing should be considered, since a product can be chosen with a composition suited to the degree of exudate present. In addition, these dressings help physically protect the wound from trauma. Wounds should be continuously monitored for secondary infection necessitating systemic antibiotics. Leg elevation and the use of compression stockings are helpful and can be encouraged. Although a wide variety of local agents have been reported to be useful in treating PG, perhaps the most reliable are intralesional corticosteroids. Triamcinolone acetonide (5 mg/cc) is usually chosen and is directed into the active border of the ulcer.

Because of the risk of pathergy, local therapy must be delivered with care. PG has been precipitated iatrogenically—following injections, incisions and drainage, even after acupuncture (60). Skin grafting risks both graft failure when placed on an inflamed wound, and pathergy at the donor site. As a result, surgical intervention (aggressive debridement, grafting) is usually discouraged. However, such a prohibition cannot and should not be absolute (61). Successful grafting has been accomplished in difficult cases following preconditioning/stabilization with systemic immunosuppressants (62). The availability of bioengineered skin equivalents provides an additional resource that obviates the potential problem of pathergy at the donor site during autologous grafting (63).

Most cases of PG require systemic therapy to effect complete healing. Myriad agents have been used in individual patients, reflecting the intransigence that many of these wounds display. An abbreviated list would include minocycline, dapsone, clofazimine, azathioprine, thalidomide, IVIG (64), and mycophenolate mofetil. When using immunosuppressive agents, consideration should be given to *Pneumocystis carinii* pneumonia prophylaxis (65).

Systemic corticosteroids have traditionally been the mainstay of therapy, and remain the treatment of choice for some physicians; oral corticosteroids are started at high doses (1 to 2 mg/kg/day), and fairly reliably relieve pain and initiate healing (66). Adjuvant steroid-sparing agents are generally added to facilitate and complete wound closure. For especially resistant lesions intravenous methyl-prednisolone may be tried.

Cyclosporine has also been recommended as a primary treatment of PG. Matis et al. reported a series of 11 patients with refractory PG, 10 of who experienced complete healing with this agent. Perhaps importantly, seven of nine patients available for follow-up maintained their healing for 5 to 36 months after discontinuation of the drug (67). Since many patients with PG continue to experience relapses in the absence of maintenance therapy, the durability of this response is noteworthy.

Tacrolimus has also been used with success in patients with PG, including those with lesions resistant to cyclosporine (68). Effective dosages range from 0.1 to 0.3 mg/kg/day. Tacrolimus has a mechanism of action similar to that of cyclosporine, inhibiting calcineurin and ultimately the production of IL-2 by T-cells. Tacrolimus also down-regulates IL-8 and its receptor (69)–an effect that is advantageous when brought to bear against a neutrophilic condition such as PG. This author considers tacrolimus to be a preferred initial therapy for PG in those patients without contraindications.

Recently the TNF-α antagonist infliximab has been reported effective against pyoderma gangrenosum (70). This agent is currently FDA-approved for the treatment of Crohn's disease and rheumatoid arthritis—two conditions, as noted above, that may be associated with PG. The published successes to date using infliximab against PG have been almost exclusively in patients with concomitant Crohn's disease. It remains to be seen whether this agent's effect on PG-will be uniform amongst patients with and without co-existing bowel and/or joint disease.

10. PROGNOSIS

Even with aggressive therapy, pyoderma gangrenosum often heals slowly, and recurrences may occur. Bennett et. al. recently published their experience treating 64 patients with "typical" PG, of whom 85% were treated with prednisone and/or a systemic immunosuppressive agent. These patients required an average of 6 months to stabilize their lesions ("no inflammation"), and 11.5 months to heal them. After 3 years, approximately 95% of patients were healed, but 2 cases were refractory and still active at 4+ years (11). Von Den Driesch followed 42 patients for a median of 27 months and noted a mortality rate of ~15% attributed directly to the PG and/or the accompanying diseases; 56% of his surviving patients required continuing therapy (2).

These data only serve to underscore the challenges posed by pyoderma gangrenosum. Physicians and patients alike should anticipate a close and lengthy interaction when contending with this condition—variably characterized by therapy, monitoring, and surveillance for extracutaneous disease.

REFERENCES

1. Brunsting LA, Qoeckerman WH, O'Leary PA. Pyoderma (ecthyma) gangrenosum. Clinical and experimental observations in five cases occurring in adults. Arch Dermatol 1930; 22:655–680.
2. Von Den Driesch P. Pyoderma gangrenosum: a report of 44 cases with follow-up. Br J Dermatol 1997; 137:1000–1005.
3. Jacobs JC, Gaffney JA, Marboe CC. Pyoderma gangrenosum in infancy. J Am Acad Dermatol 1993; 29:509–510.
4. Powell FC, Perry HO. Pyoderma gangrenosum in childhood. Arch Dermatol 1984; 120:757–761.
5. Powell FC, Su WPD, Perry HO. Pyoderma gangrenosum: classification and management. J Am Acad Dermatol 1996; 34:395–409.
6. Cairns BA, Herbst CA, Sartor BR, Briggaman RA, Koruda MJ. Peristomal pyoderma gangrenosum and inflammatory bowel disease. Arch Surg 1994; 129:769–772.
7. Callen J. Pyoderma gangrenosum. Lancet 1998; 351:581–585.
8. Khandpur S, Mehta S, Reddy BSN. Pyoderma gangrenosum in two siblings: a familial predisposition. Pediatr Dermatol 2001; 18:308–312.
9. Alberts JH, Sams HH, Miller JL, King LE. Familial ulcerative pyoderma gangrenosum: a report of 2 kindred. Cutis 2002; 69:427–430.
10. Yeon HB, Lindor NM, Seidman JG, Seidman CE. Pyogenic arthritis, pyoderma gangrenosum, and acne syndrome maps to cbipmosome 15q. Am J Hum Genet 2000; 66: 1443–1448.
11. Bennett ML, Jackson JM, Jorizzo JL, Fleischer AB Jr., White WL, Callen JP. Pyoderma gangrenosum: a comparison of typical and atypical forms with an emphasis on time to remission. Case review of 86 patients from 2 institutions. Medicine 2000; 79:37–46.
12. Koester G, Tarnower A, Levisohn D, Burgdorf W. Bullous pyoderma gangrenosum. J Am Acad Dermatol 1993; 29:875–878.
13. Hughes AP, Jackson JM, Callen JP. Clinical features and treatment of peristomal pyoderma gangrenosum. JAMA 2000; 284:1546–1548.
14. Powell FC, Schroeter AL, Su WPD, Perry HO. Pyoderma gangrenosum: a review of 86 patients. Quar J Med 1985; 55:173–186.
15. Prystowsky JH, Kahn SN, Lazarus GS. Present status of pyoderma gangrenosum: review of 21 cases. Arch Dermatol 1989; 125:57–64.
16. Vignon-Pennamen MD. The extracutaneous involvement in the neutrophilic dermatoses. Clin Dermatol 2000; 18:339–347.

17. Chanson P, Timsit J, Kujas M, Violante A, Guillausseau PJ, Derome PJ, Warnet A, Lubetzki J. Pituitary granuloma and pyoderma gangrenosum. J Endocrinol Invest 1990; 13:677–681.

18. Marie I, Levesque H, Joly P, Reumont G, Courville P, Baudrimont M, Baubion D, Cailleux N, Courtois H. Neutrophilic myositis as an extracutaneous manifestation of neutrophilic dermatosis. J Am Acad Dermatol 2001; 44:137–139.

19. Vadillo M, Jucgla A, Podzamczer D, Rufi G, Domingo A. Pyoderma gangrenosum with liver, spleen, and bone involvement in a patient with chronic myelomonocytic leukaemia. Br J Dermatol 1999; 141:541–543.

20. Mlika RB, Riahi I, Fenniche S, Mokni M, Dhaoui MR, Dess N, Dhahri ABO, Mokhtar I. Pyoderma Gangrenosum: a report of 21 cases. Int J Dermatol 2002; 41:65–68.

21. Brown TS, Marshall GS, Callen JP. Cavitating pulmonary infiltrate in an adolescent with pyoderma gangrenosum: A rarely recognized extracutaneous manifestation of a neutrophilic dermatosis. J Am Acad Dermatol 2000; 43:108–112.

22. Vignon-Pennammen MD, Zelinsky-Gurung A, Janssen F, Frija J, Wallach D. Pyoderma gangrenosum with pulmonary involvement. Arch Dermatol 1989; 125:1239–1242.

23. Kruger S, Piroth W, Takyi BA, Breuer C, Schwarz ER. Multiple aseptic pulmonary nodules with central necrosis in association with pyoderma gangrenosum. Chest 2001; 119:977–978.

24. Wilson DM, John GR, Callen JP. Peripheral ulcerative keratitis—an extracutaneous neutrophilic disorder: Report of a patient with rheumatoid arthritis, pustular vasculitis, pyoderma gangrenosum, and Sweet's syndrome with an excellent response to cyclosporine therapy. J Am Acad Dermatol 1999; 40:331–334.

25. Talansky AL, Meyers S, Greenstein AJ, Janowitz HD. Does intestinal resection heal the pyoderma gangrenosum of inflammatory bowel disease? J Clin Gastroenterol 1983; 5: 207–210.

26. Janowitz HD. Pyboerma gangrenosum. Lancet 1998; 351:1134.

27. Cox NH, Peebles-Brown DA, MacKie RM. Pyoderma gangrenosum occurring 10 years after proctocolectomy for ulcerative colitis. Br J Hosp Med 1986; 36:363.

28. Romano J, Safai B. Pyoderma gangrenosum and myeloproliferative disorders. Report of a case and review of the literature. Arch Intern Med 1979; 139:932–934.

29. Dagan O, Barak Y, Metzker A. Pyoderma gangrenosum and sterile multifocal osteomyelitis preceding the appearance of Takayasu arteritis. Pediatr Dermatol 1995; 12:39–42.

30. Ackerman AB, Ghongchitnant N, Sanchez J, Guo Y, Bennin B, Reichel M, Randall MB. Inflammatory Diseases. In: Ackerman AB, Chongchitnant N, Sanchez J, Guo Y, Bennin B, Reichel M, Randall MB. Histologic Diagnosis of Inflammatory Skin Diseases: An Algorithmic Method Based on Pattern Analysis. 2nd Baltimore: Williams & Wilkins, 1997:171–786.

31. Hurwitz RM, Haseman JH. The evolution of pyoderma gangrenosum: a clinicopathologic correlation. Am J Dermatopathol 1993; 15:28–33.

32. Su WPD, Schroeter AL, Perry HO, Powell FC. Histopathologic and immunopathologic study of pyoderma gangrenosum. J Cutan Pathol 1986; 13:323–330.

33. Magro C, Crowson AN, Mihm M Jr. Cutaneous manifestations of nutritional deficiency states and gastrointestinal disease. In: Elder D, Elenitsas R, Jaworsky C, Johnson B Jr., eds. Lever's Histopatnology of the Skin. 8th ed. Philadelphia:Lippincott-Raven, 1997; 353–368.

34. Sanders S, Tahan SR, Kwan T, Magro CM. Giant cells in pyoderma gangrenosum. J Cutan Pathol 2001; 28:97–100.

35. Rafael MR, Fernandes CM, Machado JM, Rodrigues PA, Cardoso OJ, Afonso A, Sousa AB, Pacheco FM, Proenca RM. Pyoderma gangrenosum or leukemia cutis? J Eur Acad Dermatol Venereol 2003; 17:449–451.

36. Magro CM, De Moraes E, Burns F. Sweet's syndrome in the setting of CD34-positive acute myelogenous leukemia treated with granulocyte colony stimulating factor: evidence for a clonal neutrophilic dermatosis. J Cutan Pathol 2001; 28:90–96.

37. Crowson AN, Mihm MC Jr., Magrp C. Pyoderma gangrenosum: a review. J Cutan Pathol 2003; 30:97–107.
38. Vignon-Pennamen MD, Wallach D. Cutaneous manifestations of neutrophilic disease: A study of seven cases. Dermatologica 1991; 183:255–64.
39. Shore RN. Pyoderma gangrenosum, defective neutrophil chemotaxis, and leukemia. Arch Dermatol 1976; 112:1792–1793.
40. Dwarakanath AD, Yu LG, Brookes C, Pryce D, Rhodes JM. "Sticky" neutrophils pathergic arthritis and response to heparin in pyodenna gangrenosum complicating ulcerative colitis. Gut 1995; 37:585–588.
41. Adachi Y, Kindzelskii AL, Cookingham G, Shaya S, Moore EC, Todd RF, Petty HR. Aberrant neutrophil trafficking and metabolic oscillations in severe pyoderma gangrenosum. J Invest Dermatol 1998; 111:259–268.
42. Shaya S, Kindzelskii AL, Minor J, Moore EG, Todd RF, Petty HR. Aberrant integrin (CR4; $\alpha_x\beta_2$; CD11c/CD18) oscillations on neutrophils in a mild form of pyoderma gangrenosum. J Invest Dermatol 1998; 11:154–158.
43. Bedlow AJ, Davies EG, Moss ALH, Rebuck N, Finn A, Marsden RA. Pyoderma gangrenosum in a child with congenital partial deficiency of leukocyte adherence glycoproteins. Br J Dermatol 1998; 139:1064–1067.
44. Oka M, Berking C, Nesbit M, Satyamoorthy K, Schaider H, Murphy G, Ichihashi M, Sauter E, Herlyn M. Interleukin-8 overexpression is present in pyoderma gangrenosum ulcers leads to ulcer formation in human skin xenografts. Lab Invest 2000; 80:595–604.
45. Shoham NG, Centola M, Mansfield E, Hull KM, Wood G, Wise CA, Kastner DL. Pyrin binds the PSTPIPl/CD2BP1 protein, defining familial Mediterranean fever and PAPA syndrpme as disorders in the same pathway. PNAS 2003; 100:13501–13506.
46. Montoto S, Bosch F, Estrach T, Blade J, Nomdedeu B, Nontserrat E. Pyoderma gangrenosum triggered by alpha2b-interferbn in a patient with chronic granulocytic leukemia. Leuk Lymphoma 1998; 30:199–202.
47. Murch SH, Lamkin VA, Savage MO, Walker-Smith JA, MacDonald TT. Serum concentrations of tumor necrosis factor alpha in childhood chronic inflammatory bowel disease. Gut 1991; 32:913–917.
48. Roitt I, Brostoff J, Male D. Immunology. 6th Ed. London: Mosby, 2001.
49. Rostenberg AR, Jr. The Shwartzman phenohomenon: a review with a consideration of some possible dermatological manifestations. Br J Dermatol 1953; 65:389–405.
50. Kupper TS. Interleukin 1 and cutaneous inflammation: a crucial link between innate and acquired immunity. In: Moshell AN, ed. Progress in Dermatology. Evanston: Dermatology Foundation 1999; 33(2):1–8.
51. Gangaram HB, Tan LP, Gan AT, Suraiya HH, Ganesapillai T. Pyoderma gangrenosum following treatment with isotretinoin. Br J Dermatol 1997; 136:636–637.
52. Hughes BR, Cunliffe WJ. Development of folliculitis and pyoderrma gangrenosum in association with abdominal pain in a patient following treatment with isotretinoin. Br J Dermatol 1990; 122:683–687.
53. Srebrnik A, Shachar E, Brenner S. Suspected induction of a pyodenna gangrenosum-like eruption due to sulpiride treatment. Cutis 2001; 67:253–256.
54. Ross HJ, Moy LA, Kaplan R, Figlin RA. Bullous pyoderma gangrenosum after granulocyte colony-stimulating factor treatment. Cancer 1991; 68:441–443.
55. Sams HH, Mitchell WM, Stratton CW, King LE, Jr. Culture and immunohistochemical evidence of *Chiamydia pneumoniae* infection in ulcerative pyoderma gangrenosum. J Am Acad Dermatol 2003; 48:966–9.
56. Das, KM. Relationship of extraintestinal involvements in inflammatory bowel disease: new insights into autoimmune pathogeriesis. Dig Dis Sci 1999; 44:1–13.
57. Magro CM, Crowson AN. Sterile neutrophilic folliculitis with perifollicular vasculopathy: a distinctive cutaneous reaction pattern reflecting systemic disease. J Cutan Pathol 1998; 25:215–221.

58. Weenig RH, Davis MDP, Dahl PR, Su WPD. Skin ulcers misdiagnosed as pyoderma gangrenosum. N Engl J Med 2002; 347:1412–8.
59. Lorentzen H, Gottrup F. Misclassification errors of ulcerative pyoderma gangrenosum. Wound Rep Reg 1998; 6:A475.
60. Castro-Duran J, Martin-Armada M, Jimenez-Alonso J. Pyoderma gangrenosum induced by acupuncture in a patient with ulcerative colitis. Arch Int Med 2000; 160:2394–2396.
61. Alam M, Grossman ME, Schneiderman PI, Blume RS, Benvenisty AI. Surgical management of pyoderma gangrenosum: case report and review. Dermatol Surg 2000; 26: 1063–1066.
62. Cliff S, Holden CA, Thomas PRS, Marsden RA, Harland CC. Split skin grafts in the treatment of pyoderma gangrenosum: a report of four cases. Dermatol Surg 1999; 25: 299–302.
63. de Imus G, Golomb C, Wilkel C, Tsoukas M, Nowak M, Falanga V. Accelerated healing of pyoderma gangrenosum treated with bioengineered skin and concomitant immuno-suppression. J Am Acad Dermatol 2001; 44:61–66.
64. Chow RKP, Ho VC. Treatment of pyoderma gangrenosum. J Am Acad Dermatol 1996; 34:1047–1060.
65. McGarry H, McLelland J. *Pneumocystic carinii* pneumonia in a patient on immunosuppressive drugs for pyoderma gangrenosum. Br J Dermatol 2002; 147:192–3.
66. Powell FC, Collins S. Pyoderma gangrenosum. Clin Dermatol 2000; 18:283–293.
67. Matis WL, Ellis CN, Griffiths CEM, Lazarus GS. Treatment of pyoderma gangrenosum with cyclosporine. Arch Dermatol 1992; 128:1060–1064.
68. D'Inca R, Fagiuoli S, Sturniolo GC. Tacrolimus to treat pyoderma gangrenosum resistant to cyclosporine. Ann Intern Med 1998; 128:783–784.
69. Lemster BH, Carroll PB, Rilo HR, Johnson N, Nikaein A, Thomson AW. IL-8/IL-8 receptor expression in psoriasis and the response to systemic tacrolimus (FK 506) therapy. Clin Exp Immnnol 1995; 99:148–154.
70. Tan M, Gordon M, Lebwohl O, George J, Lebwohl MG. Improvement of pyoderma ganrenosum and psoriasis associated with Crohn disease with anti-tumor necrosis factor a monoclonal antibody. Arch Dennatol 2001; 137:930–933.

22
Cutaneous Vasculitis

Lawrence E. Gibson
Department of Dermatology, Mayo Clinic and Mayo Foundation, Rochester, Minnesota, U.S.A.

1. INTRODUCTION

Cutaneous vasculitis (CV) is an uncommon but challenging problem in clinical practice. Although the presentation of vasculitis in the skin is most often palpable purpura, a multitude of patterns are possible including livedoid reticularis, nodules, ulcerations, and even urticarial lesions. In the simplest sense, CV is an inflammatory reaction centered in blood vessels resulting in damage to the skin. Mechanisms include immune complex deposition in combination with inflammatory mediators or possibly primarily thrombogenic states with or without immune complex deposition.

In the former category reside most of the more familiar types of cutaneous leukocytoclastic vasculitis (LCV) including, rheumatoid vasculitis, lupus erythematosus-related urticarial vasculitis (UV),mixed cryoglobulinemia, and Henoch–Schönlein purpura (HSP). Disorders thought to be due primarily to thrombogenic states include livedoid vasculitis (LV), with or without lupus anticoagulant, thrombocytosis, monoclonal cryoglobulinemia, and others. In this chapter, a proposed classification scheme for CV based primarily on clinical and pathologic findings is discussed as well as the proposed pathogenesis for several types of vasculitis.

Illustrative examples of CV are presented to better demonstrate the clinical patterns of disease. A proposed outline for the evaluation of patients with vasculitis is presented, followed by a brief discussion of treatment.

2. CLASSIFICATION

There is no agreed upon classification system for CV. Various classification schemes are based primarily upon the clinical pattern, whereas other classification systems are based on the proposed pathogenesis, mechanisms of disease, or underlying disorder. All "primary" cutaneous vasculitides fall into the category of small-vessel disease. The skin may demonstrate capillary inflammation even in the setting of large-vessel disease elsewhere. For example, in cranial arteritis, LCV may be seen in the capillaries of the skin. The manifestations of vasculitis in the skin can be variable, change

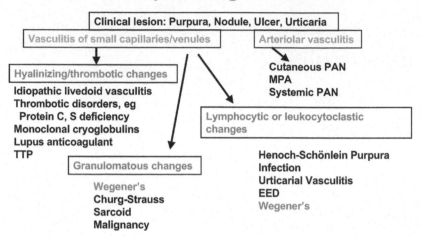

Figure 1 "Working" classification of cutaneous vasculitis based on clinicopathologic correlation.

over time, and the underlying causes numerous. For these reasons, the classification proposed in Fig. 1 is a "working system" based primarily on the combination of clinical findings correlated with pathologic findings (41,42). On the basis of the pathologic findings, one can then subclassify CV into those types involving capillaries or postcapillary venules and those types that involve primarily the arterioles. Cutaneous vasculitis can be subclassified in the skin by those types that are primarily thrombogenic, related to hypercoagulable states and those that are due to active inflammation of the blood-vessel wall resulting in leukocytoclasis or fibrinoid necrosis of the blood-vessel wall. The former cases would be typified by LV, and the latter would be typified by HSP or erythema elevatum diutinum (EED). Arteriolar vasculitis in the skin is unusual but can be seen in cutaneous polyarteritis nodosum (c-PAN) and in some cases of systemic arteritis including classic polyarteritis nodosum (PAN), systemic arteritis, lupus coagulant syndrome, and others. Lymphocytic vasculitis is more difficult to define unless one uses a strict histologic definition of blood-vessel wall damage in the setting of perivascular lymphocytic inflammation. There are many causes for lymphocytic vasculitis including drug hypersensitivity, connective tissue diseases, selected cases of UV, infectious diseases, and pityriasis lichenoides. Granulomatous vasculitis (GV) may be seen as a result of lymphocytic vasculitis or LCV or may develop de novo in the skin. Wegener's granulomatosis (WG) may present as LCV, GV or even rarely cause arteriolar inflammation in the skin (1,2).

3. PATHOGENESIS

The causes of CV include connective tissue diseases, systemic vasculitides, inflammatory disorders such as infectious diseases, sarcoid, and HSP (Table 1). At times, drug

Table 1 Approximate Precentages of Associated Disorders

Primary CV	35%
Connective tissue disease	22%
Henoch–Schönlein purpura	15%
Systemic vasculitis	12%
Miscellaneous, i.e., sarcoid, infection	11%
Malignancy	5%

Source: From Ref. 3.

eruptions can result in hypersensitivity vasculitis and vasculitis can also be the result of a paraneoplastic phenomenon. The primary and secondary lesions associated with vasculitis and the distribution of these lesions may vary depending upon the under-lying cause and the specific type of vasculitis. Even after careful medical evaluation and longitudinal follow-up, ~35% of CV cases are classified as "primary" in the sense that there is no associated systemic disorder found (1,3–6,36,38).

The pathogenesis of LCV depends initially upon antigenic stimulation of anti-bodies followed by immune complex formation. Instead of rapid clearing of these immune complexes from the circulation, other factors come into play that result in slowing of blood flow and exposure of antigen-antibody complexes to the endothelial cells, complement activation, and increased vascular permeability. Sev-eral mediators of inflammation including TNF-α, IL-2, IL-8, and other proinflam-matory chemokines and cytokines result in increased endothelial cell adhesion and upregulation of endothelial cell adhesion molecules such as intercellular adhesion molecule-1 or E-selectin (7,8). Coagulation is enhanced by factors such as plasmino-gen activator inhibitor (PAI-1) (9). Various downregulators of inflammation need to be employed to stop the pathologic process including tissue plasminogen activator that induces fibrinolysis and cytokines and chemokines produced by CD4 positive lymphocytes, macrophages, and endothelial cells. Most likely, fibrogenic or hyper-coagulable states enhance the blood-vessel damage in the presence of immune complex formation. It is also possible, under certain circumstances of vasocon-striction induced by cold temperature, trauma, or other noxious stimuli, to induce hypercoagulability. Prolonged active vasculitis with repeated recurrences may bring about granulation response and fibrosis. Erythema elevatum diutinum is the prototype of chronic fibrosing vasculitis. Thorough evaluation of CV should include all factors that may lead to immune complex formation and a thorough investigation of blood flow and coagulation.

4. ILLUSTRATIVE EXAMPLES OF CV

4.1. Livedoid Vasculitis

Livedoid vasculitis is an example of a primarily coagulative vasculitis (Fig. 1). It is known by several names including livedo vasculitis, livedo with ulcerations, seasonal (summer or winter) ulcerations, segmental hyalinizing vasculitis, and vasculitis of atrophie blanche (Fig. 2). Most often limited to the lower extremities, it is character-ized by a net-like vascular pattern with episodic ulcerations. Healing leaves white, atrophic scars usually surrounded by small punctate vascular prominences, referred

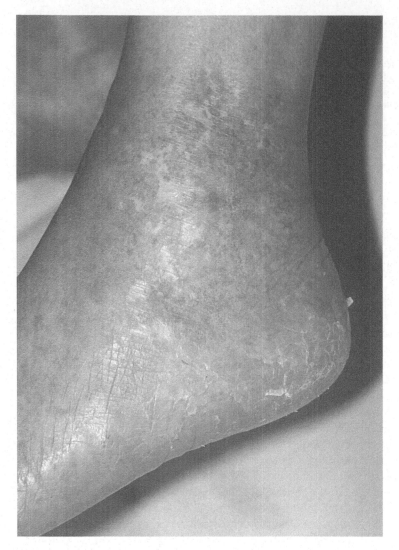

Figure 2   Healed LV with atrophie blanche-type scarring.

to as atrophie blanche and cayenne pepper-like changes (10–12). Ulcerations usually begin as linear or small chevron-shaped lesions, which then expand. Typically, the ulcerations are extremely painful, sometimes out of proportion to size. Neuropathic symptoms, as well as lower extremity or pedal edema, may be present. The differential diagnosis includes ulceration due to chronic venous disease, c-PAN, classic PAN, micropolyangiitis (MPA), lupus anticoagulant syndrome, calciphylaxis, hydroxyurea dermopathy, monoclonal gammopathy, and others. Clinicopathologic correlation is critical in differentiation of the earlier-mentioned disorders. Most often patients with uncomplicated LV do not have signs and symptoms of systemic disease to suggest PAN or MPA. Cutaneous polyarteritis nodosum generally presents with discrete areas of livedo with central nodularity (Fig. 3). Careful selection of biopsy site is critical in separating LV from c-PAN. Older, ulcerated lesions may show only granulation response on biopsy as opposed to hyalinizing changes in the blood-vessel walls

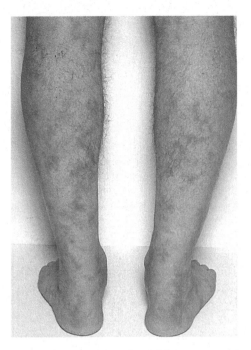

Figure 3 Prominent livedoid pattern on the legs in c-PAN.

together with capillary occlusion. Leukocytoclastic vasculitis on the biopsy would suggest an alternative diagnosis including MPA or PAN. This differential diagnosis is discussed later (see c-PAN) and is summarized in Table 2. All patients with LV need thorough vascular studies to rule out arterial or venous compromise. In addition, coagulation studies are recommended including antiphospholipid antibodies, homocysteine levels, and assay for Protein C and S activity and activated protein C resistance (9). Patients previously labeled as "idiopathic" LV may have had various disorders of coagulation. Even in the setting of thorough investigation, there remain a large percentage of patients with LV for whom no adequate explanation can be found. The treatment of these patients is challenging and may require various degrees of anticoagulation as well as supportive care plus wound healing techniques for those with ulcerations (13).

4.2. Henoch–Schönlein Purpura

Henoch–Schönlein purpura typically presents as LCV in the skin. It is distinguished from other types of necrotizing small-vessel vasculitis on the basis of clinical features and the presence of IgA in the involved tissues. First recognized by Heberden and then Schönlein as a purpuric condition in children associated with arthritis, Henoch later described abdominal pain and renal disease thus composing the diagnostic features of HSP.

The majority of the patients are less than 7 years of age with a median age of ∼4 years, and with a greater frequency in boys by a ratio of 1.5:1. Outbreaks are most common during the winter and spring months with another smaller peak in the fall. The incidence is estimated to be 18 per 100,000 population in children <14 years of age (14). The earliest sign of HSP may be acral edema, although the

Table 2 Summary Features of c-PAN, MPA, and Systemic or Classic PAN

	c-PAN	MPA	PAN
Purpura (cutaneous LCV)	+	++	++
Livedo	++	++	±
Cutaneous nodules	++	±	±
Lung involvement	−	+	−
Glomerulonephritis	−	+	−
Neuropathy	±	+	+
Aneurysm	−	±	+
ANCA	−	++(p-ANCA/MPO)	−
Hepatitis B/C	−	−	±

most specific cutaneous finding is palpable purpura, most often located on the lower extremities, buttocks, and abdomen. Purpura is the presenting sign of HSP in ~50% of cases (Fig. 4). Other characteristic findings include abdominal pain, hematochezia, and arthralgias. Hematuria and glomerulonephritis may also be seen. In most patients, < 20 years of age, the renal abnormalities are clear; however, 1–5% may have persistent renal disease. Other less common findings include orchitis, which may mimic testicular torsion, intestinal angina with intussusception, infarction or perforation, esophageal erosions, eye involvement, mononeuritis, myocardial infarction, and CNS abnormalities (15–17,19,21).

In the skin, HSP is characterized histologically by LCV located in the papillary and reticular dermis (Fig. 5). Cutaneous biopsies often show IgA vascular fluores-

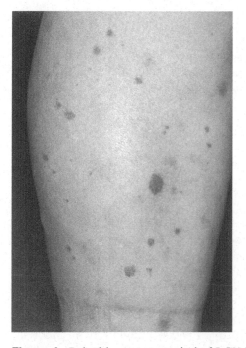

Figure 4 Palpable purpura typical of LCV including HSP.

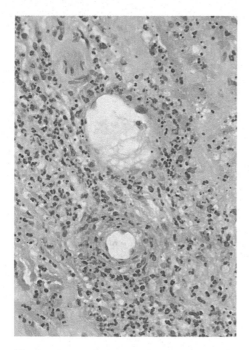

Figure 5 Leukocytoclastic vasculitis in the dermal blood vessels (H&E, 60X).

cence on direct immunofluorescence (DIF) study. The percentage of cases with vascular IgA deposition depends upon population studied but is usually >75%. Combining the finding of IgA, vascular fluorescence on cutaneous biopsy with clinical criteria improves the diagnostic specificity for HSP (18).

The etiology of HSP is unknown, but there are many associated disorders including preceding bacterial or viral infections. Various other associated problems have been reported with HSP including sensitivity to azodyes and salicylates and drug sensitivities. Henoch–Schönlein purpura has also been associated with pregnancy, cryoglobulinemia, lymphoma, and adenocarcinoma. The immunologic basis for these associations is unknown. Elevated serum IgA is seen in approximately one-half of patients with HSP. IgA complexes may be cleared less quickly in those patients susceptible to HSP. IgA1 is thought to be the major immune globulin related to renal disease in HSP. Recent studies point to a possible defect in glycosylation of the "hinge" region of IgA1 as a cause for renal damage (20,21).

4.3. Urticarial Vasculitis

Urticarial vasculitis clinically resembles urticaria, but skin lesions generally persist >24 hr and may be purpuric upon resolution. Urticarial vasculitis is generally divided into normocomplementemic and hypocomplementemic types. Patients with normal complement may have hypersensitivity reactions to various antigenic stimuli including drugs, infections, or others. Biopsies of skin lesions often show perivascular neutrophilic inflammation with eosinophils, lymphatic dilatation, and edema.

Hypocomplementemic urticarial vasculitis (HUV) is defined as the constellation of persistent urticarial skin lesions with decreased total complement levels

(Fig. 6). Most often, biopsy of characteristic skin lesions shows mild LCV combined with features of urticaria including lymphatic dilatation and edema. Eosinophils may not be as prominent in HUV when compared with normocomplement UV. Often, these patients also exhibit other symptoms and signs suggestive of connective tissue disease including joint pain, chest pain, and may have renal abnormalities including active urinary sediment and microhematuria. There are several areas of overlap with systemic lupus erythematosus (SLE) not only in the signs and symptoms of disease, but also in the laboratory abnormalities. It has been suggested that HUV may actually be a special subset of lupus erythematosus. Hypocomplementemic urticarial vasculitis may differ; in that, many HUV patients have anti-C1q antibodies. Patients with SLE less commonly exhibit these antibodies (22). The skin pathology in HUV may show dermal neutrophilia to the extent that a diagnosis of Sweet's syndrome (SS) is considered. It has been suggested that marked dermal neutrophilia in the setting of UV suggests decreased complement and HUV (23,24). In those cases where doubt exists as to the correct diagnosis, DIF can be helpful as it will often demonstrate a granular basement membrane zone fluorescence with one or more conjugates in HUV but not in SS or EED. In addition, SS should generally not show blood-vessel changes of vasculitis. Clinical input and other laboratory findings are needed to differentiate SLE from HUV.

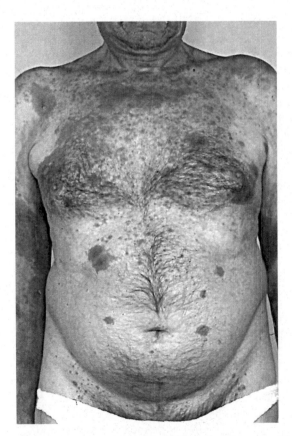

Figure 6   Urticarial lesions with purpuric residual in UV.

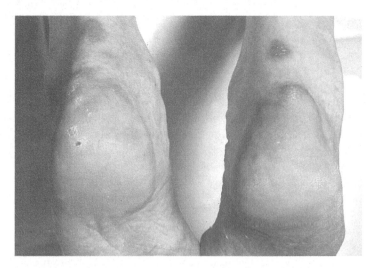

Figure 7 Nodular and fibrotic skin lesions typical of EED.

4.4. Erythema Elevatum Diutinum

Erythema elevatum diutinum typifies chronic recurring LCV followed by fibrosis. It often presents as persistent, symmetrical, firm, tender, red to reddish brown or purple papules and nodules, which then may coalesce to form larger nodules or plaques. The extensor aspects of the extremities are the preferred location for skin lesions. Most often, these lesions are located near joints such as the fingers, hands, elbows, ankles, and knees, although palmar and plantar lesions are also seen (Fig. 7). At times, the lesions may resemble vesicles, hemorrhagic nodules, ulcerations, or other vascular processes. Partial resolution may give a yellowish or brown hue to the lesions resembling xanthomata. The cause of EED is unknown but is presumed related to vascular immune complex deposition. Streptococcal infection and/or rheumatoid disease have been cited as possible causes for immune complex formation. Erythema elevatum diutinum may be associated with several autoimmune disorders including seropositive rheumatoid arthritis, ulcerative colitis, Crohn's disease, relapsing polychondritis, pyoderma gangrenosum, type I diabetes mellitus, and gluten-sensitive enteropathy. Associated infections have included bacterial, viral, tuberculous, hepatitic, as well as syphilitic. There have been several reports detailing the association of EED with HIV infection. Many of these HIV patients are also infected with hepatitis B, hepatitis C, or CMV as well as other opportunistic organisms (25,26). Erythema elevatum diutinum has been associated with hypergammaglobulinemia as well as with IgA monoclonal gammopathies (27).

The diagnosis of EED is based upon the characteristic clinical lesions in combination with supporting histopathological findings supported by appropriate laboratory investigations.

4.5. Granulomatous Vasculitis

Granulomatous vasculitis in the skin may be the result of several seemingly unlinked diseases ranging from infection to neoplasia. Several infectious agents can create GV, such as syphilis, herpesvirus, mycobacterium, and others. Granulomatous processes such as Crohn disease or sarcoid may cause GV in the skin (2,36,4,41). Systemic vasculitides such as Churg–Strauss granulomatosis and WG may bring about vasculitis in the skin. Wegener's granulomatosis is discussed in detail, as the patterns of disease in the skin are rich and overlap with presentations of other systemic vasculitides (28,36).

In general, cutaneous lesions of any type are more likely in patients with WG who have multiple organ system involvement. "Specific" lesions are directly related to WG and not due to infection, drug sensitivity, or other definable cause other than WG. Specific cutaneous lesions are seen in ~15% of WG patients (28–33).

The most common lesion in WG of the skin is palpable purpura of the lower extremities and, occasionally, the upper extremities as well as the digits. The histopathologic correlation of purpura is most often LCV, often without granuloma formation.

Ulceration with a histopathologic correlate of acute and/or granulomatosis inflammation is the second most common manifestation of cutaneous WG (29,37). Ulceration may be located on the lower extremities, upper extremities, or the head and neck area (Fig. 8). Clinically, these lesions may resemble pyoderma gangrenosum of the classic variety or may be superficial or granulomatous in appearance (36,37). The histopathologic differential diagnosis may include neutrophilic dermatoses if neutrophils predominate the infiltrate and may also be suggestive of granulomatous

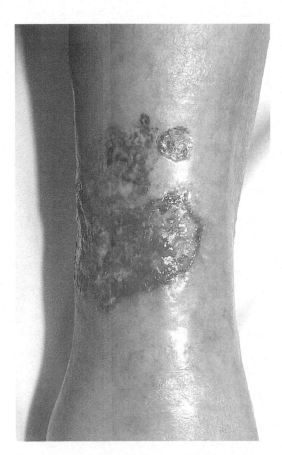

Figure 8 Leg ulceration in patient with WG.

processes including infection. In the past, a selected group of patients with facial skin ulceration and systemic complaints had been reported as "malignant facial pyoderma." This latter term is best not used as a specific diagnostic entity, as many of these patients were found to have WG or other vasculitic or inflammatory and neoplastic conditions (34,43). Ulceration over the temple may resemble cranial arteritis, requiring careful clinicopathologic correlation and serologic testing to confirm WG.

Other diagnostic entities to be considered in the differential diagnosis of WG include cutaneous Crohn's disease, especially in those patients with oral lesions. Gingival hyperplasia with a reddish to purple appearance with petechiae can also be seen in WG.

Papules when seen over the extensor joints may be a manifestation of WG. Histopathologic correlates include vasculitis (LCV or GV), acute and/or neutrophilic inflammation, or palisaded granuloma. This latter entity has been referred to as the Churg–Strauss granuloma or extravascular granuloma (47). Once again, this entity is not specific for WG and can be seen in a variety of other illnesses including Churg–Strauss granulomatosis, other systemic vasculitides, inflammatory conditions such as inflammatory bowel disease and malignancy. The Churg–Strauss granuloma may closely resemble rheumatoid nodules or papules or possibly granuloma annulare, both clinically and on biopsy (44).

The diagnosis of WG is confirmed by serologic testing in combination with clinical and pathologic findings. Antineutrophil cytoplasmic antibodies (ANCA) correlate well in those patients with active skin disease, as most of these patients also have internal organ involvement at or shortly after the time of diagnosis. Recently, direct and indirect ELISA techniques have been developed for ANCA. ELISA techniques give positive or negative results and will also differentiate c-ANCA from p-ANCA and proteinase-3 (PR-3)/c-ANCA from myeloperoxidase (MPO)/p-ANCA. The former pattern when PR-3 is positive is very suggestive of WG. p-ANCA may be an MPO or may represent some other nonspecific pattern. Myeloperoxidase is most closely associated with an MPA. Clinical correlation of these serologic tests is always required, as overlap in ANCA specificities exists and several nonspecific ANCAs can be seen. Antineutrophil cytoplasmic antibody titers may change over time and in relationship to disease activity or treatment (35,37).

4.6. Cutaneous Polyarteritis Nodosum

The concept of limited PAN was first described by Lindberg (48,49) in 1931 and 1932. Cutaneous PAN is separated from the systemic form because it remains limited and is associated with a better prognosis. The site of involvement with c-PAN is primarily the legs with over 95% of lesions located in this region (38,46,50). Lesions can be located elsewhere, including the arms, trunk, head and neck area, and buttock area in descending order of frequency. The typical primary lesion is a subcutaneous nodule. There may be numerous nodules, which are usually small (< 1 cm) and can number as many as 100. These nodules are often painful and located in dependent areas. Ulcers develop in <50% of patients. Another cutaneous pattern is livedo, which is especially likely after to accompany new nodule formation. The livedo pattern radiates out from a new lesion in a starburst pattern (Fig. 3). Acral edema may be one of the earliest signs of c-PAN. Cutaneous PAN involves both sexes approximately equally with a median age of 37 years (39,46). Systemic complaints include malaise, fever, myalgias, and sore throat.

Histologically, c-PAN is characterized by polyarteritis with inflammation involving the entire vessel wall of the small arterioles, usually located at the dermal–pannicular junction (Fig. 9). One vessel may be involved, and serial sections may be required to identify involved vessels. Leukocytoclastic vasculitis can be seen either on the same biopsy specimen or in the additional specimens from the same patients in less than one-third of patients (39,40).

Laboratory abnormalities are not common, but most often, there is an elevated erythrocyte sedimentation rate. Other findings include anemia, in 50% of patients, and increased white blood count, in ~20% of patients. Antineutrophil cytoplasmic antibodies are most often negative. c-ANCA/PR-3 and MPO should be negative. The most commonly associated noncutaneous finding is mononeuritis multiplex, which can result in various neurologic deficits, including paresthesias, dysesthesias, and foot drop. EMG studies have found that 60% of the patients with neuropathy have mononeuritis multiplex type (39,50). Systemic disorders associated with cutaneous PAN include Crohn's disease, superior and inferior vena cava thrombosis, positive antibodies to streptococci, hepatitis B antigenemia, and hepatitis C infection. Overlap may exist in the differentiation of c-PAN from classic systemic PAN or MPA. Table 2 summarizes features of these three diseases. The livedoid pattern of c-PAN may resemble early-onset calciphylaxis (Fig. 10). Adequate biopsy of

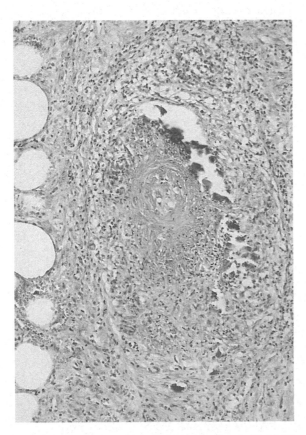

Figure 9 Histopathology of c-PAN showing arteriolar inflammation and fibrinoid damage in the deep dermis (H&E, 60X).

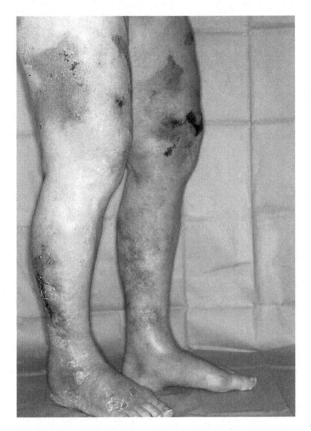

Figure 10 Vascular occlusion and purpura/ecchymoses in a patient with chronic renal failure and calciphylaxis.

the deep dermis and pannus plus clinical correlation is a key to separating these two disorders.

The course of cutaneous PAN varies from weeks to many months. Most often, acute symptoms resolve within 2–8 weeks, but these patients are at risk for recurrence.

5. EVALUATION

The evaluation of CV should follow a logical pattern beginning with assessment of the primary clinical lesions such as livedo, palpable purpura, nodules, or urticaria (Table 3). The distribution is important, as some types of vasculitis, such as LV, primarily involve the feet, ankles, and lower legs, whereas systemic processes, such as HSP, can involve other acral areas including the face and the genitalia. Notation of secondary lesions such as ulceration and impetiginization is important. The proper diagnosis and treatment of CV depends upon correlation of the clinical pattern with the histopathology. Routine microscopy is best obtained from a newer primary lesion of 24–48 hr duration if possible. In addition to routine microscopy, special stains for micro-organisms including the Gram stain, acid fast stains, and methenamine–silver stains are recommended to rule out infectious causation. In

Table 3 Proposed Evaluation of CV

Assess clinical pattern
  Primary lesion, e.g., livedo, nodules, urticaria, palpable purpura
  Distribution, e.g., limited to acral areas or upper and lower extremities
  Secondary lesions, e.g., ulceration, impetiginization
Histopathology
  Routine microscopy from newer primary lesions (<48 hr)
    Include stains for micro-organisms (Gram, acid fast, methenamine–silver, others)
    Tissue cultures in selected cases
  Direct immunofluorescence biopsy
    Most often from leading edge or just perilesional in newest lesion (<24 hr)
    Most helpful in HSP, UV, cryoglobulins
Medical evaluation
  Review of systems including thorough drug/exposure/travel history in all cases
  Routine laboratory tests such as chest x-ray, complete blood count with differential,
  sedimentation rate, urinalysis
Special serologies or tests
  May include lupus serologies, rheumatoid factor, cryoglobulins, coagulation tests, ANCA.
  Specifics based on results of evaluations and tests done above

addition, tissue cultures may also be helpful in ascertaining the role of infection and causation of the vasculitic lesion. Direct immunofluorescence biopsy is helpful in selected cases of CV, especially in disorders, such as HSP, which typically demonstrate IgA deposition in the blood vessels or UV where one may see basement membrane zone fluorescence in addition to blood-vessel fluorescence or in cryoglobulinemia where IgM deposition may be prominent. Direct immunofluorescence biopsies are best taken from a leading erythematous edge or just perilesional in the newest possible lesion, preferably < 24 hr duration.

Medical evaluation is important in all patients with CV and should include a thorough review of systems. Drug history, chemical exposures, and travel histories are all essential. The presence or absence of other connective tissue diseases or inflammatory diseases may play an important role in the manifestation of CV. Routine laboratory tests such as a complete blood count with a differential, sedimentation rate, urinalysis, and chest x-ray are appropriate in all cases of CV.

On the basis of the information gleaned from the clinical pattern, histopathology, and medical evaluation, special serologies or special tests may be indicated, including lupus serologies, rheumatoid factor, cryoglobulins, coagulation tests, ANCA, and complement studies. Most often, a combination of the clinical, laboratory, and histopathologic features noted earlier allow for a diagnosis of the subtype of CV. There are cases, however, where only longitudinal follow-up and continued close clinical monitoring are successful in confirming the correct diagnosis.

The treatment of CV depends upon a thorough understanding of the mechanisms involved in the causation of the cutaneous lesions, together with an understanding of the underlying medical illness if present. The foremost reason to treat CV is to comfort the patient. In those cases with known cause, treatment of the underlying cause may bring about an improvement in the cutaneous lesions. Examples of the latter include hepatitis C-induced mixed cryoglobulinemia where treatment of the hepatitis brings about improvement in the associated CV (38,51).

Contributing factors to tissue destruction should also be identified and eliminated as much as possible, including stress and exposure to extreme cold or heat.

Secondary infection should be treated to allow for adequate wound healing. Tobacco use is known to interfere with tissue oxygenation, as well as with the fibrinolytic pathway, and should be discouraged.

Prednisone is still the cornerstone of therapy for many patients with CV. It is the most reliable medication in relieving symptoms and for stopping progression of the cutaneous disease. Treatment of c-PAN usually requires oral prednisone. Alternative medications include dapsone, azathioprine, acetyl salicylic acid and indomethacin, sulfapyridine, nicotinic acid (39). Stanozolol has been reported to be effective in a few patients (52,55). Corticosteroid-sparing medications are sought in those cases where prednisone therapy is needed for a longer period of time (53). Immunosuppressive medications are used in those cases associated with systemic vasculitides such as WG. The treatment of systemic vasculitides is designed to stop tissue damage quickly and then alternative less toxic therapies are sought to maintain remission. There are many immunosuppressives successfully used in the treatment of vasculitis including methotrexate, azathioprine, and more recently mycophenolate mofetil (53,54). In those cases of vasculitis thought to be due primarily to thrombogenic states, various types of anticoagulation combined with vascular dilatation may be helpful.

6. SUMMARY AND CONCLUSION

In conclusion, CV remains a challenging problem in clinical practice. Owing to the multitude of clinical patterns and associated disorders, a thorough general medical evaluation, combined with histopathologic correlation, is essential in all patients. Therapeutic options can only be employed, once the possible associated disorders and complications have been identified. Close clinical observation and continuous longitudinal follow-up are the key for the successful treatment of CV.

REFERENCES

1. Sanchez NP, Van Hale HM, Su WPD. Clinical and histopathologic spectrum of necrotizing vasculitis: report of findings in 101 cases. Arch Dermatol 1985; 121:220–224.
2. Gibson LE, Winkelmann RK. Cutaneous granulomatous vasculitis: its relationship to systemic disease. J Am Acad Dermatol 1986; 14:492–501.
3. Blanco R, Martínez-Taboada VM, Rodríguez-Valverde V, et al. Cutaneous vasculitis in children and adults: associated diseases and etiologic factors in 303 patients. Medicine 1998; 77:403–418.
4. Del Rossa A, Generini S, Pignone A, et al. Vasculitis secondary to systemic diseases. Clin Dermatol 1999; 17:533–547.
5. Gyselbrecht L, De Keyser F, Ongenae K, et al. Etiological factors and underlying conditions in patients with leukocytoclastic vasculitis. Clin Exp Rheumatol 1996; 14:665–668.
6. Sanchez NP, Winkelmann RK, Schroeter AL, et al. The clinical and histopathologic spectrums of urticarial vasculitis: study of 40 cases. J Am Acad Dermatol 1982; 7:599–605.
7. Groves RW, Ross EL, Barker WN, et al. Vascular cell adhesion molecule-1: expression in normal and diseased skin and regulation in vivo by interferon gamma. J Am Acad Dermatol 1993; 29:67–72.
8. Ghersetich I, Comacchi C, Katsambas A, et al. Cellular steps in pathogenesis of cutaneous necrotizing vasculitis. Clin Dermatol 1999; 17:597–601.

9. Papi M, Didona B, De Pita O, et al. Livedo vasculopathy vs. small vessel cutaneous vasculitis: cytokine and platelet P-selectin studies. Arch Dermatol 1998; 134:447–452.

10. Nelson LM. Atrophie blanche en plaque. Arch Dermatol 1955; 72:242–251.

11. Stiefler RE, Bergfeld WF. Atrophie blanche. Int J Dermatol 1982; 2:1–7.

12. Bard JW, Winkelmann RK. Livedo vasculitis: segmental hyalinizing vasculitis of the dermis. Arch Dermatol 1967; 96:489–499.

13. Klein KL, Pittelkow MR. Tissue plasminogen activator for the treatment of livedoid vasculitis. J Invest Dermatol 1992; 98:574.

14. Nielsen HE. Epidemiology of Schönlein—Henoch purpura. Acta Paediatr Scan 1988; 77:125.

15. Gibson LE, Su WPD. Cutaneous vasculitis. Rheum Dis Clin North Am 1990; 16(2): 309–324.

16. Heng MCY. Henoch–Schönlein purpura. Br J Dermatol 1985; 112:235–240.

17. Raimer SS, Sanchez RL. Vasculitis in children. Semin Dermatol 1992; 11(1):48–56.

18. Helander SD, de Castro FR, Gibson LE. Henoch–Schönlein purpura: clinical pathologic correlation of cutaneous vascular IgA deposits and the relationship to leukocytoclastic vasculitis. Acta Dermatol Venereol (Stockh) 1995; 75:125–129.

19. Michel BA, Hunder GG, Bloch DA, Calabrese LH. Hypersensitivity vasculitis and Henoch–Schönlein purpura: a comparison between the 2 disorders. J Rheumatol 1992; 19:721–728.

20. Davin JC, Ten Berge IJ, Weening JJ. What is the difference between IgA nephropathy and Henoch–Schönlein purpura nephritis? Kidney Int 2001; 59(3):823–834.

21. Saulsbury F. Henoch–Schönlein purpura (vasculitis syndromes). Cur Opin Rheumatol 2001; 13(1):35–40.

22. Wisnieski JJ, Baer AN, Christensen J, Cupps TR, et al. Hypocomplementemic urticarial vasculitis syndrome. Clinical and serologic findings in 18 patients. Medicine 1995; 74:24.

23. Davis MDP, Daoud MS, Kirby B, Gibson LE, Rogers RS. Clinicopathologic correlation of hypocomplementemic and normocomplementemic urticarial vasculitis. J Am Acad Dermatol 1998; 38:899.

24. Mehregan DR, Gibson LE. Urticarial vasculitis: a clinicopathologic review of 72 cases. J Am Acad Dermatol 1992; 26:441–448.

25. Cockerell CJ. Noninfectious inflammatory skin diseases in HIV-infected individuals. Dermatol Clin 1991; 9:531–541.

26. Dronda F, González-López A, Lecona M, Barros C. Erythema elevatum diutinum in human immunodeficiency virus-infected patients—report of a case and review of the literature. Clin Exp Dermatol 1996; 21:222–225.

27. Yiannias JA, el-Azhary RA, Gibson LE. Erythema elevatum diutinum. A clinical and histopathologic study of 13 patients. J Am Acad Dermatol 1992; 26:38–44.

28. Schönermarck U, Lamprecht P, Csernok E, Gross WL. Prevalence and spectrum of rheumatic diseases associated with proteinase 3-antineutrophil cytoplasmic antibodies (ANCA) and myeloperoxidase-ANCA. Rheumatology 2001; 40:178–184.

29. Barksdale SK, Hallahan CW, Kerr GS, Fauci AS, Stern JB, Travis WD. Cutaneous pathology in Wegener's granulomatosis: a clinicopathologic study of 75 biopsies in 46 patients. Am J Surg Pathol 1995; 19:161–172.

30. Barnett VT, Sekosan M, Khurshid A. Wegener's granulomatosis and α_1-antitrypsin-deficiency emphysema: proteinase-related diseases. Chest 1999; 116:253–255.

31. Langford CA, Specks U. Wegener's granulomatosis and other vasclitides. Respiratory Medicine. 3rd ed. In press.

32. Walsh JS, Gross DJ. Wegener's granulomatosis involving the skin. Cutis 1999; 64: 183–186.

33. Fauci AS, Haynes BF, Katz P, Wolff SM. Wegener's granulomatosis: prospective clinical and therapeutic experience with 85 patients for 21 years. Ann Intern Med 1983; 98:76–85.

34. Lerner EA, Dover JS. Malignant pyoderma: a manifestation of Wegener's granulomatosis. J Am Acad Dermatol 1986; 15:1051–1052.

35. Daoud MS, Gibson LE, Specks U. Cutaneous leukocytoclastic vasculitis with positive anti-neutrophil cytoplasmic antibodies. Acta Derm Venereol 1998; 79:328–329.
36. Gibson LE, el-Azhary RA, Smith T, et al. The spectrum of cutaneous granulomatous vasculitis: histopathologic report of eight cases with clinical correlation. J Cutan Pathol 1994; 21:437–445.
37. Daoud MS, Gibson LE, DeRemee RA, Specks U, el-Azhary RA, Su WPD. Cutaneous Wegener's granulomatosis: clinical, histopathologic, and immunopathologic features of thirty patients. J Am Acad Dermatol 1994; 31:605–612.
38. Daoud MS, Gibson LE, Daoud S, el-Azhary RA. Chronic hepatitis C and skin diseases: a review. Mayo Clinic Proc 1995; 70:559–564.
39. Daoud MS, Hutton KP, Gibson LE. Cutaneous periarteritis nodosa: a clinicopathological study of 79 cases. Br J Dermatol 1997; 136:706–713.
40. Gibson LE, el-Azhary RA. Erythema elevatum diutinum. Clin Dermatol 2000; 18: 295–299.
41. Gibson LE. Cutaneous vasculitis: approach to diagnosis and systemic associations. Mayo Clin Proc 1990; 65(2):221–229.
42. Gibson LE, Su WPD. Cutaneous vasculitis. Rheum Dis Clin North Am 1995; 21(4): 1097–1113.
43. Gibson LE, Daoud MS, Muller SA, et al. Malignant pyodermas revisited. Mayo Clin Proc 1997; 72:734–736.
44. Hamacher KL, Gibson LE. Churg–Strauss granuloma. Int J Dermatol 2002; 41:230–231.
45. Guillevin L, Durand-Gasselin B, Cevallos R, et al. Microscopic polyangiitis: clinical and laboratory findings in eighty-five patients. Arthritis Rheum 1999; 42:421–430.
46. Diaz-Perez JL, Winkelmann RK. Cutaneous periarteritis nodosa: a study of 33 cases. Wolff K, Winkelamnn R, eds. Major Problems in Dermatology. Philadelphia: WB Saunders, 1980.
47. Finan, MC, Winkelmann RK. The cutaneous extravascular necrotizing granuloma (Churg–Strauss granuloma) and systemic disease: a review of 27 cases. Medicine (Baltimore) 1983; 62:142–158.
48. Lindberg K. Ein beitnag zur kenntsnis der periarteritis nodosa. Acta Med Scand 1931; 76:183–225.
49. Lindberg K. Uber line subkutase fur fer periarteritis nodosa mit langwierigen verlauf. Acta Med Scand 1932; 77:455–462.
50. Meyrick-Thomas RH, Black MM. The wide clinical spectrum of polyarteritis nodosa with cutaneous involvement. Clin Exp Dermatol 1983; 8:534–541.
51. Zimmermann R, Konig V, Bauditz J, et al. Interferon alpha in leukocytoclastic vasculitis, mixed cryoglobulinemia, and chronic hepatitis C. Lancet 1993; 341:561–562.
52. Gibson LE. Cutaneous vasculitis update. In: Robert E, Rakel MD, Edward T, Bope MD, eds.Conn's Current Therapy Dermatology Clinics. 53rd ed. Philadelphia: W.B. Saunders, 2001:819–822.
53. Vena GA, Cassano N. Immunosuppressive therapy in cutaneous vasculitis. Clin Dermatol 1999; 17:633–640.
54. Nowack R, Gobel U, Klooker P, et al. Mycophenolate mofetil for maintenance therapy of Wegener's granulomatosis and microscopic polyangiitis: a pilot study in 11 patients with renal involvement. J Am Soc Nephrol 1999; 10:1965–1971.
55. Atozor L, Ferreli C, Biggio P. Less common treatments in cutaneous vasculitis. Clin Dermatol 1999; 17:641–647.

23
Vasculopathy

Esperanza Welsh and Jennifer T. Trent
Department of Dermatology, University of Miami School of Medicine,
Miami, Florida, U.S.A.

Francisco A. Kerdel
Chief of Dermatology and Director of Inpatient Services, Cedars Medical Center,
Miami, Florida, U.S.A.

Vasculopathy is a term reserved for the process producing vascular damage with mild or no inflammation of the blood vessels. This is different from vasculitis that involves fibrinoid necrosis of the blood vessel and significant inflammation. Vasculopathy is caused by coagulation disorders, metabolic disorders, emboli, and other miscellaneous processes.

1. DISSEMINATED INTRAVASCULAR COAGULATION

Disseminated intravascular coagulation (DIC) is a condition caused by alteration in the patient's normal coagulation system leading to both hemorrhage and thrombus formation (1–4). Overstimulation of the intrinsic and extrinsic coagulation pathways occurs producing fibrin that disseminates throughout the body. This fibrin lodges within the microvasculature, leading to thrombus formation and results in ischemia, infarction, and necrosis of organ systems. Moreover, these fibrin thrombi trap platelets, thus worsening the ischemia. In attempts to degrade the thrombi, the fibrinolytic system releases plasmin to lyse the fibrin clots, which subsequently releases fibrin degradation products (FDPs). These FDPs in turn inhibit thrombin and platelet aggregation, leading to hemorrhage.

Disseminated intravasular coagulation can be associated with various clinical scenarios, most commonly infections and neoplasms (Table 1) (1–3). It can occur in 10% of all cancer patients, especially in patients with acute promyleocytic leukemia where it can occur in up to 85% (1). Oftentimes, DIC will arise as a consequence of treatment with chemotherapeutic agents. Although DIC may result from infection with various organisms, including gram-positive bacteria, viruses, and malaria, it is most frequently associated with gram-negative sepsis. Ten to twenty percent of patients with gram-negative sepsis will exhibit signs of DIC (1). Other etiologies

Table 1 Etiology of DIC

Infections	Vascular
Pseidomonas	Malformations
Meningococcus	Hemangiomas
Enterobacteriaciae	Vasculitis
Salmonella	Grafts
Hemophilus	Prostheses
Pneumpcpccus	LaVeen shunt
Staphylococcus	Aortic balloon assist device
Cytomegalovirus	Hepatic
Hepatitis	Obstructive jaundice
Varicella	Fulminant hepatic failure
Human immunodeficiency virus	Tissue injury
Aspergillosis	Head trauma
Postsplencetomy Sepsis	Burns
Purpura fulminans	Electric shock
Rocky mountain spotted fever	Transfusions
Malaria	Acute pancreatitis
Obstetric	Snake bite
Abruptio placentae	Heat stroke
Amniotic fluid embolism	Fat embolism
Abortion	Malignant hyperthermia
Eclampsia	Immune complexes
Retained fetus	Glomerulonephritis
Neoplasms	
Leukemias	
Pancreas	
Lung	
Prostate	
Gastric	
Colon	
Ovary	
Gallbladder	
Breast	

include obstetric complications, hepatic failure, LaVeen shunts, severe transfusion reactions, burns, and fat emboli.

Patients clinically can exhibit signs of both hemorrhage and thrombosis (1–3). In 47% of patients, cutaneous manifestations of DIC are the initial presenting signs (3). Bleeding usually occurs at three or more unrelated sites (1–3). This bleeding may present as acute hemorrhage or slow oozing from venipucture sites, surgical sites, skin, renal, gastrointestinal, or central nervous system. Cutaneous manifestations include ecchymoses, petechiae, or hemorrhagic bullae. Evidence of thrombosis may manifest in the kidneys, lungs, or skin. The areas of cutaneous hemorrhagic necrosis [purpura fulminans (PF)] may progress to gangrene and autoamputation distally.

Although there is no single laboratory test diagnostic of DIC, there is a group of tests, which, when combined, is highly suggestive of DIC (1–3). Because of the overstimulation of the clotting cascade, there is a consumption of clotting factors leading to an elevated prothrombin time (PT) and an activated partial thromboplastin time (PTT). The rapid consumption of platelets leads to thrombocytopenia. In addition, fibrinogen can be decreased, FDPs can be increased, and D-dimers can be elevated.

Critical to successful treatment is prompt intervention. Medical management includes treatment of the underlying cause (broad spectrum antibiotics for infections) and aggressive supportive care (1–3). Replacement of clotting factors with fresh frozen plasma (FFP) and replacement of platelets may be instituted in bleeding patients. The administration of continuous intravenous heparin or periodic subcutaneous low molecular weight heparin (LMWH) injections is beneficial in certain circumstances, such as transfusion reactions, malignancy with thrombosis, and continued bleeding despite massive transfusions. However, the risk of hemorrhage, especially in the central nervous system, is associated with heparin and to a lesser extent LMWH. Recently, the use of activated protein C (APC) in the treatment of patients with sepsis and DIC have resulted in significant decreases in mortality (5–8). It is believed that APC works through antithrombotic, profibrinolytic, and anti-inflammatory mechanisms.

2. PURPURA FULMINANS

Purpura fulminans is a disabling, life threatening condition characterized by fever, circulatory collapse, peripheral gangrene due to dermal vascular thrombosis, and DIC (9–13). It primarily occurs in three clinical scenarios: (1) inherited protein C or S deficiency in neonates, (2) 7–10 days after an acute infection with varicella, scarlet fever, or rubella, and (3) during an acute infectious illness with several pathogens, including *Neisseria meningitidis, Streptococcus pneumoniae,* or *Staphylococcus aureus* (Table 2). Bacterial endotoxins will cause damage to the endothelium, which activates the coagulation cascade. Disseminated intravasular coagulation subsequently develops leading to fibrin thrombi deposition in dermal vessels, especially in the subpapillary plexus, causing tissue necrosis.

Patients may complain of fever or cutaneous discomfort or present with sepsis and circulatory collapse (9–12). Attention to certain clinical signs is critical to limb salvage. First, erythema with or without edema may occur, followed by petechiae or ecchymoses. At this stage, the cutaneous changes are still reversible. If left un-noticed or untreated at this point, the lesions will progress to palpable purpuric plaques with erythematous advancing borders. Later, hemorrhagic bullae develop, followed by thick black eschar and gangrenous necrosis, which may extend to subcutaneous tissue, muscle, and bone.

Laboratory findings are consistent with DIC, including elevated PT/PTT, thrombocytopenia, hypofibrinogenemia, elevated FDPs, and reduced protein C/S and antithrombin III (9–12). Other findings include leukocytosis and anemia.

The sooner the diagnosis is made, the sooner treatment may be implemented and the lower the morbidity or mortality will be (9–12). Intravenous antibiotics, such as a third generation cephalosporin, respiratory and hemodynamic support, and nutritional supplements should be instituted immediately. Transfusions of platelets, packed red blood cells, FFP, heparin, and antithrombin III concentrates are appropriate. The role of APC may prove valuable in the treatment of PF as well. The use of prostacyclin, tissue plasminogen activator, topical nitroglycerin, plasmapheresis, hyperbaric oxygen, and medicinal leeches are controversial. Oftentimes, surgical fasciotomies, escharotomies, or amputations are necessary.

Table 2 Etiology of PF

Postinfectious
  Varicella
  Scarlet fever
  Streptococcal tonsillopharyngitis
  Viral exanthem
  Rubella
  Measles
  Upper respiratory tract infection
  Gastroenteritis
Acute infectious
  Neisseria
  Streptococus
  Hemophilus
  Rickettsia
  Staphylococcus
  Klebsiella
  Escherichia
  Proteus
  Enterobacter
  Capnocytophaga
Idiopathic
Hereditary protein C and S deficiency
Disseminated intravascular coagulation
Antithrombin III deficiency

3. THROMBOTIC THROMBOCYTOPENIC PURPURA

Thrombotic thrombocytopenic purpura (TTP) is characterized by microangiopathic hemolytic anemia, thrombocytopenia, fever, renal failure, and central nervous system dysfunction (14–16). Thrombotic thrombocytopenic purpura overlaps with hemolytic uremic syndrome (HUS); however, in HUS, renal dysfunction is more prominent while neurologic dysfunction is more associated with TTP. The incidence of TTP is 3.7 cases per million per year and appears to be increasing (15). Mortality ranges from 10% to 20%, with the majority occurring within the first 48 hr. Thrombotic thrombocytopenic purpura may occur during pregnancy/peripartum, in HIV, SLE, or in bone marrow transplant patients. It can also be due to medications, such as ticlid, plavix, mitomycin C, cyclosporin, and tacrolimus (Table 3).

Thrombotic thromhocytopenic purpura is the result of platelet aggregation with subsequent thrombi formation (14,15). Unlike DIC, there is no fibrin detected in the thrombi nor is there any endothelial damage. In addition to platelets, von willebrand factor (VWF) multimers are present, which function by increasing platelet aggregation. These diffuse platelet thrombi formation leads to consumptive thrombocytopenia, organ ischemia, and necrosis. These thrombi cause not only ischemia/necrosis, but also intravascular hemolysis of red blood cells secondary to shearing forces within the vessels. In certain patients, the VWF cleaving protease (VWF-CP) is missing, allowing for the continued circulation of the multimeric VWF, thus promoting thrombi formation. Other patients are afflicted with IgG autoantibodies against the VWF-CP.

Table 3 Etiology of TTP

Idiopathic
Familial
Infection
   Escherichia
   Human immunodeficiency virus
Autoimmune
   Systemic lupus erythematosus
Pregnancy
Postpartum
Malignancy
Chemotherapy
   Mitomycin
   Cisplatin
   Gemcitabine
Medications
   Ticlopidine
   Clopidogrel
   Quinidine
   Cyclosporin
Bone marrow transplantation

The presence of fragmented red blood cells/schistocytes is pathognomonic for TTP (14,15). In addition, thrombocytopenia, elevated reticulocyte count, elevated indirect bilirubin level, elevated LDH, and absence of haptoglobin are present. Coagulation studies are normal in TTP.

Ninety percent of patients respond to the combination of plasmapheresis and plasma infusion with FFP, whereas 78% respond to plasmapheresis alone (14,15). The plasmapheresis will remove these large multimeric VWF, whereas the plasma infusion will replace the missing VWF-CP. Other adjuvant therapies include systemic steroids, packed red blood cell transfusions, hemodialysis, supportive care, and platelet transfusion, if bleeding is profuse. In addition, if TTP is medication induced, the culprit agent must be discontinued. Cancer, chemotherapy, and bone marrow transplant-related TTP may respond to immunoadsorption with plasma perfusion over a staphylococcal protein A column. Patients with refractory TTP may benefit from vincristine, intravenous immunoglobulin, or splenectomy.

4. FACTOR V LEIDEN MUTATION

Venous leg ulcers occur in patients with venous insufficiency, 50% of which occur in patients with history of a deep venous thrombosis (DVT) (17). Among the risk factors for DVT are coagulation defects (17–21). These defects include a resistance to APC caused by a point mutation substituting glutamine for arginine in the factor V gene, which is known as the Leiden mutation. This defect has been found in 7.7–36% of post-thrombotic venous leg ulcers (18,20).

One serious consequence of factor V Leiden mutation is leg ulcers (19). Other complications include recurrent DVTs, superficial venous thrombosis, and cutaneous necrosis (17–21).

While coagulation studies, such as APTT, can be used to screen for factor V Leiden mutation, the gold standard test is polymerase chain reaction of DNA (19).

It has been suggested that compression stockings should be worn for 2 years after diagnosis of DVT (19). The use of compression stockings has been shown to reduce the rate of post-thrombotic syndrome by 50%. Long-term oral anticoagulation was effective in preventing recurrent thrombosis or post-thrombotic syndrome complications (19,21). However, LMWH and aspirin might also be effective.

5. PROTEIN S DEFICIENCY

Protein S is a vitamin K-dependent plasma protein, which works in conjunction with protein C to promote natural anticoagulation (21–23). There are homozygous and heterozygous forms of this heritable condition. Acquired forms of protein S deficiency can occur when protein S is bound to other antibodies or is consumed in DIC.

Clinically, the patient may present with extensive cutaneous necrosis, venous thromboembolic events, limb ischemia progressing to gangrene, leg ulcers, and arterial thrombosis (21,22). Recurrence rates run as high as 77%, with DVT and pulmonary embolus being the most common event to recur. These episodes usually occur in patients under 40 with a family history of thrombotic conditions.

Long-term oral anticoagulation is the treatment of choice to prevent recurrent thrombosis and to heal the ulcers (21,23). Early treatment with FFP may reverse the cutaneous necrosis caused by protein S deficiency; however, repeated infusions are necessary. Heparin and aspirin are not helpful in the treatment of this condition.

6. PROTEIN C DEFICIENCY

Protein C is a vitamin K-dependent plasma protein, which is designed to inhibit coagulation and stimulate fibrinolysis (24). Protein C deficiency is a coagulation defect, which may be inherited as an autosomal dominant or recessive trait or may be acquired (24–26).

There are many cutaneous findings associated with protein C deficiency (24–26). Homozygous patients, who inherit this trait recessively, will present shortly after birth with neonatal PF resulting in extensive cutaneous necrosis. Acquired forms of this condition result from DIC, hormones, and liver disease. In addition, 3% of patients with protein C deficiency, who are treated with Coumadin, will develop Coumadin-induced skin necrosis. Other complications include DVTs, pulmonary embolus, leg ulcers, and cutaneous necrosis.

The cornerstone of treatment is oral anticoagulation (24–26). However, some cases of recurrent thrombosis, despite anticoagulation, necessitated the use of LMWHs. Homozygous patients who present with late complications will respond to heparin, whereas those who present as a neonate will not respond. Instead, these neonates require FFP or protein C replacement. Stanazolol, anticytokines, thrombolysis, and antiendotoxins have shown some efficacy.

7. COUMADIN NECROSIS

Coumadin necrosis was first described (27–30). It is a rare but serious condition affecting 0.01–0.1% of all patients taking Coumadin (27–31). Classically, middle-aged, obese women are most at risk. Women are afflicted more than men, at a ratio of 9:1.

The majority of patients report symptoms within the first 3–5 days after beginning Coumadin for anticoagulation of DVT, pulmonary embolus, or cardiac and cerebral thrombotic events (27–31). There is a propensity for involvement of fatty areas, such as buttocks, breast, and thighs. Decreased perfusion, decreased temperature, and external pressure may account for the predilection to necrosis of these areas (31). However, there have been reports in the literature of the involvement of the face, distal extremities, and penis (27). Eighty percent of lesions are found on the lower-half of the body (27).

Initially, patients may have one or more erythematous, well demarcated, painful plaques with a peau d'orange appearance (27–31). Thirty-five percent of patients have multiple lesions (27). After 24 hr, petechiae will appear, progressing into ecchymoses and finally large hemorrhagic bullae (27–31). Oftentimes, there are islands of normal tissue within these areas of ecchymoses. With the appearance of bullae, the condition is considered irreversible. These bullae will rupture, leaving black eschar covering large defects, which extend into the subcutaneous tissue.

The pathogenesis of Coumadin necrosis is unclear (27–31). It has been proposed that a transient hypercoagulable state occurs at the initiation of Coumadin therapy, which causes to a decrease in protein C. Protein C is a natural anticoagulant, which inhibits the procoagulant clotting factor VIIIa and Xa. Protein S works in conjunction with protein C to augment this inhibition of procoagulants. Thus, patients with inherited protein C and S deficiencies are at increased risk of Coumadin necrosis. It has also been hypothesized that there is a direct toxic effect by Coumadin on the dermovascular loop at the junction of the capillary and precapillary arterioles, leading to petechiae and microthrombi (28,30). The resultant stasis occurring in the venules of the distal loop leads to thrombosis and necrosis. Histologically, there is occlusion of dermal and subcutaneous veins with fibrin thrombi, subcutaneous fat necrosis and hemorrhage, foreign body giant cell reaction, and oftentimes a neutrophilic vasculitis.

Treatment should include the discontinuation of Coumadin; however, there has been no conclusive proof that this has any impact on the mortality or clinical course (27–31). However, 10–20 mg of vitamin K, heparin (35,000 U every day for 3–4 days), and FFP must be given immediately. Activated protein C should be administered to patients who are deficient (29). Prompt intervention can prevent extensive damage. In addition, intervention prior to the appearance of hemorrhagic bullae may completely reverse the damage. The majority of patients can be restarted on Coumadin; however, there have been rare reports of relapses (31). It is recommended that loading doses of Coumadin (more than 10 mg/day) be avoided and that heparin should be started 24 hr prior to Coumadin to prevent the transient hypercoagulable state from occurring, thus preventing Coumadin necrosis. Unfortunately, over 50% of patients need surgical intervention, including debridement, grafting, amputations, or mastectomies (27,31).

8. ANTIPHOSPHOLIPID ANTIBODY SYNDROME

Antiphospholipid antibody syndrome (APS) is an immunologic disorder characterized by the presence of antiphospholipid antibodies and thrombotic events. Anticardiolipin antibodies, lupus anticoagulant, and anti-β_2-glycoprotein I antibodies are the most common findings in APS (32). There are three main subtypes of APS: primary, secondary, and catastrophic (32). Primary APS is not commonly found in conjunction with any other autoimmune diseases; however, secondary APS is associated with several autoimmune disorders, such as lupus erythematosus, Sjogren syndrome, rheumatoid arthritis, systemic sclerosis, and dermatomyositis (33). Recently described in 1992, catastrophic APS is characterized by the simultaneous failure of at least three different organs due to thrombotic events in the vascular beds, which often leads to death (34).

The precise mechanism by which thrombotic events occur in APS is not entirely known; however, several theories have been proposed. One theory is through the activation of endothelial cells (35). Another is by the cross-reaction of autoantibodies against oxidized LDL of damaged endothelial cells in vessels with atherosclerosis (36). The third theory implies that the antiphospholipid antibodies hamper the function of proteins involved in the regulation of coagulation (37). Finally, there is the theory of a "second hit" on damaged blood vessels (38).

In order to make the diagnosis of APS, certain clinical and laboratory criteria must be fulfilled. These clinical criteria include one or more visceral arterial or venous thrombotic events and/or complications of pregnancy (39). Complications during pregnancy include one or more unexplained deaths of otherwise normal fetuses at or after 10 weeks of gestation, one or more premature births at or before 34 weeks of gestation, or three or more unexplained consecutive miscarriages before the 10th week of gestation (39).

The laboratory criteria include elevated serum IgG or IgM anticardiolipin antibodies (2.0 or 2.5 times the median level) on two or more occasions at least 6 weeks apart, the presence of serum lupus anticoagulant on two or more occasions at least 6 weeks apart (39).

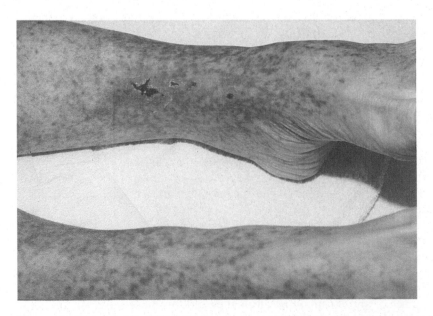

Figure 1 Patient with APS demonstrating necrotic ulcers on the lower extremity.

Table 4 Clinical Findings Associated with APS

Cutaneous	Cardiovascular	Respiratory
Thrombophlebitis	Angina	Pulmonary emboli
Splinter hemorrhages	MI	Pulmonary hypertension
Leg ulcers	Valvular vegetations	Alveolar hemorrhage
Necrosis of the skin	Thrombi	Acute respiratory distress
Blue toe syndrome	Endocarditis	syndrome
Cyanosis	Atherosclerosis	
Livedo reticularis	Myocarditis	Renal
Gangrene	Valvulopathy	Renal infarction
Purpura	Deep vein thrombosis	Renal failure
Echymosis	Arterial thrombosis	Nephrotic syndrome
Neurologic	Gastrointestinal	Endocrine
TIA	Esophageal perforation	Adrenal insufficiency
Stroke	Intestinal infarction	Pituitary infarction
Transient amnesia	Splenic infarction	Pituitary failure
Dementia	Hepatic infarction	
Encephalopathy	Gall bladder infarction	Hematologic
Migranes	Pancreatic infarction	Thrombocytopenia
Pseudotumor cerebri	Pancreatitis	Hemolytic anemia
Mononeuritis multiplex	Ascitis	HUS
Myelitis	Budd–Chiari syndrome	TTP
Seizures		
Chorea	Osteoarticular	Miscellaneous
Ataxia	Arthritis	Nose perforation
Amaurosis fugax	Arthralgia	Testicular infarction
Optic neuropathy	Avascular necrosis of bone	
Retinal artery thrombosis		
Retinal vein thrombosis		
Obstetrical		
Pregnancy loss		
HELLP syndrome		
Uteroplacental		
insufficiency		
Pre-eclampsia		
Abruptio placentae		
Premature birth		
Oligohydraminos		

Thromboembolism and thrombotic microangiopathy cause the majority of clinical findings in APS patients. Thrombosis may affect any part of the body but most commonly will manifest as DVT of the legs (32,33). The incidence of DVT in these patients was reported as 31.7% (33). In addition, superficial thrombophlebitis has been reported. Cutaneous manifestations include livedo reticularis, leg ulcers, cyanosis and necrosis of the skin, purpura, ecchymosis, splinter hemorrhages, and gangrene (Fig. 1). Obstetric complications include pregnancy loss, generally occurring after the 10th week of pregnancy and intrauterine growth retardation (39). Other sequela of APS are myocardial infarction, pulmonary emboli, renal failure, renal infarction, stroke, and adrenal infarction (Table 4).

The main goals in caring for patients with APS are the treatment of thromboses and the prevention of future thrombotic events. Risk factors, such as oral contraceptive use and smoking, should be avoided. Aspirin has been shown to be ineffective in providing protection against deep vein thrombosis and pulmonary embolism in men (40). In women, aspirin was proven to be beneficial in preventing thrombosis in APS (41). In addition, it has been reported that patients with lupus and APS may benefit from treatment with hydroxychloroquine (42). Warfarin has been shown to prevent thrombotic events when the INR is 2–3 (43).

9. CRYOGLOBULINEMIA I

Cryoglobulins are plasma proteins that precipitate at 37°C and dissolve upon rewarming. There are three types of cryoglobulinemia: types I, II, and III (Table 5). Cryoglobulinemia type I is mainly associated with a lymphoproliferative disorder. This type is mainly associated with Waldestrom's macroglobulinemia, multiple myeloma, chronic lymphocytic leukemia, and immunocytoma (44,45). Cryoglobulinemia types II and III are caused by monoclonal, monoclonal–polyclonal, and polyclonal immunoglobulins. Types II and III can be associated not only with malignancies, but also with various infectious and immunologic diseases.

It is not known what exactly causes the precipitation of the immunoglobulins, but it has been suggested that carbohydrate abnormalities decrease the solubility of the cryoglobulins (46). Another hypothesis is that the precipitation may result from varied interactions between immunoglobulin structures at decreased temperatures (47).

Classically, cryoglobulinemia is characterized by purpura, arthalgias, and asthenia (Meltzer's triad). Patients with type I cryoglobulinemia generally present with livedoid vasculitis, cold-induced acrocyanosis especially of the helices of the ears, leg ulcerations with hemorrhagic crusts, Raynaud's phenomenon, cold urticaria, arterial thromboses, and retinal hemorrhage (48,49). Types II and III cryoglobulins are associated with vascular purpura, arthritis, renal and neurologic symptoms (Figs. 2 and 3) (45).

The diagnosis is made on the basis of both the clinical and the laboratory findings. Ten to twenty milliliters of blood are needed for diagnosis. The blood is left to clot at 37°C for 30–60 min before centrifugation. Then, the serum is left at 4°C for 7 days. Cryoglobulin precipitate is generally apparent by 24 hr in types I and II; however, precipitate in type III may take up to several days to become evident. Serum cryoglobulin values are not related with the severity and prognosis of the disease. Immunoelectrophoresis, immunoblotting, and immunofixation can be done for evaluation of the cryoglobulins (45,50,51).

As type I cryoglobulinemia is often found in patients with a lymphoproliferative disorder, the treatment is mainly directed at the underlying condition. Treatment options include melphalan, chlorambucil, and prednisone (44). Plasmapheresis has been reported to be of benefit (52). Cryoglobulinemia types II and III can be treated with low antigen diet, interferon, ribavirin, steroids, plasma exchange, cyclophosphamide, chlorambucil, azathioprine, cyclosporine, and colchicine (53).

Table 5 Characteristics of Cryoglobulinemia

	Cryoglobulinemia I	Cryoglobulinemia II	Cryoglobulinemia III
Cryoglobulins	Monoclonal IgM, IgG, IgA, or free light chains	Monoclonal IgM, IgG, or IgA and polyclonal (principally IgG)	Polyclonal all isotypes
Pathology	Vasculopathy	Leucocytoclastic vasculitis	Leucocytoclastic Vasculitis
Associated diseases	Multiple myeloma, Waldenstrom's macroglobulinemia, CLL, B cell NHL, Benign monoclonal gammopathy	Hepatitis C and B, connective tissue diseases, other viral and bacterial infections, as well as lymphoproliferative disorders, but these are rare	Hepatitis C and B, connective tissue diseases, other viral and bacterial infections, as well as lymphoproliferative disorders, but these are rare
Percentage of cases	10–15%	60%	25–30%

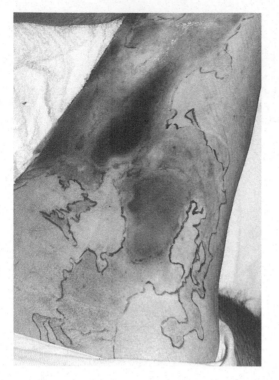

Figure 2 Patient with cryoglobulinemia manifested as purpura of the lower extremity.

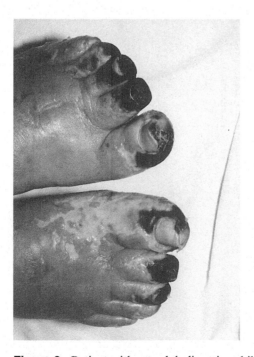

Figure 3 Patient with cryoglobulinemia exhibiting necrotic ulcers and gangrene of the toes.

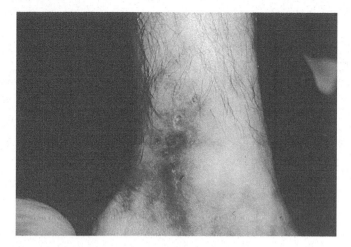

Figure 4 Patient with cryofibrinogenemia showing necrotic ulcers of the lower extremity.

10. CRYOFIBRINOGENEMIA

Cryofibrinogenemia, like cryoglobulinemia, is caused by the precipitation of certain proteins when exposed to cold temperatures. These proteins include fibrinogen, fibrin, and fibronectin (54). Cryofibrinogenemia is also associated with malignancies, multiple myeloma, B-cell lymphoma, and leukemia; pregnancy; oral contraceptive use; collagen vascular diseases; thrombohemorrhagic phenomena; and diabetes mellitus (54–56).

As with other vasculopathies, cutaneous manifestations include purpura, livedo reticularis, ecchymoses, gangrene, ulcerations, and Raynaud's phenomenon (Fig. 4) (56,57). These painful ulcerations generally occur on the legs and are often unresponsive to treatment (56).

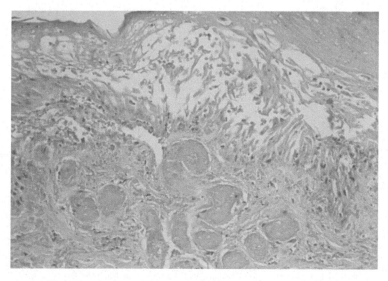

Figure 5 Skin biopsy of patient with cryofibrinogenemia stained with H&E demonstrating fibrin thrombi within the vessels of the dermis.

Skin biopsy reveals intravascular thrombi composed of an eosinophilic amorphous material without surrounding inflammation (Fig. 5). Current laboratory recommendations include the collection of serum samples in tubes prepared with citrate, oxalate, or ethylenediamine-tetra-acetic acid, because the use of heparin may lead to the formation of heparin–fibronectin cryoprecipitate complexes (58). These complexes can give false positive results.

Treatment focuses on the underlying condition and thrombosis, as well as on the prevention of future thrombotic events. Certain therapeutic modalities have been used in the treatment of cryofibrinogenemia-associated thrombosis, such as dipyridamole, heparin, warfarin, streptokinase, streptodornase, stanozolol, oral corticosteroids, immunosuppressive therapy, and plasmapheresis (56,59–61). Treatment of the underlying malignancy involves the use of agents such as chlorambucil (44).

11. CALCIPHYLAXIS

Calciphylaxis, also known as calcific uremic arteriolopathy (CUA), is a rare, often fatal disease affecting 1% of patients with end stage renal disease and 4.1% of patients on hemodialysis (62–64). It is also associated with Crohn's disease, advanced liver disease, and with extensive bowel resections (65,66). It affects patients between the ages of 6 months and 83 years (mean 48 ± 16 years) (67). Calciphylaxis carries a poor prognosis, with mortality rates as high as 80% (67).

The pathogenesis of CUA is largely unknown but likely multifactorial. It has been proposed that CUA might result from sensitization to different agents, such as elevated levels of calcium and phosphorus, which renders the patient more susceptible to subsequent inflammation upon subsequent challenges (68,69). Secondary hyperparathyroidism, as well as protein C and S deficiencies, may also play an important role in the pathogenesis of the disease (70,71). It has been suggested that a calcium–phosphorus product >70 is associated with the characteristic calcium deposition within vessels (63).

There are two clinical variants of CUA described in the literature, proximal and distal (64,69). Proximal involvement has a poorer prognosis and it generally affects the trunk, abdomen, buttocks, and arms. The cutaneous manifestations

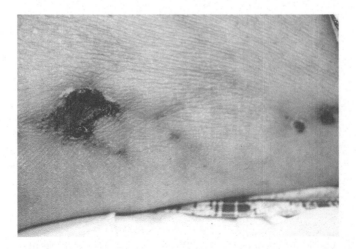

Figure 6 Necrotic ulcers of the lower extremity in a patient with calciphylaxis.

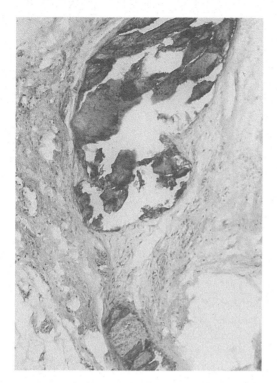

Figure 7 Skin biopsy of patient with calciphylaxis stained with H&E showing calcium within the vessels.

include reticulated violaceous patches and indurated plaques, which rapidly progress into painful bilateral necrotic ulcers, often with extension into muscle (Fig. 6) (68,69).

Diagnosis can be made on the basis of clinical findings and biopsy. Serum analysis consistent with hypercalcemia, hyperphosphatemia, and elevated parathyroid hormone levels can be associated with CUA. Radiographic studies reveal calcified vessels, known as "pipe stem" calcifications (68). Calcification of the intima and media of small and medium vessels in the dermis and subcutaneous tissue, which is readily visible on biopsy, can result in vascular compromise, ischemia, and necrosis (Fig. 7) (68,69).

The treatment of calciphylaxis involves meticulous wound care and IV antibiotics, when necessary. Serum calcium and phosphorus levels should be normalized with the use of diet, phosphate binders, low calcium dialysis, and surgery. Parathyroidectomy is recommended mainly in two settings: elevated parathyroid hormone and pain unresponsive to medications. Hyperbaric oxygen, cyclosporine, stanazolol, and cimetidine have been reported to be beneficial (68,69,72,73).

12. CHOLESTEROL EMBOLI SYNDROME

Cholesterol embolization syndrome (CES) is generally precipitated by procedures involving the manipulation of the atherosclerotic blood vessels. This leads to the dislodging of pieces of atherosclerotic plaques, and when combined with the use of

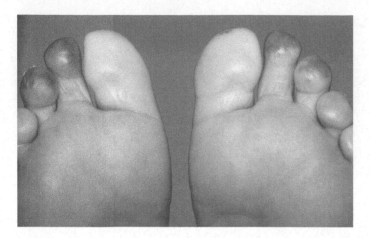

Figure 8 Purpura of the toes in a patient with CES, also referred to as "blue toe syndrome."

anticoagulation, contributes to the plaque instability. The clinical findings of CES include leg and/or foot pain, livedo reticularis, often with worsening of renal function along with the history of surgical procedures or the start of anticoagulation (74,75). Mortality rates have been upwards of 81% (76). Cholesterol embolization syndrome can also affect the central nervous system, pancreas, spleen, gastrointestinal tract, liver, and gallbladder (77,78).

The most common clinical findings present in >50% of cases of CES is livedo reticularis and "blue toe syndrome," consisting of digital mottling, ischemic changes, and gangrene (Fig. 8) (74). Ulceration, nodules, and purpura can also be present. In cases caused by surgical procedures, clinical symptoms appear rapidly, whereas cases involving anticoagulation, cutaneous manifestations may develop more slowly.

The diagnosis of CES requires a careful history of prior surgical procedures and anticoagulation, cutaneous manifestations, normal peripheral pulses, worsening of renal failure, and a positive skin biopsy. Biopsy specimens show needle-shaped clefts within the lumina of small blood vessels, which correspond to cholesterol microemboli (75,79). Other laboratory findings associated with CES include eosinophilia, increased sedimentation rate, and leukocytosis.

Treatment of CES involves discontinuation of anticoagulation and local wound care. Corticosteroids and iloprost, a prostacycline, have been beneficial to patients. The use of antiplatelet therapy, pentoxifylline, and low molecular dextran have not lead to clinical improvement in patients with CES (75,80,81).

13. ATROPHIE BLANCHE

This is a condition that affects generally female patients with a higher incidence between 30 and 60 years of age (82,83). It is associated with chronic venous insufficiency and found in up to 9–38% of the patients (82,84–87). The incidence is higher if there is recurrent venous ulceration. Atroptrie Blanche (AB) can also be associated with systemic diseases such as systemic lupus erythematosus and scleroderma (88,89).

It typically affects the ankle and dorsa of the feet with small, whitish, stellate, areas that may have peripheral telangiectasias around them. Painful ulcerations can develop and livedo reticularis can be associated (90). Often, there are associated changes from CVI with brown macules and patches, as well as the presence of varicose veins.

The differential diagnosis includes lichen sclerosus et atrophicus, malignant atrophic papulosis (Dego's disease), scleroderma, and scar formation.

Histology findings are nonspecific and include the deposition of fibrinoid material in the blood vessel lumen and wall. The overlying epithelium can become atrophic, and the dermis can show sclerotic changes. If there is inflammation this is often minimal (91).

There are three different theories proposed in the pathogenesis of this disease. The first one is the deposition of a fibrin cuff around the blood vessels, which leads to less oxygenation of the surrounding tissues and the delivery of less nutrients (92,93). The second theory is the "white-cell trapping" where the slow blood flow causes the white cells to attach to the endothelium and releases destructive proteolytic enzymes (94,95). The last theory is the deposition of microthrombi inside the blood vessels as a result of coagulation and fibrinolysis abnormalities (96,97).

Compression is the mainstay of AB therapy, as CVI is the most common associated finding (90). Other treatments that can be used, which have been proven effective, include medications that change the coagulation process such as aspirin, dipyridamole, heparin, and warfarin (90). Ethylestrenol, pentoxyfylline, sulfazalazine, nifedipine, and PUVA therapy have been reported to be useful in case reports (90,98–103).

REFERENCES

1. Maxson JH. Management of disseminated intravascular coagulation. Crit Care Nurs Clin North Am 2000; 12:341–352.
2. Colman RW, Minna JD, Robboy SJ. Disseminated intravascular coagulation: a dermatologic disease. Int J Dermatol 1977; 16:47–51.
3. Robboy SJ, Mihm MC, Colman RW, Minna JD. The skin in disseminated intravascular coagulation. Br J Dermatol 1973; 88:221–229.
4. Faust SN, Heyderman RS, Levin M. Disseminated intrasvascular coagulation and purpura fulminans secondary to infection. Baillieres Clin Haematol 2000; 13:179–197.
5. Warren HS, Suffredini AF, Eichacker PQ, Munsford RS. Risks and benefits of activated protein C treatment for severe sepsis. N Engl J Med 2002; 347:1027–1030.
6. Levi M. Pathogenesis and treatment of disseminated intravascular coagulation in septic patients. J Crit Care 2001; 16:167–177.
7. Dhainaut JF, Yan SB, Cariou A, Mira JP. Soluble thrombomodulin, plasma derived unactivated protein C and recombinant human activated protein C in sepsis. Crit Care Med 2002; 30s:s318–s324.
8. Aoki N, Matsuda T, Saito H, Takatsuki K, Okajima K, Takahashi H, Takamatsu J, Asakura H, Ogawa N. A comparative double blind randomized trial of activated protein C and unfractionated heparin in the treatment of disseminated intravascular coagulation. Int J Hematol 2002; 75:540–547.
9. Nolan J, Sinclair R. Review of management of purpura fulminans and two case reports. Br J Anesth 2001; 86:581–586.
10. Darmstadt GL. Acute infectious purpura fulminans: pathogenesis and medical management. Ped Dermatol 1998; 15:169–183.
11. Masquelet AC, Romana MC, Gilbert A, Berard J. Management of purpura fulminans at the upper extremity. Hand Clinics 2000; 16:723–731.

12. Adcock DM, Hicks MJ. Dermatopathology of skin necrosis associated with purpura fulminans. Semin Thromb Hemost 1990; 16:283–292.
13. Auletta MJ, Headington JT. Purpura fulminans: a cutaneous manifestation of severe protein C deficiency. Arch Dermatol 1988; 124:1387–1391.
14. Moake JL. Thrombotic thrombocytopenic purpura: the systemic clumping "plague". Ann Rev Med 2002; 53:75–88.
15. Elliott MA, Nichols WL. Thrombotic thrombocytopenic purpura and hemolytic uremic syndrome. Mayo Clin Proc 2001; 76:1154–1162.
16. Burniss JB, Cohen LM, Thomas HA, Callen JP. Unilateral emboli in a patient with thrombotic thrombocytpenic purpura. J Am Acad Dermatol 1993; 29:838–840.
17. Ribeaudeau F, Senet P, Cayuela JM, Fund X, Paul C, Robert C, Scrobohaci ML, Dubertret L. A prospective coagulation study including resistance to activated protein C and mutations in factors V and II in venous leg ulcers. Br J Dermatol 1999; 141:259–263.
18. Gaber Y, Siemens HJ, Schmeller W. Resistance to activated protein C due to factor V leiden mutation: high prevalence in patients with post-thrombotic leg ulcers. Br J Dermatol 2001; 144:546–548.
19. Maessen-Visch MB, Hamulyak K, Tazekaar DJ, Crombag NHCMN, Neumann HAM. The prevalence of factor V leiden mutation in patients with leg ulcers and venous insufficiency. Arch Dermatol 1999; 135:41–44.
20. Grossman D, Heald PW, Wang C, Rinder HM. Activated protein C resistance and anticardiolipin antibodies in patients with venous leg ulcers. J Am Acad Dermatol 1997; 37:409–413.
21. Hafner J, Kuhne A, Schar B, Bombeli T, Hauser M, Luthi R, Hanseler E. Factor V leiden mutation in postthrombotic and non-postthrombotic venous ulcers. Arch Dermatol 2001; 137:599–603.
22. Amster MS, Conway J, Zeid M, Pincus S. Cutaneous necrosis resulting from protein S deficiency and increased antiphospholipid antibody in a patient with systemic lupus erythematosus. J Am Acad Dermatol 1993; 29:853–857.
23. Kulthanan K, Krudum T, Pintadit P, Khonnaseam R, Kullavanijaya P. Chronic leg ulcers associated with hereditary protein S deficiency. Internat J Dermatol 1997; 36:198–212.
24. Pescatore P, Horellou HM, Conard J, Piffoux M, Van Dreden P, Ruskone-Fourmestraux A, Samama M. Problems of oral anticoagulation in an adult with homozygous protein C deficiency and late onset of thrombosis. Thromb Haemost 1993; 69:311–315.
25. Esmon CT, Vigano-D'Angelo S, D'Angelo A, Comp PC. Anticoagulation Proteins C and S. Adv Exp Med Biol 1987; 214:47–54.
26. Alberio L, Lammle B, Esmon CT. Protein C replacement in severe meningococemia: rationale and clinical experience. Clin Infect Dis 2001; 32:1338–1346.
27. DeFranzo AJ, Marasco P, Argenta LC. Warfarin induced necrosis of the skin. Ann Plast Surg 1995; 34:203–208.
28. Schleicher SM, Frisker MP. Coumadin necrosis. Arch Dermatol 1980; 116:444–445.
29. Chan YC, Valenti D, Mansfield AO, Stansby G. Warfarin induced skin necrosis. Br J Surg 2000; 87:266–272.
30. Faraci PA. Warfarin induced skin necrosis. Intern J Dermatol 1982; 21:329–330.
31. Whitaker-Worth DL, Corlone V, Susser WS, Phelan N, Grant-Kels JM. Dermatologic diseases of the breast and nipple. J Am Acad Dermatol 2000; 43:733–751.
32. Levine JS, Branch DW, Rauch J. The antiphospholipid syndrome. N Engl J Med 2002; 346:752–763.
33. Cervera R, Piette JC, Font J, Khamashta MA, Shoenfeld Y, Camps MT, Jacobsen S, et al. Antiphospholipid syndrome: clinical and immunologic manifestations and patterns of disease expression in a cohort of 1,000 patients. Arthritis Rheum 2002; 46(4):1019–1027.

34. Asherson RA, Cervera R, Piette J-C, et al. Catastrophic antiphospholipid syndrome: clinical and laboratory features of 50 patients. Medicine (Baltimore) 1998; 77:195–207.

35. Meroni PL, Raschi E, Camera M, et al. Endothelial activation by aPL: a potential pathogenic mechanism for the clinical manifestations of the syndrome. J Autoimmun 2000; 15:237–240.

36. Ames PRJ. Antiphospholipid antibodies, thrombosis and atherosclerosis in systemic lupus erythematosus: a unifying "membrane stress syndrome" hypothesis. Lupus 1994; 3:371–377.

37. Kandiah DA, Krilis SA. Beta 2-glycoprotein I. Lupus 1994; 3:207–212.

38. Arnout J. The pathogenesis of the antiphospholipid-antibody syndrome: a hypothesis based on parallelisms with heparin-induced thrombocytopenia. Thromb Haemost 1996; 75:536–541.

39. Brandt JT, Triplett DA, Alving B, Scarrer I. Criteria for the diagnosis of lupus anticoagulants: an update. Thromb Haemost 1995; 74:1185–1190.

40. Ginsgurg KS, Liang MH, Newcomer L, et al. Anticardiolipin antibodies and the risk for ischemic stroke and venous thrombosis. Ann Intern Med 1992; 117:997–1002.

41. Erkan D, Merrill JT, Yazici Y, Sammaritano L, Buyon JP, Lockshin MD. High thrombosis rate after fetal loss in antiphospholipid syndrome: effective prophylaxis with aspirin. Arthritis Rheum 2001; 441:1466–1467.

42. Petri M. Hydroxychloroquine use in Baltimore lupus cohort: effects on lipids, glucose, and thrombosis. Lupus 1996; 5(suppl 1):S16–S22.

43. Rosove MH, Brewer PMC. Antiphospholipid thrombosis: clinical course after the first thrombotic event in 70 patients. Ann Intern Med 1992; 117:303–308.

44. Dammaco F, Sansonno D, Piccoli C, Tucci FA, Racanelli V. The cryoglobulins: an overview. Eur J Clin Invest 2001; 31:628–638.

45. Ferri C, Zignego AL, Pileri SA. Cryoglobulins. J Clin Pathol 2002; 55:4–13.

46. Levo Y. Nature of cryoglobulinemia. Lancet 1980; 1:285–287.

47. Grey HM, Kohler PF. Cryoimmunoglobulins. Semin Hematol 1973; 10:87–112.

48. Gorevic PD. Cryopathies: cryoglobulins and cryofibrinogenemia. Immunological Diseases. Boston/Toronto: Little, Brown, 1978.

49. Cohen SJ, Pittelkow MR, Su WP. Cutaneous manifestations of cryoglobulinemia: clinical and histopathologic study of seventy-two patients. J Am Acad Dermatol 1991; 25:21–27.

50. Dispenzeri A, Gorevic PD. Cryoglobulinemia. Hematol Oncol Clin North Am 1999; 13(6):1315–1318.

51. Campioli D, Ghini M, Mascia MT, et al. Characterization of immunoglobulins: some remarks on methodology. Clin Exp Rheumatol 1995; 13(S):75–78.

52. Siami FS, Siami GA. Cryofiltration apheresis in the treatment of cryoprecipitate induced diseases. Ther Apher 1997; 1:58–62.

53. Dispenzieri A. Symptomatic cryoglobulinemia. Curr Treat Options Oncol 2000; 2: 105–118.

54. Beightler E, Diven DG, Sanchez RL, Solomon AR. Thrombotic vasculopathy associated with cryofibrinogenemia. J Am Acad Dermatol 1991; 24:342–345.

55. Smith SB, Arkin C. Cryofibrinogenemia: incidence, clinical correlation, and review of the literature. Am J Clin Pathol 1972; 58:524–530.

56. Kirsner RS, Eaglstein WH, Katz MH, Kerdel FA, Falanga V. Stanozolol causes rapid pain relief and healing of cutaneous ulcers caused by cryofibrinogenemia. J Am Acad Dermatol 1993; 28:71–74.

57. Brüngger A, Brülisauer M, Mitsuhashi Y, Schneider V, Bollinger A, Schnyder UW. Cryofibrinogenemic purpura. Arch Dermatol Res 1987; 279(S):S24–S29.

58. Gorevic P. Cryopathies: cryoglobulins and cryofibrinogenemia. In: Frank MM, Austen KF, Claman HN, et al. Immunological Diseases. 5th ed. Boston: Little, Brown, 1995: 951–974.

59. Copeman PWN. Cryofibrinogenemia and skin ulcers: treatment with plasmapheresis. Br J Dermatol 1979; 101:57–59.
60. Rachilimiwetz EA, Sacks MI, Zlotnik A. Essential cryofibrinogenemia: clinical, pathological, and immunological studies. Israel J Med Sci 1970; 6:32–43.
61. Mosseson MW, Coleman RW, Sherry S. Chronic intravascular coagulation syndrome: report of a case with special studies of an associated plasma precipitate ("cryofibrinogen"). N Engl J Med 1968; 278:815–821.
62. Coates T, Kirkland GSM, Dymock RB, et al. Cutaneous necrosis from calcific uremic arteriolopathy. Am J Kidney Dis 1998; 32:384–391.
63. Kang AS, McCarthy JT, Rowland C, Farley DR, van Heerden JA. Is calciphylaxis best treated surgically or medically? Surgery 2000; 128:967–972.
64. Budisavjevic MN, Cheek D, Ploth DW. Calciphylaxis in chronic renal failure. J Am Soc Nephrol 1996; 7:978–982.
65. Smiley CM, Hanlon SU, Michel DM. Calciphylaxis in moderate renal insufficiency: changing disease concepts. Am J Nephrol 2000; 20:324–328.
66. Fader DJ, Kang S. Calciphylaxis without renal failure. Arch Dermatol 1996; 132:837–838.
67. Hafner J, Keusch G, Wahl C, Sauter B, Hürlimann A, von Weizsäcker F, et al. Uremic small-artery disease with medial calcification and intimal hyperplasia (so-called calciphylaxis): a complication of chronic renal failure and benefit from parathyroidectomy. J Am Acad Dermatol 1995; 33:954–962.
68. Oh DH, Eulau D, Tokugawa DA, McGuire JS, Kohler S. Five cases of calciphylaxis and a review of the literature. J Am Acad Dermatol 1999; 40:979–987.
69. Trent JT, Kirsner RS. Calciphylaxis: diagnosis and treatment. Adv Skin Wound Care 2001; 14(6):309–312.
70. Mehta RL, Scott G, Sloand JA, Francis CH. Skin necrosis associated with acquired protein C deficiency in patients with renal failure and calciphylaxis. Am J Med 1990; 88:252–257.
71. Perez-Jijares R, Guzman-Zamudio JL, Payan-Lopez J, Rodriguez-Fernandez A, Gomez-Fernandez P, Almaraz-Jimenez M. Calciphylaxis in a haemodyalisis patient: functional protein S deficiency? Nephrol Dial Transplant 1996; 11:1856–1859.
72. Llach F. The evolving pattern of calciphylaxis: therapeutic considerations. Nephrol Dial Transplant 2001; 16:448–451.
73. Howe SC, Murray JD, Reeves RT, Hemp JR, Carlisle JH. Calciphylaxis, a poorly understood clinical syndrome: three case reports and a review of the literature. Ann Vasc Surg 2001; 15:470–473.
74. Chaudhary K, Wall BM, Rasberry RD. Livedo reticularis: an underutilized diagnostic clue in cholesterol embolization syndrome. Am J Med Sci 2000; 321:348–351.
75. Pennington M, Yeager J, Skelton H, Smith KJ. Cholesterol embolization syndrome: cutaneous histopathological features and the variable onset of symptoms in patients with different risk factors. Br J Dermatol 2001; 146:511–517.
76. Fine MJ, Kapoor WN, Falanga V. Cholesterol crystal embolization: a review of 221 cases in the English literature. Angiology 1987; 38:769–784.
77. Geraets DR, Hoehms JP, Burke TG, Grover-McKay M. Thrombolytic-associated cholesterol emboli syndrome: case report and literature review. Pharmacotherapy 1995; 14:441–450.
78. Gore I, Collins DP. Spontaneous atheromatous embolization. Review of the literature and a report of 16 additional cases. Am J Clin Pathol 1960; 33:416–426.
79. Dahlberg PJ, Frencentese DF, Cogbill TH. Cholesterol embolism: experience with 22 histologically proven cases. Surgery 1989; 105:737–746.
80. Mann SJ, Sos TA. Treatment of atheroembolization with corticosteroids. Am J Hyperten 2000; 14:831–834.
81. Elinav E, Chajek-Shaul T, Kerem E, Stern M. Improvement in cholesterol emboli syndrome after iloprost therapy. Br Med J 2002; 324:268–269.

82. Maessen-Visch MB, Neumann HAM, Koedam MI, Groeneweg DA. Repercussion de l' atrophie blanche chez les patients atteints d'un ulcua cruris venosum. Phlebologie 1996; 50:367–370.

83. Gray HR, Graham JH, Johnson W, Burgoon CF. Atrophie blanche: periodic painful ulcers of lower extremities. Arch Dermatol 1966; 93:187–193.

84. Molen van der HR. Revacularisatie van de "atrophie blanche" van Milian. Ned Tijdschr Geneesk 1953; 97:2194–2197.

85. Folescu F. Venous disease: epidemiological and clinical aspects. Scripta Phlebologica 1994; 2:42.

86. Frian-Bell W. Atrophie blanche. Transact of the St. John's Hosp Dermatol Soc 1959; 42:59–65.

87. Wesener G. Uber die klinische reversibilität der atrophie blanche. Z Haut-Geschlechtskr 1967; 42:925–927.

88. Winkelmann RK, Schroeter AL, Kierland RR, Ryan TM. Clinical studies of livedoid vasculitis (segmental hialinizing vasculitis). Mayo Clin Proc 1974; 49:746–750.

89. Stevanovic DV. Atrophie blanche, a sign of dermal blood occlusion. Arch Dermatol 1974; 109:858–862.

90. Maessen-Visch MB, Koedman MI, Hamulyak K, Neumann HAM. Atrophie blanche. Int J Dermatol 1999; 38:161–172.

91. Elder D, Elenitsas R, Jaeorsky C, Johnson B. Lever's histopathology of the skin. 8th ed. Philadelphia, PA: Lippincot-Raven, 1997.

92. Browse NL, Burnand KG. The cause of venous ulceration. Lancet 1982; ii:243–245.

93. Burnand KG, Whimster I, Naidoo A, Browse NL. Pericapillary fibrin in the ulcer-bearing skin of the leg; the cause of lipodermatosclerosis and venous ulceration. Br Med J 1982; 285:1071–1077.

94. Coleridge Smith PD, Thomas P, Scurr JH, Dormandy JA. Causes of venous ulceration: a new hypothesis. Br Med J 1988; 296:1726–1727.

95. Thomas PRS, Nash GB, Dormandy JA. White cell accumulation in dependent legs of patients with venous hypertension: a possible mechanism for trophic changes in the skin. Br Med J 1988; 296:1693–1695.

96. Bollinger A. Atrophie blanche: Hautinfarkt verschiedener Pathogenese? VASA, Zeitschrift fur Gefäßkrankheiten 1981; 10:67–69.

97. Bollinger A, Leu AJ. Evidence for microvascular thrombosis obtained by intravital fluorescence videomicroscopy. VASA, Zeitschrift fur Gefäßkrankheiten 1991; 20: 252–255.

98. Choi HJ, et al. Livedo retcularis and livedoid vasculitis responding to PUVA therapy. J Am Acad Dermatol 1999; 40:204.

99. Sauer GC. Pentoxifylline (trental) therapy for the vasculitis of atrophie blanche. Arch Dermatol 1986; 122:380–381.

100. Sams WM. Livedo vasculitis: therapy with pentoxifylline. Arch Dermatol 1988; 124:684–687.

101. Champion RH. Livedo reticularis with recurrent ulceration treated with anticoagulants. Br J Dermatol 1962; 74:195–196.

102. Purcell SM, Hayes TJ. Nifedipine treatment of idiopathic atrophie blanche. J Am Acad Dermatol 1986; 14:851–854.

103. Gupta AK, Goldfarb MT, Voorhees JJ. The use of sulfasalazine in atrophie blanche. Int J Dermatol 1990; 29:663–665.

24

Antiphospholipid Antibody Syndrome

Sarah L. Jensen and George T. Nahass
Department of Dermatology, St. Louis University Hospital,
St. Louis, Missouri, U.S.A.

1. INTRODUCTION

The antiphospholipid antibody syndrome (APS) is a multisystem disorder characterized by persistently elevated antiphospholipid antibodies (APAs) with vascular thrombosis and/or pregnancy morbidity. Anticardiolipin antibodies (ACAs), β_2-glycoprotein, and the lupus anticoagulant are different classes of APAs associated with this disorder. Various hematologic, neurologic, obstetric, and cutaneous abnormalities are manifest in this syndrome. The chapter reviews the characteristic features of the APS and the various cutaneous manifestations of this syndrome.

2. DEFINITION

Antiphospholipid antibodies are a heterogeneous group of circulating antibodies. Research over the past several years demonstrates that a large proportion of APAs do not solely recognize phospholipids; rather they are more often directed against phospholipid-binding plasma proteins, such as β_2-glycoprotein I (β_2-GPI) and prothrombin, or complexes of these proteins with negatively charged phospholipids.

Reagin, the first APA described, was discovered by Wasserman in 1907 (1). This antibody was clinically associated with syphilis and later found to be specific for a bacterial phospholipid component, which was termed "cardiolipin" (2). A modified antigen mixture composed of cardiolipin, phosphatidylcholine and cholesterol and named after the Venereal Diseases Research Laboratory (VDRL), was developed to analyze for reagin.

With increased utilization of the serologic assay for syphilis, a subset of patients with biologically false-positive serologic tests for syphilis (BFP-STS) was defined (3). Acute or transient BFP-STS were observed in patients with recent infections and found to clear as the infection dissipated (4). Long-term or chronic BFP-STS were more commonly detected in patients with autoimmune processes (e.g., systemic lupus erythematosus [SLE]) (5).

The APAs in patients with chronic BFP-STS are divided into subgroups on the basis of the laboratory methods used to identify them. The most commonly detected

Table 1 Antibodies Detected in Conventional Antiphospholipid Antibody Assays

---

Anticardiolipin ELISAs
  Anti-β_2-glycoprotein I
  Anticardiolipin
  Antibodies to other cardiolipin-binding serum proteins
  Lupus anticoagulant assays
  Antiprothrombin
  Anti-factor V
  Anti-factor X
  Antiphospholipid

---

are lupus anticoagulant antibody (LA), ACA, and anti-β_2-glycoprotein I antibody (anti-β_2-GPIA). Lupus anticoagulant antibodies are identified by coagulation assays, in which they prolong clotting times. Anticardiolipin antibodies and anti-β_2-GPIAs are identified by immunoassays that measure immunologic reactivity to a phospholipid, as with cardiolipin, or to a phospholipid-binding protein, as with β_2-GPI (6). Numerous studies have elucidated the specificity of APAs for phospholipid-binding plasma proteins, as summarized in Table 1.

In general, LAs are more specific for the APS, while ACAs are more sensitive (7). There is no particular association between clinical manifestations and particular subgroups; therefore, if APS is clinically suspected, all subgroups of APAs should be screened with appropriate testing.

Patients with APS are classically those with persistently elevated APAs with vascular thrombosis and/or pregnancy morbidity. In 1998, an international multidisciplinary group formulated preliminary classification criteria in order to better define the essential features of APS (8). These classification criteria are outlined in Table 2. Definite APS is considered to be present in a given patient when at least one of the clinical criteria and at least one of the laboratory criteria are met. Primary APS involves patients without an underlying systemic disorder, while secondary APS is associated with underlying disease, most commonly SLE (Table 3).

3. PHYSIOLOGY

While the immunoglobulin and clinical manifestations of APS are diverse, phospholipid antibodies are detected in a vast majority of cases. Phospholipids are a class of polar lipids composed of a phosphate moiety, one or more fatty acid molecules and different chemical head groups esterified to phosphate. Formed in essentially all cells in the body, 90% of phospholipids are manufactured in the liver. They function primarily as structural support of plasma membranes and are stored in small quantities.

Phospholipids are involved at several points in the extrinsic, intrinsic, and common pathways of the coagulation cascade. The phospholipids required for coagulation reactions are supplied by cells expressing tissue factor for the extrinsic pathway and by platelets for the intrinsic and common pathways. Various anticoagulant mechanisms serve to balance the intricate coagulation system. Thrombomodulin, protein C and protein S, antithrombin III, and heparin cofactor act at various

Table 2 Preliminary Criteria for the Classification of the Antiphospholipid Antibody Syndrome

Clinical criteria

1. Vascular thrombosis
   a. One or more clinical episodes of arterial, venous or small vessel thrombosis in any tissue or organ. Thrombosis must be confirmed by imaging or Doppler studies or histopathology, with the exception of superficial venous thrombosis. For histopathologic confirmation, thrombosis should be present without significant evidence of inflammation in the vessel wall.
2. Pregnancy morbidity
   a. One or more unexplained deaths of a morphologically normal fetus at or beyond the 10th week of gestation, with normal fetal morphology documented by ultrasound or by direct examination of the fetus, or
   b One or more premature births of a morphologically normal neonate at or before the 34th week of gestation because of severe preeclampsia or eclampsia, or severe placental insufficiency or
   c. Three or more unexplained consecutive spontaneous abortions before the 10th week of gestation, with maternal anatomic or hormonal abnormalities and paternal and maternal chromosomal causes excluded
   In studies of populations of patients who have more than one type of pregnancy morbidity, investigators are strongly encouraged to stratify groups of subjects according to a, b, or c above.

Laboratory criteria

1. Anticardiolipin antibody of IgG and/or IgM isotype in blood, present in medium or high titer, on two or more occasions, at least 6 weeks apart, measured by a standardized ELISA for β_2-glycoprotein I-dependent anticardiolipin antibodies.
2. Lupus anticoagulant present in plasma, on two or more occasions as least 6 weeks apart, detected according to the guidelines of the International Society on Thrombosis and Hemostasis (Scientific Subcommittee on Lupus Anticoagulants/Phospholipid-Dependent Antibodies) in the following steps:
   a. Proglonged phospholipid-dependent coagulation demonstrated on a screening test, e.g., activated partial thromboplastin time, kaolin lotting time, dilute Russell's viper venom time, dilute prothrombin time, and Textarin time.
   b. Failure to correct the prolonged coagulation time on the screening test by mixing it with normal platelet-poor plasma.
   c. Shortening or correction of the prolonged coagulation time on the screening test by the addition of excess phospholipid.
   d. Exclusion of other coagulopathies, e.g., factor VIII inhibitor or heparin, as appropriate.

Definite antiphospholipid antibody syndrome is considered to be present if at least one of the clinical criteria and one of the laboratory criteria are met.

---

points in the cascade to reverse coagulation. Fibrinolysis, or digestion of the clot, is performed by plasmin upon activation by the tissue plasminogen activator, urokinase, or neutral proteases.

Antiphospholipid antibodies, once thought to target anionic phospholipids, more often show specificity for different phospholipid-binding plasma proteins including β_2-glycoprotein (β_2-GPI), prothrombin, factor V, and factor X. The effect of APA binding to different antigenic targets is variable. For example, APAs enhance the activity of β_2-GPI (9,10) and inhibit the function of protein C (11).

Table 3 Diseases Associated with Antiphospholipid Antibodies

Immunologic diseases
   Systemic lupus erythematosus
   Autoimmune thrombocytopenic purpura
   Autoimmune hemolytic anemia
   Adult/juvenile rheumatoid arthritis
   Primary/secondary Sjogren's syndrome
   Polymyalgia rheumatica/giant cell arteritis
   Dermatomyositis/polymyositis
   Mixed connective tissue disease
   Systemic sclerosis
   Behçet's disease
   Polyarteritis nodosa
   Chronic active hepatitis

Malignancies
   Solid tumors
   Leukemia
   Hodgkin's disease/lymphoproliferative disorders
   Multiple myeloma
   Mycosis fungoides

Hematologic diseases
   Myelofibrosis
   Von Willebrand's disease
   Paraproteinemias

Infectious diseases
   Syphilis
   Leprosy
   Tuberculosis
   Mycoplasma
   Lyme disease
   HIV infection
   Viral infections (hepatitis A, varicella, mononucleosis, adenovirus, parvovirus, measles, and mumps)
   Bacterial infections (endocarditis and sepsis)

Neurologic diseases
   Sneddon's syndrome
   Myasthenia gravis
   Multiple sclerosis
   Migraine headache

Medications
   Chlorpromazine
   Phenothiazine
   Phenytoin
   Hydralazine
   Procainamide
   Quinidine
   Streptomycin
   Clozapine

Anticardiolipin antibody and lupus anticoagulant are the terms currently used to identify these immunoglobulins. Other antibodies specific for various phospholipids or phospholipid–protein complexes have been identified in association with APAs although they cannot be detected with conventional APA assays. Therefore, present information regarding their prevalence or clinical significance is limited.

β_2-Glycoprotein I, or apolipoprotein H, has been identified as the target of many ACAs. The precise hemostatic role of β_2-GPI is unclear. However, this glycoprotein has several anticoagulant properties in vitro, including the ability to inhibit the contact phase of blood coagulation, adenosine diphosphate (ADP)-dependent platelet aggregation, the prothrombinase activity of platelets, factor Xa generation by platelets and the interaction of protein S and C4b-binding protein (12). The interaction of ACAs with β_2-GPI could contribute to a hypercoagulable state by several pathways through effects on protein C, protein S, platelets, and the activity of different clotting factors (13).

The requirement of β_2-GPI for binding APA with cardiolipin is unique for patients with autoimmune disorders. Antiphospholipid antibodies associated with syphilis or other infection bind cardiolipin without β_2-GPI; this interaction is inhibited by β_2-GPI in such patients (9,14). Antiphospholipid antibodies from patients with autoimmune disorders exhibit little or no binding to the VDRL antigen, but cross-react with both cardiolipin and the other negatively charged phospholipids (15). These biochemical differences may be related to the association of APA in patients with autoimmune disorders with thrombosis, fetal loss, and thrombocytopenia.

Lupus anticoagulant antibody also requires a cofactor, such as lipid-bound prothrombin, to interact with negatively charged phospholipids. In this reaction, the LA recognizes an epitope that becomes exposed upon calcium-mediated binding of prothrombin to phospholipid. The LA, by reacting with proteins at these or other sites may interfere with the normal hemostatic system and contribute to thrombin-activated platelets by inhibiting thrombin-mediated endothelial cell prostacyclin release, or inhibiting protein C activation (16).

Several additional abnormalities have been reported that could be related to the mechanism of thrombosis involving protein C and protein S, prostacyclin, thrombomodulin, heparin sulfate, antithrombin III, annexin V, tissue factor, and platelet-activating factor (11,17–22).

Various theories have been proposed regarding the mechanism by which autoantibodies recognize phospholipid–protein complexes and contribute to coagulation abnormalities. Less is known about the origin of these autoantibodies. Theories suggest that apoptosis, or programmed cell death, may be involved in the induction of these autoantibodies associated with APS. Abnormalities in the recognition, uptake, processing, and/or presentation of self-antigen by antigen presenting cells may lead to emergence of autoimmunity (23–25).

4. CLINICAL MANIFESTATIONS

4.1. Hematologic

Recurrent venous or arterial thrombosis is a major feature of APS. Prior studies indicate the average of thrombotic events in patients with SLE is 42% (11–74%) and 12% (0–32%) in APA-positive and APA-negative patients, respectively. In these studies, thrombosis occurred in 51% of patients with LA compared with only 31% of persons with ACAs.

Thrombosis associated with APAs may occur in any anatomic location, and therefore cause a broad range of clinical manifestations. The deep leg veins are commonly affected, creating a source for secondary pulmonary embolism. Venous thrombosis affecting retinal, renal, and hepatic veins has been reported. Similarly, arterial thrombosis of the carotid, hepatic, splenic, mesenteric, and retinal arteries causing infarction has occurred.

Compromise of renal function secondary to renal artery thrombosis may occur resulting in proteinuria, mild-to-malignant systemic hypertension, cortical necrosis, thrombotic microangiopathy, and progressive renal failure requiring dialysis.

Several reports have associated ACAs with a spectrum of cardiovascular disease such as coronary artery thrombosis, intracardiac mass lesions, diastolic dysfunction, and cardiac valve vegetations (Libman–Sacks endocarditis). Elevated ACAs have been found in young patients with myocardial infarction (MI) and have been shown to be an independent risk factor for MI in middle-aged men.

Thrombocytopenia is another major feature of APS and is present in 12–89% (mean = 37%) of APA-positive cases with SLE or SLE-like disorders (26). The mechanism of thrombocytopenia is yet unknown, but may involve platelet destruction and removal of APA-coated platelets by the reticuloendothelial system.

4.2. Obstetric

Several obstetric complications have been related to APAs including recurrent fetal loss resulting from late first trimester spontaneous abortion and second or third trimester fetal death. Severe pre-eclampsia, fetal growth restriction, postpartum serositis syndrome, and the HELLP syndrome (hemolysis, elevated liver enzymes, and low platelets) have been described. Decidual vasculopathy caused by impaired prostacyclin production, placental thrombosis and infarction, and impairment of embryonic implantation have all been proposed as pathogenic mechanisms for APA-mediated obstetric complications.

4.3. Neurologic

The large and small vessels of the cerebrovasculature are frequently involved and can cause many clinical complications. Cerebral infarction followed by transient ischemic attacks is the most frequent neurologic event (27). These can involve the carotid and vertebrobasilar arteries resulting in a variety of clinical sequelae.

Multiple-infarct dementia, acute ischemic encephalopathy, and amaurosis fugax have also been associated with APAs. Other neurologic disorders such as chorea, transient global amnesia, seizures, pseudotumor cerebri, migraine headache, multiple sclerosis, and myasthenia gravis have been occasionally involved with APAs.

4.4. Cutaneous Complications

Various cutaneous lesions have been associated with APAs (Table 4). In one study, skin lesions were the first sign of APS in 41% of patients and systemic thrombosis developed in 40% of them (28). Livedo reticularis is the most recognized cutaneous finding of APS (Fig. 1). In the setting of SLE, livedo reticularis was present in 23–48% of patients and correlated with increased levels of ACA (29).

Table 4 Cutaneous Manifestations Associated with Antiphospholipid Antibodies

Livedo reticularis
Acrocyanosis
Ulceration
Necrosis
Raynaud's phenomenon
Capillaritis
Purpuric/cyanotic macules
Nodules
Digital ischemia/gangrene
Blue toe
Thrombophlebitis
Hemorrhage
Porcelain-white scars/atrophie blanche
Splinter hemorrhages

Skin ulcers and necrosis have also been reported in APS (Fig. 2). Digital ischemia and digital gangrene as a consequence of arterial or arteriolar occlusion have been described involving the hands and feet (Fig. 3). Thrombophlebitis presenting as lower leg and ankle edema and erythema was observed in 34% of 70 patients with LA (28); this was the most common cutaneous manifestation associated with APA in this series. Studies have reported thrombophlebitis affecting the popliteal, femoral, and deep veins as well as the more superficial vasculature of the lower extremities.

Acral erythematous, purpuric or cyanotic macules, painful nodules resembling vasculitis, hemorrhage, splinter hemorrhages, capillaritis, blue toe syndrome, purpura fulminans, and porcelain-white scars or atrophie blanche are additional cutaneous signs observed in APS.

5. PREVALENCE

Differences in assay standardization, population selection, and other experimental factors confound the interpretation of prevalence studies of APAs. One study found

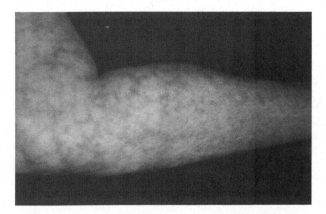

Figure 1 Violaceous reticulate pattern characteristic of livedo reticularis.

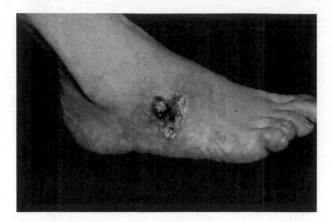

Figure 2 Skin ulcers with focal necrosis.

an abnormal value for LA and increased levels of ACAs in 8% and 5% of normal healthy blood donors, respectively (30). The LA was detected more frequently in young female patients (median age = 29.3 years) compared with the study group as a whole. One study found IgG ACAs in 51.6% of 64 clinically healthy elderly persons, while another found abnormal levels of IgG or IgM ACAs in only 12% of healthy elderly persons (31,32). The frequency of APAs in SLE ranges from 2% to 94% in different studies; upon averaging the reported frequency of APAs from these studies of approximately 2000 patients, 31% and 40% of patients were positive for LA and ACAs, respectively (33).

Elevated levels of ACAs have been associated with a variety of infectious agents and these have been recognized as a common cause for acute BFP-STS. Lupus anticoagulant antibody and ACAs have been demonstrated in HIV infection as well.

Therapeutically administered medications have been associated with APAs including procainamide, chlorpromazine, hydralazine, phenytoin, and quinidine.

Reports have addressed a familial or genetic predisposition to APS. Some studies have shown an association of LA with HLA-DQw7 (linked to HLA-DR5 and HLA-DR4 haplotypes) and ACAs with HLA-DR7. A recent study supported inheritance of a susceptibility gene for APS in an autosomal dominant pattern, however,

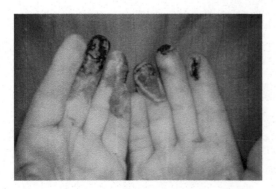

Figure 3 Digital ischemia and gangrene.

this study showed no linkage with HLA or marker for candidate genes in contrast to findings of previous studies (34).

6. DIAGNOSIS

A diagnosis of APS requires the presence of at least one of the clinical criteria and at least one of the laboratory criteria, as defined prior to the International Consensus Statement (Table 1). Clinical criteria involve vascular thrombosis or complications of pregnancy and laboratory criteria include presence of either ACAs or LA, on two or more occasions at least 6 weeks apart. While often present in clinical cases of APS, low-positive titers of IgG or IgM ACAs, IgA isotype of ACAs, and antibodies to other phospholipids or phospholipid-binding proteins, aside from those detailed in the preliminary classification, are not included in the criteria for the APS. These factors were considered to require further standardization and study and were therefore excluded from the current criteria.

A wide variety of laboratory assays have been developed to detect LA and ACAs. However, not all patients with LA have detectable ACAs and the contrary is true, as well. But LA and ACAs occur simultaneously in 75% of cases, indicating that they are distinct and unique classes of immunoglobulins that recognize different epitopes.

Several different tests are available to screen for LA activity in plasma. The APTT, kaolin clotting time (KCT), and dilute Russell viper venom time (dRVVT) are the most widely used methods. The platelet neutralization procedure, Textarin time, dilute tissue thromboplastin inhibition test, and plasma clotting time are other less frequently used assays. The LA screening tests are exquisitely sensitive to added phospholipid and, therefore, atraumatic venipuncture and immediate centrifugation are important. Traditionally, the APTT test has been the most popular and widely used screening test. Yet, it fails to detect weak inhibitors and is subject to variations in sensitivity based on the APTT reagents used. Two international standardization committees have recommended the use of the KCT and dRVVT to screen for LA.

Identifying ACAs is more direct and initially involves a solid-phase RIA. Enzyme-linked immunosorbent assays (ELISAs) are now available and more commonly used. Isotype-specific (e.g., IgG, IgM, and IgA) second- or third-generation assays should be used in analyzing for ACAs. Results should be expressed, as directed by the International Symposium of Antiphospholipid Antibodies as low positive (5–15/<6.0 GPL/MPL units), medium positive (5–80/6–50 GPL/MPL units), or high positive (>80/>50 GPL/MPL units), where GPL and MPL represent standardized units for measurement of IgG and IgM ACAs; one GPL or MPL unit is the binding activity of 1 μg/ml of affinity-purified IgG and IgM ACAs, respectively.

Laboratory assays for both LA and ACAs should be performed during analysis for the presence of APAs or the diagnosis may be missed. The KCT/dRVVT and isotype-specific assays producing semiquantitative results are the recommended screening tests for LA and ACA activities, respectively. If the diagnosis of APS is strongly suspected on clinical basis and results of the initial screening tests are negative, laboratory testing should be repeated at a later date, as the concentration of antibodies may fluctuate.

Histologic features associated with APAs reflect the hypercoagulant diathesis associated with the presence of these immunoglobulins. Characteristic microscopic findings include a noninflammatory thrombosis of vessels (Fig. 4).

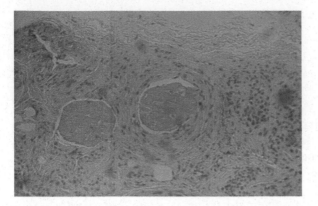

Figure 4 Photomicrograph of skin biopsy from a patient with antiphospholipid antibody syndrome showing noninflammatory thrombosis of small dermal blood vessels (H&E X400).

7. TREATMENT

Several different therapeutic agents have been tried in patients with APS. The approach depends, in part, on the clinical manifestations and the presence of underlying disease. Certainly, any factors predisposing a patient toward thrombosis should be considered and treated as able.

7.1. Prophylaxis

Studies have examined the role of aspirin at a daily dose of 325 mg as prophylaxis of thrombotic events. Aspirin failed to offer protection against deep venous thrombosis and pulmonary embolism in male physicians with ACAs. Contrary to that finding, aspirin may provide protection against thrombosis in women with APS and previous pregnancy loss (35). Hydroxychloroquine may offer prevention of thrombotic events in patients with SLE and secondary APS (36).

7.2. Therapy Post-Thrombosis

Anticoagulation is the treatment of choice for thrombotic events associated with primary and secondary APS. Benefit of anticoagulation in decreasing the rate of recurrent thrombosis has been demonstrated in three retrospective studies (37–39). Evidence has suggested adjusting anticoagulation therapy to maintain the international normalized ratio (INR) at 3 or higher (37). This level of anticoagulation may not be appropriate for all patients due to risks associated with such therapy, however, in two large series, the level of protection against venous and arterial thrombosis correlated directly with the level of anticoagulation (37,38). Among 70 patients with APS, warfarin treatment of intermediate (INR 2.0–2.9) and high intensity (INR 3.0 or greater) significantly reduced rate of thrombosis, whereas low-intensity treatment (INR 1.9 or less) did not confer significant protection (38). Recurrent thrombosis after discontinuing warfarin has been reported and, therefore, long-term anticoagulation is recommended. In patients with history of venous thromboembolic events and whose subsequent anticoagulant therapy was stopped, rate of recurrence of thrombotic events was 50% at 2 years and 78% at 8 years (39).

Warfarin combined with aspirin is not routinely used, but may be warranted in cases in which progressive thrombosis continues despite adequate anticoagulation therapy. Thrombolytic therapy and thrombectomy have been described, but are associated with rather immediate reformation of clot at the site. Overall, low-dose aspirin alone has not been shown to be of benefit in reducing the rate of recurrence of thrombosis (37,38).

Systemic corticosteroids are indicated in cases of secondary APS to manage the underlying systemic disorder. Immunosuppressive agents such as cyclophosphamide have been used successfully in conjunction with plasma exchange in SLE patients with thrombotic thrombocytopenic purpura and progressive arterial thrombosis despite anticoagulation therapy. Splenectomy has been performed in cases of severe thrombocytopenia in APS in a small number of patients with success (40).

Intravenous immunoglobulin (IVIG), plasma exchange, immunoadsorbent plasmapheresis, dapsone, and fish oil derivatives have been tried in APA patients with variable results. Studies with heparin with and without aspirin therapy have been shown to decrease complications in pregnancy of APA-positive women (41). Preliminarily positive results with the use of IVIG in APS-involved pregnancies led to a pilot study, which failed to show improvement in obstetric or neonatal outcomes beyond those achieved with heparin and low-dose aspirin regimen (42,43).

Treatment of cutaneous manifestations associated with APS reflects the general therapeutic approach to this disorder. Low-dose aspirin and dipyridamole have effectively treated purpuric lesions and necrotic ulcers. Cutaneous ulcers have been managed successfully with warfarin, heparin, and fibrinolytic agents.

Experimental murine models of APS promise potential for application in human patients, including possible utilization of anti-idiotypic antibodies, IL-3 cytokine administration, anti-CD4 antibodies, and bone marrow transplantation.

In summary, current therapy involves long-term anticoagulation and maintaining an INR at or above 3 for both primary and secondary APS. Systemic corticosteroids or other immunosuppressive agents are indicated in secondary APS to treat the underlying systemic disorder. Antiplatelet agents, fibrinolytic compounds, plasmapheresis, hydroxychloroquine, and IVIG may be considered as alternative approaches for refractory cases. While appropriate wound care to cutaneous lesions is necessary, prevention of further thrombotic events is of key importance treating this disorder.

REFERENCES

1. Wasserman A. Uber die Entwicklung und den gegenwartigen Stand der Serodiagnostick gegenuber syphilis. Klin Wochenschr (Berlin) 1907; 44:1599.
2. Pangborn MC. A new serologically active phospholipid from beef heart. Proc Soc Exp Biol Med 1941; 48:484–486.
3. Moore JE, Mohr CF. Biologically false positive serologic tests for syphilis. JAMA 1952; 150:467–473.
4. Vaarala O, PalosuoT, Kleemola M, et al. Anticardiolipin response in acute infections. Clin Immunol Immunopathol 1986; 41:8–15.
5. Moore JE, Lutz WB. The natural history of systemic lupus erythematosus: an approach to its study through chronic biological false positive reactors. J Chronic Dis 1955; 1: 297–316.
6. Roubey RAS. Immunology of the antiphospholipid antibody syndrome. Arthritis Rheum 1996; 39:1444–1454.

7. de Groot PG, Derksen RHWM. Specificity and clinical relevance of lupus anticoagulant. Vessels 1995; 1:22–26.

8. Wilson WA, Gharavi AE, Koike T, et al. International consensus statement on preliminary classification criteria for definite antiphospholipid antibody syndrome. Arthritis Rheum 1999; 42:1309–1311.

9. Galli M, Comfurius P, Barbui T, et al. Anticoagulant activity of (β2-glycoprotein I is potentiated by a distinct subgroup of anticardiolipin antibodies. Thromb Haemost 1992; 68:738–745.

10. Roubey RAS, Pratt CW, Buyon JP, et al. Lupus anticoagulant activity of autoimmune antiphospholipid antibodies is dependent upon of β2-glycoprotein I. J Clin Invest 1992; 900:110–114.

11. Oosting J, Derksen RHWM, Bobbink IWG, et al. Antiphospholipid antibodies directed against a combination of phospholipids with prothrombin, protein C, or protein S: an explanation for their pathogenic mechanism? Blood 1993; 81:2618–2625.

12. Riley RS, Friedline JF, Rogers JS. Antiphospholipid antibodies: standardization and testing. Clin Lab Med 1997; 17:397.

13. Roubey RAS. Autoantibodies to phospholipid-binding plasma proteins: a new view of lupus anticoagulants and other "antiphospholipid" antibodies. Blood 1994; 84:2854–2867.

14. Matsuura E, Igarashi Y, Fujimoto M, et al. Heterogeneity of cardiolipin antibodies defined by the anticardiolipin cofactor. J Immunol 1992; 148:3885–3891.

15. Harris EN, Gharavi AE, Asley GD, Hughes GRV. Use of an enzyme-linked immunosorbent assay and of inhibition studies to distinguish between antibodies to cardiolipin from patients with syphilis or autoimmune disorders. J Infect Dis 1998; 157:23–31.

16. Fleck RA, Rapaport SI, Rao LV. Anti-prothrombin antibodies and the lupus anticoagulant. Blood 1988; 72:512–519.

17. Malia RG, Kitchen S, Greaves M, et al. Inhibition of activated protein C and its cofactor protein S by antiphospholipid antibodies. Br J Haematol 1990; 76:101–107.

18. Carerras LO, Vermylen J, Spitz B, et al. "Lupus" anticoagulant and inhibition of prostacyclin formation in patients with repeated abortion, intrauterine growth retardation and intrauterine death. Br J Obstet Gynaecol 1981; 88:890–894.

19. Oosting JD, Preissner KT, Derksen RH, et al. Autoantibodies directed against the epidermal growth factor-like domains of thrombomodulin inhibit protein C activation in vitro. Br J Haematol 1993; 85:761–768.

20. Shibata S, Harpel PC, Ghavari A, et al. Autoantibodies to heparin from patients with antiphospholipid antibody syndrome inhibit formation of anti-thrombin III complexes. Blood 1994; 83:2532–2540.

21. Barquinero J, Ordi-Ros J, Selva A, et al. Antibodies against platelet-activating factor in patients with antiphospholipid antibodies. Lupus 1994; 3:55–58.

22. Levine JS, Branch DW, Rauch J. Medical Progress: the antiphospholipid antibody syndrome. New Engl J Med 2002; 346:752–763.

23. Casciano CA, Rosen A, Petri M, Schlissel M. Surface blebs on apoptotic cells are sites of enhanced procoagulant activity: implications for coagulation events and antigenic spread in systemic lupus erythematosus. Proc Natl Acad Sci USA 1996; 28:82–98.

24. Pittoni V, Isenberg D. Apoptosis and antiphospholipid antibodies. Semin Arthritis Rheum 1998; 28:163–178.

25. Levine JS, Koh JS, Subang R, Rauch J. Apoptotic cells as immunogen and antigen in the antiphospholipid syndrome. Exp Mol Pathol 1999; 66:82–98.

26. McNeil HP, Chesterman CN, Krilis SA. Immunology and clinical importance of antiphospholipid antibodies. Adv Immunol 1991; 49:193–280.

27. Hinton RC. Neurological syndromes associated with antiphospholipid antibodies. Semin Thromb Hemost 1994; 20:46–54.

28. Alegre VA, Gastineau DA, Winkleman RK. Skin lesions associated with circulating lupus anticoagulant. Br J Dermatol 1989; 120:419–429.

29. McHugh NJ, Maymo J, Skinner RP, et al. Anticardiolipin antibodies, livedo reticularis, and major cerebrovascular and renal disease in systemic lupus erythematosus. Ann Rheum Dis 1988; 47:110–115.

30. Shi W, Drilis SA, Chong BH, et al. Prevalence of lupus anticoagulant and anticardiolipin antibodies in a healthy population. Aust NZ J Med 1990; 20:231–236.

31. Mannoussakis MN, Tzioufas AF, Silis MP, et al. High prevalence of anti-cardiolipin and other autoantibodies in a healthy elderly population. Clin Exp Immunol 1987; 69: 557–565.

32. Fields RA, Toubbeh H, Searles RP, et al. The prevalence of anticardiolipin antibodies in a healthy elderly population and its association with antinuclear antibodies. J Rheumatol 1989; 16:623–625.

33. McNeil HP, Chesterman CN, Krilis SA. Immunology and clinical importance of anti-phospholipid antibodies. Adv Immunol 1991; 49:193–280.

34. Goel N, Ortel TL, Bali D, et al. Familial antiphospholipid antibody syndrome: criteria for disease and evidence for autosomal dominant inheritance. Arthritis Rheum 1999; 42:318–327.

35. Ginsburg KS, Liang MH, Newcomer L, et al. Anticardiolipin antibodies and the risk for ischemic stroke and venous thrombosis. Ann Intern Med 1992; 117:997–1002.

36. Petri M. Hydroxychloroquine use in the Baltimore Lupus Cohort: effects on lipids, glucose, and thrombosis. Lupus 1996; 5(suppl 1):S16–S22.

37. Khamashta MA, Cuadrado MJ, Mujic F, Taub NA, Hunt BJ, Hughes GRV. The management of thrombosis in the antiphospholipid antibody syndrome. N Engl J Med 1995; 332:993–997.

38. Rosove MH, Brewer PMC. Antiphospholipid thrombosis: clinical course after the first thrombotic event in 70 patients. Ann Intern Med 1992; 117:303–308.

39. Derksen RH, de Groot PG, Kater L, Nieuwenhuis HK. Patients with antiphospholipid antibodies and venous thrombosis should receive long-term anticoagulation treatment. Ann Rheum Dis 1993; 52:689–692.

40. Hakim AJ, Machin SJ, Isenberg DA. Autoimmune thrombocytopenia in primary anti-phospholipid syndrome and systemic lupus erythematosus: the response to splenectomy. Semin Arthritis Rheum 1998; 28:20–25.

41. Rai R, Cohen H, Dave M, Regan L. Randomized controlled trial of aspirin and aspirin plus heparin in pregnant women with recurrent miscarriage associated with phospholipid antibodies (or antiphospholipid antibodies). Br Med J 1997; 314:253–257.

42. Branch W, Druzin M, Spinnato J, et al. Randomized, placebo-controlled trial of intra-venous immune globulin (IVIG) in antiphospholipid antibody syndrome (APS) in pregnancy: a progress report. Lupus 1996; 5:553.

43. Branch DW, Peaceman AM, Druzin M, Silver RK, et al. A multicenter, placebo-controlled pilot study of intravenous immune globulin treatment of antiphospholipid syndrome during pregnancy. Am J Obstet Gyn 2000; 182:122–127.

25
Lymphedema and Wounds

John M. MacDonald

Department of Dermatology and Cutaneous Surgery, University of Miami School of Medicine, Miami, Florida, U.S.A.

1. INTRODUCTION

Lymphedema is a chronic, incurable condition characterized by an abnormal collection of fluid (lymph) resulting in swelling (edema) as a result of an anatomical alteration to the lymphatic system. Localized lymphedema secondary to trauma and wounds may be the exception and in some cases this form of lymphedema appears to be curable. Estimates state that worldwide, one person in 30 is afflicted with lymphedema. This figure does not include the millions suffering from chronic venous disease (1) nor the patients with chronic wounds and peri-wound lymphedema. Until the past decade, lymphedema has received little clinical attention. It has been termed "The Hidden Epidemic."

Understanding the pathophysiology, diagnoses and management of lymphedema is essential to the proper care of the wound care patient. This chapter is divided into two segments. The first will discuss the epidemiology, anatomy, pathophysiology, and therapy of lymphedema. The second segment will discuss the unique relationship between the chronic wound and peri-wound lymphedema. Compression, the mainstay of treatment for wound-related lymphedema, will be discussed in a separate chapter.

2. ANATOMY OF THE LYMPHATIC SYSTEM

The lymphatic system consists of lymph vessels and regional and central lymph nodes. Initial lymph vessel is the collective name given to the valveless lymphatic capillaries and the single and double valve precollectors. Lymphatic capillaries consist of flat overlapping endothelial cells surrounded by a fibrous network. Filaments fix the lymphatic vessel to the surrounding connective tissue. They prevent the narrowing of the initial vessel system and enable increased fluid influx into the lumen in the presence of edema. The initial lymphatics provide liquid resorption while the lymph collectors are transport vessels. Lymph collectors consist of three layers: intima, media, and adventitia. The lymph collectors have valves consisting of fibrous stroma lined with endothelial cells. This lymphatic vascular unit is called a lymphangion. The rhythmic pumping action of the lymphangion smooth muscle is likened to cardiac muscle. These vessels lead to lymphatic ducts that form the main parts of the transporting vessels and the thoracic duct. The lymphatic ducts do not have resorbing function. The blood supply to the lymphatic vessel wall is provided by vasa vasorum originating in the adventitia. Sympathetic nerve fibers innervate the adventitia. The extremities contain a superficial (above the fascia) and a deep (below the fascia) lymphatic system. The transport of lymph occurs not only from distal to proximal, but also from the superficial to the deep system and vice versa. The collectors generally follow the course of the blood vessels and lead to the regional lymph nodes. However, throughout the body, variations in the vessel course and directional flow are of clinical importance. As an example, the lymphatic drainage in the hand flows from the palm to the dorsum explaining the dorsal hand edema in palmer infection.

Most of the fluid filtering from the arterial capillaries perfuses the interstitium and returns to the venous circulation via the venous ends of blood capillaries. It is estimated that approximately 10% of this fluid is returned via the lymphatic system. Almost all of the lymph from the lower extremities and lower body empties into the thoracic duct and then into the left internal jugular and subclavian vein. Lymph from the left side of the head, left arm, and areas of the chest also empty into the thoracic duct prior to rejoining the venous circulation. Lymph from the right arm, right side of the neck and head, and parts of the thorax enter the right thoracic duct which then joins the right subclavian and internal jugular vein

Lymph nodes are arranged in groups or chains. Inflow of lymph occurs by afferent lymph collectors entering the node in the capsule area and exits the node in the hilar area through efferent lymphatics. Cross-connections between area lymph nodes are common as are circumvention pathways.

The body, both the deep organs and skin, is divided into a series of lymphatic drainage regions by "lymphatic watersheds." Watersheds are dividing areas free of lymph collecting vessels that contain only initial lymph capillaries. On either side of these dividing lines, the flow of lymph drains in different and generally opposite directions (Fig. 1). These lymphatic drainage areas are called "lymphotomes." Variations in lymphatic course are frequent. Knowledge of the regional anatomy of the lymphatic system enables the therapist to redirect lymphatic flow into functioning collateral circulation after lymph node removal or destruction. For example, in drainage of the lower extremity, the inguinal lymph nodes may be circumvented by lymph collectors that course along the sciatic nerve and end in the internal iliac lymph nodes. Likewise, the cephalic lymph vessels that originate in the region of the wrist anastomose with nearby lymphatic pathways and end directly in supraclavicular lymph nodes. This allows functioning collateral lymphatic circulation to be utilized after the removal of the axillary lymph nodes during the management of breast cancer.

3. PHYSIOLOGY OF THE LYMPHATIC SYSTEM

The function of the lymphatic system is the transport of interstitial fluid and its components (lymph) from the interstitium back to the venous circulation. The lymph components consist of proteins, fat, cells, organic and inorganic cell products, viruses, and bacteria. Water functions as a transport media for the lymph. High molecular weight substances such as proteins cannot be reabsorbed by the venous capillaries. The lymphatic capillary endothelial wall structure facilitates the

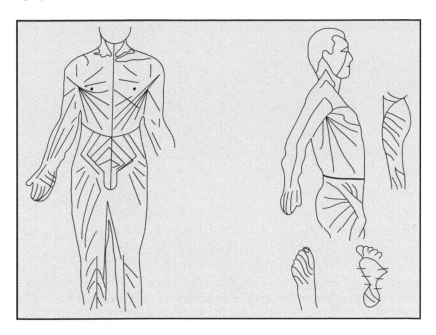

Figure 1 Lymphatic water sheds.

absorption of these substances. Resorption of excess water occurs through the venous drainage. The filtration and resorption of lymph are determined by capillary pressure tissue pressure, and colloidal osmotic pressure in capillaries and tissue fluid according to Starling's equilibrium. The lymph passes from the prelymphatic channels to the lymphatic capillaries. The continued mechanism of lymph uptake and flow is thought to be the result of several factors; the pumping action of lymphangions stimulated by vessel fluid dilatation, arterial pulsation, muscle contraction, and respiratory pressure changes. External pressure from massage and compression bandages also assists in lymph transport.

4. LYMPHEDEMA VS. EDEMA

Traditionally, the term edema/edematous is used to describe any limb or organ that becomes swollen. However, edema should be differentiated from lymphedema. Protein content defines the difference. Lymphedema is high protein edema, which is the result of damage or absence of the normal lymphatic system. Edema, in contrast to lymphedema, is mostly water.

Lymphedema is the result of a *low output failure* of the lymphatic system. Simply stated, lymphatic transport is reduced. This derangement arises from either congenital lymphatic dysplasia (primary lymphedema) or anatomical obliteration (secondary lymphedema) such as after operative dissection, from repeated lymphangitis with lymphangiosclerosis or functional deficiency (e.g., lymphangiospasm and valvular insufficiency). The result is that lymphatic transport falls below the capacity needed to handle the presented microvascular filtrate. Edema, on the other hand, is a *high output failure* of the lymph circulation (Table 1). This takes place when a

Table 1 Edema Classification

Passive hyperemia
  Chronic venous insufficiency
  Congestive heart failure
  Pregnancy
  Inactivity
Hypoproteinemia
  Malnutrition
  Malabsorbtion
  Renal disease
Active hyperemia
  Inflammation
  Allergy

normal or increased transport capacity of the intact lymphatics is overwhelmed by an excessive flow of filtrate. Common examples of edema include congestive failure, hepatic cirrhoses (ascites), chronic venous insufficiency (peripheral edema), and nephrotic syndrome (anasarca).

In some disease states, swelling may be a mixed form of edema/lymphedema. In these cases, where high output failure is chronic, a gradual deterioration of the lymphatic anatomy takes place resulting in decreased transport capacity (e.g., recurring infection).

The complications of lymphedema are secondary to the high protein content in the interstitial fluid. The persistent increase of protein and its degradation products results in chronic inflammation. This is seen by the increased number of macrophages, fibroblasts, and lymphocytes. The inflammation and resulting fibroses and sclerosis are seen in all affected tissues. Disruption of local metabolism and an increased rate of cellulites lead to hemangio-lymphangiopathy and progressive lymphostasis. Lymphatic arthropathy is common in long-standing lower extremity lymphedema. Although rare, malignant changes are a concern (Table 2).

The lymphedema associated with acute and chronic wounds is sometimes called "post-traumatic lymphedema." Perhaps, "post-traumatic lymph stasis" would be more appropriate. Acute trauma is usually followed by a transudative "low protein edema." If the lymphatic collecting anatomy is initially damaged (i.e., in an open wound), true lymphedema rapidly develops. Unless the lymphedema is pre-existing, collectors proximal and distal to the lesion are normal (2).

Table 2 Consequences of Chronic Lymphedema

Protein-rich interstitial edema
Fibrosis, sclerosis
Disturbance of local metabolism
Increased occurrence of cellulites
Progressive lymphatic damage
Lymphatic arthropathy
Chronic wounds
Malignant degeneration

5. LYMPHEDEMA CLASSIFICATION

Lymphedema is differentiated into "primary lymphedema" and "secondary lymphedema" (Table 3). Primary lymphedema is a hereditary malfunction of the lymph system resulting in impaired lymph node or lymph vessel development and accounts for 10% of all lymphedema patients. Milroy's Disease (Nonne-Milroy) is lymphedema present at birth (congenital lymphedema). This comprises 15% of primary lymphedemas. The symptoms of primary lymphedema may not be apparent until the second or third decade of life. This form of primary lymphedema may present as lymphedema praecox, appearing in adolescence and lymphedema tarda, which begins after 35 years of age. The distribution in cases of primary lymphedema between the sexes is reported to be 87% in women and 13% in men (3). Primary lymphedema occurs most often in the legs. Primary lymphedema of the upper extremities and face is rare.

Secondary lymphedema can be caused by many factors. The most recognizable are associated with lymphadenectomy, radiation, venous disease, and numerous post-surgical complications. Lymphedema secondary to vascular reconstruction, joint replacement, and venous harvesting in conjunction with with coronary by-pass comprises an ever growing problem. Peri-wound (localized) lymphedema in acute and chronic wounds is now recognized as a major inhibitory factor in wound healing (4). The most common cause of lymphedma is filariasis, a disorder caused by infection with larvae that is transmitted to humans by mosquito and infects more than 90 million people worldwide. In the Western Hemisphere, filariasis is now confined to areas of the Caribbean and South America, predominantly Haiti and Brazil.

6. DIAGNOSES OF LYMPHEDEMA

Accurate diagnoses of lymphedema, in most patients, can be made with a detailed history, physical examination, and volume measurements. Co-morbidities such as venous insufficiency, metastatic disease, morbid obesity, and repeated infections may affect the clinical presentation. Related diseases such as diabetes mellitus, congestive heart failure, and peripheral vascular occlusive disease will also influence the therapeutic approach. When presented with unilateral extremity lymphedema, venous occlusion and occult visceral tumors must be considered. It should seem obvious that informed physician input is required prior to the start of lymphedema therapy.

Table 3 Lymphedema Classification

Primary	Secondary
Birth	Surgery
Praecox-adolescent	Infection
Tarda-age 35+	Trauma
	Chronic wound
	Tumor
	Radiation
	Venous disease
	Neurological
	Filariasis

Examination of the extremities, trunk, and neck provides information as to the extent of the edematous changes and the potential areas of drainage. Papular lymph cysts, deepened natural skin creases, and lympho-cutaneous fistulas may be seen. Surgical or traumatic scars may suggest an etiology. Palpation reveals thickened skin and fibrous changes in the subcutaneous tissue. The Stemmer sign is an important diagnostic finding. This sign, considered pathgnomonic in lymphedema, shows thickened cutaneous folds on the dorsum of toes or fingers that cannot be lifted.

In the differential diagnoses of lymphedema, *lipedema* is a very important consideration. Lipedema is a chronic disease of lipid metabolism resulting in the symmetrical impairment of fatty tissue distribution and storage combined with hyperplasia of individual fat cells. This abnormal distribution of fat is usually seen between the pelvic crest and the ankle so that unless the lymphatic system has been damaged, the feet appear normal (Fig. 2). The swelling often progresses during the day as the diminished tissue resistance of fatty tissue permits the accumulation of orthostatic edema. A positive family history has been reported in 20% (5). Eventually, in many patients, mechanical insufficiency of the lymph system occurs leading to true lymphedema. Lipo-lymphedema is therefore a combination of impaired fat distribution and an impaired lymphatic system. Lipedema is seen almost exclusively in women. Men develop this pattern often in association with feminization, i.e., hepatic cirrhosis, hormonal therapy for prostatic carcinoma. In most cases, lipedema develops during puberty. Heavy hips and thighs are obvious signs. Simultaneous incidence in the upper extremities is rare, but when involved, there is often a large fold of loose hanging skin visible when the patient elevates her arm to the horizontal position.

Medical history and physical examination make the diagnoses of lipedema. Special diagnostic procedures or additional laboratory tests are rarely necessary to establish the diagnoses. The main differential consideration is lymphedema. In contrast to lymphedema, lipedema is symmetrical, often painful to palpation, susceptible to easy bruising and the patients rarely develop cellulitis. The Stemmer Sign is negative (6). The patient may show varying degrees of obesity and list many unsuccessful attempts at dieting. Often, the patient will relate that dieting resulted in weight loss only in the upper part of the body while the tissues of the lower body remained soft and rubbery as opposed to the hard and fibrotic tissue seen with Chronic Lymphedema.

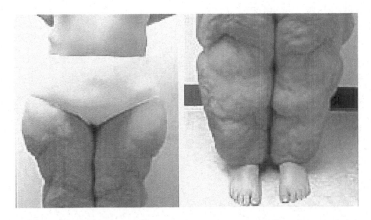

Figure 2 Lipedema.

Therapy for lipedema is for the most part palliative or directed at co-morbidities. At the present time, lipectomy and liposuction would seem to be contraindicated for fear of damage to normal lymphatic drainage. Bariatric surgery has not been found to significantly affect the abnormal fat distribution and metabolism seen in lipedema (author's personal observation).

In benign forms of lymphedema, extensive laboratory testing is usually not necessary. Most laboratory testing is performed to evaluate co-morbidities. Thyroid hormone levels are examined when thyroid dysfunction suspected. Blood chemistry may help to evaluate the degree of edema vs lymphedema.

Imaging for diagnoses can be helpful if further definition is required. Non-invasive duplex-Doppler studies, and rarely, phlebography may be required if venous disease is suspected. Computed tomography (CT), magnetic resonance imaging (MRI), and ultrasonography are also useful in selected patients. Lymphoscintigraphy (LAS) is very useful in demonstrating the detailed lymphatic pathology. LAS provides images of lymphatics and lymph nodes as well as semi-quantitative data on radiotracer (lymph) transport. However, the limited availability of experienced specialists in nuclear medicine and the ability of LAS to influence therapy would seem, at this time, to limit its usefulness to research application.

Genetic testing has been shown to define a limited number of hereditary syndromes. In the future, such testing may become routine and could hold promise for specific gene therapy.

Biopsy of enlarged regional lymph nodes in the presence of chronic lymphedema is rarely helpful and should be discouraged. Fine needle aspiration is a useful alternative if malignancy is suspected. Any invasive procedure on a lymphedematous limb has the potential to aggravate the swelling or lead to cellulitis.

7. LYMPHEDEMA STAGING

Clinical staging has proven useful for the classification of lymphedema (7):

- Stage I: spontaneous, reversible, tissue swelling leaving indentations, negative or borderline Stemmer sign, no palpable fibrous tissue.
- Stage II: spontaneous, irreversible tissue swelling with moderate or pronounced fibrosis. Indentations are difficult to produce. Stemmer sign positive, lymphostatic dermatosis.
- Stage III: lymphatic elephantiasis, usually with pronounced skin alterations.

Severity based on differences in limb volume are assessed as minimal ($<20\%$ increase), moderate (20% increase), or severe ($>40\%$ increase).

8. NON-OPERATIVE LYMPHEDEMA THERAPY

Therapy for peripheral lymphedema is divided into non-operative and operative methods. This discussion does not apply directly to wound-related lymphedema which will be detailed in a following section. The principles of modern lymphedema treatment, however, have direct application to the lymphedema/wound healing equation.

8.1. Comprehensive Decongestive Physiotherapy

Comprehensive decongestive physiotherapy (CDP), a combination of physical therapy modes, is the gold standard for the treatment of primary and secondary lymphedema (7,8). In the 1930s, Emil Vodder, a Danish physician, used a type of therapy known as manual lymph drainage (MLD) to treat lymphedema. This massage is a light, circular, superficial tissue stretching preformed with varying degrees of pressure. The effect is to increase the transport of the lymph collectors and the development of new routes for lymph drainage. Decongesting lymphotomes "upstream" from the lymphedema areas and utilizing the watershed anatomy for directional flow enhanced treatment efficiency. CDP as practiced today was introduced, applied and refined by Drs. Michael and Ethel Foldi, in Germany (9). This method has been further modified by the contribution of the Casley-Smiths in Australia (10).

CDP involves four therapy modes—Manual lymph drainage (MLD), compression bandaging, decongestive exercises, and patient education in hygiene and self-treatment (Table 4). CDP is usually divided into a two-phase treatment program. The first phase consists of daily therapy sessions of specialized manual lymph drainage/massage; range of motion exercises and compression wrapping applied with multilayered short stretch bandages. The use of short stretch bandages enables the contraction of muscles to apply pressure to a resistant force, thus mobilizing lymph with intermittent pulsations. The patient wears the bandages during the interval between therapy sessions. These sessions vary from 1 to 2 times per day and may be continued from 2 to 4 weeks or longer depending upon the severity of the disease.

Phase two, initiated immediately at the completion of phase one, is programmed to conserve and optimize the benefits achieved from the start of therapy. Phase two is a lifetime commitment by the patient. Fitted, low stretch elastic compression garments are used daily. Exercises designed to improve systemic lymphatic flow and patient self-administered MLD enable the patient to maintain the achieved lymphedema reduction. Very often, compliant patients are able to improve upon the initial reduction (11). The success of CDP depends upon the compliance of the patient and the availability of therapists trained and certified in this exacting technique. (National Lymphedema Network, 1–800–541–3259). A dramatic example of the effects of CDP carried out over four-month duration can be seen in Figure 3.

The Foldi Klinik, in Germany, has treated 2500 patients annually with CDP. Limb volume reductions averaged 50% after the completion of therapy. Greater than 50% of patients maintained their reduction during phase two (9). Casley-Smiths (12) reported volume reductions of over 60% in 618 lymphedematous limbs. The pioneering work of Boris et al. (11,13) introduced CDP to North America in the 1980s. Boris et al., in 1997, published their results in 119 consecutive patients. The affected limbs included both arms and legs. Lymphedema reduction averaged 62.6% in 56 patients with one affected arm and 68.6% in 38 patients with one affected leg. After

Table 4 Comprehensive Decongestive Physiotherapy

Manual lymph drainage (MLD)
Compression bandaging
Decongestive exercises
Education in hygiene and self treatment

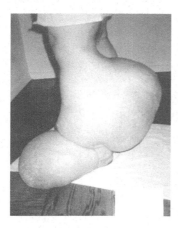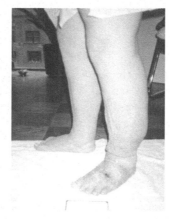

Figure 3 Results of complex decongestive physiotherapy (CDP).

36 months follow-up, the average volume reduction in the arms increased to 63.8% and remained at 62.7% in the affected legs.

8.1.1. Pneumatic Compression

Intermittent pneumatic compression by a sequential gradient pump, if prescribed, must be used with caution and under strict supervision. Inappropriately high pressures and variable time intervals must be closely monitored. The use of pneumatic pumps without the added resource of MLD can result in further lymphatic damage as well as significant pelvic, genital and opposite limb swelling (14). MLD is used to decrease fluid volume proximal to the obstructing lesion thereby improving the efficiency of lymph mobilization toward the thoracic duct and venous circulation. The role of thermal therapy and pulsed radio frequency energy in the treatment of lymphedema remains unclear.

8.1.2. Elevation

Simple elevation is an obvious first step in the treatment of the lymphedematous limb. This is especially helpful in the early stage of lymphedema. If the swelling is reduced by this means, the effect should be maintained by wearing a low stretch, elastic sleeve/stocking.

8.1.3. Drug Therapy

Diuretic agents may sometimes be useful during the early phases of CDP. However, long-term administration of diuretics in the treatment of lymphedema is of little benefit. Diuretics may induce fluid and electrolyte imbalance by decreasing the water content of the lymph fluid and increasing the viscosity, thereby hindering the mobilization of lymphedema (7).

Oral benzopyrones (coumarin) are thought to hydrolyze tissue proteins and facilitate absorption while stimulating lymphatic collectors (12).

Benzopyrines have not been approved for usage in the United States as they have been linked to liver toxicity and dosage regimens are still in question.

Antibiotics should be administered for superimposed infection (cellulitis/ lymphangitis). Skin erythema without systemic signs of infection does not necessarily imply infection and need not be treated. In severe chronic lymphedema with repeated episodes of cellulitis, appropriate prophylactic antibiotics are often indicated. Fungal infections can be treated with antimycotic drugs.

In the treatment of filariasis, drugs are used to remove microfilariae from the bloodstream. Diethylcarbamazine, ivermectin, and albendazole are recommended. Eradication of the adult nematodes by these drugs is variable and may be associated with significant side effects. These drugs have no direct effect on the limb swelling.

8.1.4. *Garment and Bandage Compression*

Garment and bandage compression are essential components in the continuous therapy for lymphedema. When therapy has resulted in volume reduction, compression prevents recurrence. The effect of continued compression results in a reduction of abnormally increased ultrafiltration and improved fluid reabsorption. Joint and muscle pump function is improved and there is a reduction of fibrosis in the limb. The studies of Mayrovitz and Larson (15) suggest that compression, within defined parameters, may actually increase arterial perfusion.

The bandage material used determines the compression effect. Short stretch bandages are the preferred bandage used in the treatment of primary and secondary lymphedema. Short stretch bandages cause a higher pressure during activity (working pressure) and relatively low pressure at rest (resting pressure). Padding using cotton and selective use of foam rubber can protect protruding bones and reduce fibrosis. The selection of compression grade and proper size is critical to the success of garment control in lymphedema. Likewise, strict attention to patient compliance and garment compatibility determines the long-term success of therapy.

9. OPERATIVE TREATMENT OF LYMPHEDEMA

Surgical approaches to alleviate extremity lymphedema have not been widely accepted. In selected patients, surgical procedures are used in combination with CDP or alone when CDP has been unsuccessful. Operative treatment for lymphedema falls within four areas: resection, drainage, reconstruction, and liposuction.

Resection or "debulking" is the most direct approach. This involves complete removal of cutaneous and subcutaneous tissue including muscle fascia. Skin from the resected area is then grafted over the resulting defect. The efficacy of this procedure is hampered by the obliteration of skin lymphatic channels, ulceration, and scar tissue. New edema peripheral to the resected and grafted regions is not uncommon. After successful CDP, redundant folds may, in selected cases, require resection in advanced elephantiasis.

Surgical drainage methods include enteromesenteric bridge procedures, skin flaps, omental transposition, and the implantation of thread or tubes. None of these procedures have demonstrated long-term benefit.

Autogenous lymph vessel transplantation or interposition vein segments have been attempted to restore lymphatic flow. Lympho-venous and lympho-nodal venous shunts have yet to confirm long-term patency.

Liposuction has recently been modified to successfully treat fibrotic upper extremity lymphedema (16). Short-term results seem encouraging but strict patient compliance is required with continued use of low stretch compression garments and supportive CDP.

10. LYMPHEDEMA AND WOUND HEALING

In order to appreciate the relationship of lymphedema to wound healing, a review of the pathophysiology of chronic venous insufficiency and venous stasis ulceration is helpful. Chronic venous insufficiency leads to venous hypertension, which results in a high filtration pressure causing increased fluid to appear in the tissues, i.e., increased lymphatic water load. When the lymphatic transport capacity is exceeded by the waterload, initially a state of low protein edema occurs as a result of this dynamic failure. Constant lymphatic hypertension causes infiltration of lymph into the perilymphatic tissue resulting in fibrosclerosis and lymphangitis. Protein permeability increases and lymphatic damage follows. Subsequently, lymphedema (high protein edema) becomes the underlying pathology that contributes to the formation of venous stasis ulcers.

Venous ulcers often exhibit many of the characteristics of the non-venous chronic wound: normal arterial blood supply, colonized bacterial contamination, and healthy granulation tissue. With compression and control of the lymphedema, these wounds will, in the majority of cases, heal. Given the exact same parameters in non-venous, acute, and chronic wounds throughout the body, controlling the peri-wound lymphedema will result in enhanced wound healing (4).

In the author's clinic, in excess of 80% of patients presenting with lower extremity, non-venous chronic wounds have demonstrated generalized or peri-wound lymphedema (data accumulated April 2000 to March 2001). The degree varied from trace to 4+ pitting. These findings were seen in multiple types of wounds, i.e., ischemic, diabetic, and traumatic (Fig. 4). In many instances, in long-standing wounds the elimination of the lymphedema enhanced the rate of healing dramatically.

11. PATHOPHYSIOLOGY OF WOUND-RELATED LYMPHEDEMA

The most obvious effect from lymphedema is swelling. This can result in abnormal function at both the tissue and cellular level. Distance between tissue channels can affect metabolic exchange causing a shift toward anaerobic metabolism. Because cells are more widely separated, the exchange of gasses between plasma membranes is likely to be affected. In chronic venous insufficiency, the removal of lymphedema results in a significant increase in intracutaneous oxygen tension (17). By capilaroscopy, it has been shown that the density of skin capillaries increases as a result of edema reduction (18).

Alterations in tissue produced by simple injections of protein are almost identical with the changes observed in sub-acute and chronic lymphedema (19). Mani and Ross (20) state "The chronic effects of edema on the viso-elastic properties of connective tissue are unknown. It is reasonable to assume that pools of edema will squash, squeeze, stretch, or affect the crimping and orientation of dermal collagen bundles."

Open wounds studied by the injection of dye have demonstrated significant reduction in lymphatic channel regeneration as compared to arterial and venous

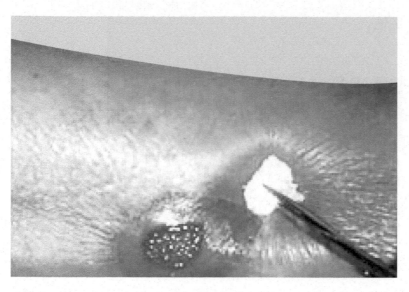

Figure 4   Peri-wound edema/lymphedema.

angiogenesis (21). Trauma increases lymphatic flow, and outflow obstruction with the accumulation of waste products generated in the wound healing process is a likely inhibitory factor in wound healing (22). Tissues surrounding acute and chronic wounds are characterized by collections of interstitial or third space fluid. This collection of fluid mechanically compromises the microvascular and lymphatic system thereby increasing capillary and venous after load. Consequently, the delivery of oxygen and nutrients and the discharge of toxins and inhibitory factors are affected (23).

Removing excess chronic wound fluid is thought to remove inhibitory factors present in the fluids. Studies have shown that fluids removed from chronic wounds suppress the proliferation of keratinocytes, fibroblasts and vascular endothelial cells in vitro (24,25). Argenta and Morykwas (26), in their investigations related to vacuum-assisted closure of wounds, have provided valuable insight into the consequences of lymph stasis and the healing wound. Their technique removes chronic lymphedema, which contributes to increased blood flow and enhanced formation of granulation tissue.

12.   LYMPHEDEMA THERAPY AND THE OPEN WOUND

Manuel lymph drainage (MLD) and continued compression are the cornerstone of treatment for non-wound-related lymphedema. However, using MLD to alleviate lymphedema associated with the open wound is neither time nor cost-efficient. After the wound has healed, CDP may be indicated if persistent swelling is a problem. In the treatment of chronic venous leg ulcers, improving the efficiency of the calf muscle pump by using compression bandages is widely accepted as essential for proper care. It is reasonable, then, to postulate that the therapy for lymphedema/lymph stasis associated with the open non-venous wound is also compression. Limb elevation, when practical, is obviously helpful. In addition to the accepted dictums of modern wound care, the reasoned use of compression with short stretch, long stretch or combinations of such bandages is designed to create a dynamic wound dressing (27). As has been mentioned, diuretics are rarely indicated as primary therapy and, in fact, can impair fluid mobilization by extracting water from the lymph (7). Diuretics are useful in treating limb swelling when a significant degree of edema superimposed on the underlying lymphedema is evident, as in chronic congestive failure.

REFERENCES

1. Casley-Smith JR. Frequency of Lymphedema. In: Casley-Smith JR, ed. Modern Treatment for Lymphedema. 5th ed. Adelaide, Australia: The Lymphedemac Association of Australia, 1997:81–84.
2. Casley-Smith JR. Pathology of Oedema-Causes of Oedema. In: Casley-Smith JR, ed. Modern Treatment for Lymphedema. 5th ed. Adelaide Australia: The Lymphedema Association of Australia, 1997:41–59.
3. Brunner V, Klinik und Farbstofftest beim primaren Lymphoderm der Beine . In: GDL, ed. I. Kongress Gesellschaft Deutchspracheiger Lymphologen. Wien: Perimed, Erlangen, 1985:39–47.
4. Macdonald JM. Wound healing and lymphedema: a new look at an old problem. Ostomy/Wound Manage 2001; 47(4):52–57.
5. Allen EV, Hines EA. Lipidema of the legs. Proc Staff Mayo Clin 1940; 15:184–187.
6. Stemmer R. Ein Klinisches Zeichen Zur Fruh-und Differential Diagnose des Lymphoderms. VASA 1967; 5:262.
7. Bernas MJ, Witte CL, Witte MH. The diagnosis and treatment of peripheral lymphedema. Draft Revision of the 1995 Consensus Document of the International Society of Lymphology Executive Committee. Lymphology 2001; 34:84–91.
8. Foldi M. Treatment of lymphedema (editorial). Lymphology 1994; 27:1–5.
9. Foldi E, Foldi M, Weissleder H. Conservative treatment of lymphedema of the limbs. Angiology 1985; 36:171–180.
10. Casley-Smith JR. Complex physical therapy; the first 200 Australian limbs. Aust J Dermatol 1992; 33:61–68.
11. Boris M, Weindorf S, Lasinski B, et al. Lymphedema reduction by non-invasive complex lymphedema therapy. Oncology 1994; 8:95–106.
12. Casley-Smith JR. Lymphedema therapy in Australia; Complex physical therapy, exercises and benzopyrones on over 600 limbs. Lymphology 1994; 27(suppl):622–625.
13. Ko D, Lerner R, Klos G, et al. Effective treatment of lymphedema of the extremities. Arch Surg 1988; 133:452–458.
14. Boris M, Weindorf S, Lasinski B. The risk of genital edema after external pump. Compression for lower limb lymphedema. Lymphology 1998; 31:15–20.
15. Mayrovitz H, Larson P. Effects of compression bandaging on leg pulsitile blood flow. Clin Physiol 1997; 17:105–117.
16. Brorson H, Svensson H, Norrgren K, et al. Liposuction reduces arm lymphedema without significantly altering the already impaired lymph transport. Lymphology 1998; 31:156–172.
17. Kolari PJ, Pekanmaki K, Pohjola RT. Transcutaneous oxygen tension in patients with post-traumatic ulcers: treatment with intermittent pneumatic compression. Cardiovasc Res 1988; 22:138–141.
18. Neumann HAM. Possibilities and limitation of transcutaneous oxygen tension measurements in chronic venous insufficiency. Int J Microcirc Clin Exp 1990; (suppl): 105:1.
19. Gaffney RM, Casley-Smith JR. Excess protein as a cause of chronic inflammation and lymphedema: biochemical estimations. J Pathol 133:243.

20. Mani R, Ross JN. The study of tissue structure in the wound environment in chronic wound healing. In: Mani R, Falanga V, Shearman CP, Sandeman D, eds. Clinical Measurement and Basic Science. Philadelphia: WB Saunders, 1999:139.

21. Eliska O, Eliskova M. Secondary healing wounds and their lymphatics. Eur J Lymphol 2000; 8(31):64.

22. Szczesny G, Olszewski WL. Lymphatic and venous changes in post traumatic edema of lower limbs. Eur J Lymphol 2000; 8(31):60.

23. Witkowski JA, Parish LC. Histopathology of the decubitus ulcer. J Am Acad Dermatol 1982; 6:1014–1021.

24. Falanga V. Growth factors and chronic wounds: the need to understand the microenvironment. J Dermatol 1992; 19:667–672.

25. Bucalo B, Eaglestein WH, Falanga. Inhibition of cell proliferation by chronic wound fluid. Wound Repair Regeneration 1993; 1:181–186.

26. Argenta L, Morykwas M. Vacume-assisted closure: a new method for wound control and treatment: clinical experience. Ann Plast Surg 1997; 38:563–567.

27. Macdonald JM, Sims N, Mayrovitz HN. Lymphedema, Lipedema, and the open wound. The role of compression therapy. Surg Clin N Am 2003; 83:639–658.

26
Malignancy and Wounds

Jennifer T. Trent and Robert S. Kirsner
Department of Dermatology and Cutaneous Surgery, University of Miami School of Medicine, Miami, Florida, U.S.A.

1. INTRODUCTION

Chronic wounds and malignancies may be related in several ways (Table 1). First, wounds may, over time, degenerate into malignancy through chronic antigenic or nonspecific stimulation. Most commonly, this is seen with squamous cell carcinoma (SCC). Second, cutaneous malignancies may present initially as ulcerated wounds. The classic example of this is a basal cell carcinoma (BCC), which by out growing its blood supply will erode and subsequently ulcerate. Also, cutaneous metastases may present as cutaneous ulcers. Third, treatment of malignancies can lead to the development of chronic wounds. For example, hydroxyurea used to treat certain leukemias may cause lower extremity ulcerations. Finally, wounds may be associated with malignancy. For example, chronic wounds resulting from vasculitis or from pyoderma gangrenosum have been linked to malignancy.

2. MALIGNANT DEGENERATION OF WOUNDS

Malignancies found within chronic wounds are rare but well documented in the literature (Table 2) (1–6). Marjolin first reported this occurrence in 1827, and, as a result, chronic wounds which develop into malignancies are referred to as "Marjolin's" ulcers. Hawkins first reported the occurrence of SCC in chronic osteomyelitis in 1835 in one of the seven "Cases of Warty Cicatrices." This finding of SCC associated with a draining sinus tract is a common clinical scenario in which SCC occurs (1–3). The incidence of chronic wounds which undergo malignant degeneration has been estimated at 1.7%. Malignant degeneration of a wound into an SCC classically affects men, 40–70 years of age, who have had osteomyelitis and chronic wounds on the lower extremities. These preexisting conditions may be present for a long time, 20–50 years, but can be present as little as 18 months (2). While SCC is the most common malignancy to present in draining sinus tracts of chronic osteomyelitis and wounds, other malignancies have been found, such as BCC, adenocarcinoma, fibrosarcoma, osteosarcoma, melanoma, lymphoma, and plasmacytoma (Fig. 1) (1–3,7).

Table 1 Types of Wounds Associated with Malignancy

Wounds that degenerate into malignancy
Malignancies that present as wounds, including cutaneous metastases
Wounds with etiologies associated with malignancies
Wounds resulting from treatment of malignancies

In addition to sinus tracts of osteomyelitis, other chronic wounds are at risk for malignant degeneration as well. One example is the chronic venous ulcer. In addition to SCC, other malignancies such as sarcomas, lymphoma, melanoma, and BCC have been reported to develop within chronic venous ulcers (4–6,8–18). The risk of developing a malignancy within a venous ulcer is 0.21% (4). It appears that SCCs occur more frequently in venous ulcers than BCC (19:1) (8,12,14). Squamous cell carcinomas associated with venous ulcers have been found to occur more frequently in women, possibly because women's legs are more often exposed to sunlight than men's (5,19). This suggests that the ulcers developing into malignancies share some of the risk associations that nonulcerated skin has. In the latter example, perhaps exposure to ultraviolet radiation was causal. In addition, the development of SCC

Table 2 Types of Wounds That Degenerate into Malignancy

Venous ulcers
Burns
Osteomyelitis
Trauma
Hidradenitis suppurativa
Radiotherapy
Diabetic ulcers
Arterial ulcers
Acne conglobata
Lupus vulgaris
Frostbite
Pilonidal sinus
Dissecting perifolliculitis of the scalp
Anogenital fistula
Lymphogranuloma venereum
Granuloma inguinale
Leprosy
Actinomycosis
Candidiasis
Herpes zoster
Onchocerciasis
Vaccination scars
Injection sites
Tattoos
Discoid lupus
Epidermolysis bullosa
Lichen sclerosis et atrophicus
Lichen planus
Acrodermatitis chronica atrophicans

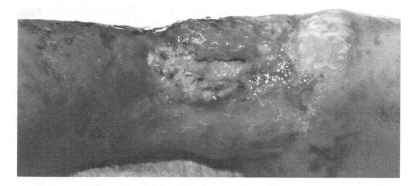

Figure 1   Squamous cell carcinoma which developed within a chronic venous leg ulcer.

has been reported to occur in other wounds such as those secondary to burns, trauma, hidradenitis suppurativa, radiotherapy, and diabetes, among others (6–8,14,20–25).

There are several theories which have been suggested to explain why malignancies develop within chronic wounds; however, the exact mechanism is unknown (Table 3). It is postulated to be an example of normal wound healing gone awry. Some believe that constant irritation and infection, chronic ulceration, repeated trauma, or exposure to noxious environmental agents lead to development of malignancies (8,17). This chronic irritation with repeated damage and attempted repair of the damaged cutaneous tissue may be a contributory factor in the initiation of carcinogenesis (26). Arons et al. (27) believed there is a sequence of events involved in wound carcinogenesis. Normal tissue, subjected to constant trauma, inevitably overwhelms the tissue's normal control of epidermal proliferation; and neoplasia results (24). Histologically, chronic trauma leads to acanthosis, followed by basal cell hyperplasia, pseudoepitheliomatous hyperplasia, basal cell atypia, and finally an epidermoid carcinoma.

Other theories suggest the induction of once dormant neoplastic cells occurs (16,28). During the initiation phase, normal cells become dormant neoplastic cells. Then, during the promotion phase, dormant cells mutate into malignant cells by the stimulation of a co-carcinogen, such as infection.

In addition, it is postulated that toxins released from damaged tissue lead to mutation of cells and eventually a tumor (29). These toxins injure the vasculature and/or the lymphatics, leading to insufficient nutritional support for the damaged cells. These cellular deficits lead to altered mitosis of the resultant scar. The scars that result from the healing of poorly nourished tissue cannot tolerate infection or future insult (26). Therefore, future damage is poorly tolerated, leading to mutagenesis and cancer. Also, since scar tissue is less organized, it may be more likely to ulcerate and degenerate into cancer (28).

Table 3   Theories to Explain Why Malignancies Develop Within Chronic Wounds

Chronic irritation with repeated damage and repair (ulceration, trauma, infection)
Induction of dormant neoplastic cells
Toxins released from damaged tissue
Implantation of epidermal cells within the dermis

It has also been suggested that trauma results in the implantation of epidermal cells into the dermis (28,29). These displaced epidermal cells cause a foreign body reaction within the dermis, which ultimately alters the normal regenerative processes of the tissue. Therefore, any future tissue insult will not be endured or treated in the same manner as normal tissue. This may result in neoplastic transformation.

There are several methods of treatment for SCC which arises within chronic wounds of osteomyelitis (1–3). In the case of small mobile tumors, wide local excision is preferred (29). However, amputation was indicated in several circumstances. These include: (1) when the cancer is adherent to underlying tissue and cannot be separated, (2) when wide local excision would leave an open articulation surface, (3) when there is uncontrollable suppuration, (4) when there is bone necrosis, (5) when there is decreased functional capacity after wide local excision, and (6) when there is erosion into a large vessel. Recently, the use of Mohs micrographic surgery has been shown to be effective (1–3). The use of Mohs is based on the concept that metastatic disease has not occurred and treatment is aimed at complex local eradication. Therefore, prior to surgery, the presence of regional or distant metastases should be excluded. Then, using the Mohs techniques, the tumor is followed microscopically through serial sections to ensure complete eradication. This technique may be limb saving. However, there are certain circumstances under which Mohs should not be done, including the presence of distant metastasis or regional lymph node involvement. Additionally, if a functional limb is not a possible outcome, amputation with subsequent use of prosthesis may be more desirable than Mohs (1).

As chronic osteomyelitis is often accompanied by lymphadenopathy (LAD), adenopathy may be from infection as opposed to metastatic disease. However, there is much controversy regarding lymph node dissection (LND) and advocates often base the need for LND on the histologic grade of the tumor (29). If LAD persists for >3 months, the node should be biopsied. For example, Grade 1, well-differentiated lesions, only need lymph node dissection if the nodes are palpable. Grade 2, moderately differentiated lesions, and grade 3, poorly differentiated lesions, more often and typically require LND.

3. MALIGNANCIES WHICH PRESENT AS CHRONIC WOUNDS

It is important that clinicians be aware that cutaneous malignancies can present as chronic wounds. The incidence of ulcerated malignancies is thought to be 3% (30). While this represents a small number and ulcerated malignancies are rare, there are more common than wounds undergoing malignant transformations (10,30). Additionally, it is often difficult to distinguish these primary malignancies that ulcerate from ulcers that undergo malignant transformation discussed above. Oftentimes, these malignancies go undiagnosed for a long time, since they are mistaken for nonmalignant ulcers.

Scattered reports describe various malignancies that present as ulcers (Table 4). These include reports of Kaposi's sarcoma (KS), lymphoma, melanoma, BCC, and SCC (Figs. 2–5) (12,19,30–36). In a study by Hansson and Andersson (30), BCC was the most common type of malignancy found to present initially as ulcers (Fig. 3). In this series, BCCs accounted for 60% of the malignancies while SCCs 15% (Fig. 4). This is in contrast to Marjolin's ulcers, which are more commonly SCC. The successful treatment of SCC or BCC that develop in venous ulcers has occurred with wide excision followed by placement of a skin graft (4–6,8).

Table 4 Types of Malignancies That Present as Ulcers

Squamous cell carcinoma
Basal cell carcinoma
Melanoma
Kaposi's sarcoma
Lymphoma

Melanoma has been found within long-standing pressure ulcers, osteomyelitis, burns, vaccine scars, and venous ulcers (7,14,23). Due to delayed diagnosis and advanced stage at presentation of these ulcers, the melanoma has likely already metastasized. Therefore, patients usually have a very poor prognosis. Melanomas, similar to SCC, have been found to appear in ulcers secondary to burns. For melanoma, the treatment depends on the depth of invasion and the size of the lesion.

Classically, KS presents as patches, plaques, or nodules, but only rarely as an ulcer (31–33). For example, in a series of KS of the penis, Schmidt et al. (31) reported that only 1 out of the 20 reported cases of penile KS presenting as an ulcer. Infection with HIV or an immunocompromised state of the patient has been linked to the unusual presentation of ulcerative KS. Kaposi's sarcoma has been successfully treated with excision, radiation, chemotherapy, or interferon (33).

Cutaneous lymphoma may present as various types of skin lesions, however, it too many rarely present as ulcers and the clinician should be alert to this (Fig. 5) (34,36,37). Unfortunately, ulcerative cutaneous lymphomas are associated with a worse prognosis. Lymphomas have been treated with excision, and appropriate chemotherapy and radiation (34).

4. ULCERS THAT DEVELOP SECONDARY TO TREATMENT OF A MALIGNANCY

Certain treatments for cancer may be associated with the development of cutaneous ulcers. Interestingly, some of these may eventuate into malignancy.

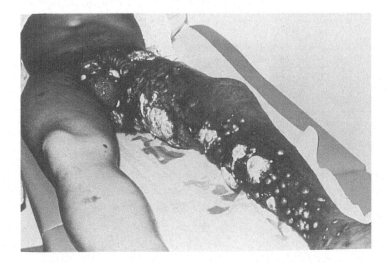

Figure 2 Kaposi's sarcoma that involved the entire lower extremity.

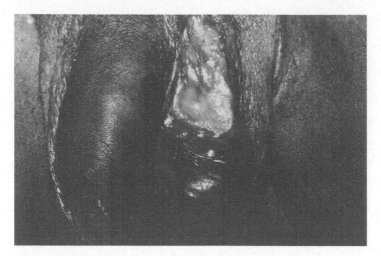

Figure 3 Lymphoma that presented as a scrotal ulcer.

Hydroxyurea (HU) is an antimetabolite used in the treatment of several malignant and nonmalignant conditions, such as chronic myelogenous leukemia, polycythemia vera, head and neck cancer, renal cell carcinoma, and breast cancer (38,39). Hydroxyurea, a ribonucleotide diphosphate reductase inhibitor, prevents conversion of ribonucleotides to deoxyribonucleotides inhibiting DNA synthesis. Inhibition of DNA synthesis is the mechanism by which HU exerts its anticancer effects. Hydroxyurea may cause several cutaneous side effects, including alopecia, difuse hyperpigmentation, poikiloderma, hyperpigmented nail bands, acral erythema and scaling, and recalcitrant ulcers. The development of painful cutaneous ulcers results from the direct effects of HU on keratinocytes (39–41). On keratinocytes, HU inhibits thymidine incorporation into DNA, impairing cell replication, inhibiting DNA repair, and inducing chromosomal damage (42). These effects lead not only to the development of ulcers but contribute to a delay in wound healing as well. Ulcers usually present in areas subject to frequent trauma, such as the malleoli (medial > lateral), tibia, dorsum of the feet and calves (39). The extent and size of

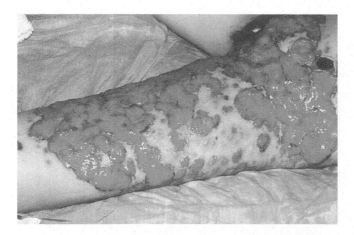

Figure 4 Lymphoma that affected the vulva and thigh.

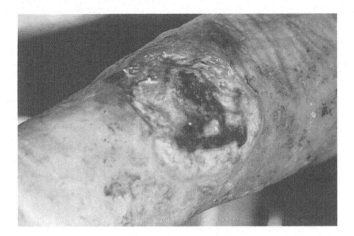

Figure 5 Mycosis fungoides which presented as an ulcer of the lower extremity.

the ulcer correlates with the dose of HU. Ulcers may develop between 1 and 15 years after beginning HU and often will not heal until the medication is discontinued, although adjuvant therapy to speed healing is often required (39,41,43,44). If HU is temporarily discontinued then restarted, the ulcers will return more rapidly than their initial presentation. Recurrence may occur in as little as 4 months (39,44).

There are also several reports of skin cancers developing within HU-induced ulcers (25,38,43). Inhibition of DNA excision repair and resultant chromosomal damage is thought to be mechanistically causal in the development of these cancers. Both SCC and BCC have been found within these ulcers (42,43). Malignant transformation is associated with sudden appearance, rapid growth, and large size. Interestingly, the malignant ulcer will decrease in size after stopping HU. Complete excision is still required.

Another chemotherapeutic agent which can lead to ulcer formation, and even the development of malignancy within that ulcer, is doxorubicin (DR). Doxorubicin acts by intercalating within the nucleotide bases to inhibit DNA replication as well as DNA and RNA polymerases (45,46). Doxorubicin is commonly used to treat lymphomas, sarcomas, and adenocarcinomas of the breast and stomach. Doxorubicin is a vesicant, and if extravasated, acts directly on the surrounding skin to cause necrosis. Doxorubicin induced ulcers usually form around the area of skin into which DR is intravenously injected. These ulcers commonly appear after 4 weeks of therapy (47). These indolent and progressive ulcers are unresponsive to most therapies (46). To effect healing, DR must be discontinued and completely removed from the surrounding tissue. As DR is retained within tissue, wide excision with closure via a flap and skin graft placement is normally required (48). To predict margins for excision, ultraviolet light (UV) light may be used. Ultraviolet light causes the tissue infiltrated by DR to fluoresce with an orange–red color (47). The use of UV light during surgical excision aids in a more complete removal of all the affected tissue. To prevent ulceration, DR should be injected into larger veins, especially avoiding areas around joints of the hand and arms.

Squamous cell carcinoma has been reported to develop within DR-induced ulcers (45). For example, one patient treated for adenocarcinoma of the stomach with adjuvant chemotherapy including DR subsequently developed an ulcer at the injection site. Ten years later, this nonhealing ulcer was found to have SCC within the wound.

Radiotherapy with conventional deep x-ray beams has been used to treat a number of cancers, such as breast, endometrial, and cervical carcinoma (49–52). The development of sarcoma, melanoma, SCC, and BCC within the radiation field many years after the treatment of the first cancer is a recognized but rare complication (49–52). Less common is the development of ulcerated second cancers within the irradiated fields. It is believed that radiation causes irreversible DNA damage, leading to gene mutations and deletions (49). On a molecular level, the proto-oncogene c-jun and the inactivation of tumor suppressor genes p53 and rb occur. A cancer is classified as radiation induced if: (1) the cancer is present within the previously irradiated field (typically this occurs 3–5 years after the initial treatment in which at least 25–80 Gy of radiation were delivered), and (2) the two cancers (the previously treated and the new cancer) must be histologically different (49). Squamous cell carcinoma and basal cell carcinoma are the most common radiation-induced carcinomas (51). Angiosarcomas are the rarest, with a risk of 0.04%. When angiosarcomas do occur, they usually present after radiation therapy to the breast (50). Surgical excision is the preferred treatment; however, chemotherapy and reirradiation may have some therapeutic benefit (49).

In several studies by Zhao et al. (53–55) evidence has been found linking several proteins to radiation-induced skin ulcers developing into malignancies. These include Telomerase reverse transcriptase (TRT) expression, c-erbB-2 and p21 oncoproteins, MDM2, p53, and NCAM.

5.   CUTANEOUS METASTASES PRESENTING AS ULCERS

There are four routes by which cancer may metastasize: via the blood (hematogenous), via the lymphatics, by direct contiguous, and by iatrogenic implantation (Table 5) (56). Unfortunately, in many cases, at the time of presentation, metastasis has already occurred (57). In 1.3% of patients, the metastases are cutaneous. While cutaneous metastases present with a frequency of 0.7–9.0%, ulcerated cutaneous metastases are uncommon as most cutaneous metastases present as nodules (56). In 0.8% of patients with internal malignancy, cutaneous mets are the first indication of cancer. Some cancers are more frequently associated with ulcerated cutaneous lesions, including primaries from the oral cavity and breast. There have been some sporadic reports of other cancers with ulcerated cutaneous mets (Table 6).

Hepatocellular carcinoma (HCC) metastasizes to skin in 2.7% of patients and usually to the scalp, chest, and shoulders (58). These metastases are more often associated in patients with underlying cirrhosis. Treatment includes local excision, chemotherapy, or local radiation.

Hodgkin's lymphoma will commonly involve the skin, especially the trunk. Reports of skin involvement range from 13 to 57% of patients (59,60). These cutaneous metastases are thought to occur due to retrograde lymphatic spread to

Table 5 Routes of Metastasis

Hematogenous
Lymphatic
Direct continguous
Iatrogenic implantation

Table 6 Types of Malignancies Associated with Cutaneous Ulcerative Metastases

Oral cancer
Breast cancer
Hepatocellular carcinoma
Hodgkin's lymphoma
Non-Hodgkin's lymphoma

regional lymph nodes. When skin metastases are present, the patient is usually in stage IV Hodgkin's. There have been reports of ulcerated cutaneous metastases appearing on the chest, scalp, and face. Ulcers have been found in 1.3–1.5% of skin mets associated with Hodgkin's. Treatment includes systemic chemotherapy and local radiation.

Similar to Hodgkin's lymphoma, the cutaneous mets of non-Hodgkin's lymphoma (NHL) usually occur in stage IV NHL (61). These ulcerated cutaneous metastases are associated with a worse prognosis and advanced systemic disease. Death is often secondary to sepsis from infection of ulcerated metastases. These ulcers are often infected with *Staphylococcus aureus*. However, infection with *Pseudomonas* and *Streptococcus* are not uncommon. After infection is treated, these lesions can be treated with chemotherapy and local radiation.

Breast cancer will metastasize to the skin in 25–60% of patients (62). They usually appear over a hard breast mass, surrounded by peau-d-orange skin changes and edema of that arm. It is thought that breast cancer metastasizes by the direct contiguous spread, which explains the frequent occurrence of skin metastases on the chest. Treatment includes excision, systemic chemotherapy, and local radiation.

Oral cancers also may metastasize commonly to the face and will present as facial ulcerations (63). Similar to breast cancer, oral cancers spread by direct contiguous method, explaining their location. Treatment with systemic chemotherapy and local radiation may be effective.

6. WOUNDS WITH ETIOLOGIES ASSOCIATED WITH MALIGNANCIES

Certain dermatologic conditions are associated with underlying malignancies. For example, pyoderma gangrenosum (PG) is frequently found in association with many diseases, such as arthritis, inflammatory bowel disease, as well as various hematologic malignancies (64–66). These hematologic malignancies include chronic myelomonocytic leukemia, Hodgkin's lymphoma, non-Hodgkin's lymphoma, myeloma, acute and chronic myelocytic leukemia, polycythemia rubra vera, and myelodysplastic syndrome. The presence of cutaneous manifestations carries a poor prognosis, and may even be the first clinical sign of disease progression (65). Oftentimes, PG, which develops in the context of underlying malignancy, will present in the bullous form. Greater than 50% of PG patients with myelodysplastic syndrome will progress to acute myelocytic leukemia. It has been postulated that this association between malignancy and PG is linked to abnormalities in cellular immunity and neutrophil function (64,65).

Vasculitis may be associated with certain medications, infections, collagen vascular diseases, and malignancies, more commonly hematologic than solid tumor (67–70). Vasculitis may also be of a paraneoplastic type. Such hematologic malignancies include myelodysplastic syndrome, myeloma, non-Hodgkin's lymphoma,

Table 7 Wound Characteristics Suggestive of Malignancy

Increase in size of wounds despite proper treatment
Malodorous wounds
Excess granulation tissue
Painful
Excess drainage
Excess bleeding
Exophytic growth
Irregular base or margins of the wound

acute and chronic myelocytic leukemias, cutaneous T cell lymphomas, Hodgkin's lymphoma, and hairy cell leukemia (70). Solid tumor malignancies, which have been found in association with vasculitis, include lung, prostate, colon, renal, breast, head and neck, and endometrial carcinomas. One to seven percent of vasculitis cases are associated with malignancy (67). Frequently, the development of vasculitis will predate the diagnosis of malignancy anywhere from 2 months to 3 years; however, vasculitis may also coexist or follow the diagnosis of malignancy. Certain characteristics should alert the physician to an underlying malignancy, such as severe constitutional symptoms, chronic and relapsing purpura, and the presence of hematologic abnormalities (70). Several mechanisms of pathogenesis have been proposed (67,69). Some believe that the tumor antigens induce the formation of immune complexes, which deposit on the vessel walls or have a direct immune reaction against the vessels. Certain antibodies against endothelial cells exist which cross react with the antigens on the leukemic cells. Tumor emboli may form. Tumor cells may release cytokines, which destroy the vessel wall.

7. DIAGNOSIS

There is considerable controversy regarding the proper time to obtain biopsies of the ulcerated wound base and margins. Some clinicians advocate performing biopsies of wounds that have been present longer than 3–4 months or have not responded to standard therapy (6,30). Some clinicians routinely biopsy all wounds regardless of the timeframe or response to treatment. Given the uncommon nature of these wounds, some authors suggest that only suspicious wounds should be biopsied (Table 7). Suspicious wounds characteristically have increased in size in spite of appropriate treatment, are malodorous, have excess granulation tissue which extends beyond the margins, are painful, have a change in the amount of or color of the drainage, have excess bleeding, have exophytic growth, or have irregularities of the base or margins (4–6,8,10,12,13,30). Any wound, which presents with the above characteristic or develops these characteristics over time, should be biopsied immediately.

REFERENCES

1. Kirsner RS, Spencer J, Falanga V, Garland LE, Kerdel FA. Squamous cell carcinoma arising in osteomyelitis and chronic wounds. Treatment with Mohs micrographic surgery vs amputation. Dermatol Surg 1996; 22:1015–1018.
2. Goldberg DJ, Arbesfeld D. Squamous cell carcinoma arising in a site of chronic osteomyelitis. J Dermatol Surg Oncol 1991; 17:788–790.

3. Kirsner RS, Garland LD. Squamous cell carcinoma arising from chronic osteomyelitis treated by Mohs micrographic surgery. J Dermatol Surg Oncol 1994; 20:133–140.

4. Baldursson B, Sigurgeirsson B, Lindelop B. Venous leg ulcers and squamous cell carcinoma: a large-scale epidemiological study. Br J Dermatol 1995; 133:571–574.

5. Franco RC. Basal and squamous cell carcioma associated with chronic venous leg ulcer. Intern J Dermatol 2001; 40:539–544.

6. Ackroyd JS, Young AE. Leg ulcers that do not heal. Br Med J 1983; 286:207–208.

7. Muhlemann MF, Griffiths RW, Briggs JC. Malignant melanoma and squamous cell carcinoma in a burn scar. Br J Plast Surg 1982; 35:474–477.

8. Liddell K. Malignant changes in chronic varicose ulceration. Practitioner 1975; 215:335–339.

9. Lanehart WH, Sanusi ID, Misra RP, O'Neal B. Metastasizing basal cell carcinoma originating in a stasis ulcer in a black woman. Arch Dermatol 1983; 119:587–591.

10. Goldman MP. Nonhealing leg ulcers: a manifestation of basal cell carcinoma. JAAD 1982; 26:791–792.

11. Black MM. Nonhealing leg ulcers. JAAD 1982; 26:792.

12. Phillips TJ, Salman SM, Rogers GS. Nonhealing leg ulcers: a manifestation of basal cell carcinoma. JAAD 1991; 25:47–49.

13. Harris B, Eaglstein WH, Falanga V. Basal cell carcinoma arising in venous ulcers and mimicking granulation tissue. J Dermatol Surg Oncol 1993; 19:150–152.

14. Kaplan RP. Cancer complicating chronic ulcerative and scarifying mucocutaneous disorders. Adv Dermatol 1987; 2:19–46.

15. Schwarze HP, Loche F, Gorguet MC, Kuchta, J, Bazex J. Basal cell carcinoma associated with chronic venous leg ulcer. Int J Dermatol 2000; 30:78–79.

16. Gan BS, Colcleugh RG, Scilley CG, Craig ID. Melanoma arising in a chronic (Marjolin's) ulcer. JAAD 1995; 32:1058–1059.

17. Andrews BT, Stewart JB, Allum WH. Malignant melanoma occurring in chronic venous ulceration. Dermatol Surg 1997; 23:594–595.

18. Dawson EK, McIntosh D. Granulation tissue sarcoma following long-standing varicose ulceration. J R Coll Surg Engl 1971; 16:88–95.

19. West JR, Berman B. Basal cell carcinoma presenting as a chronic finger ulcer. JAAD 1990; 23:318–319.

20. Kitahama A, Roland PY, Kerstein MD. Pyoderma gangrenosum with cutaneous T-Cell lymphoma manifested as lower extremity ulcers-case reports. Angiology 1991; 42:498–503.

21. Ceuppens A, Wylock P, De Raeve H. Carcinoma in a pressure sore. Br J Plast Surg 1997; 50:382–383.

22. Camisa C. Squamous cell carcinoma arising in acne conglobata. Cutis 1984; 33:185–190.

23. Ikeda I, Kageshita T, Ono T. Multiple malignant melanoma and squamous cell carcinoma in a burn scar. Dermatology 1995; 191:328–332.

24. Goldberg NS, Robinson JK, Peterson C. Gigantic malignant melanoma in a thermal burn scar. JAAD 1985; 12:949–952.

25. Yerushalmi J, Grunwald MH, Halevy DH, Avinoach I, Halevy S. Lupus vulgaris complicated by metastatic squamous cell carcinoma. Int J Dermatol 1998; 37:934–935.

26. Hill BB, Sloan DA, Lee EY, McGrath PC, Kenady DE. Marjolin's ulcer of the foot caused by nonburn trauma. S Med J 1996; 89:707–710.

27. Arons MS, Lynch JB, Rodin AE, Lewis SR. Scar tissue carcinoma. Part II: special reference to burn scar carcinoma. Surg Forum 1965; 16:488–489.

28. Arons MS, Rodin AE, Lynch JB, Lewis SR, Blocker TG. Scar tissue carcinoma. Part II: an experimental study with special reference to burn scar carcinoma. Ann Surg 1966; 163:445–460.

29. Fleming MD, Hunt JL, Purdue GF, Sandstad J. Marjolin's ulcer: a review and reevaluation of a difficult problem. J Burn Care Rehabil 1990; 11:460–469.

30. Hansson C, Andersson E. Malignant skin lesions on the legs and feet at a dermatological leg ulcer clinic during five years. Acta Derm Venereol 1997; 78:147–148.

31. Schmidt ME, Yalisove BL, Parenti DM, Elgart ML, Williams CM. Rapidly progressive penile ulcer: an unusual manifestation of Kaposi's sarcoma. JAAD 1992; 27:267–268.

32. Johnson DE, Chica J, Rodriguez LH, Luna M. Kaposi's sarcoma presenting as scrotal ulcerations. Urology 1977; 9:686–688.

33. Endean ED, Ross CW, Strodel WE. Kaposi's sarcoma appearing as a rectal ulcer. Surgery 1987; 101:767–769.

34. Cribier B, Lipsker D, Grosshans E, Duhem C, Capesius C, Dicato M. Genital ulceration revealing a primary cutaneous anaplastic lymphoma. G U Med 1997; 73:325.

35. Goldstein LJ, Williams JD, Zackheim HS, Helfend LK. Mycosis fungoides masquerading as an ischemic foot. Ann Vasc Surg 1999; 13:305–307.

36. Tnaiguchi S, Kono T, Tanii T, Yokokawa M, Kobayashi H, Nakagawa E, Furukawa M, Ishii M, Im T, Hamada T. Secondary T-cell lymphoma presenting as a giant ulcer. Clin Exp Dermatol 1992; 17:379–381.

37. Stringer MD, Melcher D, Stachan CJL. The lower limb as a presenting site of malignant lymphoma. Ann R Coll Surg Engl 1986; 68:8–11.

38. Salmon-Her V, Grosieux C, Potron G, Kalis B. Multiple actinic keratosis and skin tumors secondary to hydroxyurea treatment. Dermatology 1998; 196:274.

39. Best PJ, Daoud MS, Pittelkow MR, Petitt RM. Hydroxyurea induced leg ulceration in 14 patients. Ann Int Med 1998; 128:29–32.

40. Flores F, Eaglstein WA, Kirsner RS. Hydroxyurea induced leg ulcers treated with Apligraf. Ann Int Med 2000; 132:417–418.

41. Weinlich G, Schuler G, Greil R, Kofler H, Fritsch P. Leg ulcers associated with long term hydroxyurea therapy. JAAD 1998; 39:372–374.

42. Walsh P. Physicians Desk Reference. 55th ed. New Jersey: Medical Economics Company, Inc., 2001.

43. Callot-Mellot C, Bodemer C, Chosidow O, Frances C, Azgui Z, Varet B, De Prost Y. Cutaneous carcinoma during long term hydroxyurea therapy: a report of 5 cases. Arch Dermatol 1996; 132:1395–1397.

44. Weinlich G, Fritsch P. Leg ulcers in patients treated with hydroxyurea for myeloproliferative disorders: what is the trigger. Br J Dermatol 1999; 141:171–172.

45. Lauvin R, Miglianico L, Hellegouarch R. Skin cancer occurring 10 years after the extravasation of doxorubicin. N Engl J Med 1995; 332:754.

46. Coleman JJ, Walker AP, Didolkar MS. Treatment of adriamycin induced skin ulcers: a prospective controlled study. J Surg Oncol 1983; 22:129–135.

47. Broadbent NRG, Brown GED. Adriamycin and soft tissue injury. NZ Med J 1985; 98:71.

48. Hodgkinson DJ. Doxorubicin extravasation injuries. J Hand Surg 1983; 8:498–499.

49. Majeski J, Austin RM, Fitzgerald RH. Cutnaeous angiosarcoma in an irradiated breast after breast conservation therapy for cancer: association with chronic breast lymphedema. J Surg Oncol 2000; 74:208–213.

50. Krasagakis K, Hettmannsperger U, Tebbe B, Garbe C. Cutaneous metastatic angiosarcoma with a lethal outcome, following radiotherapy for a cervical carcinoma. Br J Dermatol 1995; 133:610–614.

51. Goette DK, Detlefs RL. Postirradiation angiosarcoma. JAAD 1985; 12:922–926.

52. Goette DK, Deffer TA. Postirradiation malignant fibrous histiocytoma. Arch Dermatol 1985; 121:535–538.

53. Zhao P, Zhijun L, Yali L, Zhang M, Gu Q, Wang D. Expression of telomerase reverse transcriptase in radiation-induced chronic human skin ulcers. J Environ Pathol Toxicol Oncol 2002; 21:67–70.

54. Zhao P, Yang Z, Wang DW, Gao Y, Li X, Li G. Overexpression of c-erbB-2 and p21 Oncoprotein in human radiation-induced skin ulcers. J Environ Pathol Toxicol Oncol 1995; 14:21–23.

55. Zhao P, Wang D, Gao Y, Yang Z, Li X. Overexpression of MDM2, p53, and NCAM proteins in human radiation-induced skin ulcers. J Environ Pathol Toxicol Oncol 1998; 17:125–127.

56. Rosen T. Cutaneous Metastases. Med Clin NA 1980; 64:885–900.

57. Cohen PR. Skin clues to primary and metastatic malignancy. Am Fam Phys 1995; 51:1199–1204.

58. Ackerman D, Barr RJ, Elias AN. Cutaneous metastases from hepatocellular carcinoma. Int J Dermatol 2001; 40:782–784.

59. Solomon BA, Goldman RJ. Ulcerated nodules and papules on the neck and chest. Arch Dermatol 1997; 133:1454–1458.

60. Sutter CD, Davis BR. Ulcerated papules, plaques, and nodules of the scalp and face. Arch Dermatol 1991; 127:405–408.

61. Helm KF, Su WPD, Muller SA, Kurtin PJ. Malignant lymphoma and leukemia with prominent ulceration: clinicopathologic correlation of 33 cases. JAAD 1992; 27:553–559.

62. Tschen EH, Apisarnthanarax P. Inflammatory metastatic carcinoma of the breast. Arch Dermatol 1981; 117:120–121.

63. Lookingbill DP, Spangler N, Sexton FM. Skin involvement as the presenting sign of internal carcinoma. JAAD 1990; 22:19–26.

64. Montot S, Bosch F, Estrach T, Blade J, Nomdedeu B, Nonserrat E. Pyoderma gangrenosum triggered by alpha 2b interferon in a patient with chronic granulocytic leukemia. Leuk Lymphoma 1998; 30:199–202.

65. Avivi I, Rosenbaum H, Levy Y, Rowe J. Myelodysplastic syndrome and associated skin lesions: a review of the literature. Leuk Res 1999; 23:323–330.

66. Vadillo M, Jucgla A, Podazamczer D, Rufi G, Domingo A. Pyoderma gangrenosum with liver, spleen and bone involvement in a patient with chronic myelomonocytic leukemia. Br J Dermatol 1999; 141:541–543.

67. Paydas S, Zorludemir S, Sahin B. Vasculitis Leuk 2000; 40:105–112.

68. Paydas S, Zorludemir S. Leukemia cutis and leukemic vasculitis. Br J Dermatol 2000; 143:773–779.

69. Odeh M, Misselevich I, Oliven A. Squamous cell carcinoma of the lung presenting with cutaneous leukocyoclastic vasculitis. Angiology 2001; 52:641–644.

70. Gonzalez-Gay MA, Garcia-Porrua C, Salvarani C, Hunder GG. Cutaneous vasculitis and cancer: a clinical approach. Clin Exp Rheum 2000; 18:305–307.

27

Pathology of Skin Ulcers

George W. Elgart
Department of Dermatology and Cutaneous Surgery, University of Miami School of Medicine, Miami, Florida, U.S.A.

Although skin ulcers are an important aspect of dermatologic practice, the histopathology of these fascinating maladies has been minimally and inadequately studied. The reasons for this are twofold. First, clinicians facing difficult skin ulcers are naturally reticent to take samples and worsen the absence of skin which defines these lesions. Second, ulcers are a common skin reaction and many (although not all) conditions which may be diagnosed in ulcers can be seen in non-ulcerated skin, often in the same patient. The natural bias of editors of pathology books and journal articles seems to prefer an illustration which demonstrates epidermis for their "textbook example." This chapter proposes to lay out general circumstances in which histopathology may be useful to the clinician treating skin ulcers and an approach to the biopsy sampling of those ulcers. In the second portion of the chapter, the emphasis will be on those particular types of ulcers most amenable to biopsy and an elucidation of the common features found therein.

In general, the same afflictions which yield to biopsy in non-ulcerated skin are amenable to skin biopsy of ulcerated skin. While many inflammatory or fibrotic conditions are "non-specific" in their histology, tumors, infections, vascular problems (vasculitis and other vasculopathic phenomena), and many immunologic conditions demonstrate pathognomonic signs or constellations of features which allow diagnosis by histopathology. Thus, as with any specimen taken for tissue analysis, assessment of the clinical circumstances is the first and critical step in the pathologic diagnosis of skin ulcers. Careful attention should be paid to the patient and the judgement that the patient suffers from "stasis" or "leg ulcers" should be appreciated as a diagnosis of exclusion. The excluded elements should include ulcers due to cancer, infection, or vasculitis. These three diagnostic categories are especially important to diagnose, as all have specific therapies available and none respond efficiently to routine measures for ulcer therapy.

Most clinicians prefer to limit their biopsies to those cases in which useful information may be gained for the care of the patient. However, even debridement specimens occasionally include useful information and it is the impression of the author that no tissue obtained from a patient should be discarded without at least some sampling for histology. This practice, while common, is far from universal and there are some clinicians who routinely jettison tissue without consideration of possible information lost. This is disappointing, as it is exactly this circumstance which obviates the first concern of clinicians to not worsen a vexing ulcer. They have already taken the tissue and may as well have it evaluated unless the clinical situation is so crystal clear that additional information from a biopsy specimen would prove superfluous. For the specific circumstances in which biopsy is clearly indicated, attention to the details of the case often guide the biopsy. The clinician is faced, as usual, with a series of important questions the answers to which will help in the selection of biopsy sites and technique.

1. HOW MANY ULCERS ARE PRESENT?

The answer to this question will impact on biopsy site since multiple ulcers may favor an infectious or inflammatory cause. In addition, multiple sites may mean that the ulcers are of various ages. While well-developed features are often the most helpful, it is sometimes useful to seek the most recent ulcer if evidence of active vasculitis, thrombi, or infection is sought.

2. WHAT IS THE DISTRIBUTION OF THE ULCERS?

Ulcers in scars or sites of prior physical, thermal, or chemical trauma raise the suspicion of a carcinomatous ulcer. Ulcers in sites of pressure may be a clue to a neuropathic ulcer. Other pressure-associated ulcers are common in bedridden patients. The typical distribution of venous ulcers on the lateral malleolus is certainly a useful clue as to causation.

3. HOW LONG HAVE THE ULCERS BEEN EVIDENT?

The age of the ulcers is a critical question, since very long-standing ulcers are less frequently associated with vasculitis, at least in the active phase. Ulcers of short duration suggest a recent insult and may favor infection or vascular compromise. Ulcers which persist and extend may be associated with cancers or indolent infections.

4. DO THE ULCERS ARISE DE NOVA, OR IS THERE SOME INITIATING OR PRE-EXISTING LESION WHICH ULCERATES?

This is an important issue as in particular, most ulcers due to vascular abnormalities may demonstrate cutaneous findings in the preulcerative phase which are diagnostic. Also, many lesions which ulcerate after a skin lesion is present may demonstrate similar findings at the periphery of even well-developed ulcers, thus allowing a biopsy in a site which may be closed following the procedure and therefore allow for a simpler and more routinely diagnostic procedure. This is particularly important in the setting of vasculitis since it allows avoidance of the situation where the pathologist must decide if the ulcer is a primary process or merely the result of vasculitis "secondary" to the presence of the ulcer.

5. WHAT ARE THE SHAPE AND CHARACTER OF THE ULCERS?

Ulcers with an unusual shape or a tendency to pathergy may favor specific diagnoses. A distribution along a vascular structure is likewise a helpful clue to a vascular component to the ulcer. Bizarre shapes or atypical ulcers may suggest a component of self-destructive behavior or secondary gain. These cases often benefit from extensive evaluation for foreign material within the affected ulcer.

6. HOW HAVE THE ULCERS RESPONDED TO CONSERVATIVE THERAPY?

Ulcers with poor response to conservative therapy are more likely to be due to infections, vascular compromise from vasculitis or cryoproteins, or carcinoma.

7. WHAT IS THE NATURE OF THE PATIENT'S GENERAL HEALTH? ARE THERE KNOWN CONDITIONS WHICH MIGHT YIELD ULCERS?

A patient with known cancer is more likely to have an ulcer as a manifestation of metastasis. Patients with autoimmune conditions including arthritis often have specific causes for their ulcers. A history of sickle cell anemia, for example, clearly pushes one toward consideration of that diagnosis as the cause, while seronegative rheumatoid arthritis or inflammatory bowel disease may be a clue to pyoderma gangrenosum.

8. IS THE PATIENT TAKING MEDICATIONS? IF SO, FOR WHAT PERIOD OF TIME?

Ulcers are rare side effects of numerous medications including methotrexate (17) and warfarin among others. This information can contribute to the evaluation of ulcers and their histopathology.

All of these questions should be considered and the results synthesized into a plan of action. That plan must include the possibility of biopsy and a clear consideration of the best strategy for obtaining the specimen. Once the decision is made to biopsy, one must also consider the information one can and should expect to obtain from the specimen. Not all cutaneous biopsies are diagnostic, but the information available may be informative by excluding some diagnostic considerations.

9. ULCERS WITH DIAGNOSTIC FEATURES

While it is true that many ulcers lack absolutely diagnostic features, some types of ulcers do lend themselves to diagnosis and should be evaluated in detail with the expectation of making a specific diagnosis. In particular, infectious ulcers, ulcers associated with tumors, and certain ulcers with specific vascular abnormalities are completely diagnosable because of pathognomonic features on microscopic evaluation.

10. INFECTIOUS ULCERS

In our practice, the most common infectious causes of skin ulcers are those caused by bacteria or viruses. However, many ulcers associated with fungi or protozoans are reported and worthy of consideration.

10.1. Bacterial Ulcers

10.1.1. Ecthyma Gangrenosum

This ulcer, most frequently the work of *Pseudomonas aeruginosa*, is a relatively common histologic diagnosis in infectious ulcers. The overlying inflamed crust and the deeper dermal structures are found teeming with Gram-negative rods (2).

More recently, interest has focused on cutaneous anthrax infections presenting as skin ulceration. In the recent anthrax outbreak associated with intentionally contaminated mail, several postal workers and recipients developed the characteristic black eschar and cutaneous ulcer associated with the malignant pustule of anthrax (3). The histology in these cases is essentially diagnostic as the Gram-positive rods are large, prominent, and quite dramatic in histologic sections. This diagnosis is worthy of consideration in animal handlers, abbatoir workers, and postal workers who may come in contact with contaminated mail.

10.1.2. Mycobacterial Ulcers

Hansen's disease (leprosy), while uncommon in the United States, generally, remains an important cause of skin ulcers worldwide. The presence of a granulomatous infiltrate in the dermis, particularly when associated with numerous foamy appearing macrophages should suggest the diagnosis of leprosy. In some subsets of leprosy patients, i.e., the reactional state of "Lucio's phenomenon," the primary feature present clinically is ulceration. These unusual patients may demonstrate extraordinarily numerous mycobacteria and numerous vascular alterations which mimic or represent cryoglobulinemia.

Tuberculosis is another cause of ulcer formation, especially in the setting of inoculation tuberculosis. In addition, scrofula, a form of extension of tuberculosis from the lung to the skin, characteristically presents with skin ulcers. The granulomas seen in this setting take on an appearance of a draining sinus.

Of course, non-lepromatous, non-tuberculous mycobacteria represent the largest portion of the mycobacterial ulcers seen in routine practice in the United States. *Mycobacterium chelonei* and M. marinum are the most frequently cited causes. However, many myobacterial species may be responsible and culture of the lesions is critical once the diagnosis is appreciated histologically. These so-called "atypical" mycobacteria are, indeed, the most typical mycobacteria we see. In many cases, the presence of at least some macrophages and giant cells is expected in cases of mycobacterial ulcers.

Few ulcers are as dramatic as those which may be seen in cases of infection with Mycobacterium ulcerans. This unusual mycobacterium is known worldwide, but is especially frequent in sub-Saharan Africa. The ulcers seen in this condition are often extraordinarily large and often show a clean base which, despite all efforts, fails to heal. The histology mainly demonstrates loss of the epidermal surface and a thin crust containing very numerous mycobacterial organisms (Fig. 1).

10.1.3. Fungal Ulcers

Many of the deep mycoses may lead to chronic cutaneous ulceration as a presentation. Notably, inoculation-induced fungi typically lead to the presence of skin ulcers. Sporothrix schenkii and chromoblastomycosis come to mind as among the most common of the fungal infections associated with skin ulceration. In both cases, the histology is absolutely diagnostic in many cases. A few examples are included

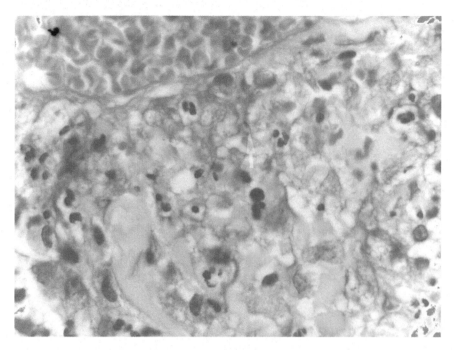

Figure 1 Buruli ulcer due to the mycobacterium *M. ulcerans*. The arrow highlights a bacterium that is generally plentiful in this condition. (Ziehl Neilson stain × 1000)

in the figures. The tiny, cigar-shaped yeasts of sporotricosis or the larger, deeply pigmented stunted hyphae of chromoblastomycosis are often quite easily seen in tissue sections. This can make a diagnostic conundrum quite simple, even in cases which have been present and unresponsive to therapy for many years (Fig. 2).

In unusual situations, other systemic fungal infections present with skin ulceration, notably in cases of Aspergillus infection or in some cases of cryptococcosis or coccidioidomycosis. While neither diagnosis is common, the diagnostic value of the histopathology cannot be overstated (Fig. 3).

10.1.4. Viral Ulcers

Viral ulcers are rare, but represent an important diagnostic category amenable to histologic evaluation (Fig. 4). In particular, herpesvirus infections are well known as causes of chronic skin ulcers, particularly in the setting of immune suppression. Both cytomegalovirus (SMV) and varicella virus are common causes in addition to the usual diagnostic consideration of herpes simplex. While the histology of these three viruses is remarkably similar in many cases, immunohistochemistry is available to readily separate these diagnoses. In instances of immunosuppression, chronic ulcers may be observed due either to herpes viruses or to CMV. Ulcers due to CMV are difficult to diagnose clinically, but histologic features and immunochemical identification of the CMV virions are essentially diagnostic (Fig. 5).

10.1.5. Protozoal Ulcers

While rare, protozoal ulcers due to amebae or leishmania are well documented. The histology is routinely useful and only close evaluation of the respective infiltrates and some use of special stains are necessary to confirm the diagnosis in most cases.

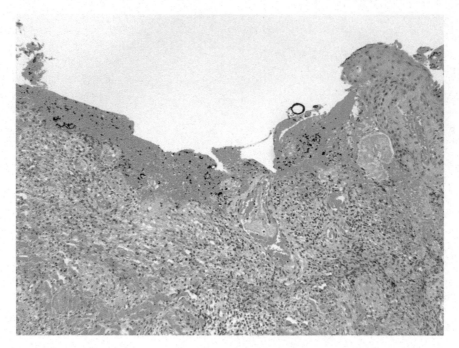

Figure 2 Ulcerated epidermis in a case of chromoblastomycosis. The stunted hyphae appear as round shapes called Medlar bodies. (H&E × 400)

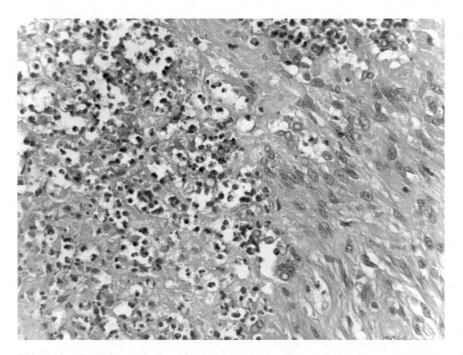

Figure 3 Organisms of *Coccidioides immitis* are diagnostic in skin sections. These lesions routinely present as ulcers. (H&E × 400)

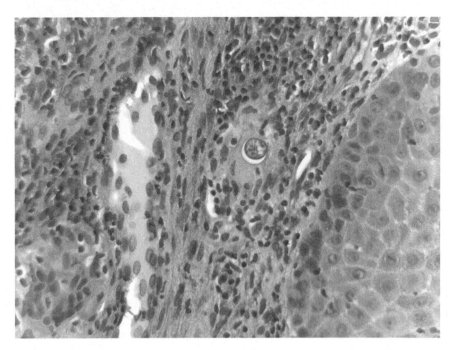

Figure 4 Chronic ulcers due to herpes viruses are common in immune suppressed hosts. (H&E × 100)

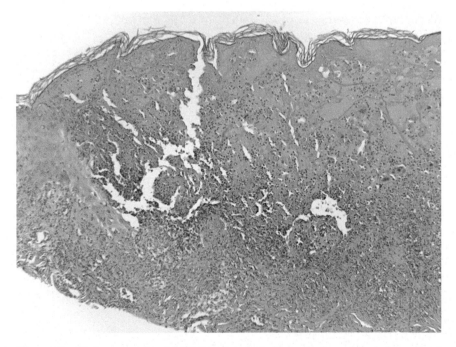

Figure 5 High power view highlights the viral giant cells in a chronic herpetic ulcer. These features often require close inspection for diagnosis although diagnosis may be aided by immunohistochemistry. (H&E × 400)

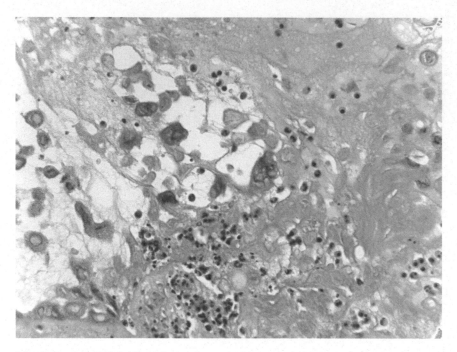

Figure 6 Marjolin's ulcer shows the typical features of squamous cell carcinoma in the base. (H&E × 400)

10.1.6. Ulcers Associated with Tumors

Malignant tumors are common causes of persistent ulceration resistant to therapy. There are two alternative settings in which malignant ulcers are seen. In the first, an ulcer occurs due to necrosis or breakdown of another malignant process. Frequently, routine skin malignancies including basal cell or squamous cell carcinoma or malignant melanoma ulcerate. In addition, less common tumors including lymphomas, sarcomas, or metastatic carcinomas may present with skin ulceration. This situation is often reason enough to obtain biopsy evaluation of unresponsive or atypical ulcers.

The second circumstance to consider is the presence of a malignancy in the late stages of a persistent ulcer. The "Marjolin's ulcer" is a typical example of this type (4,5). Ulcers that fail to granulate or persist despite appropriate therapy should be considered as potential malignant ulcers. This diagnosis, as the prognosis of these chronic irritation induced carcinomas, is said to be much worse than routine skin squamous cell carcinomas and to demonstrate a remarkably enhanced metastatic rate (6).

The histologic features are identical to those in usual SCC except for the lack of epidermis. The deep ulceration present overlies atypical squamous epithelium with mitotic figures, increased nucleus: cytoplasm ratio and other evidence of malignancy (7). Interestingly, these cases almost universally demonstrate surrounding fibrosis and cicatrix formation (Fig. 6).

11. ULCERS DUE TO VASCULAR ABNORMALITIES AND INFLAMMATORY DISEASES

Vasculitis and inflammatory diseases are important causes of cutaneous ulceration. Histology may aid in evaluating these lesions by demonstrating the presence (or absence) of vasculitis, inflammatory infiltrates, granulomas, and thrombi. Many such cases are essentially diagnostic and nearly all eventuate in the elimination of some differential diagnostic considerations.

11.1. Specific Diagnoses
11.1.1. Leukocytoclastic Vasculitis

Leukocytoclastic vasculitis (LCV) presents most commonly as palpable purpura, but in advanced or severe cases may show ulceration. The presence of fibrinous degeneration of the vascular endothelium along with other signs of vasculitis (nuclear dust, perivascular hemorrhage, and vascular destruction) is indicative of LCV and is often associated with various forms of collagen vascular disease, some severe medication reactions, and infections. Identification of this pathology is helpful in that it may lead to proper diagnosis and therapy of the inciting cause. Leukocytoclastic vasculitis is a reaction pattern, and the many causes of the condition must be sorted out. However, it is appreciated that true ulcerating lesions are rare in association with self-limited post-streptococcal and infectious causes and favor systemic involvement. Thus, histology of leukocytoclastic vasculitis in the setting of ulcers requires extensive evaluation for possible systemic involvement (Fig. 7).

11.1.2. Cryoglobuinemia and Cryofibrinogenemia

Cryoproteinemias are causes of ulceration in which the histology characteristically demonstrates features sufficiently helpful to support diagnosis (Fig. 8). In monoclonal cryoglobulinemia, the presence of an eosinophilic, pink coagulum filling dermal

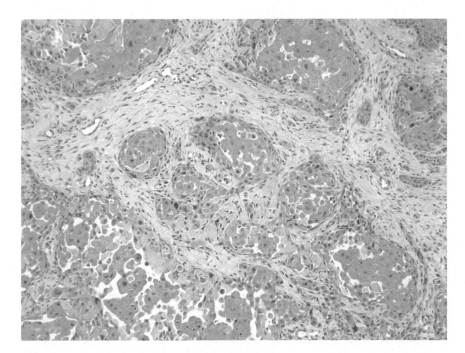

Figure 7 Impressive vascular destruction with fibrin deposition is typical of leukocytoclastic vasculitis. Care must be exercised to exclude that the vasculitis is a minor, secondary feature due to ulceration of the overlying epidermis. (H&E × 100)

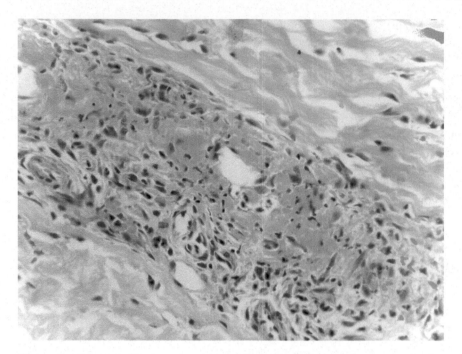

Figure 8 Cryoglobulins form an eosinophilic homogeneous collection in the dermal blood vessels evident in cases of type I cryoglobulinemia. (H&E × 100)

venules is essentially diagnostic. Other, mixed forms of cryoglobulins may demonstrate only leukocytoclastic vasculitis or may demonstrate other significant features (8). The confirmation of the presence of cryoproteins by serological tests is a demanding process, but should be done to assure appropriate diagnosis and therapy (Fig. 9).

11.2. Erythema Induratum

11.2.1. Pyoderma Gangrenosum

Controversy abounds regarding the histopathology of pyoderma gangrenosum (Fig. 10). The many and varied clinical associations and variations of the syndrome reported may support that more than one diagnosis is subsumed under this name. Considering the lack of any diagnostic test and the widespread clinical application of the term, it may be best to focus on histologic diagnosis in association with the clinical evidence of pathergy, an associated condition, and clinical response to anti-inflammatory regimens.

While pyoderma gangrenosum remains a diagnosis of exclusion, the presence of an undermined border to an ulcer with marked neutrophilic inflammation is a strong indicator of the condition (Fig. 11) (9).

11.2.2. Histological Clues

1. Follicular and perifollicular infiltrates of neutrophils (10).
2. Lymphocytic infiltrates surrounding edematous vessels at the advancing margin.
3. Lack of clear cut leukocytoclastic vasculitis.
4. Dense mixed inflammation and abscess formation at the ulcer base.

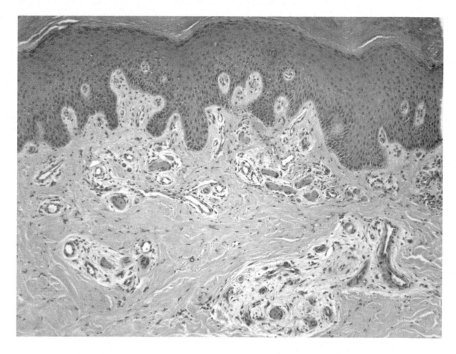

Figure 9 A high power view highlights the vessels containing cryoproteins. (H&E × 400)

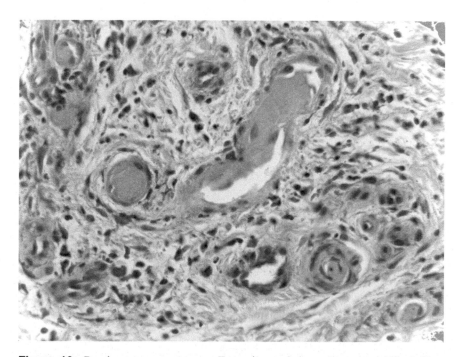

Figure 10 Pyoderma gangrenosum. Extensive and dramatic neutrophilic infiltrates at the margins of the ulcer or involving follicles favor pyoderma gangrenosum. True vasculitis with fibrin deposition should raise concern of alternative diagnoses. (H&E × 100)

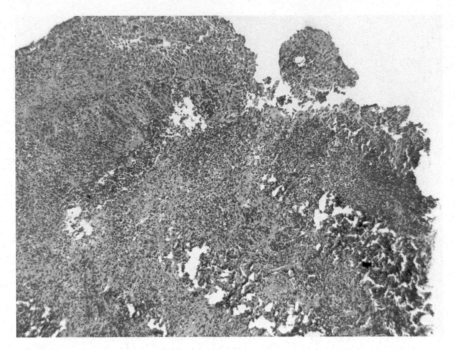

Figure 11 A case of pyoderma gangrenosum showing an undermined edge of the ulcer. Note the lack of evident vasculitis. (H&E × 100)

11.2.3. Hypertensive Ulcer (Martorell's Ulcer)

This is another example of a probably less rare problem that is not appreciated due to the rarity of biopsy of the lesion. The clinical setting is the presence of an ulcer unresponsive to compression therapy in a patient with poorly controlled hypertension. The patients characteristically complain of pain. Therapy of the hypertension resolves or improves the ulcer. The major histologic finding is markedly hyperplastic arterioles at the base of the ulcer. Vascular proliferation of the veins, fibrosis, and other findings of lipodermatosclerosis are not appreciated (Fig. 12).

11.2.4. Martorell's Ulcer

This is another example of a probably less rare problem that is not appreciated due to the rarity of biopsy of the lesion. The clinical setting is the presence of an ulcer unresponsive to compression therapy in a patient with poorly controlled hypertension (11). The patients characteristically complain of pain. Therapy of the hypertension resolves or improves the ulcer (12). The major histologic finding is markedly hyperplastic arterioles at the base of the ulcer (13). Vascular proliferation of the veins, fibrosis, and other findings of lipodermatosclerosis are not appreciated.

12. ULCERS DUE TO FIBROTIC CONDITIONS

12.1. Lipodermatosclerosis (Venous Ulcer, Sclerosing Panniculitis)

Venous disease is said to be the most common cause of ulcers, and is particularly so in the lower extremity (14). I do not favor the term "venous stasis" as it is a misnomer, but the epidermal and superficial dermal findings of "stasis dermatitis"

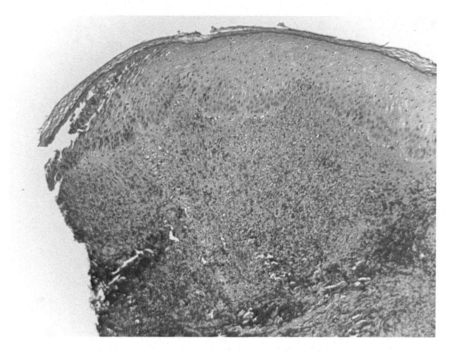

Figure 12 Hyperplastic arterioles at the base of a hypertensive (Martorell's) ulcer. (H&E × 100)

are actually common in biopsies of lipodermatosclerosis (Figs. 13 and 14). The changes seen can be divided into early and late alterations (Fig. 15).

12.1.1. Histologic clues
Early:
1. Mild chronic panniculitis at the border of the dermis and the subcutis.
2. Minimal fibrosis of the lower dermis.
3. Chronic inflammation, often with admixed eosinophils.
4. Minimal vascular changes except for pericapillary fibrin in some cases (16).
5. Lipomembranous change in the subcutis in some examples (17).

Late:
1. Almost always mild epidermal spongiosis.
2. Superficial vascular fibrosis with vascular proliferation.
3. Loss of elastic tissue on Van Gieson staining.
4. Hemosiderin deposition and perivascular hemorrhage.
5. Chronic inflammation, but no panniculitis.
6. No eosinophils in the deeper dermis.

12.2. Pressure Ulcers and Neuropathic Ulcers

These ulcers are usually sampled as part of a debridement procedure or as an evaluation for an infectious cause or neoplastic change in the ulcer. While the base of the ulcer is typically not revealing, the margins of the ulcer often demonstrate characteristic changes. Despite an appearance suggestive in many cases of verruca vulgaris, the tissue present does not demonstrate papilloma virus (Fig. 16).

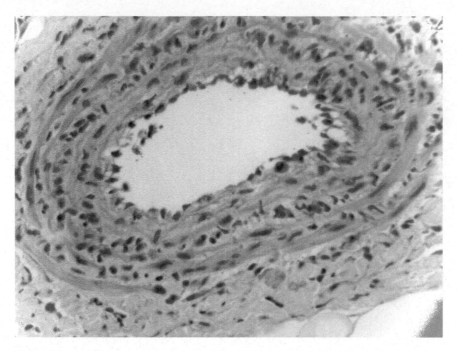

Figure 13 Lipodermatosclerosis. In this early ulcer, there is clear evidence of panniculitis at the dermal-subcutaneous interface. (H&E × 100)

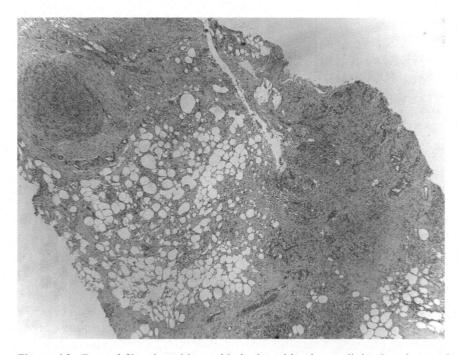

Figure 14 Dermal fibrosis and hemosiderin deposition in a well-developed example of lipodermatosclerosis. (H&E × 400)

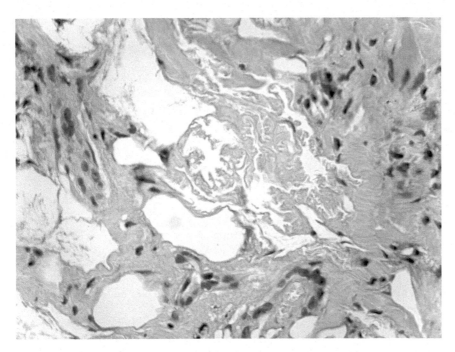

Figure 15 Lipomembranous change (panniculitis) is a frequent feature of lipodermatos-clerosis. (H&E × 400)

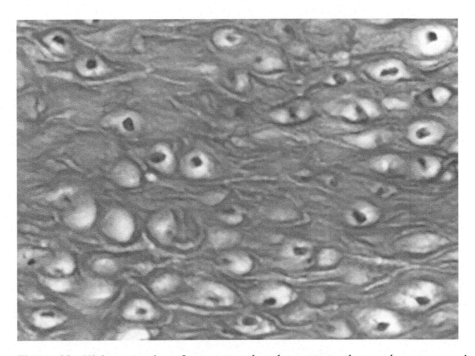

Figure 16 High power view of a pressure ulcer demonstrates the pseudo verrucous change seen at the ulcer edge. Immunohistochemistry has not demonstrated papilloma virus particles in the affected skin. (H&E × 400)

12.2.1. Histological Clues

1. The ulcer center is not diagnostic, but is often filled with necrotic debris or material.
2. Ulcer callus demonstrates remarkable hyper and parakeratosis with an alteration of the epidermis which is suggestive of the hyperkeratosis seen in verrucae.
3. Oval parakeratotic nuclei.
4. No atypia or significant hypergranulosis.

REFERENCES

1. Kazlow DW, Federgrun D, Kurtin S, Lebwohl MG. Cutaneous ulceration caused by methotrexate. J Am Acad Dermatol 2003; 49(suppl 2 case reports):S197–S198.
2. Sevinsky LD, Viecens C, Ballesteros DO, Stengel F. Ecthyma gangrenosum: a cutaneous manifestation of Pseudomonas aeruginosa sepsis. J Am Acad Dermatol 1993; 29(1): 104–106.
3. Shieh WJ, et al. The critical role of pathology in the investigation of bioterrorism-related cutaneous anthrax. Am J Pathol 2003; 163(5):1901–1910.
4. Smith J, Mello LF, Nogueira Neto NC, Meohas W, Pinto LW, Campos VA, Barcellos.
5. MG, Fiod NJ, Rezende JF, Cabral CE. Malignancy in chronic ulcers and scars of the leg (Marjolin's ulcer): a study of 21 patients. Skeletal Radiol 2001; 30(6):331–337.
6. Kirsner RS, Spencer J, Falanga V, Garland LE, Kerdel FA. Squamous cell carcinoma arising in osteomyelitis and chronic wounds. Treatment with Mohs micrographic surgery vs. amputation. Dermatol Surg 1996; 22(12):1015–1018.
7. Wu ML, Natarajan S, Lewin KJ. Peculiar artifacts mimicking carcinoma. Arch Pathol Lab Med 2001; 125(11):1473–1476.
8. Klein AD, Kerdel FA. Purpura and recurrent ulcers on the lower extremities. Essential cryofibrinogenemia. Arch Dermatol 1991; 127(1):115–118.
9. Powell FC, Schroeter AL, Su WP, Perry HO. Pyoderma gangrenosum: a review of 86 patients. Q J Med 1985; 55(217):173–186.
10. Huang W, McNeely MC. Neutrophilic tissue reactions. Adv Dermatol 1997; 13:33–64.
11. Graves JW, Morris JC, Sheps SG. Martorell's hypertensive leg ulcer: case report and concise review of the literature. J Hum Hypertens 2001; 15(4):279–283.
12. Henderson CA, Highet AS, Lane SA, Hall R. Arterial hypertension causing leg ulcers. Clin Exp Dermatol 1995; 20(2):107–114.
13. Bello YM, Falabella AF, Kirsner RS, Elgart GW, Kerdel FA. Hypertensiveulcer ulcer. Wounds 2002; 14(4):131–135.
14. Burnand KG, Whimster I, Naidoo A, Browse NL. Pericapillary fibrin in the ulcer-bearing skin of the leg: the cause of lipodermatosclerosis and venous ulceration. BMJ (Clin Res Ed) 1982; 285:1071–1072.
15. Kirsner RS, Pardes JB, Eaglstein WH, Falanga V. The clinical spectrum of lipodermatosclerosis. J Am Acad Dermatol 1993; 28:623–627.
16. Jorizzo JL, White WL, Zanolli MD, Greer KE, Solomon AR, Jetton RL. Sclerosing panniculitis: a clinicopathologic assessment. Arch Dermatol 1991; 127:554–558.
17. Chun SI, Chung KY. Membranous lipodystrophy: secondary type. J Am Acad Dermatol 1994; 31:601–605.

28
Immunosuppression and Wound Healing

Tory P. Sullivan

Department of Dermatology and Cutaneous Surgery, University of Miami School of Medicine, Miami, Florida, U.S.A.

1. INTRODUCTION

Chronic immunosuppression is an important potential barrier to wound healing. Many conditions result in relative immunosuppression including advanced age, and disease states such as diabetes. However, in these cases, immunosuppression is a secondary process and poor wound healing is a result of a number of factors. This chapter will examine wound healing in patients who have primary immunodeficiencies.

2. EPIDEMIOLOGY

Over the past several decades, wound healing in the immunosuppressed patient has become an increasingly important issue for clinicians. Improved outcomes in organ transplantation, better treatment of HIV/AIDS, advances in oncology and the aging U.S. population have caused the number of Americans living with chronic immunosuppression to swell dramatically. In 2001, over 24,000 solid organ transplants were performed in the United States, and over 80,000 patients are currently waiting to receive an organ transplant (1). Further advances such as xenotransplantation dramatically swell the number patients living with chronic immunosuppression. Although the rate of new HIV infections has slowed, improved treatment means that the number of Americans living with HIV continues to increase. The Centers for Disease Control and Prevention (CDC) estimate that 800,000 to 900,000 U.S. residents are infected with HIV (2). The number of Americans who are iatrogenically immunosuppressed as a result of therapy for malignancy or autoimmune and inflammatory disease is unknown. However, the American Cancer Society estimates that over 1,200,000 Americans will be diagnosed with cancer in 2002 (3). It is not be unreasonable to assume that many millions of Americans are currently living with chronic immunosuppression.

3. THE ACUTE WOUND

As patients live longer with chronic immunosuppression, they will require elective and/or semi-elective surgical procedures. Wound care clinicians will be asked to provide guidance to both patients and other healthcare providers as to the patient's ability to heal should a procedure be undertaken. Examples include a kidney transplant patient who may be a candidate for knee replacement surgery or a patient taking methotrexate for psoriasis who is considering cosmetic surgery. Wound care clinicians will also be called upon to treat acute wounds in these patients whether they occur as a result of elective and emergency interventions.

4. THE NEUTROPENIC PATIENT

Entry of neutrophils into the wound bed occurs within the first 24 hours of wounding and is a critical first step in the wound healing process. Reduced neutrophil infiltration postwounding results in delayed wound healing independent of the risk for infection (4). Patients with a congenital absence of or defects in neutrophil function exhibit delayed and/or absent wound healing (5–10). A number of acquired and congenital conditions have been associated with clinical and/or sub-clinical defects in neutrophilic function (Table 1). The two important groups that are likely to be encountered by the clinician are HIV+ patients and patients undergoing chemotherapy. Fortunately, neutropenia associated with chemotherapy is generally brief. Procedures can either be delayed during episodes of neutropenia or wounds managed conservatively with the knowledge that with restoration of neutrophil counts normal wound healing will proceed. In contrast, HIV+ patients may experience prolonged deficiencies in neutrophil function. Neutrophil defects including abnormalities in chemotaxis, phagocytosis, and bacterial killing can be detected at all stages of

Table 1 Conditions Causing Neutropenia or Impaired Neutrophil Function

---

Neutropenia
Congenital
  Cyclic neutropenia
Acquired
  Drug-induced: alkylating agents, antimetabolites, antibiotics
  Hematologic diseases: aplastic anemia, idiopathic myelodysplasia
  Nutritional deficiency: vitamin B_{12}, folate
  Autoimmune disorders: rheumatoid arthritis, lupus erythematosus
Impaired neutrophil function
Congenital
  Chronic granulomatous disease, Chediak-Higashi syndrome, leukocyte adhesion protein deficiency, Job's syndrome
Acquired
  Drug induced: glucocorticoids, colchicine, alcohol, ibuprofen
  Hematologic diseases: acute and chronic myelogenous leukemia
  Nutritional deficiency: malnutrition
  Autoimmune disorders: rheumatoid arthritis, lupus erythematosus
  Infection: HIV, sepsis
  Other: hemodialysis, diabetes mellitus, severe burn injury

HIV infection and absolute neutropenia is a well-recognized complication of advanced HIV infection (11–16). The level at which reduced neutrophil counts and/or function clinically impact wound healing is not known but it is reasonable to assume that more severe the patients defect in neutrophilic function the more likely delayed wound healing will occur. Early work suggests that granulocyte-macrophage colony-stimulating factor (GM-CSF) and/or granulocyte colony-stimulating factor (G-CSF) may improve wound healing in patients with defects in neutrophilic function (17,18). Case reports describe benificial effects on wound healing in surgical patients with both acquired and congenital neutropenia (6,19,20). Further controlled studies are needed to evaluate the utility of these agents in patients with impaired neutrophilic function.

5. THE HIV+ PATIENT

The role of T-lymphocytes in wound healing is complex. They appear in significant numbers in the wound around day 5 and their numbers peak around day 8 (21). Animal models have shown impaired would healing after global (CD4 and CD8) lymphocyte depletion. Wounds in these animals demonstrate significantly reduced breaking strength, and decreased collagen synthesis (22,23). However, depletion of CD4= lymphocytes alone results in no differences in wound strength and/or collagen formation and depletion of CD8+ lymphocytes resulted in increased wound strength (24). T-lymphocytes appear to act as regulators of the wound healing process and through secretion of cytokines T-lymphocytes can have both upregulatory and downregulatory effects on various aspects of the wound healing process (25).

A number of reports have suggested that reduced numbers of CD lymphocytes in HIV+ patients result in impaired healing (26–38). Lord (39) retrospectively evaluated 101 HIV+ patients who underwent a total of 106 anorectal operations. Patients with a CD4 count of less than 50 were significantly more likely to experience delayed or absent wound healing than those with higher CD4 counts. Additionally, even after complete healing scar tissue in HIV+ patients is significantly weaker as measured by several biomechanical parameters (40). Cytokines secreted by T-lymphocytes regulate fibroblast migration, fibroblast replication, and collagen synthesis. Impaired wound healing in HIV+ patients with reduced T-lymphocyte counts may be related to reduced and/or dysregulated cytokine secretion (41–44). It appears that HIV+ patients experience clinically impaired healing primarily when CD4 counts are less than 200 and that poor wound healing is linearly related to the reduction in CD4 counts. From a practical standpoint, this means that patients with CD4 counts of greater than 200 will in most cases experience clinically normal wound healing. Patients with CD4 counts of less than 200 should avoid elective procedures and when procedures are unavoidable, the clinician should consider the early introduction of advanced therapies generally reserved for recalcitrant wounds.

6. THE IATROGENICALLY IMMUNOSUPPRESSED PATIENT

The effects of immunosuppression following organ transplantation on wound healing are poorly understood. The reasons for this are multiple. First, immunosuppressive regiments involve multiple drugs with varied mechanisms of action. Second, immunosuppressive utilized and the dose administered vary depending on the organ transplanted, the patient and the preferences of the transplant surgeon. Third, some immunosuppressives may have direct effects on wound healing independent of their effects on immune function. Unlike in HIV, there is no benchmark for degree of immunosuppression equivalent to a CD4 count. For these reasons, it is best to examine separately the various immunosuppressive agents and their effects on wound healing.

6.1. Cyclosporin

Since its introduction in the early 1980s, cyclosporine has revolutionized immunosuppressive therapy. As the first relatively specific and effective immunosuppressive, it has resulted in greatly improved outcomes post-transplant. Subsequent to the development of cyclosporine, both tacrolimus and sirolimus have been introduced. Although these compounds differ structurally, their mechanisms of action are similar. These agents inhibit the activation and maturation of T cells by blocking the expression of several lymphokine genes including IL-2 (45). The effects of these agents on acute wound healing in humans have not been studied. In rats cyclosporin impairs wound healing but only when supra pharmacologic doses are administered (46). In studies of pharmacologic doses neither wound strength nor histologic appearance of the healed wound were different from control (47,48).

6.2. Glucocorticoids

Corticosteroids remain a cornerstone of immunosuppressive therapy. Clinicians have long recognized that oral corticosteroids appear to impair wound healing and increase the risk of wound complications (49,50). In vitro studies and animal models have shown that glucocorticoids slow the appearance of inflammatory cells and fibroblasts in the acute wound, decrease collagen deposition, reduce wound contraction, decrease wound tensile strength, and inhibit epithelial migration (51–55).

6.3. Azathioprine

Azathioprine inhibits purine synthesis and is cytotoxic to proliferating lymphocytes. Only animal studies of azathioprine effects on wound healing are available. When given with prednisone, retardation of early re-epithelialization is seen but wound strength and late re-epithelialization are not affected (56).

6.4. Mycophenolate Mofetil (MMF)

Mycophenolate mofetil inhibits proliferative responses of T- and B-lymphocytes to antigen stimulation. In a single prospective study of 12 renal transplant patients, where MMF was the sole immunosuppressive agent administered wound-healing disturbances were reported in two of the patients (57). It is difficult to draw any conclusions from this small uncontrolled series.

Because there are no benchmarks equivalent to the CD4 count in the HIV+ patient, or the neutrophil count in the chemotherapy patient, the clinician should consider a number of variables when assessing the patient's risk for poor wound healing. First, patients whose immunosuppressive regiments include glucocorticoids, with their known effects on wound healing, are more likely to be poor wound healers. Second, a patient with a history of opportunistic infections is probably more immunosuppressed than the patient who has experienced no opportunistic infections. Finally, good communication with the transplant surgeon is critical. The transplant surgeon can inform the wound care clinician as to whether an individual patient has had multiple rejection episodes necessitating a high degree of immunosuppression or if an individual patient has been tolerant of the transplanted organ permitting only low level immunosuppression.

6.5. Antineoplastic Agents

Treatment with antineoplastic agents can result in both neutropenia and lymphopenia with resulting deficiencies in wound healing. Additionally, many of these agents target rapidly proliferating malignant cells and as a consequence may also affect proliferating cells in the wound bed. A priori one would expect these agents to result in impaired wound healing and a number of animal studies support this assumption. Evaluations in mice of single injections of vincristine, methotrexate, actinomycin D, bleomycin, and carmustine (BCNU) revealed that all reduced wound breaking strength (58). Other animal studies have demonstrated impaired wound healing from cyclophosphamide and 5-FU (58,59). It is surprising then that studies of patients undergoing pre and/or peri-operative chemotherapy fail to demonstrate clinically impaired wound healing as measured by length of hospital stay, number of outpatient dressings, seroma formation, and post-operative infections (60,61). Similarly several studies of methotrexate for the treatment of rheumatoid arthritis have failed to demonstrate impaired wound healing (62–64). Thus, even though these agents may theoretically affect wound healing as evidenced by animal models, they do not appear to cause clinically significant impaired wound healing.

7. THE CHRONIC WOUNDS

There is currently only a limited understanding of the impact of immunosuppression on chronic wounds. Based on what is known about acute wounds, it would be expected that immunosuppression delays healing. One study of neuropathic plantar ulcers compared 9 diabetic transplant patients with 14 controls matched for age, sex, and ulcer size and depth (65). All patients achieved complete healing. However, immunosuppressed patients healed significantly more slowly, with complete healing at a mean of 111 days vs. 47 days for controls. The patients' immunosuppressive regimens were varied so it is not clear if any single agent was responsible for poor wound healing. At least one additional study has confirmed these results in transplant patients (66). At present there are no data concerning the prognosis of chronic ulcers in HIV+ patients although most clinicians believe advanced HIV infection is a risk factor for poor wound healing. It is clear that increasingly clinicians will be treating HIV+ patients with chronic cutaneous ulcers. At one time, HIV infection primarily affected young and middle aged adults; however, as care for HIV-infected patients improves the older HIV-infected patient is becoming more common. Whether chronic immunosuppression is an independent risk factor for the development of noninfectious chronic cutaneous ulcers is not known.

Based on understanding of the role of the immune system in wound healing and the data available concerning acute wound healing in the immunosuppressed patient, it is possible to draw some tentative conclusions concerning the impact of immunosuppression on chronic wound healing. First, immunosuppression negatively impacts the ability of the patient to heal. Second, the degree of impact is directly related to the degree of immunosuppression. Clearly further investigation is required as little in known about the relationship that immunosuppression plays in the development and healing of chronic wounds.

8. WOUND INFECTION

Although HIV primarily affects CD4+ lymphocytes all limbs of the immune system are impacted owing to the CD4+ lymphocytes role as immune system coordinator/regulator (67,68). Of special importance when considering the risk for wound infection are defects in neutrophil function. Defects including abnormalities in chemotaxis, phagocytosis, and bacterial killing can be detected at all stages of HIV infection; however, clinically significant impairment of function is normally only apparent at CD4 counts of less than 200/cu mm (12–15,69). A number of studies have evaluated the risk of wound infection in HIV+ positive patients undergoing surgical procedures. One retrospective review compared the rate of post-operative wound infections between 40 HIV negative and 43 HIV positive hemophiliacs (70). Together these patients underwent a total of 169 procedures. The mean CD4 level in the HIV+ group was 335/cu mm. No significant differences in post-operative wound infections were observed. Conversely, in another study wound infection was more frequent in 40 HIV+ surgical patients as compared to non-HIV-infected controls (71). However a subset of the HIV+ patients, those with a CD4 cell counts greater than 500 had no increased risk of infection. At least two additional studies have demonstrated that HIV+ patients with CD4 counts of less than 200 have significantly increased incidence of surgical wound infection (72,73). It appears that the CD4 count determines the risk of post-operative wound infection with risk of infection increased when CD4 counts are below 200. As wound infection rates are increased only when CD4 counts are below 200, it is reasonable that in the HIV+ patient with a CD4 count of over 200 only standard antibiotic prophylaxis should be used. Specific data and/or recommendations for pre- and post-surgical antibiotic therapy in patients with CD4 counts under 200 are lacking.

Recently large multicenter prospective cohort studies have reported that plasma viral load is an even better predictor of clinical outcome in HIV than CD4 counts (74). Similarly, at least one study has suggested that viral load may become an even better predictor than CD4 counts of those patients at increased risk for surgical wound infection (75).

Data regarding the effects of immunosuppressive drugs and antineoplastic agents on rates of post-operative at first appear to be contradictory. A prospective study of 4468 surgical patients determined that the rate of wound infection for patient's undergoing concomitant treatment with immunosuppressive drugs was more than double (7.8%) that of the overall infection rates (3.2%) (76). Yet as previously discussed several other studies show no increase in the rate of post-operative wound infection in patients undergoing either chemotherapy or immunosuppressive therapy for psoriasis (62,77–79). Likely these conflicting data represent a situation analogous to that of the HIV+ patient. Patients on mild or moderately immunosuppressive regiments have no or little increased risk of infection whereas profoundly suppressed patients face increased risk for infection. The challenge for the clinician to assess the degree of immunosuppression. As previously discussed, other factors can be used as surrogates for degree of immunosuppression. Does the immunosuppressive regiment include glucocorticoids, are large doses of immunosuppressives being used, does the patient have a history of opportunistic infections? As in the HIV+ patient, patients on immunosuppressive should receive only standard antibiotic prophylaxis. There are no data that additional antibiotics decrease infection rates and overuse of antibiotics increases side effects and promotes super-infection and resistance.

9. CONCLUSION

Advances in organ transplantation, better treatment of HIV/AIDS, and the aging U.S. population mean that the immunosuppressed patient has become and will continue to compose an important segment of patient for the wound care clinician. Understanding the impact of immunosuppression on wound healing prepares the clinician to communicate with patients, advised other healthcare workers and to help make informed and timely therapy decisions.

REFERENCES

1. Transplant Patient DataSource (2000, February 16) Richmond, VA United Network for Organ Sharing. Retrieved July 19, 2002 from the World Wide Web: http://www.patients.unos.org.
2. Centers for Disease Control and Prevention (CDC). Guidelines for national human immunodeficiency virus case surveillance, including monitoring for human immunodeficiency virus infection and acquired immunodeficiency syndrome. MMWR 1999; 48(RR-13):1–27, 29–31.
3. http://www.cancer.org/downloads/STT/CancerFacts&Figures2002TM.pdf.
4. Nagaoka T, Kaburagi Y, Hamaguchi Y, et al. Delayed wound healing in the absence of intercellular adhesion molecule-1 or L-selectin expression. Am J Pathol 2000; 157(1):237–247.
5. Jung LK. Association of aberrant F-actin formation with defective leukocyte chemotaxis and recurrent pyoderma. Clin Immunol Immunopathol 1991; 61(1):41–54.
6. Besner GE, Glick PL, Karp MP, et al. Recombinant human granulocyte colony-stimulating factor promotes wound healing in a patient with congenital neutropenia. J Pediatr Surg 1992; 27(3):288–290; discussion 291.
7. Kuijpers TW, Van Lier RA, Hamann D, et al. Leukocyte adhesion deficiency type 1 (LAD-1)/variant. A novel immunodeficiency syndrome characterized by dysfunctional beta2 integrins. J Clin Invest 1997; 100(7):1725–1733.
8. Ambruso DR, Knall C, Abell AN, et al. Human neutrophil immunodeficiency syndrome is associated with an inhibitory Rac2 mutation. Proc Natl Acad Sci USA 2000; 97(9):4654–4659.
9. Harris ES, Shigeoka AO, Li W, Adams RH, et al. A novel syndrome of variant leukocyte adhesion deficiency involving defects in adhesion mediated by beta1 and beta2 integrins. Blood 2001; 97(3):767–776.
10. Roos D, Kuijpers TW, Mascart-Lemone F. A novel syndrome of severe neutrophil dysfunction: unresponsiveness confined to chemotaxin-induced functions. Blood 1993; 81(10):2735–2743.
11. Tufail A, Holland GN, Fisher TC, et al. Increased polymorphonuclear leukocyte rigidity in HIV infected individuals. Br J Ophthalmol 2000; 84(7):727–731.
12. Schaumann R, Krosing J, Shah PM, et al. Phagocytosis of Escherichia coli and Staphylococcus aureus by neutrophils of human immunodeficiency virus-infected patients. Eur J Med Res 1998; 3(12):546–548.

13. Roilides E, Mertins S, Eddy J, et al. Impairment of neutrophil chemotactic and bactericidal function in children infected with human immunodeficiency virus type 1 and partial reversal after in vitro exposure to granulocyte-macrophage colony-stimulating factor. J Pediatr 1990; 117(4):531–540.

14. Kuritzkes DR. Neutropenia, neutrophil dysfunction, and bacterial infection in patients with human immunodeficiency virus disease: the role of granulocyte colony-stimulating factor. Clin Infect Dis 2000; 30(2):256–260.

15. Pitrak DL. Neutrophil deficiency and dysfunction in HIV-infected patients. Am J Health Syst Pharm 1999; 56(suppl 5):S9–S16.

16. Moore DA, Benepal T, Portsmouth S, et al. Etiology and natural history of neutropenia in human immunodeficiency virus disease: a prospective study. Clin Infect Dis 2001; 32(3):469–475.

17. Gerber A, Struy H, Weiss G, et al. Effect of granulocyte colony-stimulating factor treatment on ex vivo neutrophil functions in non-neutropenic surgical intensive care patients. J Interferon Cytokine Res 2000; 20(12):1083–1090.

18. Canturk NZ, Vural B, Esen N, et al. Effects of granulocyte-macrophage colony-stimulating factor on incisional wound healing in an experimental diabetic rat model. Endocr Res 1999; 25(1):105–116.

19. Cody DT II, Funk GF, Wagner D, et al. The use of granulocyte colony stimulating factor to promote wound healing in a neutropenic patient after head and neck surgery. Head Neck 1999; 21(2):172–175.

20. Mastroianni A, Cancellieri C. Local treatment of a chronic leg ulcer with GM-CSF in a patient with HIV infection. Sex Transm Infect 1999; 75(3):203–204.

21. Fishel RS, Barbul A, Beschorner WE, et al. Lymphocyte participation in wound healing. Morphologic assessment using monoclonal antibodies. Ann Surg 1987; 206(1):25–29.

22. Efron JE, Frankel HL, Lazarou SA, et al. Wound healing and T-lymphocytes. J Surg Res 1990; 48(5):460–463.

23. Peterson JM, Barbul A, Breslin RJ, et al. Significance of T-lymphocytes in wound healing. Surgery 1987; 102(2):300–305.

24. Barbul A, Breslin RJ, Woodyard JP, et al. The effect of in vivo T helper and T suppressor lymphocyte depletion on wound healing. Ann Surg 1989; 209(4):479–483.

25. Schaffer M, Barbul A. Lymphocyte function in wound healing and following injury. Br J Surg 1998; 85(4):444–460.

26. Davis PA, Corless DJ, Gazzard BG, et al. Increased risk of wound complications and poor healing following laparotomy in HIV-seropositive and AIDS patients. Dig Surg 1999; 16(1):60–67.

27. Wilson SE, Robinson G, Williams RA, et al. Acquired immune deficiency syndrome (AIDS). Indications for abdominal surgery, pathology, and outcome. Ann Surg 1989; 210(4):428–433; discussion 433–434.

28. Burack JH, Mandel MS, Bizer LS. Emergency abdominal operations in the patient with acquired immunodeficiency syndrome. Arch Surg 1989; 124(3):285–286.

29. Robinson G, Wilson SE, Williams RA. Surgery in patients with acquired immunodeficiency syndrome. Arch Surg 1987; 122(2):170–175.

30. Consten EC, Slors FJ, Noten HJ, et al. Anorectal surgery in human immunodeficiency virus-infected patients. Clinical outcome in relation to immune status. Dis Colon Rectum 1995; 38(11):1169–1175.

31. Puy-Montbrun T, Denis J, Ganansia R, et al. Anorectal lesions in human immunodeficiency virus-infected patients. Int J Colorectal Dis 1992; 7(1):26–30.

32. Safavi A, Gottesman L, Dailey TH. Anorectal surgery in the HIV+ patient: update. Dis Colon Rectum 1991; 34(4):299–304.

33. Burke EC, Orloff SL, Freise CE, et al. Wound healing after anorectal surgery in human immunodeficiency virus-infected patients. Arch Surg 1991; 126(10):1267–1270; discussion 1270–1271.

34. Wakeman R, Johnson CD, Wastell C. Surgical procedures in patients at risk of human immunodeficiency virus infection. J R Soc Med 1990; 83(5):315–318.

35. Wolkomir AF, Barone JE, Hardy HW III, et al. Abdominal and anorectal surgery and the acquired immune deficiency syndrome in heterosexual intravenous drug users. Dis Colon Rectum 1990; 33(4):267–270.

36. Carr ND, Mercey D, Slack WW. Non-condylomatous, perianal disease in homosexual men. Br J Surg 1989; 76(10):1064–1066.

37. Wexner SD, Smithy WB, Milsom JW, et al. The surgical management of anorectal diseases in AIDS and pre-AIDS patients. Dis Colon Rectum 1986; 29(11):719–723.

38. Nadal SR, Manzione CR, Galvao VM, et al. Healing after anal fistulotomy: comparative study between HIV+ and HIV– patients. Dis Colon Rectum 1998; 41:177–179.

39. Lord RV. Anorectal surgery in patients infected with human immunodeficiency virus: factors associated with delayed wound healing. Ann Surg 1997; 226(1):92–99.

40. Davis PA, Wastell C. A comparison of biomechanical properties of excised mature scars from HIV patients and non-HIV controls. Am J Surg 2000; 180(3):217–222.

41. Postlethwaite AE, Snyderman R, Kang AH. The chemotactic attraction of human fibroblasts to a lymphocyte-derived factor. J Exp Med 1976; 144(5):1188–1203.

42. Nielson EG, Phillips SM, Jimenez S. Lymphokine modulation of fibroblast proliferation. J Immunol 1982; 128(3):1484–1486.

43. Wahl SM, Wahl LM, McCarthy JB. Lymphocyte-mediated activation of fibroblast proliferation and collagen production. J Immunol 1978; 121(3):942–946.

44. Johnson RL, Ziff M. Lymphokine stimulation of collagen accumulation. J Clin Invest 1976; 58(1):240–252.

45. Morris R. Modes of action of FK506, cyclosporin A, and rapamycin. Transplant Proc 1994; 26:3272–3275.

46. Fishel R, Barbul A, Wasserkrug HL, et al. Cyclosporine A impairs wound healing in rats. J Surg Res 1983; 34(6):572–575.

47. Eisinger DR, Sheil AG. A comparison of the effects of cyclosporin A and standard agents on primary wound healing in the rat. Surg Gynecol Obstet 1985; 160(2):135–138.

48. Goldberg M, Lima O, Morgan E, et al. A comparison between cyclosporin A and methylprednisolone plus azathioprine on bronchial healing following canine lung autotransplantation. J Thorac Cardiovasc Surg 1983; 85(6):821–826.

49. Wood SH, Lees VC. A prospective investigation of the healing of grafted pretibial wounds with early and late mobilization. Br J Plast Surg 1994; 47:127–131.

50. Diethelm AG. Surgical management of complications of steroid therapy. Ann Surg 1977; 185:251–263.

51. Ehrlich HP, Tarver H, Hunt TK. Effects of vitamin A and glucocorticoids upon inflammation and collagen synthesis. Ann Surg 1973; 177(2):222–227.

52. Ehrlich HP, Tarver H. Effects of beta-carotene, vitamin A, and glucocorticoids on collagen synthesis in wounds. Proc Soc Exp Biol Med 1971; 137(3):936–938.

53. Ehrlich HP, Hunt TK. Effects of cortisone and vitamin A on wound healing. Ann Surg 1968; 167(3):324–328.

54. Dostal GH, Gamelli RL. The differential effect of corticosteroids on wound disruption strength in mice. Arch Surg 1990; 125(5):636–640.

55. Ehrlich HP, Hunt TK. The effects of cortisone and anabolic steroids on the tensile strength of healing wounds. Ann Surg 1969; 170(2):203–206.

56. Eisinger DR, Sheil AG. A comparison of the effects of cyclosporin A and standard agents on primary wound healing in the rat. Surg Gynecol Obstet 1985; 160(2):135–138.

57. Zanker B, Schneeberger H, Rothenpieler U, et al. Mycophenolate mofetil-based, cyclosporine-free induction and maintenance immunosuppression: first-3-months analysis of efficacy and safety in two cohorts of renal allograft recipients. Transplantation 1998; 66(1):44–49.

58. Cohen SC, Gabelnick HL, Johnson RK, Goldin A. Effects of antineoplastic agents on wound healing in mice. Surgery 1975; 78(2):238–244.

59. Morris T, Lincoln F, Lee A. The effect of 5-fluorouracil on abdominal wound healing in rats. Aust N Z J Surg 1978; 48(2):219–221.

60. Chan KW, Knowling M, Beauchamp CP. Perioperative chemotherapy for primary sarcoma of bone. Can J Surg 1989; 32(1):43–46.

61. Canavese G, Catturich A, Vecchio C, et al. Surgical complications related to peri-operative adjuvant chemotherapy in breast cancer. Results of a prospective, controlled, randomized clinical trial. Eur J Surg Oncol 1997; 23(1):10–12.

62. Perhala RS, Wilke WS, Clough JD, Segal AM. Local infectious complications following large joint replacement in rheumatoid arthritis patients treated with methotrexate versus those not treated with methotrexate. Arthritis Rheum 1991; 34(2):146–152.

63. Kasdan ML, June L. Postoperative results of rheumatoid arthritis patients on methotrexate at the time of reconstructive surgery of the hand. Orthopedics 1993; 16(11):1233–1235.

64. Sany J, Anaya JM, Canovas F, et al. Influence of methotrexate on the frequency of postoperative infectious complications in patients with rheumatoid arthritis.

65. Sinacore DR. Healing times of pedal ulcers in diabetic immunosuppressed patients after transplantation. Arch Phys Med Rehabil 1990; 80:935–940.

66. Fletcher F, Ain M, Jacobs R, et al. Healing of foot ulcers in immunosuppressed renal transplant patients. Clin Orthop 1993; (296):37–42.

67. Dobmeyer TS, Raffel B, Dobmeyer JM, et al. Decreased function of monocytes and granulocytes during HIV-1 infection correlates with CD4 cell counts. Eur J Med Res 1995; 1(1):9–15.

68. Meyer L, Miedema F. Immune dysregulation and CD4 T cell loss in HIV-1 infection. Springer Semin Immunopathol 1997; 18(3):285–303.

69. Tufail A, Holland GN, Fisher TC, et al. Increased polymorphonuclear leucocyte rigidity in HIV infected individuals. Br J Ophthalmol 2000; 84(7):727–731.

70. Buehrer JL, Weber DJ, Meyer AA, et al. Wound infection rates after invasive procedures in HIV-1 seropositive versus HIV-1 seronegative hemophiliacs. Ann Surg 1990; 211(4):492–498.

71. Savioz D, Chilcott M, Ludwig C, et al. Preoperative counts of CD4 T-lymphocytes and early postoperative infective complications in HIV-positive patients. Eur J Surg 1998; 164(7):483–487.

72. Emparan C, Iturburu IM, Ortiz J, Mendez JJ. Infective complications after abdominal surgery in patients infected with human immunodeficiency virus: role of CD4 lymphocytes in prognosis.

73. Semprini AE, Castagna C, Ravizza M, et al. The incidence of complications after caesarean section in 156 HIV-positive women. AIDS 1995; 9(8):913–917.

74. Mellors JW, Rinaldo CR Jr, Gupta P, et al. Prognosis in HIV-1 infection predicted by the quantity of virus in plasma. Science 1996; 272(5265):1167–1170.

75. Tran HS, Moncure M, Tarnoff M, et al. Predictors of operative outcome in patients with human immunodeficiency virus infection and acquired immunodeficiency syndrome. Am J Surg 2000; 180(3):228–233.

76. Gil-Egea MJ, Pi-Sunyer MT, Verdaguer A, et al. Surgical wound infections: prospective study of 4,468 clean wounds. Infect Control 1987; 8(7):277–280.

77. Canavese G, Catturich A, Vecchio C, et al. Surgical complications related to peri-operative adjuvant chemotherapy in breast cancer. Results of a prospective, controlled, randomized clinical trial. Eur J Surg Oncol 1997; 23(1):10–12.

78. Kasdan ML, June L. Postoperative results of rheumatoid arthritis patients on methotrexate at the time of reconstructive surgery of the hand. Orthopedics 1993; 16(11):1233–1235.

79. Sany J, Anaya JM, Canovas F, et al. Influence of methotrexate on the frequency of postoperative infectious complications in patients with rheumatoid arthritis. J Rheumatol 1993; 20(7):1129–1132.

80. Kuritzkes DR, Parenti D, Ward DJ, et al. Filgrastim prevents severe neutropenia and reduces infective morbidity in patients with advanced HIV infection: results of a randomized, multicenter, controlled trial. G-CSF 930101 Study Group. AIDS. 1998; 12(1):65–74.

29
Wounds in Children

Isabel C. Valencia
Department of Dermatology and Cutaneous Surgery, The University of Miami School of Medicine, Miami, Florida, U.S.A.

Lawrence A. Schachner
Department of Pediatrics, The University of Miami School of Medicine, Miami, Florida, U.S.A.

1. INTRODUCTION

In contrast to the child and adult, the embryo and fetus have the unique ability to heal a potentially scarring injury without scar formation. Unlike adult epidermal cells that resurface the wound by "crawling" across it, embryonic epidermal cells are pulled by the contraction of actin fibers that draw the wound edges together. Probable reasons for this are that fetal skin has small amounts of transforming growth factor β-1, a scar promoting cytokine; but is rather rich in metalloproteinases, which may promote scarless healing (1). For a detailed description of fetal wound repair, please refer to Chapter 2. We will describe pediatric cases where wound healing represents a therapeutic challenge.

2. APLASIA CUTIS CONGENITA

Aplasia cutis congenita (ACC) is the congenital absence of all skin layers and can occur anywhere on the body but typically involves the scalp (in about 84%) at the midline vertex. Fifteen percent of cases involve nonscalp locations and are often bilaterally symmetrical. Aplasia cutis congenita may be seen in association with other defects, including the absence of distal limbs, omphalocele, cleft deformities, cardiac defects, cutis marmorata, and less frequently fetus papyraceus. Chromosome aberrations may also be present (2). Most of the ACC wounds are small (< 2.5 cm), superficial to the skull and heal with local wound care (5). However, in 20% of patients, the defects can be larger, and occasionally extend through the skull with exposure of the underlying brain and superior sagital sinus. If left untreated, eschar formation quickly develops, and predisposes to infection and sudden lethal hemorrhage (3).

Multiple treatment modalities have been suggested, with two options, conservative vs. surgical management, usually considered. Small-size defects may be treated conservatively; left to epithelialize from the edges, or even excised and closed primarily. Conservative treatment includes daily dressing changes with saline and topical antibiotic dressings, that resist eschar drying and separation while allowing epithelization to occur (4). Surgical treatments for partial or complete wound closure include full and split thickness grafts. Grafted scalp defects may need secondary surgery using tissue-expanded local flaps, pericranial flaps, or free vascularized flap (5–7). Truncal lesions treated conservatively may also require secondary surgery due to contraction and scarring, with expanded local skin flaps or grafts. In a recent report, a large truncal defect ($130\,cm^2$) in a newborn was covered with an allogeneic dermis (immunologically inert dermal matrix Allo-Derm) and cultured epithelial autografts. The allogeneic dermis provided a dermal base for the autografts, limiting contraction, and improving functional and cosmetic results (2).

3. EPIDERMOLYSIS BULLOSA

Epidermolysis bullosa (EB) is a group of heritable skin disorders manifesting with blistering of the skin and mucosae following mild mechanical trauma. The disease is both genetically and clinically heterogeneous, and adding to the clinical complexity are the extracutaneous manifestations. Continuous blistering, erosions, chronic ulceration, and scarring characterize some forms of inherited EB. The challenge of compromised wound healing due to repetitive trauma to the skin is a major problem encountered in patients with EB. Development of emerging therapies for EB aims at preventing the occurrence of chronic wounds and at enhancement of their healing. Wound healing has also relevance to carcinogenesis in EB, as aggressive skin cancers develop at the site of chronically damaged skin. The wound healing process is also complicated by infections, malnutrition, and immunologic suppression of the host, and the standard of care of such wounds has not been established (8,9).

Any dressing routine for the EB patient must minimize further damage to the skin. Dressings should be soaked off and never forcibly removed. Only nonadherent dressings should be used and secured with soft, roller gauze bandages or elastic tube dressings. Large blisters should be opened with a sterile needle to avoid fluid accumulation and pressure build up, but the blister roof should be kept in place. Rotating different topical antimicrobials every 2–3 months is recommended, as prolonged use of the same agent encourages emergence of resistant organisms (10).

A hydrocolloid dressing was compared with paraffin gauze and a non-adherent dressing Telfa (Kendall Co, Boston) in a controlled clinical trial of three pediatric patients (44 wounds) with recessive dystrophic EB. Advantages of the hydrocolloid dressing over the paraffin gauze and the telfa included faster re-epithelization, reduction of scar tissue formation, decreased pain and discomfort, and less frequent dressing changes (11).

Autografts have been used to treat wounds of recessive dystrophic epidermolysis bullosa (RDEB). Split thickness skin grafts are difficult to harvest since the skin of these patients is extremely sensitive to shearing forces. For this reason, medium thickness split grafts have been found to be most effective, but since the entire body is involved in the disease, it may be hard to find suitable donor areas. To overcome this problem, several approaches have been tried. Eisenberg and Llewelyn reported the treatment of hand deformities with combined use of medium thickness autografts and a composite of cultured skin allografts, containing both keratinocytes and fibroblasts on a unique collagen matrix. In this study, hand contractures were released and web spaces were covered with local flaps and split thickness autografts, while adjacent sides of the digits, other areas, and donor sites were grafted with composite cultured skin allografts. The areas grafted with the allografts were judged to have morphologic and functional good to excellent results, the average time to recurrence was increased approximately twofold and smaller autografts needed to be used (12).

Of particular interest in the wound healing field of EB is the recent development of skin substitutes by tissue engineering. However, controlled comparative studies that would critically evaluate the suitability of the currently available skin susbstitute for the acute and long-term therapy of EB are still lacking. Falabella et al. first described the use of tissue-engineered skin, Apligraf (Organogenesis Inc, Canton, MA) for the treatment of a newborn with a subtype of EB. Apligraf is a bilayered human skin equivalent developed from neonatal foreskin, and is FDA approved for the treatment of venous and diabetic ulcers. In this patient, Apligraf was applied to the areas more severely eroded and was kept in place with vaseline gauze, nonadherent pads and elastic gauze bandages, without the need for sutures or staples. The areas treated with the tissue-engineered skin healed faster than the areas treated with conventional therapy (Vaseline gauze) (13). The same authors conducted an open-label uncontrolled study of 15 patients (with 78 acute and chronic wounds). In this series of patients, the tissue-engineered skin induced rapid healing mostly by clinical graft take, was not clinically rejected, and was devoid of side effects. It was felt by the patients and families to be more effective than conventional dressings for EB wounds (8).

Dermagraft (Advanced Tissue Sciences—Smith & Nephew Dermagraft Joint Venture) was used to treat refractory wounds in four patients between the ages of 5 and 21 years, with generalized recessive dystrophic epidermolysis bullosa. Dermagraft is a living human dermal skin substitute comprised of human dermal fibroblasts that are harvested from the foreskin of newborns after routine circumcision. In total, 22 body sites were treated with 25 applications of Dermagraft. After 8 weeks, the mean overall epidermal coverage for all body sites of all patients was 74% (range 20–100%). Some sites showed sustained healing at prolonged intervals of 6–12 months. One patient developed fever 5 days after the application of the skin substitute, which was attributed to an infected parenteral nutrition line. No other adverse effects were noted. Dermagraft appears to stimulate wound healing and to be well tolerated, in patients with recessive dystrophic epidermolysis bullosa (14).

Although both Apligraf and Dermagraft have proven to be safe, controlled studies with a larger patient population and longer follow-up is necessary before their widespread use is advocated.

4. STEVENS-JOHNSON SYNDROME/TOXIC EPIDERMAL NECROLYSIS

Stevens-Johnson syndrome (SJS) and toxic epidermal necrolysis (TEN) are rare, life-threatening exfoliating diseases of the skin and mucous membranes, caused by immunologic reactions to foreign antigens. Drugs are implicated in the vast majority of cases. Transitional or overlapping cases of SJS and TEN are recognized clinically, and it is believed that they represent the same disease entity, differing only by the area of involved skin. Toxic epidermal necrolysis is an acute systemic condition manifesting with extensive blistering of the skin, mucous membranes, and sometimes bowel and respiratory epithelium (15,16). Children with TEN die from sepsis and the mortality from the disease has been reported to be as high as 70% (17,18). The optimal management of SJ and TEN is controversial. Treatment with systemic corticosteroids is debated, however, in a prospective study by Kakourou et al. (19), bolus infusions of methylprednisolone compared to supportive therapy resulted in significant reduction of the period of fever, reduction of the period of acute eruption, and milder signs of prostration. Another approach for treatment is the use of immunomodulators such as cyclosporine, cyclophosphamide, or plasmapheresis, which have been successful in case of TEN. The administration of intravenous immunoglobulin showed beneficial effects on survival on adult patients (15,20). Multidisciplinary treatment with a strategy emphasizing biologic wound closure, intensive nutritional support, continuous ophtalmologic evaluation, and early detection and treatment of septic foci is necessary.

For pediatric patients and cases involving large total body surface area, some authors recommend transfer to a burn center early in the disease process. However, this is still controversial, and in general the current literature agrees that patients should be managed in facilities that are specialized to care for patients with extensive skin loss, whether a burn unit or not (15). The aim at local wound care is prevention of wound desiccation and infection. Whether early debridement of all blistered areas should be performed is still controversial, as the blister roof frequently provides excellent coverage during re-epithelization. We believe that debridement should not be performed routinely in children. To reduce the rate of infections and protect the unhealed areas as well as to reduce pain, several protocols have been suggested using different topical antimicrobials and the coverage of wounds with biological dressings. Gentle cleansing with saline or Burrow solution (aluminium acetate), compresses topical antibiotic ointments such as polymyxin-bacitracin or mupirocin and sterile nonadherent dressings such as Vaseline impregnated gauze are in general recommended. Silver nitrate 0.5% also has been reported as a useful topical agent, but sulfa containing creams are not indicated when sulfonamides have been implicated in the etiology of these disorders and if they may cause toxicity through heavy percutaneous absorption. Hydrogel dressings such as Vigilon (C.R. Bard, Inc., Murray Hill, NJ) can be applied over denuded areas (17). Heimbach et al. (21) successfully treated 19 patients including 3 children by debridement and wound coverage with porcine xenograft. The tissue-engineered skin Apligraf may have a potential role in the treatment of wounds of TEN.

5. ULCERATED HEMANGIOMAS

Hemangiomas are tumors comprised of proliferated endothelial cells and are the most common soft-tissue tumors of infancy, affecting up to 2% of full-term newborns and as many as 10–12% of infants by 1 year of age (22). They are clinically heterogeneous, with their appearance dictated by the depth, location, and stage of evolution. Despite the benign course of most cutaneous hemangiomas, they may cause functional compromise or permanent disfigurement. Ulcerated hemangiomas are commonly seen in the head and neck areas, adjacent to the lip, in the postauricular sulcus, or in the neck folds. Another common site is the perineum, particularly in the perianal skin. Lesional size appears to correlate with the frequency of ulceration (23).

Ulceration is the most common complication of deep, rapidly proliferative hemangiomas, affecting between 5% and 13% of all hemangiomas. The disruption of epithelial integrity results in the potential for infection and hemorrhage. Ulcers can be extremely painful and carry the risk of loss of function and scarring. There is a paucity of literature specifically addressing the subject of ulcerated hemangiomas. Current therapies include wet to dry dressings, povidone-iodine or saline compresses, topical antibiotics, topical lidocaine jelly, hydrocolloid dressing, pastes and gels, systemic antibiotics, systemic corticosteroids, and flashlamp pulsed-dye laser (FPDL) (24). Application of a polyurethane film (Opsite Flexigrid) was found to be effective in controlling pain and accelerating re-epithelialization of ulcerated hemangiomas (25). Laser therapy is the best documented therapy for ulcerated hemangiomas. The argon and neodinium: YAG lasers and more recently the FPDL laser have been found to promote healing, decrease pain, and accelerate involution (26).

In a retrospective study, Kim et al. (23) evaluated the clinical features, management, and therapeutic responses of ulcerated hemangiomas. The authors found that no one therapeutic modality was uniformly effective in treating these ulcerations, and most patients required concurrent therapies. The decision to use specific therapies was dependent on the patient's age, the location, size and the stage of growth or involution of the hemangioma. For the authors, the simplest intervention was local wound care either alone or as an alternative or adjuvant therapy. Of the different topical antimicrobial agents, metronidazole gel seemed to be very helpful in many cases, particularly for those lesions in intertriginous or moist areas. Occlusive dressings were also particularly useful, as they serve as barriers to outside pathogens, prevent wound dessication, and accelerate healing times. Duoderm extra thin, a hydrocolloid dressing, was particularly well suited for ulcerations in a perianal location. Other dressings such as foam dressings were helpful in both absorbing exudate and in protecting areas from minor trauma and alginate dressings were useful for highly exudative ulcers. When ulceration approached the anus or female genitalia, petroleum jelly-impregnated gauze was applied overlapping the hydrocolloid dressing because it was adherent in areas close to a mucosal surface (23). As an alternative for these ulcerated hemangiomas where the hydrocolloid dressing cannot adhere in the midline and cannot protect the wound from being soiled, a thick layer of hydrocolloid paste on the wound may be applied until sufficient re-epithelization of the boundaries is attained, subsequently allowing the placement of the hydrocolloid dressing (27). Barrier creams (e.g., zinc oxide) and hydrophilic petrolatum (e.g., Aquaphor) also seemed to be effective for small perineal ulcerations (23). A useful alternative for diaper area lesions is open-air therapy (leaving the diaper off for an hour or so after each change is recommended) (28).

In addition to local wound care, the approach to the management of ulcerated hemangiomas may include management of infection, specific therapeutic modalities (systemic and intralesional corticosteroids, flashlamp pulsed-dye laser and interferon alfa-2a), and pain control (24).

6. TRAUMATIC WOUNDS

Twelve million lacerations are repaired annually in emergency departments in the United States (29). Despite these numbers, development of alternative laceration repair techniques has remained limited. Suturing of wounds can be time consuming and painful. The cyanoacrylate-based adhesives, an alternative to suture repair, are now FDA approved and commercially available. They are topical glues that bond to the outermost layer of skin to form a seal over the apposed edges of a laceration. This procedure allows for normal wound healing and is often accomplished without the need for local anesthesia. In a recent study, 83 pediatric patients presented to an emergency department for laceration repair were randomized to receive either the tissue-adhesive 2-Octylcyanoacrylate- 2-OCA, Dermabond (Ethicon/Closure Medical Corp, Raleigh, NC), or nonabsorbable sutures/staples. The length of time for laceration repair was decreased and the parents' assessment of the pain felt by their children was less in the group treated with the tissue adhesive. Cosmesis scores were slightly lower in the tissue adhesive group, although these were not statistically or clinically significant. Complications included one wound infection in the 2-OCA group that resulted in a hypertrophic scar (30,31). The authors conclude that 2-OCA is an acceptable alternative to conventional methods of wound repair with comparable cosmetic outcome.

In a more recent retrospective and concurrent chart review study, Resch and Hick evaluated the first 100 patients on which Dermabond was used in a pediatric emergency department. Three immediate complications involved a minor dehiscence and two eyelid adhesions. Two wound infections and a patient with hematoma and keloid formation were identified as later complications. The vast majority of parents preferred tissue adhesive repair to sutures. Time in department was reduced from 106 min to 69 min on average. The authors admit that certain pitfalls occurring during early experience with these adhesives can be recognized and avoided (32). Tissue adhesives provide a safe, easy, and cosmetically equivalent alternative to sutures when properly used in selected wounds and hosts. As the insert states, "Dermabond adhesive should not be used below the skin because the polymerized material is not absored by the skin and can elicit a foreign body reaction." Lacerations ideally should be clean and without a significant crush component. The glue has not been studied for use on mucous membranes, feet, moist areas, or across joints. It is relatively contraindicated for use on hands, hair bearing areas, and abraded skin. Certain host conditions should be taken into consideration such as history of keloid formation, bleeding tendencies, prolonged steroid use, diabetes, and peripheral vascular disease (32).

Puncture wounds account for 3–5% of all traumatic injuries presenting to pediatric emergency departments. They are usually innocuous and medical care is seldom sought. The majority involve the plantar surface of the foot and are caused by nails, although they can be located at other sites and be caused by wood, metal, plastic, or glass. The history will help to determine the time and mechanism of injury, the degree of contamination with foreign matter, and whether the penetrating object may have broken off. If there is any doubt about the possibility of a retained foreign body, diagnostic imaging should be requested. Erythema, swelling, or persistent pain in the area suggests a wound infection. Determination of immunization status and appropriate immunization for patients with tetanus-prone wounds is necessary. If the dermis of the puncture site is exposed, the area and the surrounding skin should be irrigated superficially with saline, avoiding high-pressure deep wound irrigation that may cause tissue damage and push bacteria/foreign bodies deeper. Similarly, aggressive surgical debridement is not indicated. Uncomplicated wounds can then be managed with rest, elevation of the foot, and intermittent warm water soaks. For children who have a delayed presentation or signs of infection, consider the possibility of a retained foreign body, and request appropriate radiologic imaging studies and start oral antibiotics (33).

7. EXTRAVASATION INJURIES

The number of established venous lines that stop flowing in children is high. In such cases, the fluid could leak into the surrounding soft tissue, and although these extravasation events are frequently innocuous, a small number (0.24%) progress to tissue necrosis (34,35). Damage may be due to a direct toxic effect, pressure effects of the accumulated drug causing collapse of small vessels, osmotic toxicity, adverse changes in pH, and induced vasospasm (36).

Children and newborns in particular are at risk because of the fragility and small caliber of their peripheral veins, their inability to localize pain allowing the infusion to continue, and the delivery devise used to accurately pump small volumes of fluid under pressure (35).

These iatrogenic injuries can lead to full thickness skin necrosis above the affected area, but where there is little subcutaneous tissue, the agent may also precipitate scarring around tendons, nerves, and joints, causing limb contractures.

Reconstructive surgery is frequently required, although permanent scarring and functional disability can result. The back of the hand, the wrist, and the back of the foot are the most frequently affected areas since these are the preferred infusion sites in infants. The toxicity of the drug, the site of the extravasation, the amount of the agent that has leaked, and the general nutrition of the patient all influence the outcome (36). Intravenously induced skin injury can be produced by several different chemicals including nutrition solutions, hypertonic glucose, electrolytes (calcium, potassium and sodium salts, bicarbonate), chemotherapeutic agents, vasoactive drugs, contrast dyes, and antibiotics (37).

The most important step in avoiding the necrotic complication of intravenous therapy is to prevent extravasation. Particular care should be taken when administering substances that are known to have a high incidence of inducing skin necrosis. Selecting larger veins and avoiding sites with little subcutaneous tissue (e.g., dorsum of the hand, sites over joints, and bony prominences) is recommended (38). There is no standard treatment of the injury but different treatment modalities have been proposed: from simple observation to aggressive surgical debridement and skin grafting (39,40). In general, for the acute stage of this type of adverse event, once detected, emergency measures must be taken immediately: stopping the infusion and aspirating any product remaining in the blood vessels, and immobilization and elevation of the affected limb. Some authors advocate the use of specific antidotes as the mainstay of treatment. Three medications have been evaluated as effective when injected into the affected area: hyaluronidase (dilutes the toxic agent trapped in the tissues), phentolamine (effective against vasoconstrictors), and glyceryl trinitrate (vasodilates the ischemic area) (37). Also, injections of saline to dilute the drug (41) and ice or steroids creams to minimize the inflammatory reaction have been proposed (42). Gault (36) reported two techniques for this type of adverse event: injection of a hyaluronidase solution into the extravasation site, which is then flushed with saline, and gentle aspiration of the site with an atraumatic liposuction cannula, to collect most of the toxic agent remaining in the fat. He reported 86% good results with these treatments when implemented within 24 hr of the adverse event. In a recent report, Casanova et al. used Gault's procedure in 14 newborn-infant extravasations, with good results in 11 patients and skin necrosis in 3 patients that subsequently healed spontaneously. The authors recommend early treatment of toxic infusion leakage, as soon as the adverse event has been detected, before any signs of skin damage occur, to avoid or limit the damage to the patient's skin (37).

8. BURNS

Standard care of children with partial thickness burns typically involves painful dressing changes twice daily in which the burn is cleansed, a topical antimicrobial ointment is applied, and the wound is dressed with sterile nonadherent gauze (43). The most popular topical antimicrobial is silver sulfadiazine. However, silver sulfadiazine promotes the accumulation of proteinaceous debris on the wound surface, and the wound bed becomes obscured from view, limiting clinical determination of the progress of wound healing (44). The cleansing of the wound with removal of the ointment as well as the adhesion of gauze or cotton dressings can be painful (43). Daily exposure of the burn to the environment during dressing changes, predisposes to local infection (45), and in addition, topical antibiotics may cause sensitization and may promote the formation of eschar (43).

The current trend toward managed care has created a heightened need for effective and cost-efficient treatment of partial-thickness burns. An alternative to topical antimicrobial agents is the use of wound coverings. In a prospective, randomized clinical trial, 63 children with partial-thickness scalds were assigned treatment with either Mepitel (Mölnlycke Health Care) or silver sulfadiazine. Mepitel is a silicone-coated nylon net-like dressing containing no biological compounds. The authors found that burns of children treated with Mepitel exhibited less eschar formation, experienced less pain at dressing change and had significantly lower mean daily hospital charges. There was not significant difference in wound infection (43). Mepitel has proved to be an easy to-use and easy-to-remove dressing, adhering only to intact skin. In addition, the holes in the sheet allow proper drainage of fluid, preventing fluid collection or hematoma (46). Similar results were obtained when comparing a bilaminar temporary skin substitute, Biobrane (Winthrop Pharmaceuticals, New York, USA) vs. silver sulfadiazine in 20 pediatric second-degree burns. Pain, pain medication requirements, wound healing time, and length of hospital stay were significantly reduced when using the Biobrane (45). In this study, none of the patients developed infection; however, infection rates from 5% to 22.6% have been reported in the literature when using Biobrane. Wounds older than 24 hr and deeper wounds are at risk for infection and may not be suitable to treatment with Biobrane (45,47)

A new biologic covering TransCyte (Advanced Tissue Sciences, La Jolla, CA, formerly marketed as Dermagraft-Transcitional Covering) was used for the treatment of partial-thickness wounds in both children and adults. This material is composed of human newborn fibroblasts which are then cultured on the nylon mesh of Biobrane. The TransCyte was compared in a prospective, randomized, comparison study, to silver sulfadiazine. It was later evaluated in a noncomparison study. The results indicated that burns treated with TransCyte healed more quickly, with less hypertrophic scarring and in the absence of infection (44).

9. LEG ULCERS IN SICKLE CELL DISEASE

Leg ulcers are the most common cutaneous complication in sickle cell anemia. They usually occur in the younger patient population, typically between the ages of 10 and 35 years. The cause of sickle cell leg ulceration is incompletely understood. Clinical experience and epidemiologic studies support the role of three major factors: marginal blood supply to the skin, local edema, and minor trauma (48). Sickle cell ulcers frequently develop secondary infection and tend to be painful. Most of the ulcers occur in the ankle area, and less commonly over the dorsum of the foot and near the Achilles tendon. They vary in size and classically appear punched out with raised margins and a deep base. Initially, there is usually extensive necrotic eschar in the ulcer base. Ulcers may penetrate to the muscle fascia and periosteum of the underlying bone. Secondary infection is almost universal, with *Staphylococcus aureus* and *Pseudomona aeruginosa,* the most consistently cultured pathogens (48,49). The strongest predictor of risk for new leg ulceration is a history of previous leg ulcers, as recurrences occur in 25–50% of healed ulcers. Patient education about the risks of recurrence, methods of prevention, and need for repeated therapy should be emphasized. Once established, classic management of sickle cell related leg ulcers include bed rest with leg elevation, gentle debridement, control of local edema, and treatment of infection. Saline wet-to-dry dressings applied two or three times a day or conservative surgical debridement are good initial therapy for most ulcers with necrotic debris, however, the procedures are painful and have the risk of removing also newly formed, viable tissue. Not painful autolytic debridement can be effectively achieved using occlusive dressings such as hydrocolloids (DuoDERM, Convatec, Princeton, NJ). Elastic or inelastic compression bandages should be initiated immediately in combination with any debridement technique, to control edema in ambulatory patients. Zinc oxide impregnated gel boots are useful in healing leg ulcers in sickle cell and other patients, and they can be used over hydrocolloid dressings if debridement is necessary. Bed rest and leg elevation should be strongly encouraged. Topical treatment with antibiotics might be beneficial, but systemic antibiotics should be reserved for patients who have evidence of cellulitis (48). Skin grafts are advocated for ulcers that are resistant to more conservative therapy (50). Zinc deficiency is prevalent in patients with sickle cell anemia, and zinc sulfate supplements are usually recommended. Serjeant et al. (51) undertook a controlled trial of oral zinc sulfate therapy in sickle cell patients, and found significant improvement in the treated group. A number of treatment modalities have been used for sickle cell ulcers with variable success, including blood transfusions, hydroxyurea alone (52,53) or in combination with erythropoietin (54), pentoxifylline (55), hyperbaric oxygen (56), and a synthetic topical extracellular matrix (57). Larger, placebo-controlled trials are needed to further evaluate the role of these approaches in the management of sickle cell ulcers.

10. KELOIDS AND HYPERTROPHIC SCARS

Keloids and hypertrophic scars may result from both major and minor trauma. Most keloids occur sporadically, but some keloid cases are familial inherited in an autosomal dominant mode with incomplete clinical penetrance and variable expression (58). They have been described in all age groups, although they tend to occur mainly in those patients aged 10–30 years and to be uncommon in very old and very young patients (59). They are more commonly seen in black patients. Keloidal scars occur more frequently on the earlobes, sternum, back, shoulders, cheeks, and upper arms. They can be cosmetically disfiguring because of their bulk and color. Symptoms such as pain, burning, or itching have been described (60). Currently, there are three accepted methods of treatment of keloids and hypertrophic scars: intralesional steroid injections, silicone gel sheeting, or surgical excision followed by either of these treatments. Corticosteroids are thought to downregulate collagen gene expression within the keloid. It appears that intralesional corticosteroids are effective as monotherapy when given every 2–4 weeks; however, there is high level of recurrence in some studies. Silicone gel sheeting, the more easily acceptable treatment for children, is noninvasive, painless, easy to apply, and almost free of side effects. The mechanism by which silicone-based products may work and the best way to use the material is unknown. Flattening of the scar is seen after continuous use for several weeks, particularly in small lesions (61,62). However, most of the studies published so far are not controlled and involve hypertrophic rather than keloidal scars (60).

Different studies have shown the inhibitory effect of interferons on dermal fibroblast growth and the production of collagen I and III. Intralesional injection of recombinant human interferon alpha-2b or interferon gamma in keloids has given promising albeit variable results (63,64). Other treatment interventions include cryotherapy alone or in combination with corticosteroid injections, radiation with or without surgical excision, Ultraviolet A1 radiation, intralesional 5-fluouracil injection, bleomycin dripped onto the scar followed by puncture with a 25-gauge needle to allow penetration into the dermis, local pressure therapy, and laser surgery (60). Further controlled studies are required before recommending these modalities for the treatment of keloids in the pediatric population.

11. TISSUE EXPANSION AS A SURGICAL ALTERNATIVE IN CHILDREN

Tissue expansion of regional skin flaps is a surgical reconstructive alternative in a wide variety of pediatric cases that cause significant deformity and where there is insufficient regional tissue availability (e.g., congenital melanocytic nevi, sebaceous nevi, hemangiomas, burn scars, large defects of aplasia cutis congenita). Tissue expansion enables defects to be covered with tissue similar in texture, color, and type. Careful planning should always precede soft-tissue expansion. Although associated initially with a relatively high complication rate, recent studies suggest that with experience, complications become less common (65).

Cutaneous surgical reconstruction in the head and neck region of children may be difficult due to insufficient elasticity or subsequent scar spread. Also, adjacent tissue is not rotated or advanced as easily as in older populations (66) Although the effects of tissue expansion on developmental structures are not completely known, clinical experience suggests that the careful use of tissue expansion under the scalp of neonates and infants is warranted (67). Even though tissue expansion is a good alternative for pediatric patients, procedure tolerance, risks and complications, insufficient adjacent skin of like quality, and concerns about the durability of the reconstruction and its ability to grow along with the child, are some of the particular concerns in these patients. Expanded donor sites (from the groin and lower abdomen) full-thickness skin grafts maintain all the characteristics of nonexpanded full-thickness skin flaps and offer a good reconstructive alternative to overcome some of the limitations (68). There are clinical situations in which even despite the use of simultaneous multiple tissue expanders, complete coverage of a defect cannot be achieved. In this situation, serial expansion may be indicated. This technique has been used successfully for excision and/or reconstruction of large defects (e.g., giant congenital nevus, burn deformities) in the pediatric population (69,70).

REFERENCES

1. Cass DL, Meuli M, Adzick NS. Scar wars: implications of fetal wound healing for the pediatric burn patient. Pediatr Surg Int 1997; 12:484–489.
2. Simman R, Priebe CJ, Simon M. Reconstruction of aplasia cutis congenital of the trunk in a newborn infant using acellular allogenic dermal graft and cultured epithelial autografts. Ann Plast Surg 2000; 44:451–454.
3. Sargent LA. Aplasia cutis congenita of the scalp. J Pediatr Surg 1990; 25:1211–1213.
4. Wexler A, Harris M, Lesavoy M. Conservative treatment of cutis aplasia. Plast Reconstr Surg 1990; 86:1066–1071.
5. Paletta CE, Huang DB, Dehghan K, Kelly C. The use of tissue expanders in staged abdominal wall reconstruction. Ann Plast Surg 1999; 42(3):259–265.
6. Moscona R, Berger J, Govrin J. Large skull defect in aplasia cutis congenital treated by pericranial flaps: long-term follow-up. Ann Plast Surg 1991; 26:178–182.
7. Argenta LC, Dingman RO. Total reconstruction of aplasia cutis congenital involving scalp, skull and dura. Plast Reconstr Surg 1986; 77:650–653.
8. Falabella AF, Valencia IC, Eaglstein WH, Schachner LA. Tissue-engineered skin (Apligraf) in the healing of patients with epidermolysis bullosa wounds. Arch Dermatol 2000; 136:1225–1230.
9. Uitto J, Eady R, Fine J-D, Feder M, Dart J. The DEBRA international visioning/consensus meeting on epidermolysis bullosa: summary and recommendations. J Invest Dermatol 2000; 114(4):734–737.
10. Lin AN. Management of patients with epidermolysis bullosa. Dermatol Clin 1996; 14(2):381–387.
11. Eisenberg M. The effect of occlusive dressings on re-epithelizations of wounds in children with epidermolysis bullosa. J Pediatr Surg 1986; 21(10):892–894.
12. Eisenberg M, Llewelyn D. Surgical management of hands in children with recessive dystrophic epidermolysis bullosa: use of allogeneic composite cultured skin grafts. Br J Plast Surg 1998; 51:608–613.
13. Falabella AF, Schachner LA, Valencia IC, Eaglstein WH. The use of tissue- engineered skin (Apligraf) to treat a newborn with epidermolysis bullosa. Arch Dermatol 1999; 135:1219–1222.
14. Williamson D, Couts P, Sibbald RG. The role of dermal skin substitutes in the management of 'hard to heal', unusual wounds. Can J Plast Surg 2002; 10(suppl A):27A–30A.
15. Spies M, Sanford AP, Low A, Wolf SE, Herndon DN. Treatment of extensive toxic epidermal necrolysis in children. Pediatrics 2001; 108(5):1162–1168.
16. Sheridan RL, Schulz JT, Ryan CM, Schnitzer JJ, Lawlor D, Driscoll DN, Donelan MB, Tompkins RG. Long-term consequences of toxic epidermal necrolysis in children. Pediatrics 2002; 109:74–78.
17. Prendiville JS, Hebert AA, Greenwald MJ, Esterly NB. Management of Stevens-Johnson syndrome and toxic epidermal necrolysis in children. J Pediatr 1989; 115: 881–887.
18. Sheridan RL, Weber JM, Schulz JT, Ryan CM, Low HM, Tompkins RG. Management of severe toxic epidermal necrolysis in children. J Burn Care Rehabil 1999; 20:497–500.
19. Kakourou T, Klontza D, Soteropoulou F. Corticosteroid treatment of erythema multiforme major (Stevens-Johnson syndrome) in children. Eur J Pediatr 1997; 156:90–93.
20. Viard I, Wehrli P, Bullani R, Schneider P, Holler N, Salomon D, Hunziker T, Saurat JH, Tschopp J, French LE. Inhibition of toxic epidermal necrolysis by blockade of CD95 with human intravenous immunoglobulin. Science 1998; 282(5388):490–493.
21. Heimbach DM, Engrav LH, Marvin JA, Harnar TJ, Grube BJ. Toxic epidermal necrolysis. A step forward in treatment. JAMA 1987; 257:2171–2175.
22. Esterly NB. Cutaneous hemangiomas, vascular strains and malformations, and associated syndromes. Curr Probl Pediatr 1996; 26:3–39.

23. Jin Kim H, Colombo M, Frieden IJ. Ulcerated hemangiomas: clinical characteristics and response to therapy. J Am Acad Dermatol 2001; 44:962–972.

24. Frieden IJ. Special symposium: management of hemangiomas. Pedriatr Dermatol 1997; 14:57–83.

25. Oranje AP, de Waard-van der Spek FB, deVillers ACA, de Laat PCJ, Maderm GC. Treatment and pain relief of ulcerative hemangiomas with a polyurethane film. Dermatology 2000; 200:31–34.

26. Scheepers JH, Quaba AA. Does the pulsed tunable dye laser have a role in the management of infantile hemangiomas? Observations based on 3 years experience. Plast Reconstr Surg 1995; 95:305–312.

27. Enjolras O. Management of hemangiomas: special symposium. Pediatr Dermatol 1997; 14:58–60.

28. Margileth AM. Management of hemangiomas: special symposium. Pediatr Dermatol 1997; 14:63–65.

29. Stussman BJ. National Hospital Ambulatory Medical Care Survey: 1994 Emergency Department Summary: Advance Data from Vital Health Statistics. Hyattsville, Maryland: National Center for Health Statistics. 1996:275.

30. Bruns TB, Robinson BS, Smith RJ, Kile DL, Davis TP, Sullivan KM, Quinn JV. A new tissue adhesive for laceration repair in children. J Pediatr 1998; 132:1067–1070.

31. Bruns TB, Simon HK, McLario DJ, Sullivan KM, Wood RJ, Anand KJS. Laceration repair using a tissue adhesive in a children's emergency department. Pediatrics 1996; 98:673–675.

32. Resch KL, Hick JL. Preliminary experience with 2-octylcyanoacrylate in a pediatric emergency department. Pediatr Emerg Care 2000; 16(5):328–331.

33. Baldwin G, Colbourne M. Puncture wounds. Pediatr Rev 1999; 20:21–23.

34. Brown AS, Hoelzer DJ, Piercy SA. Skin necrosis from extravasation of intravenous fluids in children. Plast Reconstr Surg 1979; 64:145.

35. Harris PA. Limiting the damage of iatrogenic extravasation injuries in neonates. Plast Reconstr Surg 2001; 107(3):894–895.

36. Gault DT. Extravasation injuries. Br J Plast Surg 1993; 46:91–96.

37. Casannova D, Bardot J, Magalon G. Emergency treatment of accidental infusin leakage in the newborn: report of 14 cases. Br J Plast Surg 2001; 54:396–399.

38. Dufresne RG. Skin necrosis from intravenously infused materials. Cutis 1987; 39: 197–198.

39. Larson DL. What is the appropriate management of tissue extravasation by antitumor agents? Plast Reconstr Surg 1985; 75:397–402.

40. Linder RM, Upton J. Prevention of extravasation injuries secondary to doxorubicin hydrochloride extravasation injuries. J Hand Surg 1983; 8A:32–38.

41. Heckler FR. Current thoughts on extravasation injuries. Clin Plas Surg 1989; 16: 557–563.

42. Smith R. Prevention and treatment of extravasation. Br J Parenteral Therapy 1985; 6:114–119.

43. Gotschall CS, Morrison MIS, Eichelberger MR. Prospective, randomized study of the efficacy of Mepitel on children with partial-thickness scalds. J Bn Care Rehabil 1998; 19:279–283.

44. Noordenbos J, Dore C, Hansbrough JF. Safety and efficacy of TransCyte for the treatment of partial-thickness burns. J Burn Care Rehabil 1999; 20:275–281.

45. Barret JP, Dziewulski P, Ramzy PI, Wolf SE, Desai MH, Herndon DN. Biobrane versus 1% silver sulfadiazine in second-degree pediatric burns. Plast Reconstr Surg 2000; 105:62–65.

46. Bugmann Ph, Taylor S, Gyger D, Lironi A, Genin B, Vunda A, La Scala G, Birraux J, Le Coultre C. A silicone-coated nylon dressing reduces healing time in burned pediatric patients in comparison with standard sulfadiazine treatment: a prospective randomized trial. Burns 1998; 24:609–612.

47. Ou LF, Lee SY, Chen YC, Yang RS, Tang YW. Use of biobrane in pediatric scald burns-experience in 106 children. Burns 1998; 24:49–53.

48. Eckman JR. Leg ulcers in sickle cell disease. Hematol Oncol Clin North America 1996; 10:1333–1344.

49. Ademiluyi SA, Rotimi VO, Coker AO, et al. The anaerobic and aerobic bacterial flora of leg ulcers in patients with sickle cell disease. J Infect 1988; 17:115–120.

50. Heckler FR, Dibell DG, McGraw JB. Successful use of muscle flaps in patients with sickle cell disease. Plast Reconstr Surg 1985; 76:616–619.

51. Serjeant GR, Galloway RE, Gueri MC. Oral zinc sulphate in sickle-cell ulcers. Lancet 1970; 2:891–892.

52. Nguyen TV, Margolis DJ. Hydroxyurea and lower leg ulcers. Cutis 1993; 52:217.

53. Charache S, Terrin ML, Moore RD, et al. Effect of hydroxyurea on the frequency of painful crises in sickle cell anemia. N Engl J Med 1995; 332:1317.

54. AL-Momen AK. Recombinant human erythropoietin induced rapid healing of a chronic leg ulcer in a patient with sickle cell disease. Acta Haematol 1991; 86.46–48.

55. Frost ML, Treadwell P. Treatment of sickle cell leg ulcers with pentoxifylline. Int J Dermatol 1990; 29:375–376.

56. Heng MC. Local hyperbaric oxygen administration for leg ulcers [editorial]. Br J Dermatol 1983; 109:232–234.

57. Polarek JW, Clark RAF, Pickett MP, et al. Development of a provisional matrix to promote wound healing. Wounds 1994; 6:46.

58. Marneros AG, Norris JE, Olsen BR, Reichenberger E. Clinical genetics of familial keloids. Arch Dermatol 2001; 137:1429–1434.

59. Urioste SS, Arndt KA, Dover JS. Keloidal scars and hypertrophic scars: review and treatment strategies. Semin Cutan Med Surg 1999; 18:159–171.

60. Shafer JJ, Taylor SC, Cook-Bolden F. Keloidal scars: a review with a critical look at therapeutic options. J Am Acad Dermatol 2002; 46:S63–S97.

61. Laude TA. Skin disorders in black children. Curr Opin Pediatr 1996; 8:381–385.

62. Wong TW, Chiu HC, Chen JS, Lin LJ, Chang CC. Symptomatic keloids in two children. Arch Dermatol 1995; 131:775–777.

63. Berman B, Dunkan MR. Short term keloid treatment in vivo with human interferon-alpha 2b. Results in selected and persisted normalization of keloidal fibroblast collagen glycosaminoglycan, and collagenase production in vitro. J Am Acad Dermatol 1989; 21:694–702.

64. Granstein RD, Rook A, Floote TJ, et al. A controlled trial of intralesional recombinant interferon-gamma in the treatment of keloidal scarring. Arch Dermatol 1990; 126: 1295–1301.

65. Pisarski GP, Mertens D, Warden GD, Neale HW. Tissue expander complications in the pediatric burn patient. Plast Reconstr Surg 1998; 102:1008–1012.

66. Frodel JL Jr, Whitaker DC. Primary reconstruction of congenital facial lesion defects with tissue expansion. J Dermatol Surg Oncol 1993; 19:1110–1116.

67. Bauer BS, Vicari FA, Richard ME, Schwed R. Expanded full-thickness skin grafts in children: case selection, planning and management. Plast Reconstr Surg 1993; 92:59–69.

68. Bauer BS, Vicari FA. An approach to excision of congenital pigmented nevi in infancy and early childhood. J Pediatr Surg 1988; 13:509–514.

69. Hudson DA, Lazarus D, Silfen R. The use of serial tissue expansion in pediatric plastic surgery. Ann Plast Surg 2000; 45:589–594.

70. Gossain AK, Snatoro TD, Larson DL, Gingrass RP. Giant congenital nevi: a 20-year experience and an algorithm for their management. Plast Reconstr Surg 2001; 108(3):622–636.

30
Ulcers of Infectious Etiology

Ysabel M. Bello and Anna F. Falabella
*Department of Dermatology and Cutaneous Surgery, University of Miami
School of Medicine, Miami, Florida, U.S.A.*

Ulcers result when there is loss of all of the epidermis and at least a portion of the dermis. There are many causes of ulcers. Leg ulcers are frequently caused by chronic venous insufficiency, arterial disease, neuropathy, or a combination of factors (1). Ulcers are less commonly caused by infections. A diversity of infections may cause ulcers, and diagnosis is usually difficult without a culture or biopsy. The differential diagnosis of infectious ulcers includes bacterial, fungal, parasite, and viral etiologies (Table 1).

1. BACTERIAL

1.1. Ecthyma

Ecthyma is an ulcerative condition of the skin initiated by *Staphylococcus aureus*, *Streptococcus pyogenes*, or a combination of the two. It occurs most commonly on

Table 1 Infectious Etiology of Leg Ulcers

Bacterial	Parasite
Ecthyma	Leishmaniasis
Ecthyma gangrenosum	Amebiasis
Necrotizing fasciitis	
Mycobacterial	Viral
Anthrax	Herpes simplex
Spirochetal	Cytomegalovirus
Fungal	
Mycetoma	
Sporotrichosis	
Chromoblastomycosis	
Blastomycosis	
Histoplasmosis	
Lobomycosis	

the lower legs of children after minor trauma. Risk factors for ecthyma in adults include malnourishment, debilitation, and poor hygiene. Ecthyma typically begins with a vesicle or vesiculopustule, which becomes an ulcer covered by a gray yellow crust with a punched out appearance (2). It may spread by autoinoculation. Treatment includes cleansing with soap and water, removal of the crusts, and topical or systemic antibiotics. The lesions heal slowly, frequently leaving scars.

1.2. Ecthyma Gangrenosum

Ecthyma gangrenosum is a cutaneous ulcer caused by *Pseudomonas aeruginosa*. It occurs in debilitated patients. It begins as vesicles that quickly become hemorrhagic bluish bullae. The bullae rupture, leaving punched-out ulcers with a necrotic base and surrounding induration. Ecthyma gangrenosum is most commonly found on the legs, arms, and buttocks (3). The content of the vesicles show gram-negative bacilli on Gram stain, and cultures of the lesions are usually positive for *P. aeruginosa*. It may be associated with life-threatening systemic infection (sepsis), and blood cultures grow *P. aeruginosa*. Treatment includes early systemic intravenous antibiotics.

1.3. Necrotizing Fasciitis

Necrotizing fasciitis is a soft-tissue infection of the superficial fascia and subcutaneous tissue that may present as erythema and pain out of proportion to other clinical findings. Within hours to several days, blisters with hemorrhagic fluid are commonly present in the affected area. Fever and systemic symptoms may develop. The necrotizing fasciitis that affects the perineum and external genitalia is called Fournier's gangrene. Necrotizing fasciitis usually follows a wound, surgery, or perforating trauma, however, it may also occur de novo.

There are two types of necrotizing fasciitis, categorized by the causative organism. Type I necrotizing fasciitis is caused by anaerobic species (*Bacteroides* and *Peptostreptococcus* spp.) in combination with one or more facultative anaerobic species such as streptococci (other than group A) or one of the Enterobacteriaceae (*E. coli, Enterobacter, Klebsiella, Proteus*). Type II necrotizing fasciitis is caused by group A *Streptococci* alone or in combination with other species (most commonly *S. aureus*) (4).

When necrotizing fasciitis is suspected or confirmed, MRI may help demonstrate the extent of involvement. Early and aggressive surgical intervention is essential. Aerobic and anaerobic cultures should be taken prior to initiating antibiotic therapy. Even with appropriate treatment, this condition is associated with a 20–50% mortality (2).

1.4. Mycobacterial infections

Cutaneous ulcers can be caused by several species of mycobacteria, including the obligate human pathogens *Mycobacterium tuberculosis* and *Mycobacterium leprae*, and the facultative human pathogens or "atypical" mycobacteria such as *Mycobacterium marinum* (Table 2).

Table 2 Mycobacterial Infections Cause of Ulcers

Obligate human pathogens
  Mycobacterium tuberculosis (slow growing)
  Mycobacterium leprae (not cultivable)
Facultative human pathogens
  Mycobacterium ulcerans (slow growing)
  Mycobacterium marinum (slow growing)
  Mycobacterium avium intracellulare (slow growing)
  Mycobacterium fortuitum complex (rapid growing)

Cutaneous tuberculosis, caused by *Mycobacterium tuberculosis,* is rarely seen except in immunocompromised patients. However, cases of inoculated cutaneous tuberculosis have been described in medical professionals (3). Primary inoculation tuberculosis should be suspected in a painless indurated ulcer. The diagnosis is confirmed by acid-fast staining, culture or polymerase chain reaction. Tuberculous chancre heals spontaneously within 1 year with scarring.

Lupus vulgaris, an endogenous spread of tuberculosis, may appear clinically as serpiginous leg ulcer with granulating base and hypertrophic vegetations (2). The tuberculin test is strongly positive, and culture and histology confirm the diagnosis. Treatment includes chemotherapy with isoniazid, rifampin, pyrazinamide, and ethambutol for 2 months, followed by rifampin and isoniazid for additional 4 months (3).

Erythema induratum of Bazin is a chronic disorder that typically manifests as ulcerative and indurated lesions on the lower limbs, especially the calves. This condition most commonly affects younger women. It is believed to be caused by a hyperinflammatory response to tuberculin antigen. Erythema induratum responds favorably to antituberculous therapy.

Leprosy is caused by *M. leprae*. Two different types of ulcers can be seen in leprosy: neuropathic and leprous ulcers (3). Neuropathic ulcers, which do not contain *M. leprae*, result from repeated injuries to hyposensitive areas caused by peripheral nerve damage. Treatment includes preventive measures such as routine podiatric care, regular trimming of calluses, and well-fitting shoes. Leprous ulcer results from the breakdown of lepromatous nodules usually found in the center of heavily infiltrated areas surrounded by swelling. Smears show abundance of acid-fast bacilli. Management includes leprosy-specific treatment with three drugs: rifampin, dapsone, and clofazamine.

The slow-growing organisms *Mycobacterium ulcerans, M. marinum*, and *Mycobacterium avium intracellulare*, and the fast-growing *Mycobacterium fortuitum* complex are atypical mycobacteria that can cause cutaneous ulcers.

M. ulcerans is the causative agent of Buruli ulcer, so-called because cases were first detected in Buruli County, Uganda. After tuberculosis and leprosy, *M. ulcerans* is the third most common mycobacterial disease in immunocompetent people (5). It occurs primarily in Africa and Australia. Infection is transmitted through abraded or traumatized skin that comes in contact with water, soil, or vegetation. The incubation period is usually under 3 months. The initial clinical manifestation of *M. ulcerans* range is indurated, painless subcutaneous papules and nodules, mostly involving the extremities. Over time, skin breakdown occurs, leading to large undermined necrotic ulcers. The skin surrounding the ulcer, and in some cases the entire limb, can be swollen. Some ulcers heal slowly without treatment, leaving depressed, stellate scars. Smears, curettage, or biopsy reveal acid-fast bacilli. The treatment of choice is surgical excision of nodules at the early stage, or wide excision of ulcers. The effect of antimycobacterials on Buruli ulcer is unclear.

M. marinum infections occur in individuals with aquatic occupations or continuous contact with water from lakes, salt water, swimming pool, and fish tanks. Two to three weeks following abrasion, a violaceous papule or pustule develops and may ulcerate. It tends to be a solitary lesion, but occasionally multiple lesions can develop. Treatment includes antibiotic therapies: rifampin plus ethambutol or isoniazid, tetracycline like minocycline or co-trimazole (6).

The natural reservoirs of *M. avium intracellulare* (MAI) are infected birds and soil rich in bird droppings. Infection in humans occurs after traumatic inoculation or as a result of a disseminated infection. Skin ulcers occur along with suppurative nodules and abscesses. Surgical treatment is recommended if possible due to poor organism susceptibility to antimycobacterials (7). However, clarithromycin is the most useful antimicrobial agent against MAI. Other treatments include ethambutol, rifampin, amikacin, streptomycin, ciprofloxacin, clofazimine, azithromycin, and rifabutin.

M. fortuitum, Mycobacterium abscessus, and *Mycobacterium chelonae* are grouped to form the *Mycobacterium fortuitum* complex (6). They are commonly found in soil and water (7). Infection develops at a site of traumatic or surgical inoculation. The clinical presentation includes abscesses, violaceous nodules, and ulcers. The organisms should be identified and in vitro susceptibility should be performed before initiation of chemotherapy, because *M. fortuitum* is more susceptible to amikacin, cefoxitin, ciprofloxacin, and imipenen; *M. abscessus* to amikacin, cefoxitin, and clarithromycin; and *M. chelonae* to tobramycin and clarithromycin (6,7).

1.5. Anthrax

Anthrax is caused by a Gram-positive spore-forming rod, *Bacillus anthracis.* It is an acute infectious disease of animals, transmitted to humans by inoculation, inhalation, or ingestion. It is an uncommon bacterial disease. It was used as a biological weapon in the United States in the form of powder in October 2001, and it remains a potential threat. The cutaneous form of anthrax should be considered when a painless pruritic papule appears becomes a vesicle, undergoes necrosis, and enlarges forming an ulcer covered by black eschar (8). Gram-positive rods from scrapings of the cutaneous lesion and cultures support the diagnosis. Serologic tests may be of epidemiologic value. Treatment of cutaneous anthrax is with antibiotics: ciprofloxacin (500 mg po bid) or doxycycline (100 mg po bid) for 60 days.

1.6. Spirochetal Infection

Infrequently, ulcers can be the manifestation of syphilis (*Treponema pallidum*) or yaws (*Treponema pertenenue*) (9). Syphilis is a spirochete that infects mainly humans. Painless chronic ulcers may be a manifestation of late syphilis. They may look like venous ulcers or pyoderma gangrenosum, and demonstration of the Treponema in the lesions is difficult. Specific treponemal antigen tests are helpful in establishing the diagnosis (9).

Yaws is a non-veneral transmitted disease found in the tropical climates, where inoculation takes place at the site of minor skin injury. It begins as an erythematous papule that ulcerates, to slowly form an extensive painless papillomatous ulcer (9).

2. FUNGAL

The deep mycoses that more commonly cause leg ulcers are mycetoma, sporotrichosis, chromoblastomycosis, blastomycosis, histoplasmosis, and lobomycosis (2).

2.1. Eumycetoma

Mycetoma is caused by the introduction of bacteria or fungi by trauma with thorns, wood splinters, or solid objects. Actinomycetoma is due to bacteria, and eumycetoma refers to disease of fungal origin. The most common fungal agent isolated is *Madurella mycetomatis*. The disease is known as Madura foot or maduromycosis because of its initial description in the Madura district of India (10). It consists of small, painless, firm nodules evolving to form suppurative ulcers and sinuses with granules, which are aggregates of the causative agents. The lesions spread locally. Clinical suspicion, histopathology, and culture are needed to make the diagnosis. The treatment of eumycotic mycetomas is primarily surgical resection with cosmetic repair, since Amphotericin B has been tried with poor results (10).

2.2. Sporotrichosis

Sporotrichosis is caused by traumatic implantation of *Sporothrix schenckii* (oval, cigar-shaped yeast) into the skin from contaminated plants or soil. Several clinical presentations have been described (11). The most common presentation is lymphocutaneous sporotrichosis, which is characterized by painless nodules on the distal extremities that appear after three weeks to six months at the site of inoculation. Nodules can ulcerate, and subcutaneous secondary nodules are distributed along lymphatic vessels. A fixed cutaneous form of sporotrichosis is characterized by localized skin lesions without lymphatic involvement. Disseminated forms occur via hematogenous spread. The diagnosis is made by isolation of organism on culture.

The treatment of sporotrichosis includes oral potassium iodine starting at a dose 1 mL three times a day, gradually increasing by 1.5 mL per day until reaching a maximum of 18 mL per day for four weeks if no adverse events develop. Heat therapy, Amphotericin B, ketoconazole, itraconazole, flucytosine, and terbinafine have been tried with success (10,12).

2.3. Chromoblastomycosis

Chromoblastomycosis is caused by related fungi species including *Fonsecaea pedrosoi, Phialophora verrucosa, Fonsecaea compacta, Wangiella dermatitidis* and *Cladosporium carrionii*. The organisms are introduced traumatically into the skin from soil and wood. Clinically, asymptomatic warty papules gradually ulcerate and enlarge, forming brownish, black, dry, verrucous, hyperkeratotic plaques with lymphatic obstruction. This results in elephantiasis-like edema. Chromoblastomycosis is also known as "mossy foot" (10). The diagnosis is made by the clinical presentation, demonstration of fungus on histopathologic tissue section, and isolation of fungi on culture. The treatment includes surgical excision or cryosurgery plus itraconazole.

2.4. Blastomycosis

Blastomycosis is caused by *Blastomyces dermatitidis*, which inhabits soil in the Great Lakes and southeastern coastal region of the United States (12). It starts as a primary pulmonary disease subsequent to inhalation; however, cutaneous infection can appear after accidental exposure. Nodules that later ulcerate and regional lymphadenopathy are common in primary cutaneous blastomycosis. The diagnosis can be made with KOH preparation, or biopsy stained with PAS or Gomori stain. Primary cutaneous blastomycosis can be treated with oral potassium iodide solution.

2.5. Histoplasmosis

Histoplasmosis is caused by *Histoplasma capsulatum,* found in the eastern and central part of the United States and the Ohio and Mississippi River valleys (12). The fungus has been linked to exposure to pigeons or other birds, their feathers or droppings. Exposure is usually through inhalation of the spore. Histoplasmosis can spread from the lungs to other areas of the body. Primary cutaneous lesions are infrequent and may manifest as a chancre-type ulceration. The treatment includes amphotericin B, ketoconazole, and fluconazole.

2.6. Lobomycosis

Lobomycosis is caused by *Loboa loboi*. It is characterized by localized keloidal skin, plaques and nodules, which may ulcerate and develop fistulous tracts. It predominantly affects exposed areas and extremities (ears, buttocks, lumbosacral area, scapular area, elbows, and lower limbs). The diagnosis is made by demonstration of fungi in histopathologic section (10). The treatment includes surgical excision of localized lesions or cryotherapy.

3. PROTOZOAL

3.1. Leishmaniasis

There are three forms of leishmaniasis: cutaneous, mucocutaneous, and visceral. Cutaneous or mucocutaneous leishmaniasis can cause skin ulcers (2). Cutaneous leishmaniasis is caused in the Old World by *Leishmania aethiopica, Leishmania infantum, Leishmania tropica,* and *Leishmania major*, and in the New World by *Leishmania mexicana* and *Leishmania panamensis*. Mucocutaneous disease is associated with *L. braziliensis*. It is transmitted to humans by sandflies of the genus *Phlebotomus* in the Old World and *Lutzomyia* in the New World.

A red papule or nodule develops at the site of sandfly bite, enlarges, and later ulcerates. The ulcer is circular with raised borders. It is often solitary, but multiple ulcers can occur. The acute cutaneous infections heal spontaneously with scarring, but disseminated cutaneous leishmaniasis can occur in patients with minimal cell mediated immune response. Lesions caused by *L. braziliensis* may evolve into the mucocutaneous form, and should be treated with systemic treatment (13).

The first line of treatment for leishmaniasis includes parenteral administration of pentavalent antimonials, sodium stibogluconate (Pentostam), or *N*-methyl glucamine (Glucantime) for 10–30 days. Several drugs, such as amphotericin B, pentamidine, ketoconazole, and itraconazole, have also been used successfully.

3.2. Amebiasis

Amebiasis is caused by *Entamoeba histolytica*. It is associated with intestinal and extraintestinal infection, including liver abscess, peritonitis, pleuropulmonary abscess, and cutaneous amebic lesions. Cutaneous amebiasis is a rare complication of *E. histolytica* infection. Cutaneous lesions arise from the direct extension of gastrointestinal tract amebiasis, from surgical incision, from primary infection of the skin, from venereal transmission, or from metastasis from parasitemia (14). Lesions have been reported to occur on the trunk, buttocks, perineum, genitalia, and legs. The ulcers are oval with irregular ragged borders, and enlarge quickly. A scraping from the ulcer or biopsy from ulcer edge will demonstrate trophozoites and can confirm the diagnosis. The treatment of choice for cutaneous amebiasis is oral metronidazole.

4. VIRAL

Herpes viruses must be considered in any case of resistant erosions and ulcerations. Chronic genital ulcers have been reported to be common manifestations of viral infection caused by genital herpes in patients with HIV. Cytomegalovirus, another member of the herpes family, has been demonstrated to coexist with herpes simplex virus in painful perineal ulcers in AIDS patients, as well as in patients receiving long-term immunosuppressive therapy. Ulcers are typically large and painful (15). Suppressive therapy for genital or oral herpes includes acyclovir 400 mg twice a day, famciclovir 250 mg twice a day, or valacyclovir 500 mg to 1 g once a day. The treatment of cytomegalovirus includes ganciclovir and foscarnet.

5. CONCLUSION

An infectious etiology for ulcers should always be kept in mind. They may be difficult to diagnose, even when suspected. A thorough history is vital for the appropriate assessment of an ulcer and can frequently give clues to the likelihood of an infectious cause. Ultimately, cultures and biopsies are essential to make a definitive diagnosis.

REFERENCES

1. Phillips TJ, Dover JS. Leg ulcers [see comments]. J Am Acad Dermatol 1991; 25: 965–987.
2. Ouahes N, Phillips TJ. Leg ulcers. Curr Probl Dermatol July/August 1995:114–142.
3. Harahap M. Leg ulcers caused by bacterial infections. Clin Dermtatol 1990; 8:49–65.
4. Vujevich JJ, Kerdel FA. Bacterial infections. In: Kerdel FA, Jimenez–Acosta F, eds. Dermatology Just the Facts. McGrawHill, 2003:80.
5. Van der Werf T, Van der Graaf W, Tappero J, Asiedu K. Mycobacterium ulcerans infection. Lancet 1999; 3541:1013–1018.
6. Agarwal S, Berth-Jones J. Atypical mycobacteria. In: Lebwohl M, et al., eds. Treatment of Skin Disease. Mosby, 2002:65–68.
7. Tappeiner G, Wolff K. Tuberculosis and other mycobacterial infections. In: Freedberg IM, ed. Fitzpatrick's Dermatology in General Medicine. 6th ed. McGrawHill, 2003 1933–1949.
8. Swartz M. Recognition and management of anthrax, an update. N Engl J Med 2001; 345:1621–1626.

9. Sehgal V. Leg ulcers caused by jaws and endemic syphilis. Clin Dermatol 1990; 8: 166–174.
10. Sehgal V. Leg ulcers caused by deep mycotic infection. Clin Dermatol Leg Ulcers 1990; 3(4):157–165.
11. Davis B. Sporotrichosis. Dermatol Clin 1996; 14:69–76.
12. Trent J, Kirsner R. Identifying and treating mycotic skin infections. Adv Skin Wound Care 2003; 16:122–129.
13. Hepburn N. Cutaneous leishmaniasis. J Postgrad Med 2003; 49:50–54.
14. Majmudar B, Chaiken M, Lee K. Amebiasis of clitoris mimicking carcinoma. JAMA 1976; 236:1145–1146.
15. Colsky AS, Jegasothy SM, Leonardi C, Kirsner RS, Kerdel FA. Diagnosis and treatment of a case of cutaneous cytomegalovirus infection with a dramatic clinical presentation. J Am Acad Dermatol 1998; 38(2 Pt 2):349–351.

31

Genetic Diseases Associated with Ulceration of the Skin

Sharam Samson Yashar, Lauren Grasso, and David Fivenson
Department of Dermatology, Henry Ford Health System, Detroit, Michigan, U.S.A.

1. INTRODUCTION

Erosions and ulcerations of the skin are found in a variety of congenital skin disorders. Ulceration may be the initial clinical presentation leading to the consideration and diagnosis of a genetic disease, or it may be a secondary manifestation of an established genetic disorder (1–3). Erosions and/or ulcerations may be a manifestation of a congenital absence of the skin, incompetent barrier function from defective adhesion proteins between keratinocytes, unusual sensitivity to frictional trauma due to basement membrane protein defects, a result of self-mutilation, a secondary manifestation of an inability to sense cutaneous injuries, secondary to vesicle or bullae formation, or a predisposition to recurrent bacterial infections (Table 1) (4–7). Treatment of these skin ulcers is often a chronic process, with particular attention to localized wound care, prevention of secondary infection, along with appropriate treatment of the underlying condition (7). Other unique considerations include working with appropriate genetic counselors and with the child's parents and caretakers about the disorder and allowing for participation in the wound care of the child if possible.

2. ACRO-OSTEOLYSIS

Acro-osteolysis is an autosomal dominant disorder characterized by slowly progressive osteolysis of the phalanges in the hands and the feet, associated with recurrent ulcers of the fingers, toes, palms, and soles (2,3). Healing of the ulcers occurs with eventual loss of the fingers and toes. The age of onset is usually between 1 and 10 years of age, most frequently around the age of 6 years. The pathogenesis of the condition is unknown. In addition to the osteolysis and autoamputation that leads to gross mutilation, affected individuals are at high risk for osteomyelitis (8).

Table 1 Features of Genetic Disorders Associated with Erosions or Ulceration

Disorder	Inheritance	Clinical features of ulcers	Other clinical manifestations
Acro-osteolysis	Autosomal dominant	Recurrent ulcers of the fingers, toe, palms, and soles with eventual loss of the digits	Progressive osteolysis of the phalangtes, and higher incidence of osteomyelitis
Aplasia cutis congenita	Sporadic, autosomal dominant and recessive	Congenital localized absences of the epidermis, dermis, and subcutaneous tissue. Ulcers are sharply defined, and often are on the midline scalp	Possible underlying skeletal defects
Chediak–Higashi syndrome	Autosomal recessive	*Staphylococcus aureus* leg ulcers	Recurrent bacterial infections. Slate-gray skin, and light blond hair with a silver sheen Photophobia, strabismus Recurrent sinusitis, and pneumonia Progressive neurological deterioration
Congenital hemolytic anemias	Variable	Intractable ischemic irregularly shaped lower extremity ulcers	Hemolytic anemia
Congenital indifference to pain	Variable	Ulcers on the extremities secondary to unappreciated trauma	Muted pain sensation with or without autonomic dysfunction
Congenital localized absence of skin	Autosomal dominant	Congenital ulcers in the legs, ankles, and feet. Ulcers are mildly depressed with a glistening moist base	Onychogryphosis, or complete absence of nails. Trauma induced blistering of the extremities, and mucous membranes
Cutis marmorata telangiectatica congenita	Sporadic	Reticular vascular pattern with a marbled skin appearance, with rare epidermal atrophy and ulceration	Limb hemiatrophy Glaucoma Mental deficits
Epiderolysis bullosa	Variable	Blisters, erosions, and ulcers on trauma prone areas, with varying degrees of scarring	Variable digital fusion and joint contracture Recurrent skin infections

Disease	Inheritance	Skin findings	Associated features
Familial dysautonomia/Riley–Day syndrome	Autosomal recessive	Burns and ulceration of the hands and feet due to unrecognized injury. Self-mutilation	Blotching and mottling of the skin. Increased sweating and drooling
Flynna–Aird syndrome	Autosomal dominant	Scleroderma-like atrophy of the skin with ulceration	Nerve deafness; ocular anomalies; cerebral deficits
Focal dermal hypoplasia	X-linked dominant	Ulceration at sites of congenital absence of skin, with reddish yellow outpouching of the skin	Sparse hair, short stature. Scoliosis, syndactyly, lobster-claw deformity Osteopathia striata
Hailey–Hailey disease	Autosomal dominant	Erosions on an erythematous base involving the axial, groin, and intertriginous areas	
Homocystinuria	Autosomal recessive	Ulceration involving the legs	Malar rash; deep venous thrombosis; osteoporosis; mental deficits and seizures
Ichithyosis	Variable	Shallow erosions and ulcerations associated with ichthyosis	
Klinefelter syndrome	X-chromosome aneuploidy	Large bilateral leg ulcers associated with varicose veins, and arterial insufficiency	Tall stature, obesity. Gynecomastia, small testes, infertility
Langerhans cell histiocytosis	Sporadic	Ulcerated nodules and plagues involving the flexural ureas in infancy	Seborrheic eruption of the scalp and flexural areas. Fever, anemia, thrombocytopenia. Adenopathy, hepatosplenomegaly Increased malignancies and high mortality
Lesch-Nyhan syndrome	X-linked	Mutilation and ulceration of the lips, face, fingers, and wrists due to compulsive self-destructive behavior	Disrupted uric acid metabolism. Mental retardation, spastic cerebral palsy
Porphyria	Variable	Bullae, erosions, and shallow ulcers on sun-exposed areas, presenting at variable ages depending on sub-type	Disturbed porphyrin metabolism
Werner syndrome	Autosomal recessive	Indolent ulcers on pressure points, especially the ankles and soles	Generalized vascular disease. Loss of subcutaneous tissue, muscle wasting. Cataracts, and malignancy
Xeroderma pigmentosa	Autosomal recessive	Photodistributed erythema and vesiculation in early childhood, with ulcers and neoplasm in adolescence	Very high incidence of squamous and basal cell carcinoma, as well as melanoma

3. APLASIA CUTIS CONGENITA

Aplasia cutis congenita was first described by Campbell in 1826. Autosomal dominant as well as autosomal recessive forms of the condition have been reported (2).
The gene locus is unknown. The disorder is visible at birth with the presence of a
sharply defined skin defect most frequently involving the midline scalp. Other sites
including the trunk and extremities have also been observed. The defect in the skin
is often oval or circular, measuring 0.5–5.0 cm, with a glistening red base. The epidermis as well as the dermis may be missing, and ulceration may extend to the deep
subcutaneous tissue (9). Defects vary from a denuded ulcer with a red weeping or
granulating base to an erosion covered with a thin friable membrane. In 70% of
cases, there is a single ulceration. Multiple ulcers are less common. Histologic evaluation reveals the absence of epidermis, paucity of appendageal structures, and a
variable decrease in elastic tissues. In deeper defects, there is a complete deficit of
all layers of skin and subcutaneous tissues.

Healing occurs with atrophic or hypertrophic scarring, and the final healed
defect is usually devoid of appendages (10). Large or deep defects are predisposed
to significant secondary bacterial infections and hemorrhage. Localized wound care
and prevention of infection is the mainstay of therapy (2–4). Surgical intervention
may be indicated for more extensive lesions. It is important to recognize aplasia cutis
congenita and differentiate it from forceps or other birth injury related to delivery in
order to prevent medicolegal issues. Other diagnoses in the differential include nevus
sebaceous, heterotrophic brain tissue, localized scalp infection, meningocele, and
scarring alopecia (2). Imaging studies are required for cases with palpable bony
defects, large lesions, and defects involving the lumbosacral region. Imaging should
be performed first prior to any biopsies. The prognosis of this disorder is generally
good. Rare cases of fatal hemorrhage have been reported in cases where the defect
overlies the sagital suture and sagital sinus.

4. CHEDIAK–HIGASHI SYNDROME

Chediak–Higashi syndrome is an autosomal recessive genodermatosis characterized
by defective neurophil chemotaxis and phagocytosis (2,11). The disease usually presents a few months after birth, and patients are susceptible to recurrent bacterial
infections, particularly to *Staphylococcus aureus* (2,7). Recurrent bacterial infections
lead to lower extremity ulceration. Other clinical manifestations include slate-gray
skin, eccyhymoses, light blond hair with a silver sheen, photophobia, nystagmus,
recurrent sinusitis and pneumonia, and progressive neurologic deterioration leading
to ataxia, muscle weakness, sensory loss, and seizures (12).

5. CONGENITAL HEMOLYTIC ANEMIAS

Congenital hemolytic anemias are associated with dermatologic manifestations
(11,13). Occasionally, the presenting sign is an intractable ulcer of the lower extremity. Hereditary spherocytosis, hereditary elliptocytosis, thalassemia, hereditary
nonspherocytic hemolytic anemia, and sickle cell anemia are associated with leg
ulcers with varying incidences (11).

The cause of the ulceration is ischemic necrosis due to oxygen deprivation of the affected tissue. Ulcers can be unilateral or bilateral, single or multiple (2–5). They often have irregular shapes. The morphology of the ulcers is not specific for particular types of anemia. Ulcers associated with ischemic processes are frequently resistant to conventional therapy.

Histologic evaluation of the ulcer reveals nonspecific inflammatory changes. Treatment of the underlying hematologic disorder often improves the healing of the ulcers. Hyperbaric oxygen therapy may be of particular utility in these conditions.

6. CONGENITAL INDIFFERENCE TO PAIN SYNDROME

Congenital indifference to pain syndrome is characterized by muting of the pain sensation with or without dysautonomia (8). Patients may develop ulcers secondary to unappreciated injury, often on the lower extremities (14). The condition can be differentiated from the Riley–Day syndrome by the presence of fungiform papillae on the tongue. The genetic basis of the condition and inheritance pattern is under investigation (15).

7. CONGENITAL LOCALIZED ABSENCE OF SKIN

Congenital localized absence of skin is an autosomal dominant condition first described in 1966 by Bart et al. (16,17). Patients are born with a cutaneous defect on the lower extremities, most frequently on the medial legs, ankles, and feet (18,19). The lesions are mildly depressed ulcers with a glistening moist base (1–6). The ulcers gradually heal with regrowth of the epidermis from the boarders. The final scar is generally thin.

Other clinical manifestations include trauma-induced blistering of the extremities and mucous membranes. Nail abnormalities including onychogryphosis or complete absence of nails are also observed.

8. CUTIS MARMORATA TELANGIECTATICA CONGENITA

Cutis marmorata telangiectatica congenita—also referred to as congenital livedo reticularis, nevus vascularis reticularis, or congenital generalized phlebectasia—is defined by the presence of a persistent reticular vascular pattern at birth (1–7). It has a sporadic inheritance pattern, and the gene defect is not known (20). There is equal incidence in males and females. The reticular pattern results in a marbled skin appearance with progressive epidermal atrophy and rare ulceration. Involvement may be unilateral or bilateral. Hemiatrophy of the involved limb is seen in up to 10% of cases (2). Histopathologic findings are generally nonspecific. The epidermis may be uninvolved or may show atrophy and acanthosis. Dilated vascular spaces lined by swollen epithelial cells are found in the dermis. There may be dilated lymphatic vessels and vascular fibrosis.

Other associated abnormalities include glaucoma, mental retardation, and ipsilateral hemiatrophy or hemihypertrophy (21). The differential diagnosis includes capillary malformation, physiologic cutis marmorata, neonatal lupus erythematosus, and Rothmund–Thomson syndrome (2,22).

9. EPIDERMOLYSIS BULLOSA

There are numerous subtypes of epidermolysis bullosa, all of which are characterized by bullae, erosions, ulcerations, and varying degrees of scarring (Table 2) (2–5). The majority of lesions in these children are in trauma prone areas; thus, the term mechanobullous dermatoses is also used to describe these syndromes (24,25). Epidermolysis bullosa simplex is the most common subtype, and is an autosomal dominant disorder due to mutations in keratin 5 (chromosome 12q), and keratin 14 (chromosome 17q). Light microscopy reveals an intraepidermal bullae, while electron microscopy shows clumped tonofilaments (7).

Junctional epidermolysis bullosa is an autosomal recessive disorder due to mutations in laminin 5. Dystrophic epidermolysis bullosa is a disorder due to a defect in collagen VII, and can be inherited in an autosomal dominant or recessive manner.

The clinical features of all forms of epidermolysis bullosa include blisters, erosions, and healing with varying degrees of scarring, milia formation, distal fusion, and joint contracture. Treatment is primarily supportive and protective, with cultured skin component grafts showing promise.

10. FAMILIAL DYSAUTONOMIA

Familial dysautonomia, also known as the Riley–Day syndrome, is a rare autosomal recessive condition localized to chromosome 9q31–q33 (2–5,26). It is characterized by a lack of sensation, resulting in burns, ulcerations, and biting of the tongue. The ulcerations are usually secondary to thermal burns or trauma. Blotching and mottling of the skin, as well as increased sweating and drooling are also characteristic. There may also be loss of teeth due to inadvertent biting. An almost pathognomonic sign for this condition is the absence of fungiform papillae on the tongue.

The condition presents in infancy to early childhood. It is more common in the Ashkenazi Jewish population, and has an equal male/female incidence. Developmental arrest of the unmelinated sensory and sympathetic neurons with autonomic dysfunction is the hypothesized pathogenesis (2–6). Other clinical manifestations include short stature, recurrent bronchopneumonia, gastroesophageal reflux, hypotonia, and scoliosis (27).

11. FLYNN–AIRD SYNDROME

Flynn–Aird syndrome is an autosomal dominant disorder characterized by nerve deafness, ocular anomalies, and atrophy of the skin (1,3–6,28). The earliest manifestation is nerve deafness usually seen in the first decade of life. Cutaneous atrophy and ulceration is seen in the second decade. The atrophy is similar to scleroderma in its clinical appearance, and the histologic changes are characteristic of peripheral neuritis.

Table 2 Features of Epidermolysis Bullosa

Disease group	Inheritance	Vesicle location	Clinical features	Genes involved	Proteins involved
Generalized EB simplex	AD	Intraepidermal	Onset at birth or infancy. Bullae and erosions on hands and feet. Palmar-plantar hyperkeratosis Minimal involvement oral mucosa	KRT5, KRT14	Keratins 5, 14
Localized EB simplex	AD	Intraepidermal	Onset at childhood, adolescence, or adulthood. Traumatic bullae on the extremities. Hyperhydrosis of the palms and soles	KRT5, KRT14	Keratins 5,14
Dowling-Meara EB simplex	AD	Intraepidermal	Onset at birth. Generalized distribution of bullae and ulcers. Grouped or herpetiform blisters on the trunk Oral mucosal and nail involvement. Condition is not exacerbated by heat	KRT5, KRT14	Keratins 5,14
EB simplex muscular dystrophy	AR	Intraepidermal	Generalized blistering and erosions on the extremities. Adult onset muscular dystrophy	PLEC1	Plectin
Junctional EB lethal	AR	Basement membrane zone	Severe generalized blistering at birth. High mortality rate by age 1 year. Nails and teeth are dysplastic	LAMA3, B3, C2	Laminin 5
Junctional EB pyloric atresia	AR	Basement membrane zone	Severe mucosal and cutaneous fragility. Pyloric atresia. Urologic abnormalities	ITGA6,B4	Integrin $\alpha_6\beta_4$
Generalized atrophic benign EB	AR	Basement membrane zone	Nonlethal Small and medium bullae on the trunk and extremities. Nail and hair loss. Exacerbation with increased ambient heat	COL17A1, LAMB3	BP180, laminin
Dominant dystrophic EB	AD	Sublamina densa	Onset in infancy of adulthood. Acral blistering. Nail dystrophy	COL7A1	Type VII collagen
Recessive dystrophic EB	AR	Sublamina densa	Onset at birth. Atrophic scarring of the joints. High incidence of squamous cell carcinoma	COL7A1	Type VII collagen

Source: From Refs. 1–7, 11, 23–25.

12. FOCAL DERMAL HYPOPLASIA

Goltz syndrome, also known as focal dermal hypoplasia, is an X-linked dominant disorder localized to Xp22.31, primarily affecting females (2–7). It is characterized by asymmetric atrophic lineal streaks in Blaschko's lines on the trunk and extremities. Ulcers develop at sites of congenital absence of skin and reddish yellow outpuchings of the skin can be observed. Ulcerations heal with atrophic scars. Other manifestations include papillomas on the lips, perineum, axilla, and periumbilical area. Scoliosis, sparse hair, hyperpigmentation, syndactyly, "lobster-claw" deformities, and osteopathia striata are hallmarks of the disorder (29–31). The condition is usually diagnosed at birth due to severe skeletal abnormalities.

13. HAILEY–HAILEY DISEASE

Benign familial pemphigus or Hailey–Hailey disease is an autosomal dominant blistering disorder characterized by erosions on an erythematous base involving the axilla, groin, and intertriginous areas (7). It can present in the second to fifth decade of life. The histopathology shows a suprabasal bulla with acanthosis.

14. HOMOCYSTINURIA

Homocystinuria is an autosomal recessive disorder localized to the 21q22.3 gene locus (2–6,32). It is characterized by a malar rash, deep venous thrombosis, livedo reticularis, and leg ulcers. Other manifestations of the condition include marfanoid habitus, osteoporosis, mental retardation, and seizures (11). The disorder is due to a deficiency in cystathionine beta-synthase, leading accumulation of homocystine (32). It usually presents in early childhood. Treatment of the condition includes a low methionine, high cystine diet, and vitamin B6 supplementation (11).

15. ICHTHYOSIS

Erosions and shallow ulcerations can be found in all forms of ichthyosis. In particular, epidermolytic hyperkeratosis, lamellar ichthyosis, congenital ichthyosiform erythroderma, and harlequin fetus have marked erosions (33). Local wound care with emollients and topical antibiotics are often helpful.

16. KLINEFELTER SYNDROME

Klinefelter syndrome is a disorder of X chromosome aneuploidy due to nondisjunction during maternal or paternal meiosis leading to an XXY genotype (2,11). The condition is characterized by tall stature, obesity, gynecomastia, small testes and penis, infertility, decreased levels of testosterone, scant body hair, varicose veins, and arterial as well as venous leg ulcers (2–5,34,35). The diagnosis is made by chromosomal analysis. The leg ulcers are usually bilateral and can be rather large. Varicosities are often prominent and are associated with stasis dermatitis.

17. LANGERHANS CELL HISTIOCYTOSIS

Ulcerated nodules are often seen in the flexural areas of patients with Langerhans cell histiocytosis, or histiocytosis X (2,5–7). Infants with this condition have widespread cutaneous disease with a seborrheic rash involving the scalp and flexural surfaces. The diagnosis is made by visualization of histiocytes with Birbeck granules on histologic evaluation of cutaneous biopsy specimens. Treatment of the skin lesions is usually conservative and supportive; however, in cases with more severe lesions, topical corticosteroids and/or nitrogen mustard have been beneficial (36).

18. LESCH–NYHAN SYNDROME

Lesch–Nyhan syndrome is an X-linked disorder of purine metabolism caused by a deficiency of hypoxanthine-guanine phosphoribosyl transferase (HG-PRTase) (11). This deficiency leads to an overproduction of uric acid, which leads to the clinical manifestations of mental retardation, spastic cerebral palsy, and compulsive self-mutilating behavior (37,38). Diagnosis can be made by demonstration of increased uric acid levels in the blood and urine. The main clinical features include mutilation and ulceration of the lips, face, fingers, and wrists due self-mutilation (11). Allopurinol is the primary treatment of the metabolic abnormality.

19. PORPHYRIA

Disorders of porphyrin metabolism lead to increased levels of porphyrins in the skin, which cause photosensitization following light absorption. Patients subsequently develop bullae, erosions, and shallow ulcers on sun exposed regions (Table 3) (39–41). Congenital erythropoietic porphyria, also referred to as Gunther's disease, is an autosomal recessive disorder due to deficiency of uroporphyrinogen III cosynthetase in the bone marrow. The defect has been mapped to the gene locus 10q25 (2,5–7). It presents in infancy or early childhood (11).

Erythropoietic protoporphyria is an autosomal dominant disorder secondary to a deficiency of ferrochelatase leading to excess protoporphyrin production. The defect has been mapped to chromosome 18. Hereditary coproporphyria is an autosomal dominant disorder localized to chromosome 9 (2). It usually presents in the third or fourth decade of life. Variegate porphyria is inherited in an autosomal dominant pattern, and presents after puberty. It is localized to chromosome 14q32, and is due to a deficiency of protoporphyrinogen oxidase. Acute intermittent porphyria is an autosomal dominant disorder due to porphobilinogen deaminase deficiency (39). It presents in the third to fourth decade of life. Porphyria cutanea tarda is an autosomal dominant form, due to a deficiency in uroporphyrinogen decarboxylase (40). It often presents in the third to fourth decade as well.

Urine and blood porphyrin studies are indicated in cases of suspected porphyria. Sun protection and local wound care with topical antibiotics are often helpful.

20. WERNER SYNDROME

Werner syndrome, also known as progeria of the adult is an autosomal recessive disorder mapped to chromosome 8p12, characterized by premature aging during the

Table 3 Features of Disorders of Porphyrin Metabolism

Disease	Inheritance	Age of onset (years)	Clinical features	Enzyme involved
Erythropoietic porphyria	AR	0–10	Early manifestations: vesicles, bullae, erosions, hypertrichosis. Late manifestations: atrophic scarring, cicatrizing alopecia, sclerodermoid changes, mutilating deformities of the hands, ears, face, and nose	Urogen III cosynthase
Erythropoietic protoporphyria	AD	1–4	Early manifestation: photoinduced pruritus and burning of the skin; rare vesicles and bullae. Late manifestations: waxy thickening of the hands and face with longer sun exposure	Ferochelatase
Variegate porphyria	AD	10–20	Bullae, erosions, skin fragility. Scarring, millia, and hyperpigmentation. Hypertrichosis	Protoporphyrinogen oxidase
Hereditary coproporphyria	AD		Delayed photosensitivity. Bullae, erosions, skin fragility, and hypertrichosis. Scarring, millia, and hyperpigmentation. Neurologic symptoms are very common	Coproporphyrinogen oxidase
Porphyria cutanea tarda	Variable	30–40	Moderately severe bullae on dorsa of hands and feet. Ulcerative lesions on light exposed areas. Increase skin fragility. Scarring alopecia, hyperpigmentation, hypertrichosis	Urogen decarboxylase in liver and RBC
Hepatoerythropoietic porphyria	AD	1	Severe photosensitivity. Vesicles, bullae, erosions on sun exposed areas. Mutilating scarring, sclerodermoid changes. Scarring alopecia	Uroporphyrinogen decarboxylase

Source: From Refs. 1–7, 11, 39-41.

second and third decades (2,11). The age of presentation is in the third and fourth decades of life. Loss of subcutaneous tissue with binding down of the skin leads to sclerodermatous-like changes including shiny atrophic skin and telangiectasia are common. Ulceration of the legs and feet and calcinosis cutis are found in 1/3 of patients (2–5,42). Other abnormalities include early atherosclerosis, cataracts, glaucoma, growth restriction, osteoporosis, diabetes, and malignancies (43). Urinary hyaluronic acid and serum glucose are increased. Radiologic examination of the extremities reveals osteoporosis and calcification (11). It has been hypothesized that cutaneous fibroblasts have a reduced growth potential (2). The observance of increased urinary hyaluronic acid may reflect abnormalities in glycosaminoglycan metabolism.

21. XERODERMA PIGMENTOSUM

Xeroderma pigmentosum is an autosomal recessive disorder due to defective DNA repair (44,45). Patients present early in childhood with photodistributed erythema and vesiculation (46). Subsequently, patients develop erosions, ulcers, and neoplasm. There is a high incidence of basal cell and squamous cell carcinoma, as well as melanoma. A complete skin cancer screening is required every 3 months, and any suspicious lesions, or ulcers require a biopsy. Strict sun avoidance and protection from light is crucial.

REFERENCES

1. Mallory SB, Leal-Khouri S.An Illustrated Dictionary of Dermatologic Syndromes. Pearl River, New York: Parthenon Publishing Group, 1994.
2. Spitz JL. Genodermatoses, A Full-Color Clinical Guide to Genetic Disorders. Baltimore, Maryland: Lippincott Williams & Wilkins, 1996.
3. Der Kaloustian VM, Kurban AK. Genetic Diseases of the Skin. Berlin, Germany: Springer-Verlag, 1979.
4. Sybert VP. Genetic Skin Disorders. New York, New York: Oxford University Press, 1997.
5. Schachner LA, Hansen RC. Pediatric Dermatology. 2nd ed. New York, New York: Churchill Livingston, 1995.
6. Hurwitz S. Clinical Pediatric Dermatology. Philadelphia, Pennsylvania: W.B. Saunders, 1993.
7. Freedberg I, Eisen A, Wolfe K, Austen K, Goldsmith L, Katz S, Fitzpatrick T. Dermatology in General Medicine. New York, New York: McGraw-Hill, 1999.
8. Bockers M, Benes P, Bork K. Persistent skin ulcers, mutilations, and acro-osteolysis in hereditary sensory and autonomic neuropathy with phospholipid excretion. Report of a family. J Am Acad Dermatol 1989; 21(4 Pt 1):736–739.
9. Caksen H, Kurtoglu S. Our experience with aplasia cutis congenita. J Dermatol 2002; 29(6):376–379.
10. Frieden IJ. Aplasia cutis congenita: a clinical review and proposal for classification. J Am Acad Dermatol 1986; 14(4):646–660.
11. Behrman R, Kliegman R, Jenson H. Nelson Textbook of Pediatrics. 16th ed. New York, New York: W.B. Saunders, 2000.
12. Ward DM, Shiflett SL, Kaplan J. Chediak–Higashi syndrome: a clinical and molecular view of a rare lysosomal storage disorder. Curr Mol Med 2002; 2(5):469–477.
13. Glader BE. Hemolytic anemia in children. Clin Lab Med 1999; 19(1):87–111, vi.

14. Shahriaree H, Kotcamp WW, Sheikh S, Sajadi K. Hereditary perforating ulcers of the foot: "hereditary sensory radicular neuropathy". Clin Orthop 1979; (140):189–193.

15. Indo Y. Genetics of congenital insensitivity to pain with anhidrosis (CIPA) or hereditary sensory and autonomic neuropathy type IV. Clinical, biological and molecular aspects of mutations in TRKA(NTRK1) gene encoding the receptor tyrosine kinase for nerve growth factor. Clin Auton Res 2002; 12(suppl 1):I20–I32.

16. Bart BJ, Gorlin RJ, Anderson VE, Lynch FW. Congenital localized absence of skin and associated abnormalities resembling epidermolysis bullosa. A new syndrome. Arch Dermatol 1966; 93(3):296–304.

17. Arand AG, Ball WS, Crone KR. Congenital scalp defects: Adams–Oliver syndrome. A case report and review of the literature. Pediatr Neurosurg 1991–1992; 17(4):203–207.

18. Gharpuray MB, Tolat SN, Patki AH. Congenital localized absence of skin associated with blistering of the skin and mucous membranes: Bart's syndrome. Cutis 1989; 44(4):318–320.

19. Duran-McKinster C, Rivera-Franco A, Tamayo L, de la Luz Orozco-Covarrubias M, Ruiz-Maldonado R. Bart syndrome: the congenital localized absence of skin may follow the lines of Blaschko. Report of six cases. Pediatr Dermatol 2000; 17(3):179–182.

20. Danarti R, Happle R, Konig A. Paradominant inheritance may explain familial occurrence of Cutis marmorata telangiectatica congenita. Dermatology 2001; 203(3):208–211.

21. Gerritsen MJ, Steijlen PM, Brunner HG, Rieu P. Cutis marmorata telangiectatica congenita: report of 18 cases. Br J Dermatol 2000; 142(2):366–369.

22. Picascia DD, Esterly NB. Cutis marmorata telangiectatica congenita: report of 22 cases. J Am Acad Dermatol 1989; 20(6):1098–1104.

23. Eady RA. Epidermolysis bullosa: scientific advances and therapeutic challenges. J Dermatol 2001; 28(11):638–640.

24. Uitto J, Pulkkinen L, McLean WH. Epidermolysis bullosa: a spectrum of clinical phenotypes explained by molecular heterogeneity. Mol Med Today 1997; 3(10):457–465.

25. Lin AN. Management of patients with epidermolysis bullosa. Dermatol Clin 1996; 14(2):381–387.

26. Goldstein-Nieviazhski C, Wallis K. Riley–Day syndrome (familial dysautonomia). Survey of 27 cases. Ann Paediat 1966; 206(3):188–194.

27. Laplaza FJ, Turajane T, Axelrod FB, Burke SW. Nonspinal orthopaedic problems in familial dysautonomia (Riley–Day syndrome). J Pediatr Orthop 2001; 21(2):229–232.

28. Flynn P, Aird RB. A neuroectodermal syndrome of dominant inheritance. J Neurol Sci 1965; 2(2):161–182.

29. Kegel MF. Dominant disorders with multiple organ involvement. Dermatol Clin 1987; 5(1):205–219.

30. Mevorah B, Politi Y. Genodermatoses in women. Clin Dermatol 1997; 15(1):17–29.

31. Moore DJ, Mallory SB. Goltz syndrome. Pediatr Dermatol 1989; 6(3):251–253.

32. Cacciari E, Salardi S. Clinical and laboratory features of homocystinuria. Haemostasis 1989; 19(suppl 1):10–13.

33. Shwayder T. Ichthyosis in a nutshell. Pediatr Rev 1999; 20(1):5–12.

34. Zollner TM, Veraart JC, Wolter M, Hesse S, Villemur B, Wenke A, Werner RJ, Boehncke WH, Jost SS, Scharrer I, Kaufmann R. Leg ulcers in Klinefelter's syndrome—further evidence for an involvement of plasminogen activator inhibitor-1. Br J Dermatol 1997; 136(3):341–344.

35. Veraart JC, Hamulyak K, Neumann HA. Klinefelter's syndrome as a model for skin changes in venous insufficiency. Wien Med Wochenschr 1994; 144(10–11):277–278.

36. Wong E, Holden CA, Broadbent V, Atherton DJ. Histiocytosis X presenting as intertrigo and responding to topical nitrogen mustard. Clin Exp Dermatol 1986; 11(2): 183–187.

37. Stout JT, Caskey CT. The Lesch—Nyhan syndrome: clinical, molecular and genetic aspects. Trends Genet 1988; 4(6):175–178.

38. Nyhan WL. The Lesch–Nyhan syndrome. Annu Rev Med 1973; 24:41–60.

39. Lim HW. Porphyria update. Pediatr Dermatol 2000; 17(1):75–83.

40. Lim HW, Cohen JL. The cutaneous porphyrias. Semin Cutan Med Surg 1999; 18(4): 285–292.
41. Lim HW. The porphyrias: an introduction. Photodermatol Photoimmunol Photomed 1998; 14(2):46–47.
42. Lebel M. Werner syndrome: genetic and molecular basis of a premature aging disorder. Cell Mol Life Sci 2001; 58(7):857–867.
43. Degreef H. The Werner syndrome. Dermatologica 1971; 142(1):45–49.
44. Moriwaki S, Kraemer KH. Xeroderma pigmentosum—bridging a gap between clinic and laboratory. Photodermatol Photoimmunol Photomed 2001; 17(2):47–54.
45. Berneburg M, Lehmann AR. Xeroderma pigmentosum and related disorders: defects in DNA repair and transcription. Adv Genet 2001; 43:71–102.
46. Lambert WC, Kuo HR, Lambert MW. Xeroderma pigmentosum. Dermatol Clin 1995; 13(1):169–209.

32

Wound Bed Preparation and Debridement

Meggan R. Banta and Anna F. Falabella
Department of Dermatology and Cutaneous Surgery, University of Miami School of Medicine, Miami, Florida, U.S.A.

1. INTRODUCTION

Acute wound healing generally follows an overlapping four-step process: coagulation, inflammation, proliferation/matrix repair, and remodeling/epithelialization. Nonhealing or chronic wounds become "stuck" in one of these stages. They are characterized by defective remodeling of the extracellular matrix, a failure to re-epithelialize, and prolonged inflammation (1–3). The concept of wound bed preparation is a method to systematically approach and treat chronic wounds. Debridement is often the focus of wound bed preparation, but the broad goals are to remove necrotic and/or fibrinous tissue from the wound bed, decrease bacterial burden, increase the amount of granulation tissue, decrease exudates and edema, and reduce the number of abnormal or senescent cells within the wound or at the wound edge (4). Staging systems have been developed to compare the efficacy of interventions, taking into account wound bed appearance and the amount of wound exudates (5). In this chapter, we will review the goals of wound bed preparation with a focus on debridement.

2. HISTORY

The concept of wound bed preparation dates back to ancient times when the Incas cleaned wounds using vegetable concoctions or the eggs of certain birds then covered them with feathers or bandages made from animal skin. The ancient Egyptians used "rotten bread" and gum-impregnated linen strips to treat wounds. Two ancient Chinese medical texts were entirely devoted to the treatment of wounds. These ancient civilizations and pre-Colombian cultures commonly employed surgical approaches as well. The surgeon Hua T'o reportedly treated a wound on the arm of a famous general by "cutting his flesh and scraping the bone"(6).

    The ancient Greeks treated wounds with mineral substances and plant extracts. They commonly covered wounds with cloth, likely causing the accumulation of wound fluid. This practice may have led to the concept of "laudable pus," a popular notion in the Middle Ages. Since drainage of pus precedes the healing of boils and other wounds, healers believed that the production of pus in wounds was desirable.

Ideas changed as 13th century surgeons began to apply wine-soaked bandages in order to avoid pus formation. They also treated wounds with hot irons, boiling oil, and caustic solutions. By the 17th century, physicians commonly treated wounds by careful application of bandages soaked in hot water and healing ointments. Cauterization and blood letting were also common practices (6).

3. DEBRIDEMENT

It is commonly accepted that cleansing and debridement are critical components of wound care. Removal of nonviable tissue from the wound bed reduces the number of micro-organisms, toxins, and other substances that may inhibit wound healing by stimulating inflammation and delaying granulation and epithelialization (7–9). Debridement removes senescent cells in the wound bed and nonmigratory cells from the ulcer edge, allows for improved availability of growth factors, and removes excessive or abnormal bacteria (10,11).

Current medical practice employs several methods for debridement, including autolytic, chemical, surgical (sharp), biologic or biosurgical, and mechanical (12,13). The former four methods are considered to be selective modalities, those resulting in the removal of mainly necrotic tissue. The latter method is considered to be nonselective, removing both necrotic and viable tissue (13). In practice, the selective modalities also remove or damage healthy tissue. The most selective modality is autolytic debridement.

Autolytic debridement describes the process of inherent wound bed cleaning by phagocytic cells and proteolytic enzymes (14). A moist wound environment promotes and enhances this process (15,16). Though the easiest and most natural form of debridement, it is slower than the other methods. Autolytic debridement should be promoted in all wounds but generally is contraindicated in the setting of infection.

In chemical debridement, proteolytic enzymes that chemically digest and remove cellular debris are applied to the wound bed (17). Some of these debriding agents have intrinsic bactericidal activity. Chemical/enzymatic debridement is claimed to be effective over several days to weeks. A painless modality, it can be utilized in conjunction with the other methods of wound debridement (16). Possible side effects of chemical debridement include damage to viable tissue within or around the wound and hypersensitivity reactions to product ingredients. The enzymatic agents are affected by the pH of the wound environment and can be inactivated by heavy metals present in other commonly used topical agents.

Surgical or sharp debridement is the removal of necrotic tissue by surgical instrumentation (8,13). This is the fastest form of debridement. It is utilized commonly in infected wounds or those with significant amounts of necrotic tissue. Sharp debridement offers the added advantage of allowing the clinician to more accurately assess the severity and extent of wounds. It should be practiced only by skilled clinicians. Disadvantages include the need for anesthesia, potential damage to or removal of viable tissue, and the possibility of considerable bleeding.

Biologic debridement is an old form of debridement that is regaining popularity due to both its success and its cost. Maggots, most commonly the blowfly *Lucilia sericata*, applied to a wound bed remove only necrotic tissue. They exhibit antimicrobial properties and some believe their secretions to be active against biofilm (18,19). One fly hatches enough larvae to treat five patients, an extremely cost-effective method (20).

Methods of mechanical debridement include wet-to-dry dressings, hydrotherapy, irrigation, and dextranomers. These modalities physically and rapidly remove debris from the wound bed. Wounds with larger amounts of necrotic tissue generally receive mechanical debridement. The two main drawbacks include pain and the nonselective removal of tissue.

3.1. Autolytic Debridement

Autolytic debridement, the natural and most selective form, can be promoted and enhanced by the use of occlusive dressings. Occlusive dressings help manage wound exudates and provide a moist wound environment, which has been shown to accelerate wound healing by as much as 50% compared to air-exposed wounds (21,22). Despite a number of clinical trials that have demonstrated their efficacy, occlusive dressings are underutilized by clinicians, commonly due to lack of knowledge and the incorrect perception that a moist environment promotes infection (23). Moist occlusion is conducive to bacterial growth, but wounds re-epithelialize more rapidly in this environment than in open air despite increased bacterial counts (24,25). Occlusive dressings are contraindicated in wounds that clinically appear to be grossly contaminated. Numerous clinical trials have demonstrated that acute and chronic wounds treated with occlusive dressings are less likely to become infected than wounds treated with conventional dressings (26). Proposed reasons for this include the relative impermeability of the dressings to exogenous bacteria, increased numbers of viable neutrophils in the wound fluid, the accumulation of natural substances in wound fluid that inhibit bacterial growth, and reduction of necrotic tissue in the occluded wound (23,26–30).

3.2. Chemical Debridement

In the early stages of wound healing, autolytic debridement occurs through the action of neutrophil-derived enzymes, including elastase, collagenase, myeloperoxidase, acid hydrolase, and lysosomes (31). Bacteria play a key role by also producing proteolytic enzymes that contribute to wound debridement, such as hyaluronidase, and by stimulating neutrophils to release their proteases (33). Protease inhibitors are also released in order to restrict protease action to the wound bed and minimize potential damage to viable skin at the wound edge. Understanding the inherent properties of these enzymes and their inhibitors enables a better understanding of the commercially available products for chemical/enzymatic debridement.

Collagenase is a metalloendoproteinase produced by keratinocytes, dermal fibroblasts, macrophages, and neutrophils (32). It degrades collagen in vivo. During early wound healing, collagenase assists with clot debridement. Later, it assists with wound remodeling by degrading old collagen and allowing new collagen deposition.

Collagenase, elastase, and trypsin play a critical role in cell migration by dissolving desmosomes and hemidesmosomes thereby allowing fibroblasts and endothelial cells to detach from the basement membrane and migrate into the wound (31). Plasmin, or fibrinolysin, works in similar fashion. It has been suggested that these proteases not only "clear the path" for migrating cells but also produces fragments via degradation of cellular debris by that are chemotactic to keratinocytes, thus promoting epithelialization. However, proteases can adversely affect wound healing if present in excessive amounts by breaking down the extracellular matrix substance necessary for epithelial cell migration (33).

Cell migration is terminated when protease inhibitors are released, and the proteases are deactivated. One protease inhibitor, tissue inhibitor of metalloprotease, typically remains in balance with collagenase in intact skin, thereby preventing inappropriate cellular detachment and migration. Production of protease inhibitors by cells at the wound edge keeps healing processes confined to the wound (32).

Proteolytic enzymes have been used to promote wound healing for centuries. Christopher Columbus reported a practice among warriors in the Caribbean Islands to treat wounds with pineapple juice (34), which contains the abundant amounts of the protease bromelain. Other historical examples include the use of paw-paw juice, which contains papain and chymopapain, and the use of live maggots whose salivary fluid is rich in proteases (35). Commercially available enzymatic debriding agents include fibrinolysin/DNAse, collagenase, streptokinase/streptodornase, and papain/urea.

3.2.1. Fibrinolysin/DNAse

Fibrinolysin degrades fibrin, inactivates fibrinogen and the coagulation factors I, V, and VII, and dilates blood vessels in the wound bed. Fibrin degradation and the early wound matrix allow macrophages to enter the wound bed and debride necrotic tissue. Degradation products are not resorbed. Deoxyribonuclease, a DNAse extracted from bovine pancreas, cleaves nucleic acids and leads to liquefaction of exudates and decreased viscosity (14).

The combination agent DNAse/fibrinolysin should benefit exudative wounds since exudates consist mostly of fibrinous material and nucleoproteins. It should also improve wound tissue perfusion thus healing via fibrinolysin's vasodilatory effect on the wound bed. Several small clinical trials have reported that fibrinolysin alone is an effective cleansing agent (14).

A randomized, double-blind, placebo-controlled clinical trial tested the efficacy and safety of a commercially available fibrinolysin/DNAse, Elase®, against its component agents (DNAse and fibrinolysin) and placebo (inactive carrier) for the treatment of chronic leg ulcers. A total of 84 patients with wounds were studied. Results showed that Elase provided no long-term benefit in reducing overall purulent exudates, pain, erythema, necrotic tissue, or overall condition of chronic leg ulcers when compared to either of its two components or placebo (37). The product has since been removed from the market.

3.2.2. Collagenase

Collagenase is an enzyme isolated from *Clostridium histolyticum*. It cleaves glycine in helical regions of native collagen containing the sequence x-proline-y-glycine-proline-z. The enzyme digests collagen but is not active against keratin, fat, or fibrin. It is optimally active at pH 6.0–8.0. Theoretically, collagenase promotes wound healing by digesting native collagen bundles that bind nonviable tissue to the wound surface and by dissolving collagenic debris within the wound. None of the other commercially available proteases are active against native collagen (39).

Several clinical trials of collagenase have reported rapid cleansing and enhanced removal of necrotic debris. The majority of these trials were open and uncontrolled. A controlled clinical trail comparing collagenase vs. fibrinolysin/DNAse and streptokinase/streptodornase in 258 patients with leg ulcers showed no statistically significant difference in outcomes between the treatment groups (40). A prospective, randomized, double-blind study comparing collagenase and fibrinolysin/DNAse in 121 elderly patients with pressure ulcers showed slightly better results using collagenase with regard to the change in the yellow surface of the wound bed, but it was not statistically significant (41). Another small (30 patients) double-blind, placebo-controlled trial reported that collagenase was superior to placebo (42).

3.2.3. Streptokinase/Streptodornase

Streptokinase, a fibrinolytic enzyme used to degrade clots in acute myocardial infarction, and streptodornase, an endonuclease that decreases viscosity, are available in the combined product Varidase®. Varidase is used for the treatment of purulent disease, such as empyema, and topically for purulent/suppurating wounds (43,44). It has also been shown to be useful in *Pseudomonas aeruginosa* focal infection via biofilm removal (45). In a randomized, double-blind, controlled trial comparing Varidase in a hydrogel vs. hydrogel alone in the debridement of 21 Grade IV pressure ulcers, eschar removal occurred more quickly in the hydrogel alone group but without statistical significance (46).

3.2.4. Papain-Urea

Papain is a proteolytic enzyme derived from the fruit carica papaya. Juice of the papaya fruit has been used for centuries to treat wounds. In 1879, scientists isolated and purified the proteinase derived from papaya, and named this enzyme papain. Papain digests necrotic tissue by liquefying fibrinous debris. It has an advantage over other available debriding agents in that it is active across a wider pH range, from 3.0 to 12.0. Papain requires the presence of activators to function and is relatively ineffective when used alone; therefore, it is combined with urea. This combination serves two functions: (a) urea exposes activators of papain that are present in necrotic debris but relatively inaccessible to papain and (b) urea denatures nonviable protein matter rendering it more susceptible to proteolysis. Papain is inactive against collagen (42).

Early clinical trials evaluating the efficacy of papain were performed in the 1940s and 1950s. Trial results were consistently positive, but were uncontrolled, unblinded, and small. An in vitro study comparing papain and urea vs. papain alone showed the combination therapy to provide twice as much digestion (33). To date, large, placebo-controlled, blinded trials studying the efficacy of papain/urea have not been done.

3.3. Biological Debridement

Also known as biosurgery or maggot debridement therapy (MDT), biological debridement with larva has three effects on wounds: debridement, disinfection, and promotion of wound healing (47). Maggots not only liquefy dead tissue via secretion of proteases, but also ingest the remaining debris. Recent laboratory studies confirm prior reports of the antimicrobial properties in maggot secretions (18) and demonstrate their bactericidal effect against multidrug resistant strains of *Staphylococcus aureus* and clinical isolates of pathogenic *Streptococcus* sp. (19)

In the clinical arena, prospective controlled studies comparing maggot therapy to conventional treatments for managing pressure ulcers in spinal cord injury patients showed that MDT debrided wounds faster than any of the other modalities used, and it accelerated overall wound healing (48).

3.4. Mechanical Debridement

There are several methods of mechanical debridement, including application of wet-to-dry dressings, hydrotherapy, irrigation, and dextranomers (12,49). Despite the routine use of these modalities, they have not been studied in a randomized trial. Mechanical debridement provides a rapid way to remove nonviable tissue. A potential drawback to mechanical debridement is that it is nondiscriminatory and can remove viable tissue along with necrotic material (13). Mechanical debridement is usually reserved for larger, highly exudative wounds by moistening necrotic eschars and facilitating their removal.

3.4.1. Wet-to-Dry Dressings

In this nonselective debridement, a wet gauze dressing is applied to the wound bed and allowed to dry. Necrotic debris becomes embedded in the gauze and is mechanically stripped from the wound bed when the gauze is removed (50). This method can be painful, so adequate analgesia should be provided to the patients. It should not be used on clean, granulating wounds, since it can be traumatic to granulation tissue and new epithelium (50).

This method of debridement is rarely used. Even those who advocate it often actually use a modified version of wet-to-wet dressing removal. The pain and damage to healthy tissues make wet-to-dry dressings rather obsolete.

3.4.2. Hydrotherapy and Irrigation

With these modalities, wounds are cleansed and debrided using whirlpool therapy (Fig. 1) or by irrigation with saline or a cleansing agent. Wound irrigation can be done with a number of devices that supply low, intermediate, or high pressures. As with mechanical debridement, these modalities are nonselective. Low pressure may be ineffective, while higher pressures can damage viable tissue. Devices that deliver an irrigation pressure of 8 psi effectively clean wounds while largely avoiding wound trauma.

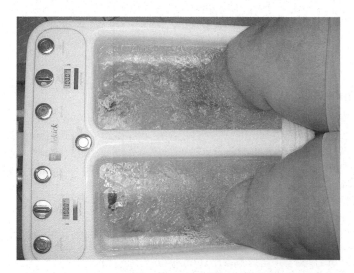

Figure 1   Mechanical debridement. Whirlpool therapy in a patient with venous ulcers.

Hydrotherapy and irrigation are best used on wounds with thick exudates, slough, or necrotic debris, and should not be used when the ulcer already has a clean granulating base. Potential drawbacks of these treatments include dehydration of the wound bed and maceration of surrounding tissues (51). In general, there are no studies indicating that whirlpool or irrigation actually enhance wound healing, although many clinicians would argue that they are helpful.

3.4.3. Dextranomer Therapy

A dextranomer is a high-molecular-weight derivative of dextran manufactured as dry, insoluble spherical beads measuring 0.1–0.3 mm in diameter. The beads are three-dimensional networks of dextran polymer cross-linked with epichlorhydrin. This structure is very hydrophilic and has a high absorptive capacity. One gram of dextranomer can absorb up to 4 g of fluid (52,53). Dextranomer absorbs exudates, bacteria, and other debris. There are potential drawbacks to its use: difficulty of application, painful dressing removal, wound bed dehydration, and periwound tissue irritation (53).

A product that combines iodine with a dextranomer has been marketed, cadexomer iodine, and will be discussed in the bacterial wound colonization section.

3.5. Surgical Debridement

Sharp debridement describes the use of sharp instruments such as curettes, scalpels, or scissors to remove nonviable tissue. As with mechanical debridement, experts routinely recommend sharp debridement despite the absence of randomized trials proving its efficacy vs. other treatment modalities. Sharp debridement is recommended for removal of thick, adherent eschars and devitalized tissue in large ulcers (Fig. 2a–c). It is also used to remove necrotic tissue rapidly when there is evidence of infection or sepsis. In diabetic foot ulcers, aggressive sharp debridement, or "excision of the wound," leads to improved outcomes when used with topically applied platelet-derived growth factor (54).

4. BACTERIAL WOUND COLONIZATION

All wounds are colonized with bacteria. The controversial issue is what role they play in wound healing. While bacteria contribute to debridement by producing proteolytic enzymes, it is commonly accepted that colonization should be kept to a minimum. High tissue bacterial counts are known to interfere with graft take (55), and small bacterial counts of specific organisms are known to impair wound healing (56). The recent attention to groups of genotypically and phenotypically altered bacteria that form colonies termed biofilm create particular difficulty in controlling pathogenic flora.

Surgical debridement is effectively used to reduce the bacterial burden. Some topical therapies combine antimicrobial effects with control of wound exudates and improvement in granulation tissue appearance. Maggot debridement therapy resorbs small amounts of exudate as described above and promotes granulation. Silver dressings that deliver silver ions act as antiseptics and share with cadexomer iodine the advantage of slow release, thereby decreasing the chance of cellular and tissue toxicity (4).

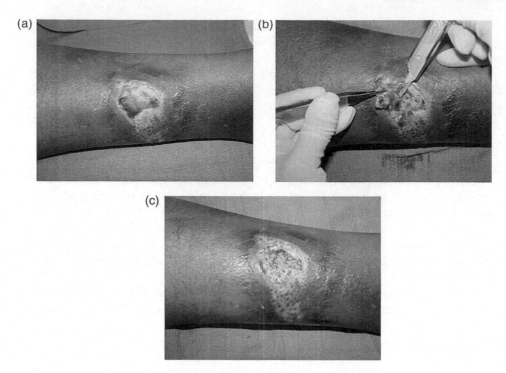

Figure 2 Surgical debridement. Lower extremity arterial ulcer with black eschar (a) before, (b) during, and (c) after sharp debridement.

Cadexomer iodine (Iodosorb®, Iodoflex®) is an antiseptic and antimicrobial that releases iodine at low concentrations while absorbing exudates (see Fig. 3). It is composed of a three-dimensional starch lattice, arranged into microspheres which contain physically immobilized 0.9% iodine. When applied to an exudative wound, the starch lattice swells as it absorbs exudates and debris thus increasing the size of its micropores and slowly releasing iodine into the wound bed (57). Cadexomer iodine has been shown to be effective in vivo against *S. aureus* and methicillin-resistant *S. aureus* (58,59). Over 40 clinical trials comparing cadexomer iodine to

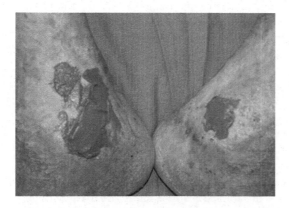

Figure 3 Cadexomer iodine applied to bilateral venous leg ulcers.

other methods of debridement in the treatment of wounds consistently have shown cadexomer iodine to be as effective or more effective than standard treatments.

5. EDEMA AND WOUND EXUDATE CONTROL

Edema impedes healing most likely due to impaired blood flow causing interstitial fluid accumulation and a rising bacterial burden. Leg elevation and compression therapy are the basis for edema control.

Chronic wound fluid differs from acute wound fluid in that it blocks the activity and proliferation of fibroblasts, keratinocytes, and endothelial cells (60). Matrix metalloproteinases (MMP) and other proteases are abundant in this fluid and out of balance with their inhibitors, tissue inhibitors of metalloproteinases (TIMP). They break down extracellular matrix materials and growth factors (61). The ratio of MMP-9 to TIMP-1 has been found to be predictive of healing in some chronic wounds (62). Dressings aimed at absorbing proteases (Promogran™) and highly absorptive dressings such as foams (Allevyn®) and hydrofibers (Aquacel Ag®) are commercially available. A prospective trial evaluating venous leg ulcers treated with Promogran vs. Adaptic in 73 patients showed statistically significant accelerated healing in the Promogran group (41%) vs. the Adaptic group (31%) (63).

6. CELLULAR SENESCENCE

Cellular aging that results in a reduced growth capacity, morphologic changes, and overexpression of certain matrix proteins such as cellular fibronectin is termed cellular senescence. These changes can be detected by increased activity of beta-galactosidase as a pH of 6.0 (64). Senescent cells are less responsive to growth factors (2). Chronic wound fluid may induce cellular senescence and cellular aging. Thus, the removal of chronic wound fluid as above and the removal of senescent cells via debridement logically follows.

7. CONCLUSION

Wound bed preparation is important for chronic wounds unable to progress through the stages of normal healing. It provides a systematic clinical approach to clinical problems with a basic science foundation. Understanding the chronic wound environment as more than an extrapolation of an acute wound is essential to the concept of wound bed preparation. Optimization of the wound bed via modalities such as debridement is essential to the success of advanced and expensive wound care techniques.

REFERENCES

1. Hasan A, Murata H, Falabella A, Ochoa S, Zhou L, Badiava E, Falanga V. Dermal fibroblasts from venous ulcers are unresponsive to action of transforming growth factor-beta I. J Dermatol Sci 1997; 16:59–66.
2. Agren MS, Steenfos HH, Dabelsteen S, Hansen JB, Dabelsteen E. Proliferation and mitogenic response to PDGF-BB of fibroblasts isolated from chronic venous leg ulcers is ulcer-age dependent. J Invest Dermatol 1999; 112:463–469.

3. Cook H, Davies KF, Harding KG, Thomas DW. Defective extracellular matrix reorganization of chronic wound fibroblasts is associated with alterations in TIMP-1, TIMP-2, and MMP-2 activity. J Invest Dermatol 2000; 115:225–233.
4. Kirsner R. Wound bed preparation. Ostomy Wound Manag 2003; suppl:2–3.
5. Falanga V. Classifications for wound bed preparation and stimulation of chronic wounds. Wound Repair Regen 2000; 8(5):347–352.
6. Lyons AS, Petrucelli RJ. Medicine: an illustrated history. New York: Henry A. Abrams, Publications, 1987.
7. Fowler E, van Rijswijk L. Using wound debridement to help achieve the goals of care. Ostomy/Wound Manag 1995; 41:23S.
8. Berger MM. Enzyme debriding preparations. Ostomy Wound Manag 1993; 39:61.
9. Fowler E. Instrument/sharp debridement of non-viable tissue in wound. Ostomy/Wound Manag 1992; 38:26.
10. Mulder GD, Vande Berg JS. Cellular senescence and matrix metalloproteinase activity in chronic wounds. Relevance to debridement and new technologies.. J Am Podiatr Med Assoc 2002; 92:34–37.
11. Trengrove NJ, Stacey MC, MacAuley S, Bennett N, Gibson J, Burslem F, Murphy G, Schultz G. Analysis of the acute and chronic wound environments: the role of proteases and their inhibitors. Wound Repair Regen 1999; 7:442–452.
12. Kennedy KL, Tritch DL. Debridement. In: Krasner D, Kane D, eds. Chronic Wound Care 2nd ed. Wayne, PA: Health Management Publications, 1997:227–234.
13. Donati L, Magliano E, Colonna M. Surgical versus enzymatic debridement. In: Westerhof W, Vanscheidt W, eds. Proteolytic Enzymes and Wound Healing. New York: Springer-Verlag, 1994:38–39.
14. Hellgren L, Vincent J. Debridement: an essential step in wound healing. In: Westerhof W, ed. Leg Ulcers: Diagnosis and Treatment. Amsterdam: Elsevier Science Publishers, 1993:305–312.
15. Ovington LG. The well-dressed wound: an overview of dressing types. Wounds 1998; 10(suppl A):1A–11A.
16. Kerstein M. Moist wound healing: the clinical perspective. Ostomy/Wound Manag 1995; 41(7A):375.
17. Levine N, Seifter E, Connerton C, Levenson SM. Debridement of experimental skin burns of pigs with bromelain, a pineapple stem enzyme. Plast Reconstruct Surg 1973; 52:413.
18. Friedman E, Shaharabany M, Ravin S, Golomb E, Gollop N. Partially purified antibacterial agent from maggots displays a wide range of antibacterial activity. 3rd International Conference on Biotherapy, Jerusalem, Israel, 1998.
19. Thomas S, Andrews AM, Hay NP, Bourgoise S. The antimicrobial activity of maggot secretions: results of a preliminary study. J Tissue Viability 1999; 9(4):127–132.
20. Church J. The Third Annual John Boswick Memorial Award and Lectureship. 17th Annual Symposium on Advanced Wound Care, Orlando, FL, May 2–5, 2004.
21. Nemeth AJ, Eaglstein WH. Wound dressings and local treatment in leg ulcers: diagnosis and treatment. In: Westerhof W, ed. Leg Ulcers: Diagnosis and Treatment. Amsterdam: Elsevier Science Publishers, 1993:325–333.
22. Geronemus RG, Robins P. The effect of two new dressings on epidermal wound healing. J Dermatol Surg Oncol 1982; 8:850–852.
23. Eaglstein WH. Occlusive dressings. J Dermatol Surg Oncol 1993; 19:716–720.
24. Mertz PM, Ovington LG. Wound healing microbiology. Dermatol Clin 1993; 11(4):739–747.
25. Mertz PM, Eaglstein WH. The effect of a semiocclusive dressing on the microbial population in superficial wounds. Arch Surg 1984; 119:286–289.
26. Hutchinson JJ. Prevalence of wound infection under occlusive dressings: a collected survey of reported research. Wounds 1989; 1:123–133.
27. Laurence JC. Dressings and wound infection. Am J Surg 1994; 167(1A):215–245.

28. Hutchinson JJ, Lawrence JC. Wound infection under occlusive dressings. J Hosp Infect 1991; 17:83–94.

29. Lawrence JC. What material for dressings? Injury. Br J Accident Surg 1980; 13:500–512.

30. Mertz PM, Marshal DA, Eaglstein WH. Occlusive wound dressings to prevent bacterial invasion and wound infection. J Am Acad Dermatol 1985; 12:662 668.

31. Sinclair RD, Ryan TJ. Types of chronic wounds: indications for enzymatic debridement. In: Westerhof W, Vanscheidt W, eds. Proteolytic enzymes and wound healing. New York: Springer-Verlag, 1994:7–20.

32. Krane SM. Collagenases and collagen degradation. J Invest Dermatol 1982; 79:83–86.

33. Stone LL. Bacterial debridement of the burn eschar: the in vivo activity of selected organisms. J Surg Res 1980; 29:83–92.

34. Bicherstaff CR. Hidden powers of the pineapple. New Sci 1998; 118:46–48.

35. Sherman RA, Tran JM, Sullivan R. Maggot therapy for venous stasis ulcers. Arch Dermatol 1996; 132:254–256.

36. Westerhof W, Jansen FC, DeWit FS. Controlled, double-blind trial of fibrinolysin-deoxyribonuclease (Elase) solution in patients with chronic leg ulcers who are treated before autologous skin grafting. J Am Acad Dermatol 1987; 17:32–38.

37. Falabella AF, Carson P, Eaglstein WH, Falanga V. The safety and efficacy of Elase in the treatment of chronic ulcers of the lower extremity. J Am Acad Dermatol 1998; 39:737–740.

38. Peter FW, Li-Pwuser H, Vogt PM, Muehlberger T, Homann HH, Steinau HU. The effect of wound ointments on tissue microcirculation and leucocyte behaviour. Clin Exp Dermatol 2002; 27(1):51–55.

39. Alteres WV. Debriding enzymers. J Enterostam Ther 1984; 11:122–123.

40. Van Scheid TW, Weiss JM. Types of enzymes on the market. In: Westerhof W, Vanscheidt W, eds. Proteolytic Enzymes and Wound Healing. New York: Springer-Verlag, 1994:59–72.

41. Pullen R, Popp R, Volkers P, Fusgen I. Prospective randomized double-blind study of the wound-debriding effects of collagenase and fibrinolysin/deoxyribonuclease in pressure ulcers. Age Ageing 2002; 31:126–130.

42. Shapira E, Giladi A, Neiman Z. Use of water insoluble papain for debridement of burn eschar and necrotic tissue. Plast Reconstruct Surg 1973; 52:279.

43. Simpson G, Roomes D, Reeves B. Successful treatment of empyema thoracis with human recombinant deoxyribonuclease. Thorax 2003; 58(4):365–366.

44. Rutter PM, Carpenter B, Hill SS, Locke IC. Varidase: the science behind the medicament. J Wound Care 2000; 9(5):223–226.

45. Nemoto K, Hirota K, Murakami K, Taniguti K, Murata H, Viducic D, Miyake Y. Effect of Varidase (Streptodornase) on biofilm formed by Pseudomonas aeruginosa. Chemotherapy 2003; 49:121–125.

46. Martin SJ, Corrado OJ, Kay EA. Enzymatic debridement for necrotic wounds. J Wound Care 1996; 5(7):310–311.

47. Sherman RA, Hall MJR, Thomas S. Medicinal maggots: an ancient remedy for some contemporary afflictions. Annu Rev Entomol 2000; 45:55–81.

48. Sherman RA, Wyle F, Vulpe M. Maggot debridement therapy for treating pressure ulcers in spinal cord injury patients. J Spinal Cord Med 1995; 18:71–74.

49. Clinical Practice Guideline, Number 15, Treatment of Pressure Ulcers. U.S. Department of Health and Human Services, Public Health Service. Agency for Health Care Policy and Research, 1994.

50. Hulten L. Dressings for surgical wounds. Am J Surg 1994; 167:521–524.

51. Rodeheaver GT. Wound cleansing, wound irrigation, wound disinfection. In: Krasner D, Kane D, eds. Chronic Wound Care. 2nd ed. Wayne, PA: Health Management Publications, 1997:97–108.

52. Hell RC, Morton P, Brogden RN, Speight TM, Avery GS. Dextranomer: a review of its general properties and therapeutic efficacy. Drugs 1979; 18:89–102.

53. Weber DC, Parish LC, Witowski JA. Dextranomer in chronic wound healing. Clin Dermatol 1984; 2:116–120.

54. Steed DL. The diabetic ulcer study group. Clinical evaluation of recombinant human platelet-derived growth factor for the treatment of lower extremity diabetic ulcers. J Vasc Surg 1995; 21:71–81.

55. Baccheta CA, Magee W, Rodeheaver G, Edgerton MT, Edlich RF. Biology of infections of split thickness skin grafts. Am J Surg 1975; 130:63–67.

56. Robson MC, Stenberg BD, Heggers JP. Wound healing alterations caused by infection. Clin Plast Surg 1990; 17:485–492.

57. Sundberg J, Meller R. A retrospective review of the use of cadexomer iodine in the treatment of chronic wounds. Wounds 1997; 9:68–86.

58. Mertz PM, Davis SC, Brewer L. Can antimicrobials be effective without impairing wound healing? The evaluation of cadexomer iodine ointment. Wounds 1994; 6:184–193.

59. Oliveira-Gandia MF, Davis SC, Mertz PM. The evaluation of a cadexomer iodine dressing (Iodoflex) in preventing the multiplication of methicillin resistant *Staphylococcus aureus*. J Invest Dermatol 1995; 104:654.

60. Schultz GS, Sibbald RG, Falanga V, Ayello E, Dowsett C, Harding K, Romanelli M, Stacey M, Teot L, Vanscheidt W. Wound bed preparation: a systematic approach to wound management. Wound Repair Regen 2003; 11:1–28.

61. Kirsner RS, Orsted H, Wright JB. Matrix metalloproteinases in normal and impaired wound healing: a potential role for nanocrystalline silver. Wounds 2001; 13(suppl 3): S4–S13.

62. Ladwig GP, Robson MC, Liu R, Kuhn MA, Muir DF, Schultz GS. Ratios of activated matrix metalloproteinase-9 to tissue inhibitor of matrix metalloproteinase-1 in wound fluids are inversely correlated with healing of pressure ulcers. Wound Repair Regen 2002; 10:26–37.

63. Vin F, Teot L, Meaume S. The healing properties of Promogran in venous leg ulcers. J Wound Care 2002; 11(9):335–341.

64. Mendez MV, Stanley A, Park HY, Shon K, Phillips T, Menzoian JO. Fibroblasts cultured from venous ulcers display cellular characteristics of senescence. J Vasc Surg 1998; 28(5):876–883.

33

Compression Therapy

Harvey N. Mayrovitz and Nancy Sims
*College of Medical Sciences, Nova Southeastern University, Ft. Lauderdale,
Florida, U.S.A.*

Therapeutic limb compression is used to prevent edema formation, to reduce existing edema, and to prevent reaccumulation of edema once it is reduced. Forms of therapeutic compression for limb edema, lymphedema, and venous ulcers include compression bandaging, pneumatic compression, and compression garments (stockings/sleeves). Of these, compression bandaging is usually applied as an initial therapeutic intervention to reduce edema during a "decongestive" phase (obtain a result) and compression garments are used for maintenance (sustain the result) or preventatively as with chronic venous insufficiency. Pneumatic compression may be used in conjunction with bandages or garments. This chapter describes major relevant aspects and offers some practical pearls and guidelines.

1. COMPRESSION BANDAGING

1.1. Bandage Features and Function

Differences in bandage materials and structure give rise to functional differences. A bandage material that contains a high proportion of elastic fibers is referred to as a "long-stretch" bandage. These behave in a manner similar to stretched springs; the more you stretch it, the greater is the recoil force. Long-stretch bandages can be stretched to a length two to three times their zero tension length, as they are applied to a limb. The reactive tension in the bandage causes a sub-bandage pressure (SBP), which is the basis for an inward radial directed "resting pressure." Here the term "resting" is used to distinguish an SBP in a muscularly relaxed limb from one in which muscular contraction is occurring resulting in a dynamic pressure (Fig. 1). A "short-stretch" bandage has few, if any, elastic fibers; so, it exerts much less recoil tension on the limb. During bandaging, a small amount of stretch is made possible by the weave of the bandage fabric and this feature is used to allow the bandage to be molded to the shape of the limb. As the recoil force is low, so is the resting pressure. At the limit of the short-stretch type is the "zero-stretch" or inextensible bandage. Typically, these consist of open-weave cloth or gauze impregnated with a zinc oxide gel that may be applied directly over wounds and skin irritations. These bandages are applied without tension and are molded to the leg while wet to form a cast-like

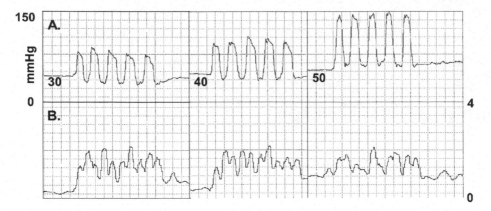

Figure 1 Effect of increased compression on sub-bandage resting and dynamic pressures. A subject was exposed to increasing levels of calf compression (30–40–50 mmHg) as they stood flat-footed. Sub-bandage pressure (A) was monitored with static and dynamic sensors and blood perfusion (B) was monitored with laser-Doppler at the posterior calf during rest and during a sequence of five calf contractions by consecutive heel-up maneuvers. As pressure increases, resting counter-pressure increases and, as radial expansion is restricted, dynamic pressures also increase. Time lines are 1 sec.

bandage. In the case of short-stretch and zero-stretch bandage, additional layers of bandaging can be used to increase pressures (Fig. 2). Padding may be used to protect bony prominences and to make pressures more uniform over irregular-shaped limb contours. Another bandage is a cohesive type that does not stick to the skin, but its individual layers adhere to each other. This material contains some elastic fibers, but the amount of extension has not been determined when the layers cohere. Clinical experience suggests they act like short-stretch bandages as applied to the limb.

Another feature that distinguishes bandages is their "stretchability" when exposed to radial-directed outward forces caused by muscular contraction. A

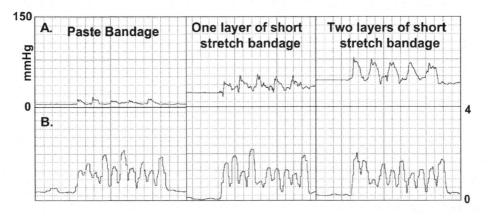

Figure 2 Effect of increasing the number of bandage layers. Same measuring conditions as with Fig. 1. Application of a paste bandage with very low recoil has little effect on resting pressure. Adding one and then two layers of bandaging raises resting pressures somewhat and increases dynamic pressures because of the short-stretch feature of the bandage.

bandage material that has little or no elastic fibers (short stretch) will stretch less than a material with many elastic fibers (long stretch). The most widely known "inelastic" bandage is Unna's boot, which after hardening, may act as a near-rigid shell around the limb. With muscle contraction, the reduced expansion of the bandage results in larger dynamic pressure ("working pressure") than would occur with highly elastic bandage types (Fig. 3).

Thus, under static conditions (muscles relaxed), SBPs generated by bandage compression depend on bandage structure and manner of wrapping. A low-stretch bandage made to form fit a limb without additional tension results in a low SBP (low resting pressure). In contrast, a high-stretch bandage that is applied with some amount of initial stretch results in an SBP that depends on the bandage restoring force and on limb contour and properties.

Under resting conditions, a portion of the bandage-related SBP is transmitted interiorly and serves to raise interstitial/tissue pressures (P_T), which thereby reduces vascular transmural pressures. Direct passive effects of this serve to reduce vessel diameters and reduce transcapillary filtration into tissue. Under dynamic conditions, internal pressures assume much greater values when low- or no-stretch bandages are used. This is explained by the fact that the effective dynamic compliance of the limb to volume expansion is less due to the relatively more rigid surface covering. Thus, rather than significant limb radial expansion, as in the case of a high-stretch bandage, expansion is limited with the short stretch, resulting in much higher dynamic or "working pressures" as shown in Figs. 2 and 3. These dynamic pressures play an important role in controlling edema/lymphedema via their favorable effects on interstitial fluid movement which, together with lymphatic activation, help reduce localized tissue edema.

1.2. Rationale for Compression

A basic goal of compression for treating venous ulcers is to try to normalize altered venous and microcirculatory hemodynamics that contribute to ulcer development and prolongation. Normal lower extremity venous hemodynamics and volumes rely

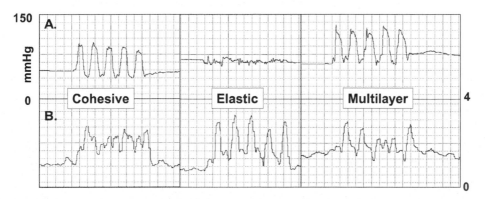

Figure 3 Low dynamic pressures with pure long-stretch bandages. Same measuring conditions as with Fig. 1. The cohesive bandage is associated with a low resting pressure but significant dynamic pressure. The pure elastic and multilayer bandages both are associated with higher resting pressures, but for the elastic bandage, there is virtually no dynamic pressure as the limb radial expansion has little restriction.

on valve competency of superficial, perforating, and deep venous systems that protect against both gravitational and muscle pump pressures. Normal venous return for muscle is via the deep system and via the superficial system for skin and subcutaneous structures. Properly functioning valves in perforating veins prevent superficial veins from being exposed to high pressures developed in deep veins, as they compress against fascia during calf contraction. They also permit unidirectional flow from superficial to deep during relaxation. Normally functioning deep veins, with competent valves, provide a unidirectional, low-resistance pathway for venous return, resulting in adequate blood volume ejection fraction to keep venous and leg volumes at normal levels.

Valve dysfunction alters this situation. If perforator vein valves are dysfunctional, some deep vein volume at high pressure is transmitted to the superficial system with each calf contraction. This may have at least three major effects: (1) effective ejection fraction for venous return from the deep system is reduced; (2) excessive pressures in the superficial system may further compromise valve competency; and (3) the sustained increase in venous volume effects microcirculation resulting in endothelial cell changes and an increase in outward flux of fluids and materials from capillaries and venules. Resultant changes in capillary hemodynamics, nutritional blood flow, and interstitium content and volume then follow.

Although the precise sequence whereby initiating hemodynamic changes end in skin ulceration is not fully worked out, there is strong evidence implicating a reduction in nutritional capillary density and degradation of capillary function (1). These changes may be due to retrograde dynamic pressures that are transmitted to nutritive capillaries (2), likely causing trauma and inflammatory-like responses (3). The venous hypertension may result in vessel rarefaction in a manner akin to that seen in systemic hypertension. Surprisingly, in spite of increased leg-blood flow in the ulcer region (4) and in periulcer subcutaneous microcirculation (5), transcutaneous oxygen is reduced. Normalization of microcirculatory parameters (6) is a positive feature of compression bandaging. In addition to microcirculatory effects, limb compression augments arterial flow pulsatility (7), which likely stimulates interstitial fluid and lymphatic dynamics and ulcer healing (Fig. 4). Thus, appropriate compression therapy may pre-empt ulcer formation in cases of chronic venous insufficiency and significantly aid in the healing of ulcers in part due to combined hemodynamic effects.

A basic goal of compression in the treatment of edema and lymphedema is to prevent further limb swelling and to facilitate limb-volume reduction. The form of bandaging/compression needed here may differ in detail from that needed for therapy related to venous ulcer treatment. A difference in bandaging approach relates to the importance here of achieving high dynamic pressures during the active treatment phase. Whereas static pressure enhancement is important in venous ulcer therapy to sustain vascular compression during resting conditions, in the case of lymphedema, elevated resting tissue pressures may in fact inhibit lymphatic function and thereby interstitial fluid removal. However, sufficient resting pressure is still needed to sustain gains made in decongestion.

1.3. Compression Bandaging Mechanisms of Action

Compression bandaging causes a "counter pressure" that is directed in such a fashion so as to reduce abnormally elevated transmural pressures of veins that may be caused by combined valve incompetence, gravitational forces, and muscular dynamics.

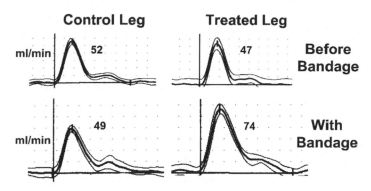

Figure 4 Compression bandaging augments pulsatile blood flow. Nuclear magnetic resonance was used to measure pulse blood flow at mid-calf with and without multilayer compression bandaging of one lower extremity (treated leg). Each flow pulse is the ensemble average of 30 beats and numbers indicate average flow per pulse in mL/min. Scales are the same for all pulses. Before bandaging, flow was similar in both limbs. With the bandage in place, pulsatile flow significantly increased resulting in a greater "dynamic" flow pattern. It is likely that this enhances tissue and lymphatic fluid movements.

The amount of counter pressure that is functionally effective depends on the type of bandage material that is used (highly extensible or relatively inelastic), the manner of wrapping (tightness of wrap), and whether the limb is relaxed (static conditions) or muscle is contracting (dynamic conditions). For a given set of conditions, the counter pressure needs to be sufficient to reduce abnormally elevated superficial venous volume by reducing overload volume entering the superficial system during muscular contraction and to maintain a lessened volume during static conditions. The resultant lessened average venous pressure tends to reduce excessive transcapillary outward filtration into interstitial spaces, which in turn reduces tissue edema. Simultaneously, a greater dynamic tissue pressure promotes greater tissue fluid movement and its uptake and removal by the lymphatic system, which adds to the edema-lessening process. Deep vein volume is also reduced because its effective ejection fraction is returned toward normal concomitant with the reduction in venous reflux.

The literature is replete with reports demonstrating the efficacy of compression bandaging as a main component in the treatment of venous ulcers (8–10). Most small ulcers, present for short durations (<6–9 months), tend to heal with good standard wound care combined with compression bandaging (11–13). However, questions still remain about the optimum approach to compression bandaging and the precise mode of action. One issue concerns the relative efficacies of long-stretch, short-stretch, or multilayer bandaging systems (14). A benefit has been suggested for multilayer when compared with short stretch (15), whereas others have found both to be equally effective (16,17). Still, others have advocated short-stretch bandaging to achieve therapeutically effective graduated compression (18). Other questions relate to achieving verifiable and appropriate compression pressures and gradients. Still, other questions relate to possible direct effects of the compression on the wound bed (19).

1.4. Bandage Compression Pressures (Sub-bandage and Tissue)

Limb bandaging with either single layer or multilayer combinations achieve SBPs between skin and bandage that depend on bandage material properties, extent of bandage stretch as applied, number of layers used, wrapping pattern, and the structure, physical features, shape, and dimensions of the limb. As a simplified estimate to describe SBP dependency on limb size, the law of Laplace is often applied. Accordingly, for the same amount of tension in the bandage, SBP is inversely proportional to the circumference of the limb to which it is applied. As a consequence, if a bandage is applied to a lower extremity with equal bandage stretch along the limb length, then in theory, SBP varies along the limb, being greatest at limb sites with the least circumference. Actual pressure dependencies differ from this due to many factors including the fact that a limb is not a true cylinder and it has many nonuniformities in its contour and physical properties. Local regions, with small radii of curvature such as at the malleolus, have larger pressures. Shape distortions, as with significant lymphedema, also lead to unexpected pressure gradients (20). Nonetheless, it is useful to keep in mind that all else being equal, SBP tends to be greater, the smaller the circumference for the same bandage tension.

A direct outcome of this "principle" is that an ankle-to-knee bandage applied at uniform tension will result in an SBP gradient, with pressure being greatest at the ankle and least at the calf site with the maximum circumference. This is a fortuitous result with respect to the ability of a bandage to counteract gravitational dependencies of lower extremity intravascular pressures under resting conditions. However, the effect of such graduated pressures with respect to impacts of dynamic pressures is less clear. In fact, it is unclear which aspect—static or dynamic pressure gradients—is the most relevant parameter vis-à-vis ulcer healing potential. Considerable differences in both pressures have been observed with different bandage systems, as applied ostensibly in the same manner by experienced practitioners (21), although training improves the variability (22).

A part of the effectiveness of compression therapy depends on an increase in compression-related subcutaneous tissue pressure (P_T) to diminish transcapillary fluid filtration and promote vascular resorption and removal of interstitial fluids. Local or generalized reduction in such edema or microedema allows better oxygen and nutrient delivery to, and chemical byproduct removal from, skin, subcutaneous tissues, and the wound bed. It should be noted that tissue pressure is already elevated in edematous limbs. For example in untreated lymphedema of the arm, P_T differences between affected and nonaffected arms averaged 4.6 cm H_2O (23) with even larger differences reported for the leg (24). This component of elevated P_T is due to excess tissue fluid and is diminished as compression therapy reduces fluid volume. However, promotion of fluid resorption by the compression-induced increase in P_T is not as great as would be indicated by the amount of P_T increase. This is because capillary pressure simultaneously increases by about 80% of the P_T increase (25). There is also evidence that SBP in the range of 20–40 mmHg may blunt the normal veno-arterial constriction response in dependent limbs (26,27). This effect would tend to maintain capillary pressure higher and thus detract from the desired decrease in capillary filtration.

If compression-induced tissue pressures become too large for too long, there is a negative impact on blood vessels and perfusion (28) and on lymphatic vessels and their lymph flow. Optimal tissue pressures have not been defined and there is little direct information as to relationships between surface SBPs and associated tissue pressures (29). Subdermal pressure measurements under compression garments give some idea of surface-to-subsurface radial pressure gradients to be expected at different sites (30). Absolute pressures are greater at bony prominences, but gradients are larger for soft tissue. For example, at the posterior mid-calf, an SBP of 66 mmHg resulted in a subdermal pressure of 24 mmHg, whereas at medial mid-calf, an SBP of 36 mmHg resulted in a subdermal pressure of 21 mmHg.

2. PNEUMATIC COMPRESSION

Intermittent pneumatic compression (IPC) devices deliver controlled sequential pressures to a limb. Parameters of such systems include absolute pressures achieved, rate of pressure development, and for sequential systems, the timing. Considerable variation in parameters has been reported (31). Regarding IPC applications to venous ulcer treatment, a recent review of the literature (32) indicates that available evidence for IPC effectiveness is inconclusive. Thus, although some studies showed no benefit, others showed benefit if IPC was used in patients with long-standing, previously intractable ulcerations (33). As of this writing, IPC is covered only for patients with sustained edema and significant remaining ulceration after a 6-month trial of standard therapy. The potential therapeutic value of IPC for venous ulcers in immobile patients has been suggested but not established (34). An aspect not previously considered in this connection is the possible effects of IPC on promoting wound healing via direct nitric oxide pathways or related vasodilatory processes. Experimental studies (35) have shown that IPC upregulates eNOS mRNA and induces vasodilation of arterioles in noncompressed tissues. Variability in effectiveness of IPC therapy in venous ulcer patients may have roots in differences in these aspects among patients. In addition, greater IPC-induced vasodilatory effectiveness has been shown to be related to greater inflation velocity (36); so, variability in effectiveness may be due to differences in IPC-device parameters. In addition, there is evidence that IPC-related limb edema reduction in venous ulcer patients causes an increase in periwound oxygen tension (37). This may be unrelated to how the edema is reduced.

The possible utility of IPC as an adjunctive therapy for breast cancer treatment-related lymphedema is suggested by recent work in which IPC was added to standard decongestive lymphedema therapy and compared to standard therapy alone (38). Effectiveness of initial and maintenance phases of therapy improved with respect to limb-volume reductions in this small group of patients. It is unclear whether the mechanism of action is related to improved lymph fluid transport or reduction in capillary filtration into interstitial spaces (39). Sophisticated dynamic lymphoscintigraphy tests suggest an immediate IPC effect that facilitates tracer transport within edematous tissue in patients with lymphedema (40). This would be consistent with known IPC-related lymph flow augmentation in experimental animals (41). Use of IPC therapy in patients with filarial lymphedema has also been reported (42). However, IPC per se has not shown itself to improve limb-volume reductions when compared with complete decongestive physiotherapy (43) nor has a beneficial effect of IPC always been demonstrated (44). The IPC effectiveness for limb-volume reduction is inversely related to the extent of fibrosis present (45,46). There are also significant concerns about using pump therapy to treat lower extremity lymphedema, especially with regard to risk of causing genital lymphedema (47). Such risks do not often justify pump use for lower extremity lymphedema.

A retrospective study of patients with lower extremity critical ischemia and nonhealing ulcers suggests a positive benefit as measured by wound healing and limb salvage (48,49). These effects may be related to the improvement in arterial blood flow associated with a very rapid rise in compression pressure (50,51). Other aspects of IPC clinical applications have been recently reviewed (52).

3. COMPRESSION GARMENTS

Maintenance of limb-volume reductions achieved during decongestive phases and prevention of reoccurrence of healed ulcers are aided or dependent on the use of compression garments. Elastic stockings provide an elevated resting pressure that mainly acts on superficial veins to help prevent gravitational overload and deep-to-superficial reflux. Both standard and custom stockings are specified by class/grade corresponding to calf–ankle pressures (20–30, 30–40, 40–50 mmHg) they produce. Larger pressures project pressures to a greater depth and are associated with greater dynamic pressures.

However, even with the use of compression hosiery after healing, there may be a significant recurrence of venous ulceration. For example, of 502 ulcer legs initially treated with compression bandaging, 75% healed by 24 weeks but 44% recurred within 3 years (53). With respect to recurrence, patient compliance in using the compression stockings is an important factor; better compliance—less recurrence. In another study (54), of 62 patients initially treated with compression bandaging and subsequent maintenance compression hosiery, about two-third experienced venous ulcer recurrence at 4 years posthealing. Careful attention to stocking fit, absolute pressure levels achieved, ankle-to-calf pressure gradient, and patient compliance may improve this situation.

In addition to elastic-graded compression garments, inelastic sleeves and leg compression devices are available. They use inelastic fabric straps secured with Velcro to produce a graded compression. The amount of SBP produced is determined by how tightly the straps are pulled. Some types incorporate foam padding inner layer, whereas others can be worn over a separate padding layer or over compression garments to provide additional compression and support. Because of their inelasticity and adjustability, these devices have the benefits of short-stretch bandages and the convenience of easy application and removal. Their low resting pressures allow them to be worn at night to prevent reaccumulation of edema in patients who require constant compression.

4. ARTERIAL AND MICROCIRCULATORY BLOOD-FLOW CONSIDERATIONS

The potential impact of all forms of limb compression on arterial and microcirculatory flow needs to be considered from both functional and safety perspectives. Compression-induced pressures if too large, or in some cases even at levels therapeutically needed, may compromise blood circulation. This possibility is of particular concern if long-stretch compression is used, as elastic restoring forces are sustained under resting conditions. This is an issue in persons with normal limb circulation but of greater concern in persons with compromised circulation. In supine persons, skin-blood perfusion decreases with increasing levels of limb compression (55,56). Comparisons of the effects of various leg compression pressures on blood perfusion in skin overlying bone and in skin distal to leg compression (57) show significant reductions in both at therapeutically used pressures (Fig. 5).

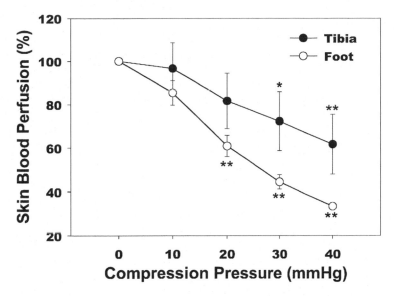

Figure 5 Compression-induced skin-blood perfusion reductions. Skin-blood perfusion using laser-Doppler was simultaneously measured overlying the anterior tibia and foot dorsum, as compression was applied from ankle-to-knee. Relative flow reduction was greater at the foot, but both regions demonstrated significant effects ($^*p < 0.05$, $^{**}p < 0.01$, when compared with no compression).

It is important to note that increases in tissue pressure, whether edema-induced or compression-related, are transmitted to veins and arteries, increasing their intravascular pressures. Because the pressure increase is greater in veins, the effective perfusion pressure (arteriovenous pressure difference) that drives blood flow through the compressed limb region is thus reduced. When edematous legs are elevated, venous pressure tends to decrease, but it cannot go below the abnormally increased tissue pressure. In contrast, intravascular pressures in arteries are reduced in proportion to the amount of leg elevation. Thus, under these circumstances, perfusion pressure is further reduced with a greater potential for blood-flow compromise. Such tendencies have been experimentally demonstrated (58).

In contrast to limb elevation, limb dependency causes a blood-flow reduction that is partly due to the increased venous volume, which reflexively induces an arteriolar vasoconstriction (27). Compression bandaging, even in normal subjects, helps reverse this blood-flow reduction and the associated tissue oxygen decrease (55). The bandage effect is due in part to unloading of venous stretch receptors and in part due to reduced arteriolar transmural pressure that results in a myogenic vasodilation in persons with normal vasodilatory capacity (59). However, similar compression pressures reduce blood flow when a person is supine (55) in both subcutaneous and skeletal muscle blood flow (60).

It is expected that in persons with micro- or macrocirculatory dysfunction, including blunted or absent vasodilatory reserve, compression-related flow decrements would be greater. These facts have led to the adage that compression bandaging should generally be withheld in patients with ABIs <0.80 and used with extreme care in patients with possible microcirculatory deficits such as in diabetes. It should also be recognized that the combination of edema, limb compression, and limb elevation might introduce further blood-flow reductions.

5. ASSESSING OUTCOMES

For venous ulcers, the effectiveness of compression therapy is measured by the rate and extent of healing, which is linked to the effectiveness in reducing the edema component. The effectiveness of compression therapy in lymphedema is measured by the lymphedema/edema reduction and by changes in tissue properties. The deformability of the tissue can be measured by applying a fixed amount of pressure for a specific amount of time and by determining the depth of penetration and/or the rate of tissue recovery. In very fibrotic tissues, even prolonged pressure will produce only minimal indentation. In normal tissues, the elasticity of the skin produces recoil and there is no prolonged indentation. Changes in depth and rate of recoil are indicators of the amount of fibrosis and edema in tissues. Edema reduction can be documented by calculating and tracking limb-volume changes. The size of a limb at selected points (i.e., ankle, calf) may change as compression is applied to those areas, whereas the total volume of the limb remains constant. When compression of the lower part of the limb produces a movement of edema into the upper part of the limb, more extensive compression and decongestive therapy is necessary. Therefore, it is important to determine the total limb volume. The effectiveness of home maintenance programs and patient compliance can also be monitored by tracking limb-volume changes.

Several methods are available for determining limb volume, such as water displacement, mathematical models based on circumferential measurements, and photoelectric instruments (61). Of these, the circumferential measurements are the easiest to use and require minimal equipment and staff time. Computer programs that automatically calculate, track, and graph limb volumes from circumferential measurements are available and are very useful (62). Professional reports and graphs provide a visual record of treatment progress and are valuable tools for communicating the effectiveness of treatment to referring physicians and other members of the medical team, to patients to enhance compliance with treatment, and to insurance companies to help assure reimbursement for treatment.

REFERENCES

1. Junger M, Hahn M, Klyscz T, Steins A. Microangiopathy in the pathogenesis of chronic venous insufficiency. Curr Probl Dermatol 1999; 27:124–129.
2. Steins A, Hahn M, Junger M. Venous leg ulcers and microcirculation. Clin Hemorheol Microcirc 2001; 24:147–153.
3. Hahn J, Junger M, Friedrich B, Zuder D, Steins A, Hahn M, Klyscz T. Cutaneous inflammation limited to the region of the ulcer in chronic venous insufficiency. Vasa 1997; 26:277–281.
4. Mayrovitz HN, Larsen PB. Leg blood flow in patients with venous ulcers: relationship to site and ulcer area. Wounds 1994; 6:195–200.
5. Mayrovitz HN, Larsen PB. Periwound skin microcirculation of venous leg ulcers. Microvasc Res 1994; 48:114–123.
6. Junger M, Steins A, Hahn M, Hafner HM. Microcirculatory dysfunction in chronic venous insufficiency (CVI). Microcirculation 2000; 7:S3–S12.
7. Mayrovitz HN, Larsen PB. Effects of compression bandaging on leg pulsatile blood flow. Clin Physiol 1997; 17:105–117.
8. Moffatt CJ, O'Hare L. Venous leg ulceration: treatment by high compression bandaging. Ostomy Wound Manage 1995; 41:16–18, 20–22.
9. Fletcher A, Cullum N, Sheldon TA. A systematic review of compression treatment for venous leg ulcers. BMJ 1997; 315:576–580.

10. Palfreyman SJ, Lochiel R, Michaels JA. A systematic review of compression therapy for venous leg ulcers. Vasc Med 1998; 3:301–313.
11. Mayberry JC, Moneta GL, Taylor LM Jr, Porter JM. Fifteen-year results of ambulatory compression therapy for chronic venous ulcers. Surgery 1991; 109:575–581.
12. Margolis DJ, Berlin JA, Strom BL. Which venous leg ulcers will heal with limb compression bandages? Am J Med 2000; 109:15–19.
13. Phillips TJ. Current approaches to venous ulcers and compression. Dermatol Surg 2001; 27:611–621.
14. Macdonald J, Sims N, Mayrovitz HN. Lymphedema, lipedema, and the open wound: the role of compression therapy. Surg Clin N Am 2003; 83:639–658.
15. Ukat A, Konig M, Vanscheidt W, Munter KC. Short-stretch versus multilayer compression for venous leg ulcers: a comparison of healing rates. J Wound Care 2003; 12: 139–143.
16. Scriven JM, Taylor LE, Wood AJ, Bell PR, Naylor AR, London NJ. A prospective randomised trial of four-layer versus short stretch compression bandages for the treatment of venous leg ulcers. Ann R Coll Surg Engl 1998; 80:215–220.
17. Partsch H, Menzinger G, Mostbeck A. Inelastic leg compression is more effective to reduce deep venous refluxes than elastic bandages. Dermatol Surg 1999; 25:695–700.
18. Hampton S. Venous leg ulcers: short-stretch bandage compression therapy. Br J Nurs 1997; 6:990–992, 994, 996–998.
19. Roberts G, Hammad L, Collins C, Shearman C, Mani R. Some effects of sustained compression on ulcerated tissues. Angiology 2002; 53:451–456.
20. Williams AF, Williams AE. 'Putting the pressure on': a study of compression sleeves used in breast cancer-related lymphoedema. J Tissue Viability 1999; 9:89–94.
21. Wertheim D, Melhuish J, Williams R, Harding K. Measurement of forces associated with compression therapy. Med Biol Eng Comput 1999; 37:31–34.
22. Hafner J, Luthi W, Hanssle H, Kammerlander G, Burg G. Instruction of compression therapy by means of interface pressure measurement. Dermatol Surg 2000; 26: 481–486; discussion 487.
23. Bates DO, Levick JR, Mortimer PS. Subcutaneous interstitial fluid pressure and arm volume in lymphoedema. Int J Microcirc Clin Exp 1992; 11:359–373.
24. Christenson J, Shawa N, Hamad M, Al-Hassan H. The relationship between subcutaneous tissue pressures and intramuscular pressures in normal and edematous legs. Microcirc Endothelium and Lymphatics 1985; 2:367–384.
25. Mellander S, Albert U. Effects of increased and decreased tissue pressure on haemodynamic and capillary events in cat skeletal muscle. J Physiol 1994; 481:163–175.
26. Nielsen HV. Effects of externally applied compression on blood flow in the human dependent leg. Clin Physiol 1983; 3:131–140.
27. Mayrovitz HN. Posturally induced leg vasoconstrictive responses: relationship to standing duration, impedance and volume changes. Clin Physiol 1998; 18:311–319.
28. Matsen FA III, Krugmire RB Jr, King RV. Increased tissue pressure and its effects on muscle oxygenation in level and elevated human limbs. Clin Orthop 1979; 144:311–320.
29. Hargens AR, McClure AG, Skyhar MJ, Lieber RL, Gershuni DH, Akeson WH. Local compression patterns beneath pneumatic tourniquets applied to arms and thighs of human cadavera. J Orthop Res 1987; 5:247–252.
30. Giele HP, Liddiard K, Currie K, Wood FM. Direct measurement of cutaneous pressures generated by pressure garments. Burns 1997; 23:137–141.
31. Rithalia SV, Heath GH, Gonsalkorale M. Evaluation of intermittent pneumatic compression systems. J Tissue Viability 2002; 12:52–57.
32. Berliner E, Ozbilgin B, Zarin DA. A systematic review of pneumatic compression for treatment of chronic venous insufficiency and venous ulcers. J Vasc Surg 2003; 37:539–544.
33. Smith PC, Sarin S, Hasty J, Scurr JH. Sequential gradient pneumatic compression enhances venous ulcer healing: a randomized trial. Surgery 1990; 108:871–875.

34. Vowden K. The use of intermittent pneumatic compression in venous ulceration. Br J Nurs 2001; 10:491–509.

35. Chen LE, Liu K, Qi WN, Joneschild E, Tan X, Seaber AV, Stamler JS, Urbaniak JR. Role of nitric oxide in vasodilation in upstream muscle during intermittent pneumatic compression. J Appl Physiol 2002; 92:559–566.

36. Liu K, Chen LE, Seaber AV, Urbaniak JR. Influences of inflation rate and duration on vasodilatory effect by intermittent pneumatic compression in distant skeletal muscle. J Orthop Res 1999; 17:415–420.

37. Kolari PJ, Pekanmaki K, Pohjola RT. Transcutaneous oxygen tension in patients with post-thrombotic leg ulcers: treatment with intermittent pneumatic compression. Cardiovasc Res 1988; 22:138–141.

38. Szuba A, Achalu R, Rockson SG. Decongestive lymphatic therapy for patients with breast carcinoma-associated lymphedema. A randomized, prospective study of a role for adjunctive intermittent pneumatic compression. Cancer 2002; 95:2260–2267.

39. Miranda F Jr, Perez MC, Castiglioni ML, Juliano Y, Amorim JE, Nakano LC, de Barros N Jr, Lustre WG, Burihan E. Effect of sequential intermittent pneumatic compression on both leg lymphedema volume and on lymph transport as semi-quantitatively evaluated by lymphoscintigraphy. Lymphology 2001; 34:135–141.

40. Baulieu F, Baulieu JL, Vaillant L, Secchi V, Barsotti J. Factorial analysis in radionuclide lymphography: assessment of the effects of sequential pneumatic compression. Lymphology 1989; 22:178–185.

41. McGeown JG, McHale NG, Thornbury KD. Effects of varying patterns of external compression on lymph flow in the hindlimb of the anaesthetized sheep. J Physiol 1988; 397:449–457.

42. Manjula Y, Kate V, Ananthakrishnan N. Evaluation of sequential intermittent pneumatic compression for filarial lymphoedema. Natl Med J India 2002; 15:192–194.

43. Johansson K, Lie E, Ekdahl C, Lindfeldt J. A randomized study comparing manual lymph drainage with sequential pneumatic compression for treatment of postoperative arm lymphedema. Lymphology 1998; 31:56–64.

44. Dini D, Del Mastro L, Gozza A, Lionetto R, Garrone O, Forno G, Vidili G, Bertelli G, Venturini M. The role of pneumatic compression in the treatment of postmastectomy lymphedema. A randomized phase III study. Ann Oncol 1998; 9:187–190.

45. Raines JK, O'Donnell TF Jr, Kalisher L, Darling RC. Selection of patients with lymphedema for compression therapy. Am J Surg 1977; 133:430–437.

46. Pappas CJ, O'Donnell TF Jr. Long-term results of compression treatment for lymphedema. J Vasc Surg 1992; 16:555–562; discussion 562–554.

47. Boris M, Weindorf S, Lasinski BB. The risk of genital edema after external pump compression for lower limb lymphedema. Lymphology 1998; 31:15–20.

48. Montori VM, Kavros SJ, Walsh EE, Rooke TW. Intermittent compression pump for nonhealing wounds in patients with limb ischemia. The Mayo Clinic experience (1998–2000). Int Angiol 2002; 21:360–366.

49. van Bemmelen PS, Gitlitz DB, Faruqi RM, Weiss-Olmanni J, Brunetti VA, Giron F, Ricotta JJ. Limb salvage using high-pressure intermittent compression arterial assist device in cases unsuitable for surgical revascularization. Arch Surg 2001; 136:1280–1285; discussion 1286.

50. Eze AR, Cisek PL, Holland BS, Comerota AJ Jr, Verramasuneni R, Comerota AJ. The contributions of arterial and venous volumes to increased cutaneous blood flow during leg compression. Ann Vasc Surg 1998; 12:182–186.

51. Eze AR, Comerota AJ, Cisek PL, Holland BS, Kerr RP, Veeramasuneni R, Comerota AJ Jr. Intermittent calf and foot compression increases lower extremity blood flow. Am J Surg 1996; 172:130–134; discussion 135.

52. Chen AH, Frangos SG, Kilaru S, Sumpio BE. Intermittent pneumatic compression devices—physiological mechanisms of action. Eur J Vasc Endovasc Surg 2001; 21:383–392.

53. Barwell JR, Taylor M, Deacon J, Ghauri AS, Wakely C, Phillips LK, Whyman MR, Poskitt KR. Surgical correction of isolated superficial venous reflux reduces long-term recurrence rate in chronic venous leg ulcers. Eur J Vasc Endovasc Surg 2000; 20:363–368.

54. McDaniel HB, Marston WA, Farber MA, Mendes RR, Owens LV, Young ML, Daniel PF, Keagy BA. Recurrence of chronic venous ulcers on the basis of clinical, etiologic, anatomic, and pathophysiologic criteria and air plethysmography. J Vasc Surg 2002; 35:723–728.

55. Gaylarde PM, Sarkany I, Dodd HJ. The effect of compression on venous stasis. Br J Dermatol 1993; 128:255–258.

56. Mayrovitz HN, Delgado M, Smith J. Compression bandaging effects on lower extremity peripheral and sub-bandage skin blood perfusion. Ostomy Wound Manage 1998; 44: 56–65.

57. Mayrovitz HN, Sims N. Effects of ankle-to-knee external pressures on skin blood perfusion in the compressed leg and non-compressed foot. Adv Skin Wound Care 2003; 16: 198–202.

58. Matsen FA III, Wyss CR, Krugmire RB Jr, Simmons CW, King RV. The effects of limb elevation and dependency on local arteriovenous gradients in normal human limbs with particular reference to limbs with increased tissue pressure. Clin Orthop 1980; 150:187–195.

59. Nielsen HV. External pressure–blood flow relations during limb compression in man. Acta Physiol Scand 1983; 119:253–260.

60. Nielsen HV. Effects of externally applied compression on blood flow in subcutaneous and muscle tissue in the human supine leg. Clin Physiol 1982; 2:447–457.

61. Mayrovitz HN, Sims N, Macdonald J. Limb volume measurement in patients with edema. Adv Skin Wound Care 2000; 113:272–276.

62. Software. Bioscience Research Institute (bioscience-research.net) offers an excellent and inexpensive software package called Limb Volumes Professional 4.0 software. Available from Bioscience Research Institute at http://bioscience-research.net/lymphedema.html.

34

Pearls of Compression

Dot Weir, RN, CWOCN, CWS.
Orlando Regional Healthcare, Lucerne Wound Healing Center
Orlando, Florida, U.S.A.

Compression of the lower extremity is widely accepted as the cornerstone of management of patients with chronic venous insufficiency (CVI), and treatment of ulcers associated with CVI (1–4). Appropriate compression therapy reduces edema, helps prevent recurrence of edema once eliminated, and enhances venous return of blood to the heart. Comprehensive understanding of the disease, local and supportive management are essential in the treatment of these patients. Previous chapters have addressed the pathophysiology and management of CVI as well as the science of compression therapy. This chapter will further address the clinical perspective and approach to the patient requiring compression.

1. MAKING THE DIAGNOSIS

As previously described, longstanding venous insufficiency will cause characteristic changes to the lower extremity including edema, lipodermatosclerosis (a "woody" consistency to the skin), varicose veins and telangiectasia, and red-brown pigmentation caused by hemosiderin deposits in the dermis (5). Coupled with a history which includes risk factors for venous insufficiency (including previous leg injury, obesity, pregnancy, history of phlebitis or deep vein thrombosis, varicose veins or sedentary lifestyle) (4), a diagnosis of CVI in many cases is readily apparent. While venous insufficiency is the most common cause of lower-leg ulcers, accounting for nearly 80% of all cases (4), not all ulcers in patients with venous disease are of venous etiology. Differential diagnosis may need to be made to exclude other conditions causing the ulcer such as malignancy, vasculitis, pyoderma gangrenosum, or an infectious process.

Additionally, as arterial disease can exist in up to 30% of cases (3), the standard of care for patients with venous disease requires assessment of the arterial flow prior to consideration for compressive therapy (3,4,6–9). The most common bedside assessment of arterial flow is the ankle/brachial index (ABI). The ABI compares the brachial arterial flow to that of the flow at the ankle of the same side. A hand-held Doppler should be utilized for the exam, as the palpation of the pulses is less reliable (10). The ankle systolic pressure is divided by the brachial systolic

Table 1 Calculating the Ankle/Brachial Index

Ankle systolic pressure	⟶	80
Brachial systolic pressure	⟶	100
80/100 = 0.80		
ABI = 0.8		

pressure to reveal a number (see Table 1). Extent of compression therapy may need to be modified for patients with an abnormal ABI and in some cases contraindicated due to arterial disease. Conversely, patients with diabetes and/or renal disease may have calcification making their vessels noncompressible, causing their ABI to be falsely elevated and higher than one (the ankle pressure will be higher than the brachial pressure). The patient with either low or high indices should be referred for further limb perfusion workup prior to initiation of compression therapy. In settings where an ABI is not possible, the patient should be referred for a vascular assessment so that the appropriate diagnostic workup can be accomplished.

2. OPTIONS FOR COMPRESSION

Earlier chapters have dealt with the science of compression, bandage pressures, and the effect on limb fluids, both of venous and lymphatic etiology. The basic, readily available compression wraps and garments will be addressed here along with practical guidelines for use, emphasizing patient education that should be included in the plan of care.

2.1 Tubular Bandages (Figs. 1 and 2)

Available in rolls or individual unit dose type of packaging, these bandages provide ease of use along with the convenience of being relatively inexpensive as well as being semi-disposable. The rolls are ideal for clinic use as they can be cut to fit to the length needed. These devices can provide minimal to moderate levels of compression, 8 mmHg as a single layer, 16 mmHg when doubled (11). Even when applied as a

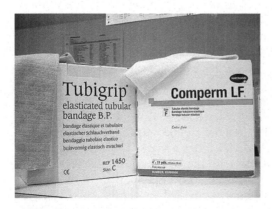

Figure 1 Tubular bandages, both latex and latex free.

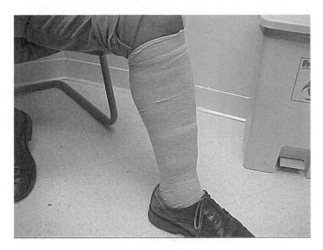

Figure 2 Double layer tubular bandage over dressings.

single layer, tubular bandages can provide enough mild compression to effect a change. They are especially helpful for those with exudative ulcers or legs, when frequent dressing changes are desired, or when arterial flow is being assessed. They can also be washed in cold soapy water, allowed to hang dry, and re-used.

Tubular bandages are sized specific to the manufacturer. Specialized measuring tapes are available to determine the size needed for low, medium, or high compression. Latex rubber content should be noted for those patients with allergies or sensitivities.

2.2 Paste Bandages (Figs. 3 and 4)

Commonly referred to as an "Unna's boot," paste bandages are rolls of gauze commonly impregnated with zinc oxide, gelatin, and, in some cases, calamine lotion to counteract itching (resulting in a pink color). Traditionally, these bandages were wrapped from the toe to the knee and secondarily wrapped with a gauze bulky bandage. Before the advent of longer wearing moist wound healing products, the

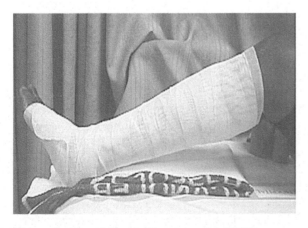

Figure 3 Unna's boot. (Courtesy of AAWC.)

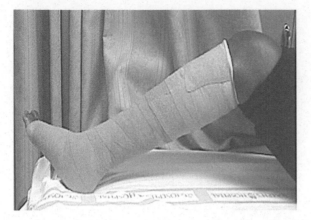

Figure 4 Unna's boot with cohesive wrap. (Courtesy of AAWC.)

paste bandage also served as the local wound dressing. The disadvantage was that when they dried, they tended to loosen, thus reducing the compression effectiveness. Additionally, exudate was trapped under the wrap resulting in problems with the skin surrounding the ulcer. In more recent years, clinicians have added a second layer of cohesive type of bandage [i.e., Coban® (3M, St, Paul, MN)] to enhance compression once wrapped. The wraps are changed once or twice a week. Application should begin just above the toes and proceed smoothly up the leg to just below the knee. Wrapping should be in a spiral with 50% overlap of each layer, and care taken to exert no tension on the bandage. Care should be taken to cut the wrap at the curves of the heel and ankle to avoid folds and seams, which could be a source of irritation, and actually create new skin breakdown. Prominent bone and tendon areas can be padded with foam prior to application.The secondary cohesive wrap is applied in a similar fashion (though cutting is not necessary) with 50% or less tension depending on the patient tolerance and perfusion status. The leg should be washed thoroughly and moisturized between wraps. The choice of primary wound dressing should be one that provides the appropriate level of moisture or exudate absorption, and suitably left in place for the duration of the time the wrap is left in place.

The paste bandage/cohesive wrap is more beneficial in the patient who is ambulatory, though the nonambulatory patient may receive some benefit. The wrap, being less elastic, will enhance blood flow and movement of fluid by providing more rigid resistance to the calf muscle during ambulation.

2.3 Multilayer Wraps (Figs. 5–8)

Developed in more recent years, the concept of the multiple layers of elastic wraps has enhanced the clinician's ability to provide constant, sustained compression whether the patient is lying, sitting, standing, or walking. Provided by manufacturers in prepackaged kits, these bandages may consist of two, three or four layers. The common component of all of the systems is a skin contact layer of a soft cotton-like material that is applied in a spiral, overlapping wrap. This layer provides several advantages including padding of bony and tendon prominences, equalizing the shape of the leg (particularly around the heel, post-tibial area, and ankle) providing more consistent and even pressures, and absorption of some moisture. One to two more

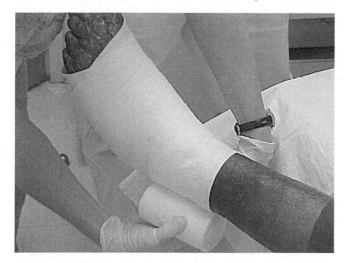

Figure 5 Cotton layer of multilayer wrap.

additional layers provide elastic compression and commonly an outer layer of cohesive wrap is used. Most manufacturers recommend that one of the inner elastic wraps be applied in a circle of eight fashion, which provides two layers overlapping in different directions at any one place on the leg, further enhancing the compressive force, even when the leg is at rest. Additionally most of the elastic layers are marked with objects that change to a particular shape (i.e., rectangle to a square) to let the clinician know that the proper amount of stretch is being applied.

As with the Unna's boot, the choice of wound contact layer can be left to the discretion of the clinician to meet the needs of the individual wound. Again, the wound dressing choice would be one that can be left in place for the duration of the wrap, generally 4–7 days. Experience educates us that the first time this type

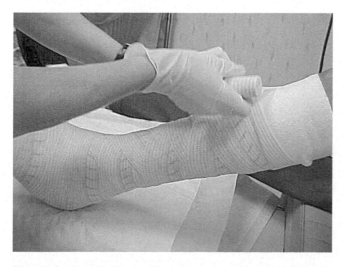

Figure 6 Stretch layer of multilayer wrap showing circle of eight wrap.

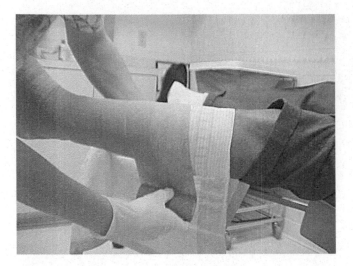

Figure 7   Cohesive layer of multilayer wrap.

of wrap is used, it would ideally be changed for the first time after 3 or 4 days of wear to assess the patient's tolerance and to examine the leg for any areas of pressure or rubbing that may need to be addressed. Because these wraps are thicker and tend to move as one piece once applied, gravity may cause them to slip down the leg and cause wrinkles, which may cause areas of pressure. Should this occur, these may then be padded further with foam for comfort and protection. Additionally, it is important to warn the patient that the layers of wrap will add a great deal of thickness to the foot, and shoe wear may need to be adjusted. The wrap also may need to be changed more frequently in warmer seasons and climates due to perspiration and odor concerns. And again, latex-free options are available for those with latex allergies or sensitivities.

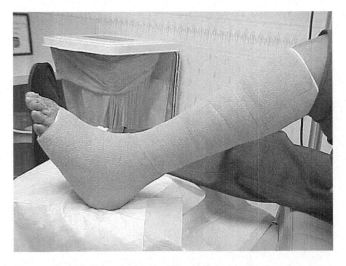

Figure 8   Final appearance of multilayer wrap.

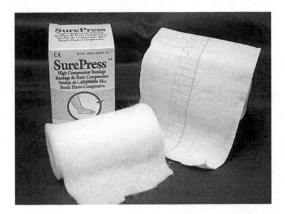

Figure 9 Single layer, long stretch wrap shown with cotton roll.

2.4 Single Layer, Long Stretch Wraps (Fig. 9)

For the patient who is able to participate in their care, the single layer, long stretch wrap is a cost-effective option. Packaged as a single component, these wraps would remind one of a higher quality sport-type wrap, with higher tension when stretched. Most of the available products are also marked with guides to indicate the appropriate amount of stretch. They are relatively easy to teach to a patient or caregiver who has good hand dexterity and strength and the ability to grasp the concept. They are manufactured of a relatively dense material, so padding of bony prominences and tendons may be necessary. The manufacturers recommendations should be followed as to the method of application, but generally they are applied as a spiral from the toes to the knee. Because of the tendency to slip and separate, these wraps are generally reapplied once or twice daily, and can be laundered in cold soapy water when soiled and reused.

The use of standard sport-type wraps [i.e., Ace Wraps® (BD, Franklin Lakes, NJ)] is generally saved as a last resort because of the vast differences in quality and density of the fabric and elasticity. If availability and cost constraints make them the only option obtainable, they may provide some level of useful compression, but will need to be reapplied and replaced more frequently.

2.5 Orthotic Devices (Fig. 10)

For long-term management of edema for the patient unable to apply stockings or wraps, orthotic devices are available which consist of inelastic straps that overlap each other and are secured with velcro. These devices are easier to apply for the patient with arthritis or who lack the strength to apply other types of compression. They are primarily for longer term use and are much more durable than stockings or wraps, consequently making them more cost effective.

2.6 Compression Pumps

Mechanical pumps which involve the use of a limb sleeve connected to a pneumatic pump are available for the patient unable to wear or ideally, in addition to compression stockings, or as an adjunct to stockings in severe edema. They are also

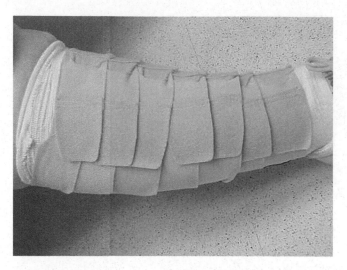

Figure 10 Orthotic wrap with Velcro® straps.

frequently used in the management of lymphedema, which has been addressed in another chapter. The sleeves are generally knee or thigh length, and are usually sequential (multiple chambers which inflate and deflate proximally to facilitate movement of fluid) and gradient (gradually decreasing levels of compression beginning at the foot proximally). These devices are quite costly, and specific criteria must usually be met in order for the pumps to be reimbursed by payers.

2.7 Stockings

Though also used for treatment of existing ulcers, the ultimate goal for the patient with chronic venous insufficiency is use of compression stockings for lifelong management of the disease. Worn faithfully, they can mean the difference between remaining healed and recurrence of ulcers for most patients. Ready-to-wear garments are available for purchase, but should accompany a prescription from a healthcare practitioner recommending the appropriate level of compression, size, and style appropriate for their leg. Many options are available with differing ankle to calf size differences, availability of zippers and liners, fabrics (i.e., stocking vs. sock), and a sheer appearance vs. a denser look to the stocking. They too are available latex free for the patient who is latex allergic or sensitive.

For the patient who does not fall into the range of sizing available in the ready-to-wear stockings, custom fit garments may be required. These need to be fit and ordered by a certified fitter who can measure the leg, usually in 1-in. increments, and custom made for the individual. It is generally recommended that the patients have several pair, which can be carefully washed and maintained, and that the stockings be replaced every six months. The patient should be counseled to return for follow-up visits to assure that sizing or compression needs have not changed.

Aids to assist in application of compression stockings in the form of frames or other donning devices to facilitate application of the stockings are available for patients who experience difficulty in putting on compression stockings. Medical supply dealers who provide the stockings can show patients options that might be best for them. Clinicians should make themselves aware of local dealers in their treatment area, variety and brands available, level of expertise of local fitters, as well as level of reimbursement assistance offered for their patients.

3. CHOICE OF COMPRESSION MANAGEMENT—CONSIDER THE PATIENT

Lifestyle and occupation should always be considered when choosing a method of compression for the patient with venous insufficiency . The most therapeutically appropriate compression therapy is useless if the patient is unable or unwilling to apply or wear it. Prior to initiation of therapy, extensive education and counseling should take place providing a detailed description of the therapy including the pros and cons, comforts and discomforts, and impact on the patient's day to day life. Many patients are branded as "noncompliant" if they return for follow-up care not wearing the prescribed stocking or wrap. Before clinicians label patients in this manner, discussion should take place to ascertain the reason for the nonadherence to the treatment plan.

4. HYPOTHETICAL SCENARIOS

Consider the patient who normally would wear a fitted business or dress shoe to work. Sending them out in a multilayered wrap which adds up to an inch to the diameter of their foot makes wearing their normal shoe impossible, thus leading them to alter or cut the wrap off in order to go to work (Fig. 11). Possible solution is: first, always prepare them for this possibility at the onset. Second, providing the patient with an inexpensive postoperative shoe to wear for the duration of their compressive therapy may enable them to wear the wrap.

Next consider the patient who works in a construction, landscaping or other vocation requiring them to work outside. Applying a wrap that we would expect to stay on for a full 7 days may be unrealistic. Both perspiration from the skin

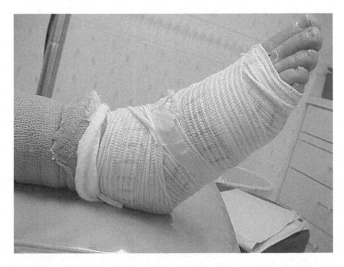

Figure 11 Patient "self-altered" three-layer wrap in order to fit into work shoe comfortably.

and dirt from the outside could make the wrap unbearable to live with after a few days. Additionally, offering this patient the option of "bathing at the sink" is unacceptable. Possible solutions could include altering the wrap to a stocking or other modality that the patient can control or change as needed, or offering twice weekly clinic or home visits to change the wrap. Clinic or home visits for changes of the wrap may be another alternative. Additionally, the use of commercially available protective extremity bags for the shower can enable them to shower normally without risk of wetting the wrap. Patients can also get creative at home with plastic bags and tape. Teaching should always include warnings of shower safety with any of these devices to avoid slipping.

Lastly, consider the elderly patient with arthritis or weakness of the hands. While preventing recurrence in the healed legs would perhaps be best managed with therapeutic compression stockings of 30–40 mmHg, if they are unable to get them on or off, even with the use of assistive devices, the likelihood of wearing them consistently if at all is slim. While the higher level of compression is ideal, an alternative plan of lesser compression coupled with frequent leg elevation may need to be considered.

5. WHO SHOULD COMPRESS?

Application of lower extremity compression wraps is a learned skill that can be taught safely to both clinical and nonclinical caregivers. Of extreme importance, though, is that it is also a procedure that can cause discomfort, irregular swelling (Fig. 12), and even damage if done incorrectly. Simply reading an instruction sheet is not adequate preparation in a novice to the concept. Much of the finesse in wrapping, for example, is in the feel and the stretch of the particular wrap being used. Common mistakes include wrapping too tightly, too loosely, or in a pattern more appropriate for a sport wrap (i.e., heel and post-tibial areas left open).

Once one has mastered the basic concept and feels confident in the principles guiding compression wraps, variations on different wraps should pose no significant challenge. Several options are available for learning and obtaining the skill level to feel proficient in wraps of various types. Larger conferences and symposia on wound management often include a pre- or postconference workshop on venous ulcers,

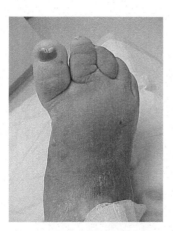

Figure 12   Swollen toes from tight wrap.

which include both didactic and hands on learning experiences. Locally, in-services can be made available through the local sales representative of the companies who market the compression systems available for use either in person or on video or DVD, with the opportunity to practice on each other in your group. Additionally, one can check locally for a certified wound nurse, vascular nurse, or physical therapist that would come to your facility or office to provide hands on education and practice.

Teaching nonclinical caregivers such as spouses or family members is not impossible but must be done in a relaxed, nonrushed setting with ample opportunity for return demonstration. Most likely, it will require more than one session to adequately teach the procedure. If the caregiver can visualize the goal of the compression, understand the basic principles, and possess the manual dexterity to accomplish the wrap, then teaching them is a realistic goal.

No matter who does the wrapping, or how skilled one is at the techniques, there will be patients who either cut the wraps off or call in for emergent appointments to have them changed due to discomfort. Considering gravity and the contours and prominences of the feet and ankles, the potential for discomfort, shifting, and wrinkling of the bandages is high. See Table 2 for troubleshooting tips.

6. ASSESSING EFFICACY

How does one assess that compression management in any one individual is effective? The obvious answer is in the assessment of the wound. Improvement or healing of the wound noted by reduction in size, lessening, or elimination of wound exudate or build-up of fibrinous tissue on the surface of the wound may be factors by which adequacy of the compression can be judged. In the patient in whom ulcers are minimal or nonexistent, serial measurements of calf and ankle circumference can provide a reliable basis for evaluating and documenting successful compression.

7. COMPRESSING THE INFECTED LEG

Recommendations for the utilization of compression in the presence of infection are difficult to impossible to find in the literature, and without question must be considered on a patient-by-patient basis. Clearly, the infected ulcer or limb with cellulitis present should be able to be observed and inspected frequently to ascertain the effectiveness of antibiotic therapy and to observe for worsening of the infection. While it stands to reason that reduction of edema and improvement of perfusion to the skin would enhance antibiotic therapy, use of compression during this time must be approached with extreme caution and certainly utilization of a management method allowing visualization of the ulcer and the leg would be prudent in the initial treatment phase.

8. PATIENT EDUCATION

Education of the patient and caregivers of the patient utilizing compression therapy of any type is ongoing and vitally important to increase the likelihood of success.

Table 2 Pearls for Troubleshooting Compression Wraps

Challenge	Possible solutions
Sliding down of entire multilayer wrap	1. Add increased bulk or soft wrap at ankle to enhance fit and decrease sliding 2. Wrap with increased tension, increasing slightly with each subsequent wrap to assess tolerance 3. Add something to top of leg below knee to make skin "tacky" and cause the cotton layer to stick 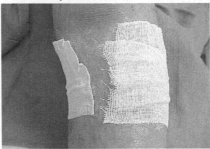 *Use of non-circumferential Unna boot-wrap to provide tacky layer.*
Discomfort and rubbing of prominent tendons, bony prominence	Add padding, such as gauze or ABD pad, or ideally foam over areas of discomfort or concern 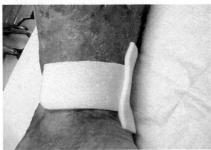 *Use of foam padding on prominent areas of leg.*
Generalized itching Stasis dermatitis Contact dermatitis	1. Apply moisturizer, barrier cream or ointment, antipruritic, or mild- to mid-potency topical steroid cream prior to application. Decision should be made on causative agent of skin condition or patient allergies 2. Change type of compression

(Continued)

Table 2   Pearls for Troubleshooting Compression Wraps (*Continued*)

Challenge	Possible solutions

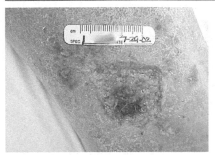

Dermatitis pretreatment.

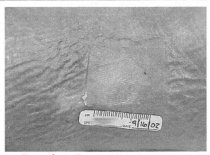

Same leg: Deramitis post-treatment.

Complaint of "sticking" of cohesive outer layer of multi-layer wrap.
- It may be found to be most bothersome at night, with wrap catching on sheets
- Slacks worn during the day may ride up or adhere to wrap when going from sitting to standing position

1. Apply loose layer over outer wrap to enable leg to slide over sheets or garments
- Stockinet or queen-sized ladies knee-high stocking (nonsupport) with the top band split to avoid constriction

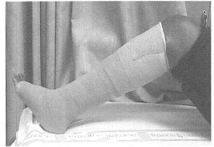

Leg with outer cohesive wrap.

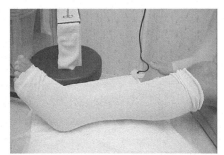

Wrap covered with stockinet material.

High level of exudate saturating dressings, wraps, clothing, and causing peri-wound skin irritation/breakdown.

1. Deep tissue culture, antibiotics if warranted
2. If not cellulitic or clinically infected, consider topical antimicrobial dressing to reduce bioburden, which may be causing increased exudate
3. If adequate perfusion, high-level compression to eliminate edema. Wraps would most likely be best changed at least twice weekly until exudate under control
4. Protection/treatment of peri-wound skin with barrier such as a protective cream or ointment

(*Continued*)

Table 2 Pearls for Troubleshooting Compression Wraps (*Continued*)

Challenge	Possible solutions
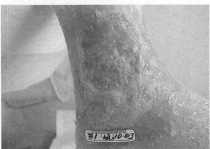 *Weepy denued leg caused by exudate from ulcers.*	*After one-month of treatment with twice weekly multi-layer wraps, absorptive silver dressings, and barrier ointment: Note moderate improvement in ulcer but dramatic reduction in exudate and improvement of peri-wound skin.*

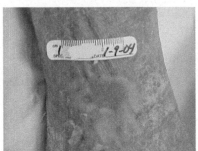

Two months of treatment:
Successful control of exudate, reduction in edema (as evidenced by wrinkles in skin), and progressive healing of ulcer.

Information about their disease, the goals of compression, and lifelong management are essential. Although teaching is continuous and repetitive during the course of treatment, certain facts should be shared before they leave the healthcare setting with a new wrap or bandage on to maintain safety and comfort. Points to be covered and provided in written form should include:

- Recommendation for frequent rest periods with the legs elevated above the level of the heart.
- Exposed areas of the toes should be checked frequently for warmth, coolness, or discoloration.
- If numbness, tingling, pain, or swelling of the toes or the knees above the wrap should occur, remove the wraps and notify your physician, nurse, therapist, or clinic.
- Wraps should not be allowed to get wet. Bathe at the sink or carefully shower with a plastic protective bag or device over the wrap to prevent

wetting. A rubber shower mat should be utilized to prevent slipping in the shower. Wet wraps will need to be removed, call the nurse or clinic to have it replaced.

- If wound exudate should penetrate through the wrap and this is unusual or unexpected, notify your physician, nurse, therapist, or clinic.
- For patients with a history of congestive heart failure, onset of congestion or difficulty breathing should be reported immediately and the wraps should be removed.
- Sections of the wraps or layers should not be removed or replaced. If the wraps become dislodged or uneven, remove and notify your physician, nurse, therapist, or clinic.

9. SUMMARY

In the final analysis, successful compression therapy is dependent upon accurate diagnosis, patient tolerance, adherence to the treatment plan, and product availability. Combined with removal of local barriers to healing, ulcers caused by chronic venous insufficiency can usually be resolved successfully. While compression management may be somewhat of an art form, when combined with attention to the science of wound healing, by and large it will result in an improved quality of life, body image, and well being of our patients, as well as reduced morbidity in this large population of patients.

REFERENCES

1. Cullum N, Nelson EA, Fletcher AW, Sheldon TA. Compression for venous leg ulcers (Cochrane Review). The Cochrane Library. Issue 2. 2003.
2. Nelson EA, Bell-Syer SEM, Cullum NA. Compression for preventing recurrence of venous ulcers (Cochrane Review). The Cochrane Library. Issue 2. 2003.
3. Ennis WJ, Meneses P. Standard, appropriate, and advanced care and medical–legal considerations: part two—venous ulcerations. Wounds 2003; 15(4):107–122.
4. de Araujo T, Valencia I, Federman DG, Kirsner RS. Managing the patient with venous ulcers. Ann Intern Med 2003; 138(4):326–324.
5. Lopez AP, Phillips TJ. Venous ulcers. Wounds 1998; 10(5):149–157.
6. Sibbald, RG. Venous leg ulcers. Ostomy/Wound Manage 1998; 44(9):52–64.
7. Lorimer KR, Harrison MB, Graham ID, Friedberg E, Davies B. Venous leg ulcer care: how evidence-based is nursing practice? Wound Ostomy Continence Nurs 2003; 30(3):132–142.
8. Eagle M. Compression bandaging. Nurs Stand 2001; 15(38):47–52.
9. Goldstein AB, Mureebe L, Kerstein MD. Differential diagnosis: assessment of the lower-extremity ulcer—is it arterial, venous, neuropathic? Wounds 1998; 10(4):125–131.
10. Bjellerup M. Does dorsal pedal pulse palpation predict hand-held Doppler measurement of ankle–brachial index in leg ulcer patients? Wounds 2003; 15(7):237–240.
11. Faria D, Fowler E, Carson S. Understanding edema and managing the edematous lower let. In: Drasner DL, Rodeheaver GT, Sibbald RG. Chronic Wound Care: A Clinical Source Book for Healthcare Professionals. 3rd ed. Wayne, PA: HMP Communications, 2001:537.

35
Electrical Stimulation

Luther C. Kloth
Department of Physical Therapy, College of Health Sciences, Marquette University, and Department of Plastic Surgery, The Medical College of Wisconsin, Milwaukee, Wisconsin, U.S.A.

1. INTRODUCTION

It is interesting to note that among the chapters of this section there are seven topics each of which represent a physical form of energy that is employed to enhance wound healing. The delivery of electrical current into recalcitrant wounds for the purpose of accelerating tissue repair is not new. Reports from the seventeenth and twentieth centuries describe the application of electro-statically charged gold leaf to skin lesions associated with smallpox (1) and wounds of various etiologies, however, findings from these studies are inconclusive (2–7). In 1850, the first report of the use of electrical stimulation (ES) to treat bone fractures was published (8). More recent research related to the use of ES to augment bone repair (9,10) has lead to FDA approved electromagnetic devices that are labeled for treatment of nonunion and delayed union fractures (11,12). Still other investigators have demonstrated that ES augments the healing and increases the breaking strength of severed tendons (13,14). Since the mid-1960s much research has been directed at evaluating the effects of ES on healing of chronic wounds, that unlike acute wounds are wounds that do not heal spontaneously within a predictable time frame and are frequently resistant to many standard treatment procedures.

Today, treatments available to patients with chronic wounds are largely influenced by Medicare authorities who increasingly base reimbursement decisions on treatment efficacy, which they in turn establish by ascertaining the strength of evidence derived from clinical research trials.

This chapter will: (a) define basic terminology related to ES and identify types and characteristics of therapeutic electrical currents, (b) review experimental research and discuss putative mechanisms by which ES accelerates wound healing, (c) review clinical research evidence that supports ES as an efficacious intervention for healing chronic wounds, (d) describe clinical methods of applying ES to facilitate wound healing, (e) identify precautions and contraindications to the use of ES for wound healing. This chapter will present an evidence-based approach to assessing basic science research and clinical trials that provide strength of evidence for the clinical use of ES in augmenting the healing of chronic wounds.

2. ELECTRICAL STIMULATION TERMINOLOGY AND TYPES OF THERAPEUTIC CURRENTS

Reviewers of the wound healing literature related to ES often express that they are confused by the diverse types of current and stimulation parameters reported in research studies which makes it difficult to compare studies and draw conclusions related to efficacy. It appears that the primary reason for this confusion may stem from a lack of standardization of ES terminology. Recognizing that ES treatments and research studies can neither be clearly understood nor replicated because of the terminology confusion, the Section on Clinical Electrophysiology of the American Physical Therapy Association (APTA) has published a document (15) that is intended to clarify ES terminology and types of therapeutic currents among clinicians and researchers. Hopefully, the following terminology modified from the APTA document will relieve some of the confusion related to the use of ES in wound healing.

2.1. Terms and Definitions

1. *Charge*: Electrical charge is a fundamental property of matter. Matter either has no net charge (electrically neutral) or is negatively or positively charged. The fundamental particle of negative charge is the electron (e–). Charge is measured in specific quantities of electrons called coulombs (Q). The quantity of charge delivered to tissues by ES is measured in micro-coulombs (μQ).

2. *Charge density*: This is a measure of the electrical charge of a treatment electrode's surface area and is inversely related to electrode size. For wound treatment, since the amount of charge on the electrode surface area is relatively small, charge density is likely to be expressed as μQ/cm^2.

3. *Electrodes*: Electrodes are the conductive elements of an electrical circuit that are applied to the body for the purpose of transferring electrical charge into the tissues. For current to flow through a circuit, a minimum of two electrodes are required. The negative electrode called the cathode (–) attracts positive ions (cations), while the positive electrode or anode (+) attracts negative ions (anions) in the tissues. Electrodes consist of carbonized silicon, conductive polymers, or aluminum foil placed in contact with saline moist gauze.

4. *Polarity*: Polarity is the property of having two oppositely charged poles or electrodes. At any given time while current is flowing, one electrode is relatively more positive while the other is relatively more negative. When the cathode and anode have sufficient charge they may cause undesirable electrochemical burning of healthy tissues due to formation of NaOH and HCl, respectively.

5. *Electrical circuit*: An electrical circuit used for wound healing applications consists of at least two leads, one of which is connected to the cathode terminal and the other connected to the anode terminal of an ES device. The patient end of each lead is connected to an electrode that is applied to the patient.

6. *Voltage*: The electrical force capable of moving electrons or ions between two points of a conductor is the voltage or potential difference between the two points. The voltage between the two points (e.g., two electrodes on the body) is created by the separation of charges between them such that one electrode has an excess of negatively charged electrons or ions compared with the other. The two electrodes are "polarized" with respect to one another, one being negative and the other positive.

7. *Electric current*: The rate of flow of charged particles (electrons or ions) through a conductive medium past a specific point in a specific direction constitutes electrical current. Current is produced in a conductor (metal wire) by the voltage or potential difference between two points. Current flow in a metal wire occurs as a result of the flow of electrons, whereas current flow in tissues is carried by ions (e.g., Na^+, K^+, Cl^-). The unit of measure of current is the ampere (A) that represents the movement of 1 coulomb of charge per second. Exogenous currents used for wound treatment that are intended to mimic bioelectric tissue currents may be delivered to the tissues either in the milliampere (mA) or microampere (μA) range of current amplitude. When a unidirectional current flows in the circuit, positive charge carriers in the tissues (Na^+, K^+, or H^+) and cells (fibroblast and activated neutrophil) migrate toward the cathode, while negative charge carriers (Cl^-, HCO_3^-, P^-) and cells (epidermal, macrophage, neutrophil) migrate toward the anode.

8. *Resistance*: As electrons and ions (charged particles) flow in metallic and biological conductors, respectively, their movement is impeded by collisions with other charged carriers and by the inherent properties of the substance. Thus, resistance is the opposition to the flow of current. A conductor's resistance is 1 ohm if a potential difference of 1 V causes 1 A to flow through it. This is one form of Ohm's Law, which states $R = V/I$.

9. *Waveform*: A waveform is a visual representation of voltage or current on an amplitude–time plot. A waveform represents a picture of an electrical event that begins when the current or voltage leaves the zero (isoelectric) baseline in one direction, then after a finite time either returns to and stops at the same baseline (monophasic waveform) or crosses the baseline in the opposite direction, and ends when the voltage or current returns again to the baseline (biphasic waveform).

10. *Phase*: This term describes an electrical event that begins when the current (or voltage) leaves the isoelectric line and ends when it returns to the baseline.

11. *Phase/pulse duration*: Phase duration is the time in microseconds or milliseconds between the beginning and the end of one phase of a pulse. Pulse duration is the time in microseconds or milliseconds between the beginning of the first phase and the end of the second phase that may include the inter-phase interval within one pulse.

12. *Pulse frequency*: This term describes the number of pulses per second (pps) for a pulsed current or the number of cycles per second for alternating current.

2.2. Types and Characteristics of Therapeutic Currents

Although there are two basic types of currents that include direct current (DC) and alternating current (AC), a third type of current (pulsed current [PC]) has been adopted by the Section on Clinical Electrophysiology (SCE) of the APTA (15) as an additional "therapeutic current." The reason the SCE adopted PC is to provide clearer descriptions of "pulsed" waveforms that are delivered by the majority of electrotherapeutic devices used by clinicians. The adoption of PC is not meant to imply that there is an additional type of basic current.

1. *Direct current*: DC (sometimes referred to as galvanic current) is the continuous, unidirectional flow of charged particles for one second or longer (Fig. 1). In the tissues, the direction of DC flow is determined by the polarity selected, with negatively charged ions moving toward the anode and positively charged ions moving toward the cathode (15). Once selected, electrode polarity remains constant until it is changed manually on the ES device. Continuous DC has no pulses and

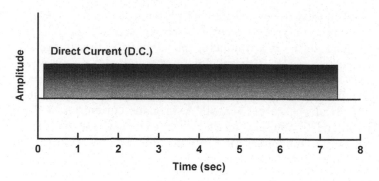

Figure 1   Graphic representation of direct current (DC). (From Ref. 131.)

therefore no waveform. When DC is delivered to a solution or to tissues containing electrolytes, the charged ions (Na^+, K^+, Cl^-) are attracted to the cathode and anode, respectively. At the cathode, Na^+ reacts with H_2O to form NaOH and H_2, while at the anode Cl^- reacts with H_2O to form HCl and O_2. The caustic products of NaOH and HCl that form at the tissue surface of the cathode and anode, respectively, can cause electrochemical burning seen as blistering. When DC is used to treat wounds care must be taken to avoid undesirable responses by delivering less than 1.0 mA to the electrodes. Current amplitudes under 1.0 mA are in the micro-amperage (μA) range.

Later in this chapter results will be discussed for several clinical trials that reported accelerated healing of chronic wounds treated with DC at 50–1000 μA (16–19).

2.   *Alternating current*: AC is the continuous bidirectional flow of charged particles in which a change in direction of flow occurs at least once every second. An AC waveform is represented by one cycle which describes an electrical event that begins when the current or voltage leaves the zero (isoelectric) baseline in one direction then crosses the same baseline in the opposite direction to end when the current or voltage returns again to the baseline. When available from an ES device, the most common AC waveform is the sine wave, in which both phases of the cycle are charge balanced so there is no electrode polarity. Unlike PC, AC has no off time interval between phases of adjacent cycles.

Some authors have erroneously indicated that current delivered by transcutaneous electrical nerve stimulation (TENS) devices represents AC (20–27). In reality, ES modalities classified as TENS devices by the US Food and Drug Administration deliver trains of isolated electrical events (pulses) that are either monophasic or biphasic PC not AC (15). Since only DC and PC have been used in clinical wound healing studies, AC will not be discussed in this context.

3.   *Pulsed current*: PC is the brief unidirectional or bidirectional flow of charged particles (electrons or ions) in which each pulse is separated by a longer off period of no current flow. Thus, each pulse is an isolated electrical event separated from each of a series or train of pulses by a finite off time. PC is described by its waveform, amplitude, duration, and frequency. PC can have two waveforms: monophasic or biphasic. A monophasic pulse (Fig. 2A) represents a very brief movement of electrons or ions away from the isoelectric line, returning to the zero line after a finite period of time (less than 1.0 sec). When the duration of a monophasic pulse is less than 1.0 sec, the current is not DC because it does not cause electrochemical

Pulsed Current (P.C.)

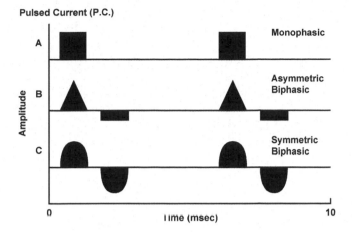

Figure 2 Graphic representation of pulsed current (PC) showing (A) monophasic PC, (B) asymmetric biphasic PC, and (C) symmetric biphasic PC. (From Ref. 131.)

changes in the tissues. Monophasic PC waveforms that have been described in the clinical wound healing literature include the rectangular waveform (28–32) and the twin-peaked waveform of high voltage PC (33–36). High voltage PC (HVPC) typically has very short duration (2–20 μsec) twin triangular pulses that have single-phase charges on the order of 1.6 μQ (34) (Fig. 3). Because HVPC is unidirectional, one may incorrectly assume that this type of current is "galvanic" or DC that causes caustic skin and wound tissue damage secondary to pH changes. However, investigators have demonstrated that pH changes do not occur in human skin following 30 min of HVPC stimulation (37).

The biphasic PC waveform also represents a very brief duration of movement of electrons or ions. However, in this case the pulse is bidirectional and consists of

High Voltage Pulsed Current (HVPC)

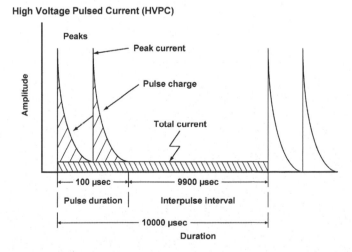

Figure 3 Graphic representation of monophasic high voltage PC. (Courtesy of the American Physical Therapy Association, Alexandria, VA.)

two phases. One phase leaves the isoelectric line, and after a brief finite time returns to baseline. Then without delay (or in some waveforms, a few microseconds delay), the second phase leaves the isoelectric line in the opposite direction, and after a brief time returns to baseline. The biphasic waveform may be asymmetric or symmetric about the isoelectric line (Fig. 2B and C). In the symmetric biphasic waveform, the phase charges of each phase are electrically equal or balanced, therefore there is no polarity. Asymmetric biphasic waveforms may be electrically balanced or unbalanced. Biphasic symmetrical (charge balanced) (38,39) and asymmetrical (charge balanced) (38,40) waveforms have been described in recent clinical wound healing literature.

3. RESEARCH REVIEW—THE EVIDENCE

Considerable experimental research has contributed to the expanding body of knowledge that provides insights into the mechanisms by which ES augments wound healing. In addition, numerous clinical studies have shown that ES enhances the healing of chronic wounds. This section will address the research that has led to the advancement of theories that in turn have influenced the development of protocols for the use of ES in the treatment of chronic wounds.

3.1. Experimental Research In Vitro and In Vivo
3.1.1. *Effects of Electric Fields on Tissue Cells In Vitro*
Numerous studies have investigated how cells respond when exposed to electrical currents of different amplitudes and frequencies. Some studies have reported changes in cell synthesis and metabolism, while others have observed migratory effects of cells exposed to electric fields.

a. *Protein synthesis*: Bourguignon et al. (41,42) stimulated human fibroblasts growing in cell culture with HVPC. They reported that the fibroblasts were induced to increase their rate of DNA and protein synthesis, the latter of which increased by 160% over controls. Maximum synthesis occurred at 50 and 75 V and 100 pps with the cells positioned close to the cathode. Voltages in excess of 250 V inhibited both protein and DNA synthesis. In another study, the same ES parameters triggered an increase in Ca^{2+} uptake followed by upregulation of insulin receptors on the fibroblast membrane during the second minute of stimulation (43). The significance of the latter finding is that if insulin is available to bind the additional receptors, the fibroblasts will significantly increase both protein and DNA synthesis. The ES has also been shown to increase the expression of fibroblast receptors for transforming growth factor-beta (44). Other investigators have noted that fibroblasts in a 3-dimensional collagen matrix that were exposed to an electric field responded by increasing the intake of ^{3}H-thymine (45).

b. *Cell migration*: Several studies (Table 1) have reported migration of cells involved in wound healing toward the anode or cathode of an electric field delivered into the tissue culture (46–54). This phenomenon known as galvanotaxis is the attraction of positively or negatively charged cells toward an electric field of opposite polarity. For example, macrophage cells that play important roles during the inflammatory phase of healing migrate toward the anode (46), whereas neutrophils migrate toward both the anode and cathode (47,48). However, Dineur (49) and Monguio (47) have reported that leukocytes migrate toward the cathode in regions where there

Table 1 Putative Cellular Galvanotaxis During Wound Healing Phases.

Phase of healing	Biological effects	Cells and their polarity	Current/polarity	Investigator (Ref.)
Inflammatory	Phagocytosis and autolysis	Macrophage (−)	DC (+)	Orida and Feldman (46)
		Neutrophil (−)	DC (+)	Fukushima et al. (48)
		Neutrophil (−)	PC (+)	Eberhardt et al. (57)
		Activated neutrophil (+)	DC (−)	Dineur (49)/Monguio (47)
Proliferative	Fibroplasia	Fibroblast (+)	PC (−)	Bourguignon and Bourguignon (41,42)
			DC (−)	Canaday and Lee (50)
			DC (−)	Erickson and Nuccitelli (51)
			DC (−)	Yang et al. (52)
Remodeling	Wound contraction	Myofibroblast (+)	PC (−)	Stromberg (55)
	Epithelialization	Keratinocyte (+)	DC (−)	Nishimura et al. (53), Sheridan et al. (54)
		Epidermal (−)	DC (−)	Cooper and Schliwa (56)
			PC (−/+)	Mertz et al. (58)
			PC (+)	Greenberg et al. (109)

DC = direct current; PC = pulsed current.
Source: From Ref. 131.

is infection or inflammation, which suggests a link between chemically mediated events and electrical responsiveness. There is considerable evidence that the fibroblast migrates toward the cathode (41,42,50–52). With respect to healing of the skin, investigators have recently shown that electric fields of the same magnitude as those found in mammalian wounds, direct the migration of human keratinocytes toward the cathode (53,54). Two other studies have also provided information related to galvanotaxis of cells involved in wound repair (55,56).

3.1.2. Effects of Electric Fields on Tissue Cells In Vivo

A literature review revealed two studies that investigated the indirect effect of ES on cell migration in vivo. Eberhardt et al. (57) evaluated the effects of exogenous ES on cell composition in human skin and found that 69% of 500 cells counted 6 hr post-stimulation were neutrophils compared to 45% found for control wounds. The authors proposed that the 24% difference in neutrophil percentage was due to the galvanotaxic effect created by the exogenously applied currents to periwound skin. Mertz et al. (58) assessed epidermal cell migration macroscopically for seven days following two 30-min sessions of monophasic pulsed current stimulation of induced wounds in an ovine model. They observed that wounds treated with the cathode on day zero followed by the anode on days 1–7, demonstrated 20% greater epithelialization compared to wounds treated with either positive (+9%) or negative (–9%) polarity alone. In addition, they observed that alternating polarity daily, inhibited epithelialization by 45%.

   There are several possible mechanisms by which galvanotaxis may guide cell migration in vivo. A cell may detect an electric field by electrophoretic movement of proteins within the plasma membrane. For instance, epidermal growth factor receptors have been shown to move to the cathode side of keratinocytes exposed to a DC electric field (59). Other intracellular sites the electric field may perturb to effect galvanotaxis are localized membrane depolarizations that result in changes in calcium ion fluxes (60), changes in cell shape, and cytoskeletal reorganization (61–65) and activation of protein kinases (66,67). It is tempting to speculate that the weak electric fields used to cause galvanotaxis of cells in tissue culture may mimic the natural electric fields found in mammalian wounds that guide migration of keratinocytes (53,54). As a matter of fact cell migration findings from some of the in vitro and in vivo studies previously cited have been used as the basis for selecting the anode or cathode in the clinical treatment of wounds with ES.

   The natural electric fields present as ionic currents in injured tissues were first demonstrated in 1830 (68). Fourteen years later DuBois-Reymond (69) demonstrated the existence of wound currents which in the early 1980s were recorded up to $35\,\mu A/cm^2$ from the amputated fingers of children (70) and $10-30\,\mu A/cm^2$ from induced wounds in guinea pigs (71). This "current of injury," measurable in wounded amphibian skin (72,73) where it likely contributes to wound healing, is sustained in a moist wound environment and is shut off when a wound dries out (74). Cheng et al. (75) have demonstrated that an occlusive dressing applied to human wounds, sustained the injury current at over $29.6 \pm 8.6\,mV$ for four days compared to a significantly lower potential of $5.2 \pm 12.6\,mV$ recorded from wounds exposed to air during the same time period. In addition, trans-epithelial potentials sustained by a skin battery (Fig. 4) have been recorded in human skin at amplitudes between 10 and 60 mV (skin surface negative, wound positive) (74). Apparently, these potentials are produced by the inward transport of Na^+ through the epithelial cell membrane

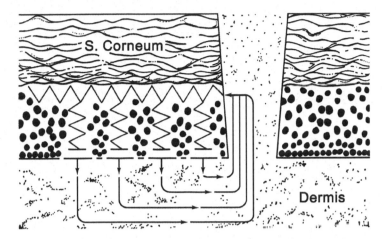

Figure 4 Generation of skin wound electric fields. Intact skin maintains a skin battery that drives Na$^+$ ions inward to generate a transepithelial potential. When wounded, the battery drives current through the low resistance hydrated wound, generating an electric field that is positive with respect to the negatively charged, intact periwound skin. This current continues until epithelialization covers the wound. (From Ref. 74).

Na$^+$/K$^+$ ATPase pumps (72). When a wound occurs in the skin, the measurable injury current flows out of the wound and is also measurable in a 2–3 mm margin of periwound skin. This lateral voltage gradient falls from a high of 140 mV/mm at the wound edge to 0 mV/mm just 3 mm lateral to the wound edge (74). McGinnis and Vanable (72) have shown that currents escaping through healing wounds and their accompanying lateral voltage gradients are gradually reduced and ultimately become nonexistent due to the resistance created by the new epithelium.

3.1.3. Antibacterial Effects of ES In Vitro and In Vivo

Recently in chronic wound management greater emphasis has been placed on reducing the bacterial burden that may lead to infection and impede or inhibit healing. Results from in vitro and in vivo studies suggest that ES either has a bacteriostatic or bactericidal effect on microbes that commonly colonize or infect wounds (Table 2). Rowley (76) and coworkers have reported in vitro bactericidal effects on *Escherichia coli* B growth rates using microamperage levels of cathodal. They demonstrated a similar effect using 1.0 mA of cathodal DC on rabbit skin wounds infected with *Pseudomonas aeruginosa* (77). Barranco et al. (78) delivered cathodal DC to infected rat and rabbit femurs and demonstrated a bacteriostatic effect on *Staphylococcus aureus*, which they attributed to a shift in pH owing to electrochemical changes. In other in vitro studies investigators found that 100 μA of DC delivered to the culture via a silver wire anode had a bacteriostatic effect on Gram-positive bacteria, whereas the same current and polarity produced a bactericidal effect on Gram-negative bacilli (79,80). Interestingly, commercial dressings containing ionic silver are now available for treating wounds that have a high bacterial burden. Other investigators have compared in vitro antibacterial effects of HVPC and DC and found that HVPC applied at 50–800 mA and 100 pps for 30 min had no inhibitory effects on *S. aureus*, whereas both anodal and cathodal continuous DC applied at 1, 5, and 10 mA did inhibit *S. aureus* growth (81). The findings from this study

Table 2 In Vitro and In Vivo Studies on the Antibacterial Effects of Electrical Stimulation

Author (Ref.)	Study type	Pathogen(s)	Current type	Stimulation parameters	Polarity/effect	Electrode type	Growth rate
Rowley (76)	In vitro	E. coli	DC[a] AC[b]	mA = 1.0, 14, 140 Frequency = 1, 10, 30, 60	Cathode none	Platinum Platinum	Inhibited Not inhibited
Rowley et al. (77)	In vivo rabbit	P. aeruginosa	DC	mA = 15 or 30 mA = 1.0	Cathode	Copper mesh in gauze	Bacteriostatic
Baranco et al. (78)	In vitro	S. aureus	DC	μA = 0.4 to 4.0	Anode (negligible gas and pH)	Silver	Inhibited
Ong et al. (79)	In vitro	S. aureus P. aeruginosa	DC	μA = 26, 100, 300, 500, 800	Anode	Silver wire	Bactericidal Bacteriostatic Bacteriostatic
Laatsch et al. (80)	In vitro	Gram + Gram −	DC	μA = 100	Anode and cathode	Silver wire Silver nylon	Bactericidal No ± inhibition
Guffey and Asmussen (81)	In vitro	S. aureus	HVPC[c] DC	mA = 50–800 Frequency = 100 pps mA = 1, 5, 10 Frequency = 100 pps	Anode and cathode Anode and cathode	Stainless steel Stainless steel	Inhibited
Kincaid et al. (82)	In vitro	S. aureus E. coli P. aeruginosa	HVPC	V = 150, 200, 250, 300 Frequency = 120 pps	Anode	Stainless steel	No inhibition
Szuminsky et al. (83)	In vitro	E. coli Klebsiella P. aeruginosa S. aureus	HVPC	V = 500 Frequency = 120 pps	Cathode Anode (gas and pH) Cathode (gas and pH)	Stainless steel Stainless steel	Inhibition All inhibited at both poles

[a] DC = direct current.
[b] AC = alternating current.
[c] HVPC = high voltage pulsed current.

suggest that the mechanism by which DC kills bacteria is through electrochemical pH changes that occur at both poles. Electrochemical pH changes have not been shown to occur at the anode or cathode when HVPC is applied to human tissues for 30 min (37). However, when Kincaid and Lavoie (82) evaluated antibacterial effects of HVPC in vitro, they observed pH changes only at the cathode at a dosage of 500 V and at both the anode and the cathode at 250 V. Szuminsky et al. (83) attempted to identify the mechanisms by which HVPC applied at 500 V causes bacterial killing in vitro. They observed bactericidal effects at both poles but were unable to determine whether the killing effect was due to the direct action of the current on the organisms, electrophoretic recruitment of antimicrobial factors, local heat generation, or pH changes. Although both of the latter studies demonstrated antimicrobial effects in vitro, it is unlikely that the high voltages used would be tolerated if applied to wounds of human subjects.

In summary, in vitro studies have reported that growth of common wound pathogens is more likely to be inhibited with microamperage levels of cathodal DC.

3.1.4. Experimental Research on Acute Wounds in Animals

Numerous studies involving a variety of animal models have reported tissue and cellular effects following treatment of traumatically induced wounds with ES. While the evidence from these studies adds to our understanding of how acute wounds respond to ES, extrapolation of the findings to chronic wounds in humans should be made with guarded optimism because of species differences and because healing of chronic wounds does not follow the acute wound model.

3.1.4.1. Effect of ES on Wound Scar Tensile Strength. The effect of ES on wound scar tensile strength has been evaluated in several studies. In three studies investigators delivered between 10 and 300 mA of DC to acute induced wounds. In all three studies wounds treated with the cathode had greater tensile strength than control wounds in two studies (84,85) or wounds treated with the anode in a third study (86). Three other studies (87–89) also reported increased wound tensile strength following treatment with DC, but polarity was not specified in two of the studies (88,89).

The results of the first three of these five studies contradict the expected findings based on the empirical assumption that the cathode from DC should decrease wound tensile strength because cathodal DC creates an alkaline pH that is known to be sclerolytic and capable of softening or solubilizing necrotic tissue (89). Conversely, anodal DC creates an acid pH which causes a sclerotic effect (89) that would be expected to increase rather than decrease wound scar tensile strength as was observed in the studies previously mentioned (84–86).

Apart from the electrochemical effects on wound tensile strength, other studies have demonstrated an increase in fibroblast proliferation (90–92) within the wound and an increase in collagen synthesis (93–96) that may also improve wound tensile strength.

Other animal studies have evaluated the effects of HVPC on acute wound closure and tensile strength. In two studies, Brown et al. (97,98) and coworkers reported that neither cathodal nor anodal HVPC had a significant effect on wound closure or tensile strength. However, histologic examination revealed that epithelialization advanced more rapidly in wounds treated with the anode (98). They also found that when polarity was changed every 3–4 days, wound closure was 100% for HVPC-treated wounds and 87% for control wounds (99).

The tensile strength response found in these studies is the response one would anticipate with cathodal DC not cathodal PC, since it has been demonstrated that HVPC does not create acid and alkaline pH changes on the skin at the anode and cathode, respectively (37). Thus, the finding that epithelialization advanced more rapidly in wounds treated with anodal HVPC (58,97,98) may be attributed to galvanotaxis of epithelial cells that may be negatively charged (56). More research is needed to definitively answer this question.

3.1.4.2. Responses of Surgical Wounds to ES. Seven studies were found that investigated the effects of ES on edema formation, skin grafts, donor sites, skin and musculocutaneous flaps, and angiogenesis. Three of these studies demonstrated that submotor levels of cathodal HVPC limited edema formation by blocking macromolecular leakage from microvessels (100–102). Evidence from the other four studies showed that microampere levels of anodal DC speed re-epithelialization and limits dermal fibrosis (103) and graft necrosis (104), whereas milliampere levels of PC increased survival of ischemic flaps (105,106). Interestingly, in a case series that involved four human subjects, investigators evaluated the effect of anodal PC on the thickness of donor site scars and found that ES reduced scar thickness and hypertrophic scar formation (28). They also showed from scar biopsies that there was a marked reduction in mast cells (107) that are associated with fibrosis (107,108). Also interesting is the finding that increased angiogenesis occurred following treatment of wounds with PC (32,109).

3.2. Clinical Research Involving Chronic Wounds

Previously cited studies have shown that human epidermis contains a skin battery capable of driving currents of significant amplitude into wounds (70–75). In both guinea pigs and humans, the skin battery is powerful enough to maintain transcutaneous voltages of up to 80 mV (inside positive) and has the capacity to drive a current of 1 µA per millimeter along the wound leading edge of epithelium (74). On the premise that electrical signals contribute to wound healing, then delivery of exogenous currents to wound tissue via ES could be expected to facilitate wound healing (110).

In reviewing the clinical studies related to treatment of human wounds with ES, one finds that virtually all of them are designed to compare healing of wounds treated with active ES plus standard care, against healing of control wounds treated with placebo ES plus standard care. In these studies, both the active and placebo ES treatment was applied to wounds only for 30–60 min, five to seven days per week. During the remaining 23 or 23.5 hr of each protocol day, investigators were ethically bound to provide wound treatment, which consisted of standard wound care alone. The clinical studies that provide evidence-based support for ES as an efficacious treatment of chronic wounds are reviewed next according to whether the type of therapeutic current used in the study was DC or PC.

3.2.1. Direct Current Clinical Studies

Three case series and two randomized-controlled trials (RCT) report using microampere levels of DC to assess healing of wounds of various etiologies. In three of these studies, wounds were initially treated with the cathode followed by periodic polarity reversal (17–19). In the other two studies, the cathode (16) and the anode (111) were used exclusively as the treatment electrodes (Table 3). In the three studies that initially used the cathode polarity selection was not arbitrary. Rather, it was based on the finding that initial application of the cathode to the ulcer slowed healing but had an antibacterial effect, while application of the anode enhanced healing but allowed bacterial replication (17,75). As previously mentioned, in vitro studies have shown that cathodal DC has an antibacterial effect on select wound pathogens (76,77). Thus, in the study of Wolcott et al. (17), the cathode was applied over the ulcer for three days or until the wound was clinically noninfected, then the anode was applied to stimulate healing. They reported that for 75 patients with one ulcer, 34 (45%) wounds closed completely over 9.6 weeks at a mean healing rate of 18.4% per week. The mean healing rate of the other 41 wounds was 9.3% per week and these wounds closed an average of 64.7% over 7.2 weeks. Results were also provided for eight patients with bilateral size-matched ulcers of the same etiology. One ulcer on each of these patients was treated with ES and the other control ulcer received standard care alone. Of the eight wounds treated with ES, six closed completely and the other two closed to 70% of their baseline size. The eight control wounds healed less well with three showing no healing, three others healed less than 50% and the remaining two healed less than 75%. Notably, 71% of all the patients in this study were paraplegics whose rate of tissue repair was about 40% slower than that for patients with other primary diagnoses. Despite the overall slower rate of wound healing for the spinal cord injured patients, the ES protocol was successful in producing an 81.8% wound volume decrease at a healing rate of 13.4% per week for the 75 treated ulcers combined. In this study if a growth plateau occurred at any time, the investigators reversed the polarity which based on the results appears to have had a beneficial effect. However, since there are no reports of multiple polarity reversals during the healing process in nonregenerating species, there appears to be no scientific explanation for reversal of polarity on reaching growth plateaus.

In a similar trial with similar results Gault and Gatens (18) treated 76 patients with 106 ischemic skin ulcers with the same ES device and protocol used by Wolcott et al. (17). Six patients with 12 bilateral size-matched ulcers served as the control group. The six control ulcers that received standard wound care healed at a rate of 14.7% per week compared with 30% per week for the six ES-treated ulcers. Three of the six ES-treated ulcers healed completely, whereas two of the control wounds increased in size during the 4-week treatment period. For the 100 single ulcers in the study, the healing rate was 28.4% per week, with complete healing of 48% of the ulcers in 4.7 weeks, which is an improvement over the single wound results reported by Wolcott et al. (17).

The RCT of Carley and Wainapel was modified so patients received 20 hr (19) rather than 42 hr (17,18) of ES per week. They enrolled 30 patients with chronic dermal ulcers and paired them according to age, diagnosis, wound location, etiology, and size. One member of each pair was randomly assigned to have their wound treated with 300–700 µA DC plus standard care; the control member received only standard care. As in the previous two studies described, ES was applied directly to the wound via the anode following cathodal stimulation for the first 3 days. Polarity was reversed for 3 days if measurable healing stopped. The healing rate of wounds treated with ES increased from 1.5–2.5 times faster than control wounds over weeks 3, 4, and 5 of the study. In all three of these cathode first studies, ES combined with standard wound care promoted faster rates of healing than standard care alone.

Table 3 Clinical Wound Healing Studies with Direct Current (Adapted from Ref. 20 Ojingwa and Isseroff 2002)

Author (Ref.)	DC dosage and polarity	Study design	Wound diagnosis	Patient study group(s)	Number of patients or wounds	% Patients or wounds healed/time	Other results
Assimacopoulos (16)	50–100 μA/cathode	Case series	Venous	DC[a]	8	100/30 days	Biopsy 1 year after healed: dense hyalinized collagen
Wolcott et al. (17)	200–800 μA 6 hr/day for 0.8–15.4 weeks; switched polarity, cathode anode, cathode	Case series	Mixed	DC	75	40/9.6 weeks	Healing rate/week: 53 paraplegics = 9.3% 5 venous disease =14.4% 15 arterial disease =14.0% other = 100 %
		Embedded RCT	Mixed	DC Control	Bilateral wounds 8 8	95/15.4 weeks 32/15.4 weeks	Healing rate/week: 13.4% 5.0%
Gault and Gatens (18)	Protocol similar to Wolcott et al. except polarity changed only once	Case series	Mixed	DC	100	48/4.7 weeks	Healing rate/week: 28.4%
		Embedded RCT	Mixed	DC Control	Bilateral wounds 6 6	50/4 weeks 0/4 weeks	Healing rate/week: 30.0% 14.7%

Study	Treatment	Type	Indicated	Control	n	Weeks	Healing rate/week
Carley and Wainapel (19)	300–700 µA 4 hr/day for 5 weeks; polarity switching same as Wolcott et al.	RCT	Not indicated	DC	15	Not reported	Healing rate/week: 18.0%
				Control	15		9.0%
Cukjati et al. (111)	600 µA DC 0.5 hr, 1.0 hr or 2 hr/day via anode or 15–20 mA PC 1 hr or 2 hr/day until wound closure	RCT	Mixed	DC or Balanced biphasic	42 181	90/60 weeks	Healing rate/week: not reported
				PC[b] Standard care	54	72/60 weeks	Healing rate/week: not reported
				Sham ES	230	70/60 weeks	Healing rate/week: not reported

[a] DC = direct current.
[b] PC = pulsed current.
Source: Adapted from Ref. 20.

Another case series involved eight venous leg ulcers in existence from 8 months to 5 years that were treated with 50–100 μA of only cathodal DC (16). All wounds closed in an average of 30 days and none recurred over a 3-year follow-up period. Note that the use of cathode polarity alone in this latter study does not agree with the polarity protocol used in the three studies that used polarity reversal. Nevertheless, healing may have advanced secondary to a reduction in wound bacterial burden owing to the antibacterial effects of cathodal DC or to galvanotactic attraction of fibroblasts by the same polarity, which would favor connective tissue formation in the proliferative phase.

In the RCT of Cukjati et al. (111), 214 patients with 300 wounds were enrolled. The most frequent primary diagnosis was spinal cord injury (71.7%). The majority of wounds were pressure ulcers (82.7%) along with wounds of other etiologies that included arterial insufficiency (1%), diabetic neuropathy (6.3%), trauma (6.1%), and venous insufficiency (3.9%). Wounds were randomly assigned to be treated with standard wound care ($n = 54$), sham ES ($n = 230$), charge balanced biphasic PC ($n = 181$), and anodal DC ($n = 42$). Wounds treated with DC either had the anode applied over the wound surface with the cathode placed on healthy skin or both the anode and cathode were placed on healthy skin on opposite sides of the wound along its margin. Their rationale for using both electrode placements and pooling the data from both was based on the fact that both methods have been shown to accelerate wound healing (19,24,34,39,40). The DC was delivered at 600 μA for 0.5, 1, or 2 hr per day until wound closure. Both electrode placement methods were also used for PC that was delivered at 15–20 mA for 0.5, 1, or 2 hr daily until wound closure. Results from the pooled ES data showed that over 90% of ES-treated wounds closed within 60 weeks, whereas during the same time period only 70% of sham-treated wounds and 72% of wounds treated with standard care closed. They also found that wounds treated with PC healed significantly faster than wounds treated with sham ES or standard care. Despite the fact that there was no significant difference in the healing rates between wounds treated with PC and DC, the difference in healing rate between the DC-treated wounds and wounds treated with sham ES and standard care was highly in favor of DC but not statistically significant.

3.2.2. Pulsed Current Clinical Studies

The voltage output of PC devices is divided into two ranges: low voltage (LVPC) devices that provide both monophasic and biphasic waveforms and high voltage (HVPC) devices that only provide a monophasic waveform. The LVPC devices deliver pulses with durations up to 1.0 ms (1000 μsec), which require lower driving voltages between 0 and 150 V. The HVPC devices deliver pulses with durations that are typically 20–60 μsec long and, therefore, require higher driving voltages between 150 and 500 V.

3.2.2.1. Low Voltage Monophasic PC. Between 1989 and 1997 five clinical wound healing studies were published that used the same monophasic PC device (Varapulse®, manufactured by Staodyn, Inc., Longmont, CO—no longer in business) with a pulse duration between 140 and 150 μsec, a peak pulse amplitude of 30–35 mA and a pulse frequency of either 64 or 128 pps (28–32). In these studies (Table 4), the accumulated pulse charge was between 250 and 500 μQ/sec that equates to between 0.89 and 1.78 Q/day delivered to the wound. Note that the characteristics of this current do not fit the definition of DC, therefore, it would be misleading to refer to it as pulsed low intensity direct current.

Table 4 Clinical Wound Healing Studies with Pulsed Current (Adapted from Ref. 20 Ojingwa and Isseroff 2002)

Author (Ref.)	Dressing PC dosage polarity	Study design	Wound diagnosis	Current type and patient study group(s)	Number of patients or wounds	% Patients or wounds healed/time	Other results provided by authors
Feedar et al. (29)	Moist wound therapy plus 29.2 mA, 128 pps, 132 μs duration for 30 min BID × 7 days × 4 weeks. Cathode initially then polarity switched to anode and pps to 64	Double-blind RCT	Mixed: 70% pressure ulcers, 18% surgical, 2% vascular, 10% traumatic	LVMPC[a]	26	0/4 weeks	Healing rate/week: 14–44 % initial size
				Control: standard wound care plus sham ES	24	0/4 weeks	8.25–67 % initial size
				Sham cross-over wounds	14	0/4 weeks	2.9% while sham to 88% of initial size; 12.8% while active to 49% of size at cross-over
Gentzkow et al. (30)	Moist wound therapy plus 35 mA, 128 pps for 30 min BID × 7 days × 4 weeks. Cathode initially then polarity switched to anode and pps to 64	Double-blind RCT	Pressure ulcers Stages II–IV	LVMPC	21	0/4 weeks	Healing rate/week: 12.5–49.8% initial size

(Continued)

Table 4 Clinical Wound Healing Studies with Pulsed Current (Adapted from Ref. 20 Ojingwa and Isseroff 2002) (*Continued*)

Author (Ref.)	Dressing PC dosage polarity	Study design	Wound diagnosis	Current type and patient study group(s)	Number of patients or wounds	% Patients or wounds healed/time	Other results provided by authors
				Control: standard wound care plus sham ES	19	0/4 weeks	5.8–23.4% initial size
				Sham cross-over wounds	15	0/4 weeks	Healed 13.4% of initial size while sham; healed 47.9% after 4 weeks active stimulation
Junger et al. (32)	Compression bandaging plus 42 mA, 128 pps for 30 min/day for up to 60 days. Cathode initially then polarity switched to anode and pps to 64	Case series	Venous ulcers	LVMPC	15	0/8 weeks	Initial ulcer size = 15.9 cm^2; end ulcer size = 5.8 cm^2 (63% decrease); beginning capillary count = 8.05/mm^2; end capillary count = 11.55/mm^2 (+ 43.5%)
Wood et al. (112)	Moist wound therapy (assumed) plus 3 applications of 300 µA at	Double-blind RCT	Pressure ulcers Stages II–III	LVMPC	74	58/8 weeks	Decrease wound size > 80%: 73%

Reference	Parameters	Design	Wound	Comparison	n	Duration	Outcomes
	0.5 pps for 1 min and 600 µA for 3 min 3 ×/ week for 8 weeks. Polarity not reported			Sham		3/8 weeks	13 %
Kaada (22)	Monophasic pulses 100 pps, 15–30 mA, 30–40 min, 3 ×/day	Case report	Mixed	LVMPC	10	70/22 weeks	None reported
Baker et al. (38)	Moist wound therapy (assumed) plus: A. Asymmetric biphasic PC, Sub-motor paresthesia, 50 pps, 100 µs PD. B. Symmetric biphasic PC, sub-motor paresthesia, 50 pps, 300 µs PD. C. Micro-current, 1 mA, 1 pps, 10 µs PD.	RCT	Diabetic Ulcers	LVBPC[b] A B C Control	29 24 20 19	Not Reported	Healing rate/week: 11 ulcers were treated under both control and ES protocols. 9.7% as controls
							43.3% with ES

(Continued)

Table 4 Clinical Wound Healing Studies with Pulsed Current (Adapted from Ref. 20 Ojingwa and Isseroff 2002) (Continued)

Author (Ref.)	Dressing PC dosage polarity	Study design	Wound diagnosis	Current type and patient study group(s)	Number of patients or wounds	% Patients or wounds healed/time	Other results provided by authors
Kaada and Emru (23)	Moist wound therapy (assumed) plus biphasic pulses at 25 mA, 100 pps, 200–300 µs for 30 min BID via cathode 5–6 days/week	Case series	Hanson's disease ulcers	LVBPC	32	59/12 weeks	Mean healing time 5.2 weeks
Lundeberg et al. (25)	Biphasic pulses at 80 pps, 1 ms PD, Current amplitude to paresthesia for 20 min BID	Double blind RCT	Diabetic ulcers	LVBPC	32	42/12 weeks	% ulcers healed: 2 weeks = 0% ES vs. 4% sham 4 weeks = 12% ES vs. 7% sham 8 weeks = 25% ES vs. 11% sham 12 weeks = 42% ES vs. 15% sham
	Controls: moist wound therapy			Control	32	15/12 weeks	
Karba and	Biphasic PC at 15–20 mA; 250 µs	Case series	Pressure	LVBPC	14	95% of all ulcers healed (time not	100% of pressure ulcers healed in

Author	Design	Intervention	Wound type	Group	N	Healed/weeks	Results
Vodovnik (24)		PD, 40 pps, 1 hr/day	Vascular Traumatic		82 17	reported)	5.5 weeks. 90% of vascular ulcers healed in 10 weeks.
Frantz (113)	Double blind RCT	Moist wound therapy plus biphasic pulses (parameters not reported) applied for 30 min 3 ×/day for 8 weeks Controls: moist wound therapy	Pressure ulcers	LVBPC (TENS)	19	42/8	All ulcers in LVBPC group healed by 20 weeks
				Control	15	20/8	
Kloth and Feedar (34)	Single blind RCT	Moist wound therapy plus 100 V, 105 monophasic pps, 45 min/5 days/week via anode. Controls: moist wound therapy	Pressure ulcers Stage IV	HVPC[c]	9	100/7.3 weeks	Healing rate /week 45%
				Control (sham) Crossover	7 3	0/17 weeks	11.6% larger 38%
Franek et al. (117)	RCT	Three groups: A. Moist wound therapy plus 100 V, 100 monophasic pps, 50 min/day × 6 days × 7 weeks.	Venous leg ulcers	HVPC A	33	41/7 weeks	After 2 weeks granulation tissue development was significantly greater for group

(Continued)

Table 4 Clinical Wound Healing Studies with Pulsed Current (Adapted from Ref. 20 Ojingwa and Isseroff 2002) (*Continued*)

Author (Ref.)	Dressing PC dosage polarity	Study design	Wound diagnosis	Current type and patient study group(s)	Number of patients or wounds	% Patients or wounds healed/time	Other results provided by authors
	Cathode 3 weeks, Anode 4 weeks						A than for groups B and C
	B. Topical medications 6 weeks			B	32	65/6 weeks	
	C. Unna's boot 5.5 weeks			C	14	76/5.5 weeks	
Houghton et al. (118)	Two groups: A. Standard wound care based on wound etiology plus active HVPC at 150 V, 100 pps, 45 min. 3 ×/week for 4 weeks.	Double blind RCT	Diabetic venous arterial ulcers of the lower extremity				% decrease in wound size:
	Cathode on wound. B. Sham HVPC plus standard wound therapy based on wound etiology			HVPC Sham HVPC	21 22	0/4 weeks 0/4 weeks	44.3%/4 weeks 8.9%/4 weeks
Peters et al. (119)	Two groups:	Double blind RCT	Diabetic foot ulcers	HVPC	18	65/12 weeks	Stratification by compliance:

				N	Duration	
	A. Off-loading plus HVPC active HVPC at 50 V and 80 pps for 10 min followed by 8 min of 8 pps repeated for 8 hr at night for 12 weeks. B. Sham HVPC plus off-loading		Sham HVPC	17	35/12 weeks	Significantly more compliant patients in both groups healed than noncompliant patients
Goldman et al. (124)	Standard wound care plus 80–330 V to sensory threshold, 80–100 pps, 1 hr/day, 7 days/week for between 1 and 9 months	Case series; historical controls	Diabetic ischemic foot ulcers	HVPC	6	4/7.2 months 2 had amputation	Mean $TcPO_2$ before HVPC was 2 mmHg; after HVPC began it was 33 mmHg indicating increased perfusion

LVMPC = low voltage monophasic pulsed current.
[b] LVBPC = low voltage biphasic pulsed current.
[c] HVPC = high voltage pulsed current.
Source: Adapted from Ref. 20.

As mentioned earlier, Weiss et al. (28) found that one month after a seven-day treatment regimen of partial-thickness donor sites with positive polarity ES from the Varapulse®, the surgically induced wounds had softer and flatter scars compared with hypertrophic contra-lateral control scars. Histological findings from bilateral punch biopsies confirmed that electrically treated scars were reduced in thickness by a mean of 46% compared with control scars. Biopsies also showed that the ES-treated scars had a marked reduction in mast cells, which suggests that ES can decrease fibrosis, conceivably by reducing the number of mast cells.

In another study with the low volt PC device, investigators reported the results of a four-week prospective, randomized, double-blind multi-center trial, in which 26 chronic dermal ulcers of different etiologies were treated with standard wound care plus 30 min twice daily of active cathodal ES at an initial pulse frequency of 128 pps and a peak amplitude of 29.2 mA (500 µQ/sec) (29). Thirty-five (70%) of the wounds were stage II, III, and IV chronic pressure ulcers. When the ulcer was debrided or exuded serosanguinous drainage, the treatment electrode polarity was reversed every 3 days until the wound progressed to a partial-thickness ulcer. Maintaining the same amplitude, the pulse frequency was then reduced to 64 pps (250 µQ/sec) and the polarity of the treatment electrode was changed daily until the wound closed. The 24 patients randomized to the control group were treated with standard wound care and sham ES 30 min twice daily. After 4 weeks, wounds in the treatment and control groups averaged 44% and 67% of their initial size ($P < 02$). The weekly healing rates were 14% and 8.25%, respectively. None of the wounds treated with ES increased in size, compared to five wounds in the control group. After being assigned to the control group for four weeks, 14 wounds were crossed over to the ES protocol. After 4 weeks of sham ES treatment, the mean wound size reduction was 11.3% at a healing rate of 2.9% per week. After 4 weeks of active ES, these wounds were 49% of their size at crossover and had healed at a rate of 12.8% per week. The authors concluded that the results of the study support the use of low voltage monophasic PC as an effective intervention for healing chronic dermal ulcers.

Using the same low volt PC device (Dermapulse® formerly called Varapulse®, Staodyn, Inc., Longmont, CO) parameters and protocol used in the study just cited, Gentzkow et al. (30) conducted a double-blind, randomized multi-center trial on 37 patients with 40 pressure ulcers. Nineteen ulcers were treated with standard wound care plus sham ES and 21 were treated with standard care plus active ES. After E4 weeks, the ES-treated wounds had healed more than twice that of sham-treated ulcers (49.8% vs. 23.4%, $P = 0.042$) at weekly healing rates of 12.5% and 5.8%, respectively. At the end of the 4-week study period, 15 patients who had received sham ES crossed over to receive active ES. In the 15 crossover patients, 4 weeks of active ES produced three and a half times as much healing as had occurred during the 4 weeks of sham treatment (47.9% vs. 13.4%, $P = 0.012$). Intriguingly, the average healing after 4 weeks of active ES for the 15 crossover ulcers (49.9%) was almost identical to the healing after the first 4 weeks of the 21 ulcers in the active ES group (49.8%), which indicates a reliable treatment effect.

Two years later Gentzkow et al. (31) again used the same ES device (Dermapulse®), ES parameters, and protocol in a prospective, baseline-controlled study on pressure ulcers in three health-care facilities over a mean of 8.4 weeks. In this study, a cohort of 61 stage III or IV pressure ulcers served as their own control. As in the previous study, the first four weeks was a controlled phase during which all wounds received carefully documented standard wound care, consisting of dressings that maintained a moist wound environment, a 2-hr turning/repositioning schedule, a pressure reducing bed surface, infection control, and nutritional support. Only wounds that did not demonstrate measurable progress toward closure or regressed during the control period were enrolled in the second phase of the study. After 4 weeks of optimal standard wound care, 61 wounds in 51 patients met the inclusion criteria for enrollment in phase two in which patients continued to receive the same standard wound care. In addition, two 30-min sessions of active ES were added to their daily wound care program. With this research design, the authors surmised that subsequent changes in wound measurements and select characteristics could be attributed to the effects of ES. Progress toward wound healing as defined by the authors was a reduction of at least one wound stage or two wound characters. In the last week of the study (mean 7.3 weeks) 50 of 61 wounds (82.0%) had improved two or more wound characters and 45 of 61 wounds (73.8 %) had improved one or more stages toward wound closure.

In one other study with the Dermapulse® researchers investigated the effect of ES on wound healing and angiogenesis (32). They treated 15 venous leg ulcers that had failed to show significant evidence of healing with standard compression therapy over a mean period of 79 months. After a mean of 38 days of wound treatment with daily ES for 30 min, the mean ulcer area decreased by 63% ($P < 0.01$) from 16 to 6 cm^2. Prior to commencing ES when they examined these wounds with light microscopy to determine capillary density, they counted a mean of 8.05 capillaries per mm^2 compared with 11.55 capillaries per mm^2 post-ES ($P < 0.039$). The latter findings agree with those of other investigators who used the same ES device and observed prominent neovascularity following stimulation of burn wounds in pigs (107).

In an additional study that used low voltage PC, authors described the current as "pulsed low intensity direct current" that was delivered to the periwound tissue at 0.5 pps (110). The investigators referred to the current as being DC thus, the assumption is that it was monophasic but not DC because the definition of DC is the continuous flow of charged particles for 1.0 sec or longer. That means the current used in the study, which was delivered at 0.5 pps and a pulse duration of 500 μsec, falls into the monophasic PC category. The authors described the trial as a multi-center, double-blind placebo study in which 71 patients with 74 chronic stage II and III pressure ulcers were treated with either an active or a sham "pulsed DC" device after showing no significant improvement after 5 weeks of standard wound care. Active devices were used to treat 43 ulcers and sham devices were used to treat 31 ulcers, three times a week for 8 weeks. Neither the patient nor the clinician knew the identity of active or sham devices. Both groups also received standard wound care. The active devices initially delivered 300 μA of PC at 0.5 pps through negatively charged probe electrodes for 1 min to each of three different periwound sites on opposite sides of the ulcer, followed by 600 μA for 3 min at each site. After 8 weeks, 25 of the 43 ulcers (58%) closed in the active device group, whereas only 1 of 31 ulcers (3%) closed in the sham (placebo) group. A statistical analysis revealed a highly significant difference for the decrease in ulcer surface area of the 43 wounds treated with the active device compared with the 31 wounds treated with the sham device ($P < 0.0001$). In summary, three of the five studies (29,30,112) showed statistically significant decreases in the surface areas of wounds treated with ES over an average of 4.6 weeks.

3.2.2.2. Low Voltage Biphasic PC. The two phases of biphasic PC may be symmetrical and charge balanced which means the phase charge of each phase is equal and there is zero net DC (no electrochemical effect on tissues). On the other hand, the two phases may be asymmetrical and either charge balanced or unbalanced. If charge balanced there is also zero net DC, but if charge unbalanced there will be some net DC effect on tissues. Studies that report using biphasic PC do not always indicate whether the pulse phases are charge balanced or charge unbalanced. Transcutaneous electrical nerve stimulators (TENS) are ES devices that are labeled for pain suppression applications by the United States Food and Drug Administration. Most of these devices are intentionally designed to deliver biphasic charge balanced pulses so there is zero net DC, which eliminates the possibility of electrochemical skin irritation. Several clinical studies in the literature investigated the effects of "TENS" (i.e., biphasic PC) on wound healing. These studies will be reviewed in this section (Table 4).

Numerous studies have reported the effects of low voltage biphasic PC on wound healing. Six of the studies exclusively used the indirect electrode placement method of applying the treatment electrodes on the periwound skin adjacent to the wound (23,24,27,38,39,111). One study used both the direct placement method of applying the treatment electrode directly over the wound and the indirect electrode application method (111). In the latter study, the rationale for using both electrode placements and pooling the data from both was based on the authors recognizing that both methods have been shown to accelerate wound healing (19,24,34,39,40). An additional study was a case series (24) and another was a nonrandomized-controlled trial (27). In two other studies that only used the indirect electrode placement method, the authors stated they purposely wanted to stimulate cutaneous nerves rather than deliver current directly into the wound tissue where there are no cutaneous nerves, (38,39) as has been done in previous studies. They reasoned that stimulation of the cutaneous nerves near the wound could enhance wound healing through activation of the peripheral nervous system. In these two randomized-controlled studies (38,39), the same low voltage PC device (Ultrastim; Henley International, Houston, TX—no longer in business) and ES parameters were used. In both studies the investigators treated wounds with one of four ES interventions: biphasic asymmetric waveform (charge balanced), biphasic symmetric waveform (charge balanced), micro-current stimulation, or an ES sham protocol. Because the patients in these studies had impaired protective sensation in periwound skin secondary to spinal cord injury (38) or diabetes (39), the authors stated that one purpose of both studies was to evaluate the efficacy of ES in enhancing wound healing in patients with neurologically impaired skin, while minimizing adverse electrochemical effects of the stimulation on the skin. In the 4-week study involving dermal ulcers in patients with spinal cord injury, wounds were treated to closure. Thirty-five wounds treated with the biphasic asymmetric waveform closed, 32 treated with the biphasic symmetric waveform closed, 18 with micro-current closed and 19 treated with sham ES closed. A statistically significant difference was found between the group that received the biphasic asymmetrical waveform and the combined micro-current and sham ES groups that served as controls. No significant difference was found between the combined groups treated with micro-current and sham ES and the group treated with the symmetric biphasic waveform. No adverse electrochemical effects were observed on the skin of patients in this study. Interestingly, 11 control patients treated with standard wound care for four weeks had a mean weekly healing rate of 9.7%. When these 11 patients were crossed-over to be treated with active ES, their mean healing rate was statistically greater during the ES protocol (43.3% per week) and seven of the 11 wounds closed during the time they received the ES protocol. The findings of this study agree with those of Stefanovska et al. (27)

and with Cukjati et al. (111), who also compared wounds treated with biphasic asymmetric ES, with DC stimulated and control wounds. In the second study by Baker et al. (39) the increased healing rate of diabetic foot ulcers treated with the biphasic asymmetrical waveform plus standard wound care, enhanced healing by almost 60% over control wounds treated only with standard wound care, but there was no statistical difference between the group treated with symmetrical biphasic ES and the group treated with asymmetrical biphasic ES.

In six other clinical studies that investigated the effects of ES on wound healing, TENS devices were used to deliver biphasic PC. One of these studies was a case report (21) and two were uncontrolled case series (22,26) in which ulcers of various etiologies including neuropathic lesions were treated by placing the electrodes over cutaneous nerves in the periwound skin. As in other studies (24,27,38,39,112) the rationale for using the indirect stimulation method (22,26) was based on the premise that a neuronally triggered mechanism would augment wound healing. Kaada and Emru (23) also reported using "TENS" (biphasic PC) in a case series to treat 32 patients with leg ulcers secondary to Hansen's disease that had failed to heal during extended periods of standard care. Using the indirect method ES was delivered to the wounds at 25 mA and 100 pps with pulse durations of 200–300 μsec for 30 min BID, 5–6 days a week. Twelve weeks after the study terminated, wounds in 59% of patients closed and wounds of all those who completed therapy closed in a mean of 5.2 weeks. In a randomized-controlled trial, Lundeberg et al. (25) evaluated the effect of "TENS" (biphasic asymmetric PC) on wound healing. Sixty-four patients with chronic diabetic foot ulcers were randomized to either receive active ES (parameters not given) or sham ES (controls) for 20 min BID for 12 weeks in addition to standard wound care. Polarity of the treatment electrode was changed each session. After 12 weeks there was a statistically significant treatment effect based on closure of 42% of wounds in the active ES group compared to 15% of the controls ($P < 0.05$). In a randomized, double-blind clinical trial, Frantz (113) used a "TENS" device to deliver biphasic PC to chronic wounds. Thirty-four patients, each with one pressure ulcer that had been resistant to healing for at least 3 months, were randomized to one of two wound treatment groups. All ulcers in both groups were treated with saline-moist gauze that was changed three times a day and remoistened at 4-hr intervals. In one group this was combined with active ES applied to the wound for 30 min three times a day. The same protocol was used on the second group except they received sham ES. During the 8-week protocol eight wounds closed with active ES compared with three that closed with sham ES, however, all wounds treated with active ES closed by 20 weeks. In summary, several of the studies that evaluated the effect of low voltage biphasic PC on wound healing have demonstrated statistically significant enhancement of healing rate compared to controls (38,39) and number of wounds closed compared to controls (25).

3.2.2.3. High Voltage Monophasic PC. High voltage PC (HVPC) is characterized by its "twin pulses" of short duration (typically 20–60 μsec) and a voltage range of 150–500 V (Fig. 3). Because of the common misconception that all monophasic pulses are DC, HVPC is frequently referred to as HVPGC, which implies that there is a DC component that will create electrochemical effects on tissues. However, research has shown that HVPC does not cause pH changes on human skin (37). Twelve publications including an experimental animal study, three case reports, one small noncontrolled comparative trial, one case series, and six clinical trials have evaluated the effects of HVPC on wound healing. Some of these studies are summarized in Table 4.

The use of HVPC to enhance tissue healing dates back to 1966 when a veterinarian applied this form of current to the hind limbs of eight dogs whose hind limb circulation was compromised for 12 hr by proximal tourniquet application (114). Twenty-four hours after tourniquet removal the hind limbs of four dogs were treated with HVPC for 5 min daily for 14 days, while four control dogs did not receive HVPC treatment. After the 14-day study period control dogs developed severe gangrene, whereas dogs treated with HVPC walked without limping and had no observable differences between their normal and traumatized limbs. Three case reports have also reported favorable outcomes following HVPC treatment of patients with infected wounds (36,115,116). However, in two of these studies (36,115) patients were treated simultaneously with HVPC and antibiotics so no conclusion can be drawn regarding a treatment effect from HVPC. A study by Akers and Gabrielson (33) reports the results of a noncontrolled comparative trial in which 14 patients had their pressure ulcers treated with one of three treatment protocols. The three treatment groups were whirlpool therapy once daily, whirlpool therapy plus HVPC twice daily, and HVPC alone twice daily. There was no mention of the numbers of patients in the three groups, the number or duration of treatments or the ES parameters. Also, patients in the three groups were not comparable in that those who received ES alone had sensory loss while those in the other groups had some sensation. Based on a comparison of wound pretreatment size with weekly wound surface area measurements, patients treated with ES alone showed the greatest change in wound size followed by the combined ES and whirlpool therapy group and the group treated with whirlpool alone. There were no statistical differences between the three groups because of the small sample size and the wide variability within the groups.

Five clinical studies all of which are randomized-controlled trials have investigated the effects of HVPC on chronic wound healing. In two of the studies, the authors mentioned that the charge quantities delivered to the wound tissues were 342 (34) and 500 (35) $\mu Q/sec$. These charge values or dosages of electrical current coincide with the range of charge values previously reported in the five low voltage PC studies (28–32). In a controlled study, Kloth and Feedar (34) randomly assigned 16 patients with stage IV dermal ulcers to either an experimental (active ES) or control (sham ES) group. Wounds of both groups received standard care 24 hr a day. In addition, 45 min of HVPC was delivered five days a week directly into the nine wounds of the experimental group at 105 pps and the current amplitude set to just below that which produced a visible muscle contraction. Initially, the anode was placed over the wound but in four patients whose wounds were treated with active ES, the wound electrode polarity was alternated daily when there was no change in measurable progress toward wound closure. Seven patients in the control group received 45 min of placebo ES plus standard care to the ulcer 5 days per week. The wounds of patients in the treatment group healed completely in a mean of 7.3 weeks at a rate of 45% per week. Patients in the control group experienced a mean increase in wound size of 29% during a mean period of 7.4 weeks. The wounds of three patients assigned to a control subgroup treated with standard wound care, increased in area by 1.2% over 8.7 weeks. However, when these three patients were reassigned to a treatment crossover group, their wounds healed at an average rate of 38% a week with complete healing occurring in an average of 8.3 weeks.

In a single-blind RCT, Griffin et al. (35) evaluated the efficacy of HVPC for healing stage II, III, or IV pressure ulcers in men with spinal cord injury. Of 17 patients with pressure ulcers in the pelvic region, eight were randomly assigned to the active HVPC group and nine to the placebo HVPC group. All wounds were treated daily with standard care. In addition, wounds in the HVPC group received ES for 60 min on 20 consecutive days with the cathode applied to deliver current directly into the wound. The stimulator was set to deliver 100 pps and 200 V, which produced 500 μQ/sec at the treatment electrode. Ulcer surface area was measured before and after ES treatment on days 5, 10, 15, and 20. Percentage of change from pretreatment ulcer size was calculated for each measurement interval. On days 5, 15, and 20 ulcers in the HVPC group had significantly greater mean wound area reductions relative to their pretreatment size than ulcers in the placebo group.

In several RCTs (17,18,29,30,34,35,112), ES has been shown to improve the healing rates of chronic pressure ulcers. Recent studies have reported that ES with HVPC also enhances healing of chronic leg ulcers. Franek et al. (117) enrolled 79 patients into a study that compared the effects of HVPC, topically applied medications and Unna's boot on healing of chronic venous leg ulcers. In addition to being treated with one of these interventions, wounds of all patients were treated with dressings and compression bandaging. They randomized 65 patients to have their ulcers treated either with HVPC ($N = 33$) or topical medications ($N = 32$). A subset of 14 patients who served as controls had their ulcers treated with Unna's boot. At the outset of the study all groups were identical with respect to patient and wound characteristics. The HVPC was delivered directly to wounds through saline-moist gauze for 50 min 6 days per week for an average of 7 weeks. Initial polarity of the treatment electrode was negative (1–3 weeks) to rid the wound of slough and pus, after which the polarity was switched to the anode. All groups showed a significant decrease in wound size compared to baseline measurements ($P < 0.001$). The rate of wound area change was greatest in the group treated with HVPC but there were no statistically significant differences between the groups. The rate of pus clearance and the degree of granulation tissue development after two weeks were significantly greater for wounds treated with HVPC ($P < 0.003$). The authors concluded that HVPC was an efficient treatment for enhancement of venous leg ulcer healing. In another recent study designed as a randomized, double-blind prospective clinical trial, Houghton et al. (118) separated 27 subjects with 42 chronic leg ulcers (wound age longer than 3 months) into subgroups according to primary etiology of the wound (diabetic, venous insufficiency, arterial insufficiency). They then randomly assigned them to wound treatments with active HVPC (150 V, 100 pps, 100 μsec pulse duration) or sham HVPC for 45 min, three times weekly for 4 weeks. Negative polarity of the active electrode placed on saline-moist gauze over the wound was maintained throughout the 4-week treatment period. During the days when wounds were not treated with ES and when ES was not applied to the wounds they were treated with standard care based on wound etiology. The results for all wounds demonstrated that active HVPC applied over the 4-week period reduced wound surface area to nearly one-half of initial size which was over two times greater than occurred in wounds treated with sham ES ($P < 0.05$). After the 4-week protocol, in seven patients with bilateral venous ulcers there was also a statistically significant difference in wound size between ulcers treated with active ES and sham ES ($P < 0.05$). Using the Pressure Sore Status Tool (PSST), the investigators also compared wound appearance between pretreatment, post-treatment and a 1-month follow up assessment. They found that active ES produced a statistically significant improvement in wound appearance compared with sham-treated wounds ($P < 0.05$). One other randomized, double-blind, placebo-controlled, 12-week trial investigated the effect of HVPC as an adjunct to healing diabetic foot ulcers (119). Forty patients with diabetic foot ulcers and loss of sensation due to neuropathy were randomized to active HVPC and sham HVPC. At the outset of the study there were no significant differences between active and sham ES groups in patient characteristics and clinical variables. Active (subsensory) ES was delivered to the ipsilateral lower extremity at 50 V, 80 pps, and pulse duration of 100 μsec via a Dacron-mesh silver nylon stocking nightly for 8 hr. Compliance was stratified into compliant patients who used the ES device for 20 hr or more a week on average and noncompliant patients who used the ES device less than 20 hr per week. Following 12 weeks of the research protocol, 65% of the wounds in the active ES group closed compared with 35% of wounds in the sham ES group ($P = 0.058$). Regarding compliance, significant differences were found among patients in the active ES group (71% closed) compared with 50% closed among noncompliant patients in the same group. In the sham ES group, 39% of compliant patient wounds closed compared with 29% of noncompliant patient wounds ($P = 0.038$). The authors concluded that ES enhances healing of Ediabetic foot ulcers when used adjunctively with weight off-loading and local wound care.

Other clinical studies with HVPC have provided important information regarding possible mechanisms by which ES enhances wound healing. Several studies have reported that delivery of HVPC to the skin of individuals with spinal cord injury (120,121) and diabetes (122,123) significantly increased the transcutaneous partial pressure of oxygen (TcPO_2) compared to prestimulation baselines. In the study by Peters et al. (123), diabetic patients with impaired vascular function in the lower extremity had a significant increase in perfusion after 5 min of ES as indicated by Doppler flowmetry results. Mawson et al. (121) also demonstrated a significant ($P < 0.00001$) increase (35%) in TcPO_2 in skin over the sacrum in paraplegics following 30 min of HVPC delivered at 75 V and 10 pps. They theorized that ES may help prevent development of pressure ulcers by restoring sympathetic tone and vascular resistance below the level of the spinal cord lesion, thereby increasing perfusion to the cutaneous capillary beds. Most recently, Goldman et al. (124) used HVPC to treat critically ischemic (TcPO_2 less than 10 mmHg) foot wounds in six patients with diabetes and a mean TcPO_2 of 2 ± 2 mmHg. They reported that cutaneous Emicrocirculation improved secondary to a statistically significant increase in TcPO_2 of periwound skin to 33 ± 18 mmHg and that four of six wounds healed after 207 days of ES.

3.3. Strength of Evidence of Wound Healing with Electrical Stimulation

For the healing of chronic wounds by ES, the strength of evidence is substantial. The criteria used to rate the strength of evidence for ES are based on clinical and animal trials, case or descriptive studies, or expert opinion. The criteria presented here are modified from the strength of evidence rating published in 1994 by the Agency for Health Care Policy and Research (AHCPR, now known as the Agency for Healthcare Research and Quality) which rated the efficacy of numerous wound interventions according to the following scale of A, B, C (125).

A: Results of two or more randomized, controlled, clinical trials on chronic wounds in humans provide support.

B: Results of two or more controlled clinical trials on chronic wounds in humans provide support, or when appropriate results of two or more controlled trials in an animal model provide indirect support.

C: Requires one or more of the following: (1) results of one controlled trial; (2) results of at least two case series / descriptive studies on chronic wounds in humans; or (3) expert opinion.

In 1994, the AHCPR Guideline recommended ES as the only "adjunctive therapy" with sufficient evidence to warrant recommendation by the panel (125). The panel recommended "a course of treatment with electrotherapy for stage III or IV pressure ulcers that have proved unresponsive to conventional therapy. Electrical stimulation may also be useful for recalcitrant stage II ulcers." In that 1994 document, the strength of evidence rating assigned to ES was "B" based on five "clinical trials," involving 147 patients (19,29,30,34,35). However, in the January 1999 issue of the journal *Ostomy and Wound Management*, Ovington (126) categorized these same five "clinical trials" as randomized-controlled trials (RCT), updating the 1994 AHCPR literature review through April 1998 for dressings and adjunctive therapies used to treat pressure ulcers. In her review, Ovington (126) indicated that one additional RCT involving the use of ES on pressure ulcers had been published by Wood Eet al. (112) after the AHCPR Guideline was disseminated at the end of 1994. With this additional RCT, Ovington suggested that the 1999 strength-of-evidence rating for ES "should perhaps advance from B to A, based on the five original randomized-controlled trials plus the 1994 trial."

More recently, the Paralyzed Veterans of America published a Clinical Practice Guideline entitled: Pressure Ulcer Prevention and Treatment Following Spinal Cord Injury (127). In this publication, ES was assigned a stand-alone recommendation (number 17) that no longer classifies it as an adjunctive therapy. The recommendation, based on strong strength of evidence from three RCTs (27,35,38) reads: "Use electrical stimulation to promote closure of stage III or IV pressure ulcers combined with standard wound care interventions."

The most compelling evidence of the efficacy of ES for enhancing the rate of wound healing is supported by a meta-analysis of 15 ES studies on chronic wound healing published by Gardner et al. (128). The studies they selected for the meta-analysis included nine RCTs and six nonrandom-controlled trials. Data analyzed from these studies included 24 ES samples (591 wounds) and 15 control samples (212 wounds). They calculated the average rate of healing per week for the ES and control samples and found that the rate of healing per week was 22% for the ES samples and 9% for control samples. This difference represents an increase of 144% in healing rate of ES-treated wounds over control wounds. Based on 95% confidence intervals for ES and control samples, the analysis revealed a 90% probability that the net healing effect of ES is 3.7% per week or more, which conservatively represents an increase of 40% or more over the control rate. More recent studies could be included in a new meta-analysis (117–119).

That sufficient evidence exists to support ES as an adjunctive wound healing treatment has convinced the Centers for Medicare and Medicaid Services (CMS) to issue a national coverage policy for this intervention for the treatment of chronic Stage III and IV pressure ulcers, arterial ulcers, diabetic ulcers, and venous ulcers. On July 23, 2002 CMS released a coverage memorandum announcing their intent to issue a positive national coverage decision on *"Electrical Stimulation for Wound Healing"* (129). The official memorandum (Section 35–102 Electrical Stimulation for the treatment of Wounds Effective for services on or after April 1, 2003) published November 8, 2002 (130) provided the following detail regarding coverage:

"For services performed on or after April 1, 2003. Medicare will cover electrical stimulation for the treatment of wounds only for chronic Stage III or IV pressure ulcers, arterial ulcers, diabetic ulcers, and venous stasis ulcers. All other uses of electrical stimulation for the treatment of wounds are not covered by Medicare. Electrical stimulation will not be covered as an initial treatment modality. The use of electrical stimulation will only be covered after appropriate standard wound care has been tried for at least 30 days and there are no measurable signs of healing. If electrical stimulation is being used wounds must be evaluated periodically by the treating physician, but no less than every 30 days by a physician. Continued treatment with electrical stimulation is not covered if measurable signs of healing have not been demonstrated within any 30-day period of treatment. Additionally, electrical stimulation must be discontinued when the wound demonstrates a 100% epithelialized wound bed.''

4. WOUND TREATMENT METHODS WITH HVPC: PRECAUTIONS AND CONTRAINDICATIONS

In the clinical studies described above investigators used a variety of ES devices and stimulation parameters which resulted in faster rates of healing in wounds treated with ES plus standard care than occurred in wounds treated with standard care alone. However, critics of ES clinical trials related to wound healing have correctly pointed out that there is a lack of consistency in the type of current and stimulation parameters reported. Apparently, what has not been recognized by most reviewers of the literature is that there is the common denominator of electrical charge "dosage" delivered into the wound tissues that has been reported in several of the RCTs E(29–32,34,35). The dosage falls within a narrow range of 250–500 μC/sec. To achieve this dosage the following parameters for HVPC and guidelines for treatment are recommended:

4.1. HVPC Parameter Settings

1. Voltage: 75–150 V (set voltage within this range to allow the sensate patient to perceive a moderately strong, submotor, tingling paresthesia in or around the wound).
2. Pulse frequency: 100 pps.
3. Polarity of wound treatment electrode: Polarity is changed according to the wound phase and/or the clinical needs of the wound as follows:
   a. Positive for re-epithelialization (facilitate migration of negative epithelial cells across granulation tissue).
   b. Positive for autolysis and re-activation of inflammatory phase (facilitate migration of negative neutrophils and macrophage into wound area).
   c. Negative for granulation (facilitate migration of positive fibroblasts) and increase perfusion.
   d. Treatment duration: 60 min, 7 days a week until the wound closes.

4.2. Delivery of Current to Wound Tissues

1. Application of electrodes.
   a. Monopolar (direct) application: One (treatment) electrode placed directly over the wound and one nontreatment or dispersive electrode placed on intact skin 15–30 cm from wound (Fig. 5).
   b. Bipolar (indirect) application: Two (treatment) electrodes placed on intact skin 2–5 cm from the wound edges on opposite sides of the

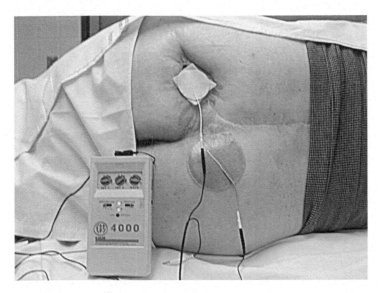

Figure 5 Monopolar or direct application of one treatment electrode directly to saline-moist conductive gauze packing placed into the wound. Polarity of this electrode will be based on whether the wound needs autolysis, granulation tissue, or epithelialization. The nontreatment (dispersive) electrode that completes the circuit is applied (adhesive surface) to the intact peri-wound skin 10–15 cm from the wound edge.

wound cavity (i.e., 6–12 or 3–9 o'clock). One nontreatment (dispersive) electrode placed on intact skin E15–30 cm away from wound border (Fig. 6).

Note: both methods of electrode application have been reported to be effective in accelerating wound healing (34,35,38,39).

2. Type of electrode for monopolar arrangement

   a. Treatment electrode: Remove wound dressing, irrigate wound cavity and fill it with clean saline-moist or hydrogel-moist gauze to enhance electrical conductivity. Select a commercial ES electrode that is at least 0.5 cm smaller than the wound opening or fold a piece of heavy-duty aluminum foil 3–4 layers thick and is at least 0.5 cm smaller than the wound perimeter. Apply the electrode or foil in contact with the moist gauze in the wound and connect it to the stimulator lead wire having the polarity that will facilitate migration of the desired cell(s) to the wound. Secure the electrode or foil to the gauze with an appropriate commercial adhesive product. After the 60 min ES treatment remove the electrodes or foil (dispose the latter properly) and either leave the saline/hydrogel-moist dressing in the wound and secure it with a secondary dressing or replace it with another standard dressing that maintains a moist wound environment.

   b. Nontreatment (dispersive) electrode: Apply a commercial, self-adhering, well-hydrated polymer electrode to the intact periwound skin 15–30 cm from the wound (the electrode should be approximately the same area as the wound surface area). When possible on subsequent ES treatments, apply this electrode at 12, 3, 6, and 9 o'clock

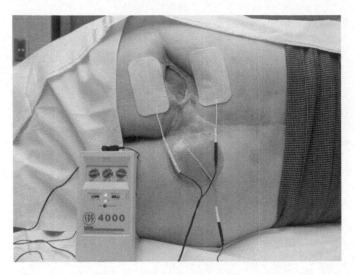

Figure 6 Bipolar or indirect application of two treatment electrodes (adhesive surface) to the intact periwound skin 2–5 cm from the wound edges on opposite sides of the wound cavity (i.e., 6–12 or 3–9 o'clock). Polarity of both of these electrodes will be based on whether the wound needs autolysis, granulation tissue, or epithelialization. One nontreatment (dispersive) electrode that completes the circuit is applied to the intact periwound skin (adhesive surface) 15–30 cm away from wound border.

around the wound perimeter so the current travels through different tissues of the wound. At the end of the treatment, remove and discard the electrode and inspect the skin.

3. Type of electrode for bipolar arrangement

    a. Treatment electrodes: If necessary remove the soiled dressing, irrigate the wound cavity and fill it with saline-moist or hydrogel-moist gauze to enhance electrical conductivity. Connect each end of a bifurcated lead wire having appropriate polarity to individual commercial, self-adhering, well-hydrated polymer electrodes that are each one-half the area of the wound opening. Apply these electrodes to intact periwound skin at 6–12 or 3–9 o'clock immediately adjacent to the wound perimeter. On subsequent ES treatments, alternate the position of these treatment electrodes around the wound clock. After the 60-min ES treatment, remove these electrodes from the patient, inspect the skin and apply them to their plastic mounting for use during the next treatment or discard them properly. After treatment, leave the saline/hydrogel-moist dressing in the wound and secure it with an appropriate secondary dressing or replace it with another standard dressing that maintains a moist wound environment.

    b. Nontreatment (dispersive) electrode: Apply a commercial, self-adhering, well-hydrated polymer electrode to the intact periwound skin about 30 cm from the wound (the electrode should be approximately the same area as the wound surface area). Remove this electrode after the treatment and inspect the skin.

4.3. Precautions

Clinicians not familiar with the electrochemical effects that may occur with any therapeutic current that delivers a net DC charge into tissues, should first determine whether the current type or waveform generated by the electrical stimulation device is DC or asymmetrical PC. If the device generates DC (even though the current output between 100 and 800 µA) the possibility exists that skin irritation or small blisters may occur especially if the nontreatment electrode applied to the periwound skin has high current density due to the electrode size being too small. This can be avoided when DC is used if the nontreatment electrode is twice the surface area of the treatment electrode. If the device delivers monophasic PC that generates a pulse with a duration between 10 and 500 µS, there will be insufficient charge accumulation to cause electrochemical injury to the skin. For example, HVPC shown in Fig. 3 typically has a pulse duration less than 100 µS.

4.4. Contraindications

The following conditions are considered to be contraindications to the use of ES for wound healing:

1. Basal cell or squamous cell carcinoma or melanoma in the wound or periwound tissues because ES may cause mitogenic activity of cancer cells (131).
2. Untreated osteomyelitis present in bone in the base of the wound, because premature closure of the wound may lead to abscess formation. If osteomyelitis is responding to antibiotic treatment, ES may be used to enhance wound closure concurrent with resolution of the osteomyelitis (131).
3. Electronic pacing devices: Positioning ES electrodes in a manner that allows current to flow through tissues in which any type of electronic pacing device is implanted is contraindicated (131). However, it is reported that when ES was applied to 10 patients who had had 20 different cardiac pacemakers no adverse effects occurred (132).
4. Passage of current into vital organs and other sensitive anatomic structures: application of ES to the thorax or neck such that current may flow through the cardiac area, carotid sinus, phrenic nerve, parasympathetic nerves and ganglia, or musculature of the larynx should be avoided (131).
5. Residues of metallic ions in wound tissues: residues of metallic ions left behind in a wound from topical agents or dressings (e.g., zinc, crystalline silver, silver sulfadiazine, cadexomer iodine) should be flushed thoroughly from the wound prior to treatment with ES. This will avoid possible irritation of tissues from iontophoresis caused by the current (131).

5. SUMMARY

Basic science research has demonstrated that ES can enhance wound healing by directing neutrophils, macrophage, epithelial, endothelial, and fibroblast migration into wound tissues, can increase DNA and collagen synthesis, increase wound scar tensile strength, and inhibit or suppress growth of some wound pathogens. Fourteen randomized-controlled clinical trials have demonstrated positive wound healing outcomes and a meta-analysis that included data from several of these studies showed that the rate of healing per week was 22% for the ES samples vs. 9% for control samples (128). Further support of this intervention that has been practiced primarily by Physical Therapists since the early 1980s is the recent decision of the Centers for Medicare and Medicaid Services to allow reimbursement of ES as an adjunctive treatment of chronic wounds. Certainly, more research evidence is needed to support ES as an efficacious treatment of chronic wounds, but the same can be said for all other interventions currently being used for chronic wound management.

REFERENCES

1. Robertson WS. Digby's receipts. Ann Med Hist 1925; 7(3):216.
2. Kanof N. Gold leaf in the treatment of cutaneous ulcers. J Invest Dermatol 1964; 43:441–444.
3. Wolf M, Wheeler PC, Wolcott LE. Gold-leaf treatment of ischemic skin ulcers. JAMA 1966; 196:105–108.
4. Smith KW, Oden PW, Blaulock WK. A comparison of gold leaf and other occlusive therapy. Arch Dermatol 1967; 96:703–705.
5. Chick N. Treatment of ischemic and stasis ulcers with gold leaf and polyethylene film. J Am Geriatric Soc 1969; 17:605–608.
6. Risbrook AT, Goodfriend SS, Reiter JM. Gold leaf in the treatment of leg ulcers. J Am Geriatric Soc 1973; 21:325–329.
7. Harris DR, Keefe RL. A histological study of gold leaf treated experimental wounds. J Invest Dermatol 1969; 52:487–491.
8. Lente FD. Cases of united fractures treated by electricity. NY State J Med 1850; 5:5117–5118.
9. Fukada E, Yasuda I. On the piezoelectric effect in bone. Nippon Seirigaku Zasshi 1957; 12:1158–1162.
10. Becker RO, Spadero JA, Marino AA. Clinical experiences with low intensity direct current stimulation of bone growth. Clin Orthop 1975; 124:75–83.
11. Bassett CAL. The development and application of pulsed electromagnetic fields (PEMFS) for un-united fractures and arthrodeses. Orthop Clin North Am 1984; 15(1):61–87.
12. Brighton CT, Pollak SR. Treatment of recalcitrant nonunion of the tibia with a capacitively coupled electric field. A preliminary report. J Bone Joint Surg 1985; 67(4): 577–585.
13. Stanish WD, Rubinovich M, Kozey J, MacGillvary G. The use of electricity in ligament and tendon repair. Phys Sports Med 1985; 13:109–116.
14. Owoeye IO, Spielholz NI, Fetto J, Nelson AJ. Low intensity pulsed galvanic current and the healing of rat Achilles tenotomized tendons: preliminary report using load-to-breaking measurements. Arch Phys Med Rehabil 1987; 68:415–418.
15. American Physical Therapy Association: Electrotherapeutic Terminology in Physical Therapy. Alexandria, VA. Copyright © 2001, Section on Clinical Electrophysiology of the APTA.
16. Assimacopoulos D. Low intensity negative electric current in treatment of ulcers of leg due to chronic venous insufficiency: preliminary report of three cases. Am J Surg 1968; 115:683–687.
17. Wolcott LE, Wheeler PC, Hardwicke HM, Rowley BA. Accelerated healing of skin ulcers by electrotherapy: preliminary clinical results. South Med J 1969; 62:795–801.
18. Gault WR, Gatens PF. Use of low intensity direct current in management of ischemic skim ulcers. Phys Ther 1976; 56(3):265–269.
19. Carley PJ, Wainapel SF. Electrotherapy for acceleration of wound healing: low intensity direct current. Arch Phys Med Rehabil 1985; 66:443–446.

20. Ojingwa JC, Isseroff RR. Electrical stimulation of wound healing. Dermatol Foundation: Prog Dermatol 2002; 36(4):1–12.

21. Westerhof W, Bos JD. Trigeminal trophic syndrome: a successful treatment with transcutaneous electrical stimulation. Br J Dermatol 1983; 108(5):601–604.

22. Kaada B. Promoted healing of chronic ulceration by transcutaneous nerve stimulation (TNS). Vasa 1983; 12(3):262–269.

23. Kaada B, Emru M. Promoted healing of leprous ulcers by transcutaneous nerve stimulation. Acupunct Electrother Res 1988; 13(4):165–176.

24. Karba B, Vodovnik L. Promoted healing of chronic wounds due to electrical stimulation. Wounds 1991; 3(1):16–23.

25. Lundeberg TC, Eriksson SV, Malm M. Electrical nerve stimulation improves healing of diabetic ulcers. Ann Plast Surg 1992; 29(4):328–331.

26. Barron JJ, Jacobson WE, Tidd G. Treatment of decubitus ulcers. A new approach. Minnesota Med 1985; 68(2):103–106.

27. Stefanovska A, Vodovnik L, Benko H, Turk R. Treatment of chronic wounds by means of electric and electromagnetic fields. Part 2. Value of FES parameters for pressure sore treatment. Med Biol Eng Comput 1993; 31(3):213–220.

28. Weiss DS, Eaglstein WH, Falanga V. Exogenous electric current can reduce the formation of hypertrophic scars. J Dermatol Surg Oncol 1989; 15:1272–1275.

29. Feedar JA, Kloth LC, Gentzkow GD. Chronic dermal ulcer healing enhanced with monophasic pulsed electrical stimulation. Phys Ther 1991; 71(9):639–649.

30. Gentzkow GD, Pollack SV, Kloth LC, Stubbs HA. Improved healing of pressure ulcers using Dermapulse, a new electrical stimulation device. Wounds 1991; 3(5):158–170.

31. Gentzkow GD, Alon G, Taler GA, Eltorai I, Montroy RE. Healing of refractory stage III and IV pressure ulcers by a new electrical stimulation device. Wounds 1993; 5(3):160–172.

32. Junger M, Zuder D, Steins A, Hahn M, Klyscz T. Treatment of venous ulcers with low frequency pulsed current (Dermapulse): effects on cutaneous microcirculation. Der Hautartz 1997; 18:879–903.

33. Akers TK, Gabrielson AL. The effect of high voltage galvanic stimulation on the rate of healing of decubitus ulcers. Biomed Science Instrum 1984; 20:99–100.

34. Kloth LC, Feedar JA. Acceleration of wound healing with high voltage, monophasic, pulsed current. Phys Ther 1988; 71(4):503–508.

35. Griffin JW, Tooms RE, Mendlus RA, Clifft JK, Zwaag RV, El-Zeky F. Efficacy of high voltage pulsed current for healing of pressure ulcers in patients with spinal cord injury. Phys Ther 1991; 71(6):433–442.

36. Fitzgerald GK, Newsome D. Treatment of a large infected thoracic spine wound using high voltage pulsed monophasic current. Phys Ther 1993; 73(6):355–359.

37. Newton RA, Karselis TC. Skin pH following high voltage pulsed galvanic stimulation. Phys Ther 1983; 63(10):1593–1596.

38. Baker LL, Rubayi S, Villar F, DeMuth SK. Effect of electrical stimulation waveform on healing of ulcers in human beings with spinal cord injury. Wound Rep Reg 1996; 4:72–79.

39. Baker LL, Chambers, DeMuth SK, Villar F. Effects of electrical stimulation on wound healing in patients with diabetic ulcers. Diabetes Care 1997; 20(3):405–412.

40. Debreceni, L, Gyulai M, Debreceni A, Szabo K. Results of transcutaneous electrical stimulation (TES) in cure of lower extremity arterial disease. Angiology 1995; 46:613–618.

41. Bourguignon GJ, Bourguignon LYW. Electric stimulation of protein and DNA synthesis in human fibroblasts. FASEB 1987; 1(5):398–402.

42. Bourguignon GJ, Bergouignan M, Khorshed A, Bourguignon LYW. Effect of high voltage pulsed galvanic stimulation on human fibroblasts in cell culture. J Cell Biol 1986; 103:344a.

43. Bourguignon GJ, Wenche JY, Bourguignon LYW. Electric stimulation of human fibro-blasts causes an increase in Ca2+ influx and the exposure of additional insulin recep-tors. J Cell Physiol 1989; 140(2):397–385.

44. Falanga V, Bourguignon GJ, Bourguignon LY. Electrical stimulation increases the expression of fibroblast receptors for transforming growth factor-beta. J Invest Derma-tol 1987; 88:488–492.

45. Cheng K, Goldman RJ. Electric fields and proliferation in a dermal wound model: cell cycle kinetics. Bioelectromagnetics 1998; 19:68–74.

46. Orida N, Feldman J. Directional protrusive pseudopodial activity and motility in macrophages induced by extra-cellular electric fields. Cell Motil 1982; 2:243–255.

47. Monguio J. Uber die polare wirkung des galvanischen stromes auf leukozyten. Z Biol 1933; 93:553–559.

48. Fukushima K, Senda N, Inui H, Miura H, Tamai Y, Murakami Y. Studies of galvano-taxis of leukocytes. Med J Osaka Univ 1953; 4(2–3):195–208.

49. Dineur E. Note sur la sensibilities des leukocytes a l'electricite. Bulletin Seances Soc Belge Microscopic (Bruxelles) 1891; 18: 113–118.

50. Canaday DJ, Lee RC. Scientific basis for clinical application of electric fields in soft tis-sue repair. In: Brighton CT, Pollack SR, eds. Electromagnetics in Biology and Medi-cine. San Francisco: San Francisco Press, 1991.

51. Erickson CA, Nuccitelli R. Embryonic fibroblast motility and orientation can be influ-enced by physiological electric fields. J Cell Biol 1984; 98:296–307.

52. Yang W, Onuma EK, Hui SW. Response of C3H/10T1/2 fibroblasts to an external steady electric field stimulation. Exp Cell Res 1984; 155:92–97.

53. Nishimura KY, Isseroff RR, Nuccitelli R. Human keratinocytes migrate to the negative pole in direct current electric fields comparable to those measured in mammalian wounds. J Cell Sci 1996; 109:199–207.

54. Sheridan DM, Isseroff RR, Nuccitelli R. Imposition of a physiologic DC electric field alters the migratory response of human keratinocytes on extracellular matrix molecules. J Invest Dermatol 1996; 106(4):642–646.

55. Stromberg BV. Effects of electrical currents on wound contraction. Ann Plast Surg 1988; 21(2):121–123.

56. Cooper MS, Schliwa M. Electrical and ionic controls of tissue cell locomotion in DC electrical fields. J Cell Physiol 1985; 103:363.

57. Eberhardt A, Szczypiorski P, Korytowski G. Effect of transcutaneous electrostimula-tion on the cell composition of skin exudate. ACTA Physiol Pol 1986; 37(1):41–46.

58. Mertz PM, Davis S, Cazzaniga AL, Cheng K, Reich JD, Eaglstein WH. Electrical stimulation: acceleration of soft tissue repair by varying the polarity. Wounds 1993; 5(3):153–159.

59. Fang KS, Ionides E, Oster G, Nuccitelli R, Isseroff RR. Epidermal growth factor recep-tor relocalization and kinase activity are necessary for directional migration of kerati-nocytes in DC electric fields. J Cell Sci 1999; 112:1967–1978.

60. Bedlack RS Jr, Wei M, Loew LM. Localized membrane depolarization and localized calcium influx during electric field-guided neurite growth. Neuron 1992; 9(3):393–403.

61. Soong HK, Parkinson WC, Sulik GL, Bafna S. Effects of electric fields on cytoskeleton of corneal stromal fibroblasts. Curr Eye Res 1990; 9(9):893–901.

62. Onuma EK, Hui SW. Electric field-directed cell shape changes, displacement, and cytos-keletal reorganization are calcium dependent. J Cell Biol 1988; 106(6):2065–2067.

63. Onuma EK, Hui SW. The effects of calcium on electric field-induced cell shape changes and preferential orientation. Prog Clin Biol Res 1986; 210:319–327.

64. Onuma EK, Hui SW. A calcium requirement for electric field induced cell shape changes and preferential orientation. Cell Calcium 1985; 6(3):281–292.

65. Luther PW, Peng HB, Lin JJ. Changes in cell shape and actin distribution induced by constant electric fields. Nature 1983; 303(5912):61–64.

66. Baker LP, Peng HB. Tyrosine phosphorylation and acetylcholine receptor cluster formation in cultured Xenopus muscle cells. J Cell Biol 1993; 120(1):185–195.

67. Peng HB, Baker LP, Dai Z. A role of tyrosine phosphorylation in the formation of receptor clusters induced by electric fields in cultured Xenopus muscle cells. J Cell Biol 1993; 120(1):197–204.

68. Matteucci C. Lectures on the physical phenomena of living beings. In: Pereira J, ed. Carlo Matteucci, 1811–1868. London: Longman, Brown, Green and Longmans, 1847:435.

69. DuBois-Reymond E. Vorlaufiger abrifs einer untersuchung uber den sogenanten frosch-strom and die electromotorischen fische. Ann Phys U Chem 1843; 58:1.

70. Illingsworth CM, Barker AT. Measurement of electrical currents emerging during the regeneration of amputated finger tips in children. Clin Phys Physiol Meas 1980; 1: 87–89.

71. Barker AT, Jaffe LF, Vanable JW. The glabrous of caries contains a powerful battery. Am J Physiol 1982; 242:358–365.

72. McGinnis ME, Vanable JW Jr. Voltage gradients in newt limb stumps. Prog Clin Biol Res 1986; 210:231–238.

73. Stump RF, Robinson KR. Ionic current in Xenopus embryos during neurulation and wound healing. Prog Clin Biol Res 1986; 210:223–230.

74. Jaffe LF, Vanable JW. Electrical fields and wound healing. Clin Dermatol 1984; 2(3):34–44.

75. Cheng K, Tarjan PP, Oliveira-Gandia MF, Davis SC, Mertz PM, Eaglstein WH. An occlusive dressing can sustain natural electrical potential of wounds. J Invest Dermatol 1995; 104(4):662–665.

76. Rowley BA. Electrical current effects on *E. coli* growth rates. Proc Soc Exp Biol Med 1972; 139:929–934.

77. Rowley BA, McKenna JM, Chase GR, Wolcott LE. The influence of electrical current on an infecting microorganism in wounds. Ann NY Acad Sci 1974; 238:543–551.

78. Barranco SC, et al. In vitro effect of weak direct current on *Staphylococcus aureus*. Clin Orthop 1974; 100: 250–255.

79. Ong PC, Laatsch LJ, Kloth LC. Antibacterial effects of a silver electrode carrying microamperage direct current in vitro. J Clin Electrophysiol 1994; 6(1):14–18.

80. Laatsch LJ, Ong PC, Kloth LC. In vitro effects of two silver electrodes on select wound pathogens. J Clin Electrophysiol 1995; 7(1):10–15.

81. Guffey JS, Asmussen MD. In vitro bactericidal effects of high voltage pulsed current versus direct current against *Staphylococcus aureus*. J Clin Electrophysiol 1989; 1:5–9.

82. Kincaid CB, Lavoie KH. Inhibition of bacterial growth in vitro following stimulation with high voltage, monophasic pulsed current. Phys Ther 1989; 69(8):651–655.

83. Szuminsky NJ, Albers AC, Unger P, Eddy JG. Effect of narrow, pulsed high voltages on bacterial viability. Phys Ther 1994; 74(7):660–667.

84. Assimacopoulos D. Wound healing promotion by the use of negative electric current. Am Surg 1968; 34(6):423–431.

85. Bigelow JB. Effect of electrical stimulation on canine skin and percutaneous device–skin interface healing. In: Brighton CT, Black J, Pollack SR, eds. Skin Interface Healing and Electrical Properties of Bone and Cartilage. New York: Grune & Stratton, 1979:289.

86. Carey LC, Lepley D. Effect of continuous direct electric current on healing wounds. Surg Forum 1962; 13:33–35.

87. Konikoff JJ. Electrical promotion of soft tissue repairs. Biomed Eng 1976; 4:1–5.

88. Smith J, Romansky N, Vomero J, Davis RH. The effect of electrical stimulation on wound healing in diabetic mice. J Am Podiatr Assoc 1984; 74(2):71–75.

89. Kahn J. Electrical stimulation. In: Kahn J, ed. Principles and Practice of Electrother-apy. New York: Churchill Livingstone, 1994:83.

90. Castillo E, Sumano H, Fortoul TI, Zepeda A. The influence of pulsed electrical stimula-tion on the wound healing of burned rat skin. Arch Med Res 1995; 26(2):185–189.

91. Cruz NI, Bayron FE, Suarez AJ. Accelerated healing of full-thickness burns by the use of high voltage pulsed galvanic stimulation in the pig. Ann Plast Surg 1989; 23(1):49–55.

92. Taskan I, Ozyazgan I, Tercan M, Kardas KY, Balkanli S, Saraymen R, Zorlu U, Ozugul Y. A comparative study of the effect of ultrasound and electrostimulation on wound healing in rats. Plast Reconstr Surg 1997; 100:966–972.

93. Dunn MG, Doillon CJ, Berg RA, Olson RM, Silver FH. Wound healing using a collagen matrix: effect of DC electrical stimulation. J Biomed Mater Res 1988; 22 (A2 suppl):191–206.

94. Alvarez OM, Mertz PM, Smerbeck RV, Eaglstein WH. The healing of superficial skin wounds is stimulated by external electrical current. J Invest Dermatol 1983; 81:144–148.

95. Cheng N, Van Hoof, Bockx E, Hoogmartens MJ, Mulier JC, De Dijcker FJ, Sansen WM, De Loecker W. The effects of electric currents on ATP generation, protein synthesis, and membrane transport in rat skin. Clin Orthoped Related Res 1982; 171: 264–272.

96. Bach S, Bilgrav K, Gottrup F, Jorgensen TE. The effect of electrical current on healing skin incision. Eur J Surg 1991; 157:171–174.

97. Brown M, Gogia PP. Effects of high voltage stimulation on cutaneous wound healing in rabbits. Phys Ther 1987; 67:662–667.

98. Brown M, McDonnell MK, Menton DN. Electrical stimulation effects on cutaneous wound healing in rabbits. Phys Ther 1988; 68:955–960.

99. Brown M, McDonnell MK, Menton DN. Polarity effects on wound healing using electrical stimulation in rabbits. Arch Phys Med Rehabil 1989; 70:624–627.

100. Reed BV. Effect of high voltage pulsed electrical stimulation on microvascular permeability to plasma proteins: a possible mechanism in minimizing edema. Phys Ther 1988; 68:491–495.

101. Taylor K, Mendel FC, Fish DR, Hard R, Burton HW. Effect of high voltage pulsed current and alternating current on macromolecular leakage in hamster cheek pouch microcirculation. Phys Ther 1997; 77(12):1729–1740.

102. Thornton RM, Mendel FC, Fish D. Effects of electrical stimulation on edema formation in different strains of rats. Phys Ther 1998; 78(4):386–394.

103. Chu C-S, McManus AT, Mason AD Jr, Okerberg CV, Pruitt BA Jr. Multiple graft harvestings from deep partial-thickness scald wounds healed under the influence of weak direct current. J Trauma 1990; 30(8):1044–1049.

104. Politis MJ, Zanakis MF, Miller JE. Enhanced survival of full-thickness skin grafts following the application of DC electrical fields. Plast Reconst Surg 1989; 84(2):267–272.

105. Im JM, Lee WPA, Hoopes JE. Effect of electrical stimulation on survival of skin flaps in pigs. Phys Ther 1990; 70(1):37–40.

106. Kjartansson J, Lundeberg T, Samuelson U. Transcutaneous electrical nerve stimulation (TENS) increases survival of ischaemic musculocutaneous flaps. Acta Physiol Scand 1988; 134:95–99.

107. Atkins FM, Clark RAF. Mast cells and fibrosis. Arch Dermatol 1987; 123:191–193.

108. Choi KL, Clamen HN. Mast cells, fibroblasts and fibrosis: new clues to the riddle of mast cells. Immunol Res 1987; 6:145–152.

109. Greenberg J, Hanly AJ, Davis SC, Mertz PM, Cazzaniga AL. The effect of electrical stimulation (RPES) on wound healing and angiogenesis in second degree burns. 13th Annual Symposium on Advanced Wound Care, Dallas, TX, Apr 1–4, 2000.

110. Weiss DS, Kirsner R, Eaglstein WH. Electrical stimulation and wound healing. Arch Dermatol 1990; 126:222–225.

111. Cukjati D, Robnik-Sikonja M, Rebersek S, Kononenko I, Miklavcic D. Prognostic factors in the prediction of chronic wound healing by electrical stimulation. Med Biol Eng Comput 2001; 39:542–550.

112. Wood JM, Evans PE, Schallreuter KU, Jacobson WE, Sulfit R, Neuman J, White C, Jacobson M. A multi-center study on the use of pulsed low intensity direct current for healing stage II and III decubitus ulcers. Arch Dermatol 1992; 129:999–1009.

113. Frantz RA. The effectiveness of transcutaneous electrical nerve stimulation (TENS) on decubitus ulcer healing in adult patients. In: Funk SG, Tornquist EM, Champagne MT, Copp LA, Wiese RA, eds. Key Aspects of Recovery: Improving Nutrition, Rest, and Mobility. New York: Springer, 1990:197–205.

114. Young GH. Electric impulse therapy aids wound healing. Mod Vet Prac 1966; 47(14):60–64.

115. Jacques PF, Brogan MS, Kalinowski D. High-voltage electrical treatment of refractory dermal ulcers. Phys Assistant 1997:84–97.

116. Thurman BF, Christian EL. Response of a serious circulatory lesion to electrical stimulation: a case report. Phys Ther 1971; 51:1107–1110.

117. Franek A, Polak A, Kucharzewski M. Modern application of high voltage stimulation for enhanced healing of venous crural ulceration. Med Eng Phys 2000; 22:647–655.

118. Houghton PE, Kincaid CB, Lovell M, Campbell KE, Keast DH, Woodbury MG, Harris KA. Effect of electrical stimulation on chronic leg ulcer size and appearance. Phys Ther 2003; 83(1):17–28.

119. Peters EJ, Lavery LA, Armstrong DG, Fleischli JG. Electric stimulation as an adjunct to heal diabetic foot ulcers: a randomized clinical trial. Arch Phys Med Rehabil 2001; 82:721–724.

120. Gagnier KA, Manix NL, Baker LL, Rubayi S. The effects of electrical stimulation on cutaneous oxygen supply in paraplegics. Phys Ther 1988; 68:835–839.

121. Mawson AR, Siddiqui FH, Connolly BJ, Sharp CJ, Summer WR, Biundo JJ. Effect of high voltage pulsed galvanic stimulation on sacral transcutaneous oxygen tension levels in the spinal cord injured. Paraplegia 1993; 31:311–319.

122. Dodgen PW, Johnson BW, Baker LL, Chambers RB. The effects of electrical stimulation on cutaneous oxygen supply in diabetic older adults (abstr). Phys Ther 1987; 67(5):793.

123. Peters EJ, Armstrong DG, Wunderlich RP, Bosma J, Stacpoole-Shea S, Lavery LA. The benefit of electrical stimulation to enhance perfusion in patients with diabetes mellitus. J Foot Ankle Surg 1998; 37(5):396–400.

124. Goldman RJ, Brewley BI, Golden MA. Electrotherapy reoxygenates inframalleolar ischemic wounds on diabetic patients. Adv Skin Wound Care 2002; 15(3):112–120.

125. Agency for Healthcare Policy and Research. Treatment of Pressure Ulcers. US Department of Health and Human Services, Public Health Service, Rockville, MD, AHCPR Publication 1994, 95–0652: 1–154. "http://hstat.nim.nih.gov/hquest/db/46/screen/DocTitle/odas/1/s/63378."

126. Ovington LG. Dressings and adjunctive therapies: AHCPR guidelines revisited. Ostomy/Wound Manage 1999; 45(suppl 1A):94S–106S.

127. Clinical Practice Guideline: Pressure Ulcer Prevention and Treatment Following Spinal Cord Injury. Copyright 2000, Paralyzed Veterans of America, Washington, DC 2005.

128. Gardner SE, Frantz RA, Schmidt FL. Effect of electrical stimulation on chronic wound healing: a meta-analysis. Wound Rep Regen 1999; 7(6):495–503.

129. Centers for Medicare and Medicaid Services, Department of Health and Human Services, Medicare Coverage Policy ~ NCDs. July 23, 2002. "http://www.cms.hhs.gov/coverage/8b3-ii3.asp."

130. Centers for Medicare and Medicaid Services, Department of Health and Human Services, Program Memorandum Intermediaries/Carriers, Transmittal AB-02-161, CMS-Pub. 60AB, November 8, 2002 and Medicare Coverage Issues Manual, Transmittal 161, CMS –Pub. 06, November 8, 2002.

131. Kloth LC. Electrical stimulation for wound healing. In: Kloth LC, McCulloch JM, eds. Wound Healing Alternatives in Management. Philadelphia: F.A. Davis, 2002.

132. Rasmussen MJ, Hayes DL, Vlietstra RE, Thorsteinsson G. Can transcutaneous electrical nerve stimulation be safely used in patients with permanent cardiac pacemakers? Mayo Clin Proc 1988; 63:443–445.

36
Lasers and Wound Healing

James Spencer
Department of Dermatology and Cutaneous Surgery, The Mount Sinai School of Medicine, New York, New York, U.S.A.

1. INTRODUCTION

The advent of lasers has revolutionized the field of dermatology. Cutaneous disorders including vascular and pigmented lesions, tattoos, and scars such as hypertrophic and keloidal scars can now be successfully treated. The term laser is an acronym for *l*ight *a*mplification by *s*timulated *e*mission of *r*adiation that succinctly describes its functions. Lasers have transformed the field of cosmetic dermatology in that they provide a treatment modality for cutaneous lesions that were once difficult to manage. Lasers, also for the past 30 years, have been used to improve the treatment of wounds. Low-level laser irradiation has gained acceptance in certain areas of medicine due to its ability to assist in the management of pain, treatment of ulcers especially in diabetics, and various wounds from different etiologies (1,2). There are, however, controversial results obtained to date on lasers and their effects on wounds. Some authors feel that there is truly an acceleration of the healing process, while others have not witnessed any beneficial results. When interpreting the data, it is quite difficult due to the variation in animal and clinical studies, treatment protocols, laser parameters, and culture mediums used. Furthermore, many of the authors who have tried to reproduce similar results have found conflicting findings. However, there is some evidence that may suggest that lasers can improve the wound healing process.

2. LASER PRINCIPLES

The unique abilities of lasers stem from Einstein's principles on electromagnetic radiation. Einstein proposed that a photon, which is a quantum of electromagnetic energy, could stimulate an excited atom to emit another photon with the same energy (3). Within the laser, there is a medium, which comprises of either gas, solid, or liquid (Table 1), that contains atoms in a resting state. Once an energy source is applied, the atoms reach an excited state, which increases the degree of population inversion. A precondition for laser action, population inversion is the number of atoms in the excited state vs. the number in the ground state. Now that the lasing medium

Table 1 Types of Laser Media

Solids	Gases	Dyes	Other
Ruby crystal: composed of aluminum oxide with scattered atoms of chromium replacing some aluminum atoms in the crystal lattice	Carbon dioxide (CO_2)	Fluorescent liquid dye	Electrical diodes
Nd:YAG (neodymium: yittrium-aluminum-garnet) with scattered atoms of meodymium replacing some yttrium atoms in the crystal lattice	Argon (Ar)		
Er:YAG (erbium: yittrium-aluminum garnet) with scattered atoms of erbium replacing some yttrium atoms in the crystal lattice	Copper (Cu)		

contains a collection of atoms with electrons in the excited state, the atoms that return to the ground state will emit energy in the form of a photon. Stimulated emission takes place in the state of population inversion. Stimulated emission involves a photon of light entering an atom with an excited electron, so that two identical photons are generated. Eventually, this process repeats itself producing a multiplication of photons that are identical. If significant population inversion exists, then stimulated emission can produce significant light amplification (4).

The light produced has inherent features such as coherence, collimation, and monochromaticity. Coherence describes the organization of the light, meaning that light travels in phase with respect to both time and space. Monochromaticity, in contrast, suggests that all the light has the same wavelength. This wavelength of light is determined by the amount of energy released when the electron drops to a lower orbit. Lastly, collimation indicates that all of the light is parallel and will not diffuse over distances, allowing the laser to be focused on small spot sizes (5). In addition to the properties of the laser light, the wave mode of a laser can be either pulsed or continuous. Continuous waves, such as the argon laser, deliver a constant beam of light; whereas with pulsed light, there is a set of surges separated by a distinct amount of time. Q-switched lasers, for example, produce short, powerful pulses of laser radiation that are frequently used in the removal of tattoos (4,5).

Laser light's monochromaticity is responsible for its selective effect on biologic tissue. Once the laser reaches the skin surface, it can be absorbed, scattered, or reflected. The effects of the laser are appreciated when the light is absorbed. When photons are absorbed, they are absorbed by chromophores, which are biological structures within the skin with a specific absorption spectrum. The goal is to match peak absorption wavelength with the wavelength of the laser. The three main endogenous chromophores targeted in the skin are water, melanin, and hemoglobin, whereas tattoos are considered exogenous chromphores (6). While melanin is localized primarily to the epidermis, oxyhemoglobin and deoxyhemoglobin are found in the capillary, arteriolar, and venular networks of the papillary and reticular dermis (7). Effective absorption of melanin occurs within the range of 600–1100 nm. Wavelengths under 600 nm are strongly absorbed by blood microvessels, and those wavelengths above 1100 nm are strongly absorbed by water in tissue. Absorption in the dermis is not easily achieved because collagen fibers scatter light. The amount of scattering is inversely proportional to the wavelength. Therefore, light scatter is greatest at shorter wavelengths and minimal at longer wavelengths, allowing greater penetration in the skin (5,6).

As the laser penetrates the skin, it produces three basic effects that cause tissue destruction. Photomechanical effect is a rapid thermal expansion that produces acoustic or stress waves that disrupt the cell permeability. This is commonly seen with q-switched lasers that are employed to treat tattoos and certain pigmented skin lesions. The other less intense reactions that occur are photothermal and photochemical. A photothermal reaction, which is another commonly observed reaction, occurs when the chromophore absorbs the energy, which is dissipated into heat, and causes destruction within the target. Inversely, a photochemical reaction, which is not observed in current cutaneous laser surgery, occurs when the laser energy can react chemically with specific molecules within tissue. This is the basis of photodynamic therapy (4).

In order to achieve the controlled destruction of targets, the theory of selective photothermolysis was developed. It assumes that the laser light will pass through tissue until it targets the specific chromophore with an absorption spectrum corresponding to the wavelength of the laser. The target then absorbs the light, generating heat in the target tissue. The determination of the necessary amount of time the laser should operate to destroy the target, but not the surrounding tissue, involves the concept of thermal relaxation. Thermal relaxation is the amount of time necessary for 50% of the peak heat to diffuse out of the target. Each chromphore and each vessel have a specific thermal relaxation time. It is important for a laser to not exceed the thermal relaxation time, or the heat will diffuse out into surrounding tissue, causing damage and possibly scarring. Moreover, this damage can be minimized through the use of skin cooling techniques such as precooling, parallel cooling, and postcooling. A number of parameters control the laser–tissue interactions and can be modified specifically to certain cutaneous disorders to achieve maximum therapeutic effects (5,6).

There are many types of lasers used for various dermatologic disorders. Table 2 illustrates the various lasers used today along with their indications. In addition to the lasers indicated, lasers can now be used as a substitution for phototherapy to treat psoriasis, dyspigmentation, and acne vulgaris. Although additional studies need to be conducted in this area, this treatment may exceed the current treatment of UV phototherapy. Despite the advancing area, there are some complications that can arise from the use of lasers. To name a few, there may be some postoperative erythema, bacterial and viral infections, and pigment alterations, especially in darker skin types (8). To avoid such complications, laser parameters and taking a thorough history are particularly important for maximizing the efficacy while limiting the risk of side effects.

3. WOUND HEALING

Wound healing is a complex interaction of biochemical and physiological events. An injury activates a cascade of chemoattractants that recruit cells, such as

Table 2 Lasers and Their Applications

Laser	Wavelength (nm)	Mode	Cutaneous applications
Argon	488/514	CW	Vascular lesions
Argon-pumped tunable dye	577/585	Quasi-CW	Vascular lesions
Copper vapor	512	Quasi-CW	Pigmented lesions, vascular lesions
Potassium-titanyl-phosphate	532	Quasi-CW	Pigmented lesions, vascular lesions
Ruby	694	Pulsed/QS	Pigmented lesions (birthmarks), blue/black/green tattoos, hair removal
Pulsed dye	585–600	Pulsed	Pigmented lesions (birthmarks)
Alexandrite	720–850	Pulsed/QS	Pigmented lesions, blue/black/green tattoos, hair removal, leg veins
Diode	800	CW	Hair removal, leg veins
	1450	Long-pulsed	Nonablative dermal remodeling, acne
Nd:YAG	1064	CW	Pigmented lesions, blue/black tattoos
	1064/1320	Long-pulsed	Nonablative dermal remodeling, hair removal, leg veins
Carbon dioxide	10,600	CW	Actinic chelitis, verrucae, rhinophyma
		Pulsed	Ablative skin resurfacing, epidermal/dermal lesions
Erbium:YAG	1540	Pulsed	Nonablative dermal remodeling

platelets, phagocytes, and fibroblasts, to the site. There are three phases of wound healing: the inflammatory, proliferative, and maturation phase. During the substrate or inflammatory phase, leukocytes and macrophages, in essence, debride the wound and produce molecules that stimulate the release of growth factors, which further enhance the inflammatory response to remove bacteria. The proliferative stage of wound healing is characterized by the production of collagen by fibroblasts. The final stage is known as remodeling or maturation. It is distinguished from the other phases by the intermolecular cross-linking of collagen (9). Nowadays, there are various modalities to promote and expedite wound healing such as mechanical and proteolytic debridement, skin grafts, vacuum-assisted closure techniques, hyperbaric oxygen, and lasers (10).

4. PROPOSED MECHANISMS OF ACTION

The actual mechanism in the enhancement of lasers on wound healing has not been reported. However, several theories have been suggested. One theory involves the activation of photo-receptors within the mitochondria. Light energy is absorbed by the respiratory chain, triggers a biochemical reaction that initiates the electron transport to increase the amount of ATP, which eventually increases the cellular metabolism and functions in the cells. However, this can only occur if there is sufficient amount of light energy to elicit changes in cell physiology. This effect was demonstrated with a helium–neon laser set at 632.8 nm and also at 760 nm (11,12). Another theory suggested that hemoglobin uses light energy at 660 nm to activate the Fenton reaction, which is a free radical reaction initiated by iron and hydrogen peroxide. A study by Stadler et al. demonstrated that the application of laser light irradiation on both whole blood and cell free suspension with hemoglobin increased anti-oxidant mediators. They concluded that hemoglobin after laser application increased the amount of reactive oxygen species, and that these intermediates may induce a stimulatory effect to enhance proliferation and the healing process or may be detrimental to wound repair (13). While another theory involves the activation of calcium channels, which increases its influx, and ultimately leads to cell proliferation (14). All these potential pathways most likely occur simultaneously. However, the conclusion drawn is that ample light energy is imperative to initiate biological reactions, but if the parameters are not adequate, i.e., increased wavelength or pulse duration, too much energy may produce an overwhelming amount of reactive oxygen species and possibly calcium, which will have negative results in the healing process. Perhaps this is the discrepancy being seen amongst the various studies reported in the literature.

5. LASER IRRADIATION ON THE CELLULAR MEDIATORS IN THE HEALING PROCESS

Fibroblasts are essential in the wound healing process due to their deposition of collagen, and secretion of growth factors. Many studies have proposed that there is a proliferation of these cells after light exposure. Pereira et al. investigated the ability of a Ga-AS diode pulsed laser at 904 nm on cell growth and procollagen synthesis of cultured fibroblasts. The results obtained showed that at smaller doses of 3 and $4 \, J/cm^2$, there was significant increase in the cell numbers compared to higher doses, but there was no effect on procollagen synthesis at any of these energy densities. This leads to the conclusion that cellular proliferation is enhanced by lasers at specific parameters, but procollagen synthesis may need another specific combination of parameters to appreciate production in collagen (15). In the work of Almeida-Lopes et al., their study compared the effect of fibroblasts on a range of wavelengths (670–786 nm) at a fixed dose of $2 \, J/cm^2$. The results from this study had similar findings to the previous study in that low level laser therapy can increase the rate of proliferation. This investigation also illustrated that culture mediums only supplemented by 5% fetal bovine serum without any other nutritional benefits had significant cell growth compared to ideal medium supplemented with 10% fetal bovine serum. This demonstrates that lasers can improve cellular functions either by increasing the amount of growth factors or other cellular mediators in stressful conditions (16).

Tang et al. used a 830 nm diode laser and studied the modifications of the collagen with microscopy after irradiation. They suggested that various types of collagen respond differently when irradiated, and it is mostly likely due to the biochemical composition which is predominately hydroxyproline (17). Reddy et al. also investigated the biochemical makeup of collagen after irradiation by a helium–neon beam at wavelength of 632.8 nm on diabetic rats. It was found that total collagen production was significantly increased compared to controls. It was further demonstrated that neutral salt soluble collagen and insoluble collagen were increased vs. pepsin soluble collagen, which showed a decrease in the wounds after light exposure. The results suggested that soluble collagen becomes insoluble after laser treatment, and this type of collagen improves the overall integrity of the wound by enhancing its biomechanical properties (18). There is, however, conflicting evidence on the effects of lasers on collagen. Some studies have shown that there is an increase in procollagen synthesis after the application of lasers, and some have said that there is absolutely no effect collagen proliferation (12,19). More investigations on laser therapy and collagen need to be conducted. Studies need to determine which collagen fiber bundles are affected, whether collagen is truly affected by laser therapy, and ultimately the mechanism that this occurs.

There are only a handful of studies on the effects of endothelial cells after laser applications. Schindl et al. demonstrated that there is a dose-dependent effect after the application of 670 nm diode laser on endothelial cell proliferation. It was also noted that at a constant dose of 8 J cm^{-2} with various light intensities, there was still a significant cellular proliferation compared to the controls. Others have also reported a dose-dependent proliferation after laser irradiation at similar wavelengths (11). Yu et al. observed keratinocyte proliferation and migration after the use of helium–neon laser. Their results also showed an increase with interleukin-1-α and interleukin-8 production in the laser-treated group vs. control, which plays a significant role healing process (20). Grossman et al. observed proliferation on normal human keratinocytes following 780 nm diode laser between 0.45 and 0.95 J/cm^2, and this stimulatory effect was suppressed by anti-oxidants, which illustrates that reactive oxygen species are involved in the proliferative response (21).

Thus far, a number of studies have reported that when living cells are exposed to elevated temperatures, there is a physiological reaction called the heat shock response, which is associated with a cellular defense mechanism. During the heat shock response, there is a production of heat shock proteins (HSP). HSP are chaperone proteins that facilitate in the folding and assembly of polypeptides, particularly heat shock protein 70, and appear to play a large role in the inflammatory reaction process and possibly wound healing, as well, because they appear to offer resistance to thermal injury (22). Capon et al. illustrate that there is a logarithmic relationship between duration and temperature for an equivalent HSP expression. As a result, overexpression of these proteins has been demonstrated in human keratinocytes and fibroblasts, and theses proteins have shown thermotolerance to thermal injury. In a previous study, they provided evidence to show that, after diode laser irradiation ($\lambda = 815$ nm) under specific parameters, the acceleration of healing was observed histologically, which resulted in a thinner scar. They further illustrated via immunocytochemistry that there was a markedly increased expression of heat shock protein as compared to that of control skin in epidermal cells as well as a dense labeling in dermal cells. Capon et al. suggested that increased production of the molecular chaperones might potentially decrease synthesis of other proteins during the heat shock response and possibly the inflammatory phase in the wound healing process, which would ultimately decrease the amount of cell proliferation. Overall, this may assist in the repair process by reducing the amount of scar tissue formation (23).

In addition to the heat shock proteins, another mediator in the cascade of wound healing has been considered. Takenaka and Hightower have shown that transforming growth factor-beta (TGF-β) appears to upregulate the synthesis of molecular chaperones in cultured chicken embryo cells. It is thought that this cytokine, which is seen in the inflammatory phase, stimulates fibroblast chemotaxis and collagen and fibronectin synthesis, as well as induces the heat shock protein (24). This evidence is supported within a study by Danno et al. that has illustrated similar findings through the discovery that near-infrared irradiation can enhance wound healing. Their light source was used on cultured human keritinocytes, endothelial cells, and fibroblasts, and it increased the secretion of TGF-β1 and upregulated a matrix metalloproteinases, which is involved in the remodeling phase (25). Research by Yu et al. found that the biostimulatory effects of the argon lasers at wavelengths ranging from 630 to 660 nm released TGF and platelet-derived growth factor. The exact mechanism in which lasers enhance inflammatory phase mediators, such as TGF-β and HSP as well as other growth factors, have not been elucidated; yet, the studies illustrate that the wound healing process is a complex series of interactions, and there appears to be a positive effect of lasers on wounds.

6. CLINICAL STUDIES

Unfortunately, well-controlled clinical trials of laser irradiation are lacking. For example, Franek et al. reported no clinical significance with a GaAlAs diode laser ($\lambda = 810$ nm, $P = 65$ mW, $p = 4$ J/cm^2) during any stage of crural ulcer healing. This was a small sample study ($n = 65$) where patients received either laser treatment along with standard therapy, sham therapy with standard treatment, or standard therapy. Irradiation occurred once a day, five times a week for five weeks. The results showed a reduction in wound area and volume in all groups, but no statistical difference in enhanced healing was measured in the laser-treated group. The authors contribute the lack of significance to the amount of pus prior to treatment in the irradiated group, the distance in which the irradiation was performed, and the output of the laser (26). Another study with similar results examined low intensity therapy (diode laser GaAlAs) with postsurgical wounds, i.e., partial and total nail avulsion and electrosurgery wounds. The physical parameters used by Lagan et al. included a $\lambda = 830$ nm, $P = 30$ mW, $p = 9$ J/cm^2 (27). This study had a total of nine patients where five patients received laser irradiation once a week for a total of 11 weeks. Healing was similar in both groups, but there were no statistical differences noted in wound closure between the two groups. As a matter of fact, the control group had greater reduction in wound size and complete healing by week 8 vs. week 11 in the treatment group. The aforementioned studies have similar results; however, the physical parameters of the lasers, types of wounds, and the size of the wounds are different, which make it difficult for comparisons. In addition, these studies lack statistical power to demonstrate any statistical significance. On the other hand, other accounts have shown significance in other areas of the healing process such as skin microcirculation, the proliferation of lymphocytes, improvement in appearance kelods, and hypertrophic scars (13,28,29).

7. CONCLUSION

The effect of lasers on wound healing still needs further investigation. Many of the animal studies are not well controlled and lack specific details in regard to physical parameters, mediums used, treatment parameters, wound sizes which make it difficult to compare results. The evidence in vivo also appears unconvincing as well secondary to the lack of statistical power in each study and the conflicting results. If standard guidelines or treatment protocols were implemented, there may be more convincing evidence that lasers do indeed accelerate wound healing by proliferating the constituents in the healing cascade. The exact mechanisms have yet to be elucidated, but once it is determined lasers will revolutionize the field of medicine once again.

REFERENCES

1. Schindl M, Kerschan K, et al. Induction of complete wound healing in recalcitrant ulcers by low-intensity laser irradiation depends on ulcer cause and size. Photodermatol Photoimmunol Photomed 1999; 15(1):18–21.
2. Schindl A, Schindl M, Schindl L. Successful treatment of persistent radiation ulcer by low power laser therapy. J Am Acad Dermatol 1997; 37:646–648.
3. Einstein A. Zur Quantentheorie der Strahlung. Physiol Z 1917; 18:121–128.
4. Lipper G, Anderson RR. Laser in Dermatology. Fitzpatrick.
5. Hirsh R, Anderson RR. Principles of laser–skin interactions. In: Bolognia J, Jorizzo J, Rapini R, eds. Dermatology. Elsevier, 2003:2143–2151.
6. Tanzi E, Lupton J, Alster T. Lasers in dermatology: four decades of progress. J Am Acad Dermatol 2003; 49(1):1–31.
7. Zonios G, Bykowski J, Kollias N. Skin melanin, hemoglobin, and light scattering properties can be quantitatively assessed in vivo using diffuse reflectance spectroscopy. J Invest Dermatol 2001; 117(6):1452–1457.
8. Stratigos A, Dover J, Arndt K. Laser therapy. In: Bolognia J, Jorizzo J, Rapini R, eds. Dermatology. Elsevier, 2003:2153–2175.
9. Robbins S. Pathologic Basis of Disease. Philadelphia, Pennsylvania: W.B. Saunders Company, 1999.
10. Bello Y, Falabella A, Eaglstein W. Wound healing modalities.
11. Schindl A, Merwald H, Schind L, et al. Direct stimulatory effect of low-intensity 670 nm laser irradiation on human endothelial cell proliferation. Br J Dermatol 2003; 148(2): 334–336.
12. Conlan M, Rapley J, Cobb C. Biostimulation of wound healing by low-energy laser irradiation: a review. J Clin Periodontol 1996; 23(5):492–496.
13. Stadler I, Evans R, Kolb B, et al. In vitro effects of low-level laser irradiation at 660 nm on peripheral blood lymphocytes. Lasers Surg Med 2000; 27:255–261.
14. Smith KC. The photobiological basis of low level laser radiation therapy. Laser Ther 1991; 3:19–24.
15. Pereira AN, Eduardo CP, Matson E, Marques MM. Effect of low-power irradiation on cell growth and procollagen synthesis of cultured fibroblasts. Lasers Surg Med 2002; 31:263–297.
16. Alemida-Lopes L, Rigau J, Zangaro R, et al. Comparison of the low level laser therapy effects on cultured human gingival fibroblasts proliferation using different irradiance and same fluence. Lasers Surg Med 2001; 29:179–184.
17. Tang J, Godlewski G, Rouy S, Delacretaz G. Morphologic changes in collagen fibers after 830 nm diode laser welding. Lasers Surg Med 1997; 21:438–443.
18. Reddy GK, Stehno-Bittel L, Enwemeka C. Laser photostimulation accelerates wound healing in diabetic rats. Wound Rep Reg 2001; 9:248–255.
19. Van Breugel HHFI, Dop Bar PR. Power density and exposure time of he–ne laser irradiation are more important than total energy dose in photo-biomodulation of human fibroblasts in vitro. Lasers Surg Med 1992; 12:528–537.
20. Yu HS, Chang KL, Y CL, et al. Low-energy helium neon laser irradiation stimulates interleukin-1-alpha and interleukin-8 release from cultured human keratinocytes. J Invest Dermatol 1996; 107(4):593–596.
21. Grossman N, Schneid N, Reuveni H et al. 780 nm low power diode laser irradiation stimulates proliferation of keratinocyte cultures: involvement of reactive oxygen species. Lasers Sugr Med 1998; 22:212–218.
22. Capon A, Mordon S. Can thermal lasers promote skin wound healing? Am J Clin Dermatol 2003; 4(1):1–12.
23. Capon A, Souil E, Gauthier B et al. Laser assisted skin closure (LASC) by using a 815-nm diode-laser system accelerates and improves wound healing. Lasers Surg Med 2001; 28:168–175.

24. Takenaka I, Hightower L. Transforming growth factor-beta 1 rapidly induces hsp70 and hsp90 molecular chapersones in cultured chicken embryo cells. J Cell Physio 1992; 152:568–577.

25. Danno K, Mori N, Toda K, Kobayashi T, Utani A. Near-infared irradiation stimulates cutaneous wound repair: laboratory experiments on possible mechanisms. Photoderm Photoimmun Photomed 2001; 17:261–265.

26. Franek A, Krol P, Kucharzewski M. Does low output laser stimulation enhance the healing of crural ulceration? Some critical remarks. Med Eng Phys 2002; 24(9):607–617.

27. Lagan K, Clements BA, McDonough S, Baxter D. Low intensity laser therapy (830 nm) in the management of minor postsurgical wounds: a controlled clinical study. Lasers Surg Med 2001; 28(1):27–32.

28. Schindl A, Heinze G, Schindl M, Pernerstorfer-Schon H, Schindl L. Systemic effects of low-intensity laser irradiation on skin microcirculation in patients with diabetic microangiopathy. Microvasc Res 2002; 64(2):240–246.

29. Manuskiatti W, Fitzpatrick R, Goldman M. Energy density and numbers of treatment affect response of keloidal and hypertrophic sterntomy scars to the 585-nm flashlamp-pumped pulsed-dye laser. J Am Acad Dermatol 2001; 45:557–565.

37

Growth Factor Therapy to Aid Wound Healing

Martin C. Robson, MD and Wyatt G. Payne
Department of Surgery, University of South Florida, Tampa, Florida, U.S.A.

It is clear that certain proteins (polypeptides) directly regulate many of the processes crucial for normal wound healing, including chemotactic migration of inflammatory cells, mitosis of fibroblasts, keratinocytes, and vascular endothelial cells, neovascularization, and synthesis and degradation of extracellular matrix components (1). These regulatory peptides known as cytokines include such polypeptides as the interleukins, hematopoietic colony-stimulating factors, and tissue necrosis factors (2). They also include the various growth factors. Growth factors are synthesized and secreted by many types of cells involved in tissue repair including platelets, inflammatory cells, fibroblasts, epithelial cells, and vascular endothelial cells (3). They may act on the producer cell (autocrine stimulation), adjacent cells (paracrine stimulation), or distant cells (endocrine stimulation). Substances such as cytokines that are chemotactic to inflammatory cells, such as neutrophils and macrophages, or mitogenic to cells, such as fibroblasts, endothelial cells, and keratinocytes, should benefit wound healing (4). Certainly, the literature is replete with examples of effects of exogenous application of cytokines and/or growth factors for animal models of both acute and chronic wounds (5–7). In all of those animal models, it has been suggested that wound healing would be enhanced by topical application of growth factors.

1. RATIONALE FOR THE USE OF GROWTH FACTORS TO MANIPULATE WOUND HEALING TRAJECTORIES

In impaired wound healing from whatever cause, the time to healing is delayed, and the wound healing trajectory slows. This may be due to the wrong amount, the wrong sequence, or the wrong time course of the necessary growth factor activity. Certainly, exogenous application of growth factors would seem to be indicated if there was a deficiency of such substances in a wound. Evidence is mounting that such is the case in chronic wounds. This deficiency could be absolute or relative due to decreased production or secretion, more rapid breakdown, or a trapping or binding of the cytokines to prevent their effective use in the healing processes (8). Using an

491

ELISA technique on retrieved chronic wound fluid, it was demonstrated that plate-let-derived growth factor (PDGF), bFGF, epidermal growth factor (EGF), and transforming growth factor beta (TGF$_\beta$) levels were markedly decreased compared with acute wounds (9). Even when growth factors are not lacking, they may not be effectively available to the wound for healing (6). In venous stasis ulcers, macro-molecular leakage, specifically fibrinogen, α macroglobulin, and albumin, leads to binding of these substances to growth factors making them unavailable to the repair process (10). This type of trapping has also been reported for diabetic ulcers (6).

In addition to the decreased availability of growth factors and the trapping of those that are present in chronic wounds, there is a problem with the bacterial bur-den (11,12). The ever-present tissue level of bacteria in chronic wounds produce higher levels of proteases and other matrix metalloproteases (MMPs) that further degrade the growth factors (13). It is clear that degradation of growth factors and their receptors limits the progression of the wound healing cascade by eliminating the mediators of the various cellular processes.

Many of the problems listed for chronic wounds are not as significant a problem for acute wounds. Bacterial loads and protease levels are much lower. Optimizing the cellular and/or molecular wound environment by topical application of growth factors is just beginning to be explored in an effort to shift the gain in wound strength toward shorter times for incisional healing of both dermis and fascia (6,14,15).

Although most surgeons observe that acute wounds heal "normally" most of the time, most surgical patients view the acute healing process as a long one that is simultaneously physically limiting and often psychologically upsetting. This time is spent limited by pain, mechanical weakness, functional loss, and cosmetic changes (8). It is therefore important to develop strategies for reducing the time of acute wound healing in order to minimize the acute wound burden and shorten the period of disability when normal healing occurs. Molecularly, this can theoretically be done by identifying and modifying the timing and/or sequence of delivery of potent cytokine and/or tissue growth factor signaling peptides believed to be most important for regulating each phase of acute wound healing.

2. TOPICAL APPLICATION OF GROWTH FACTORS TO MANIPULATE HEALING OF CHRONIC WOUNDS

Recombinant technology has allowed production of many growth factors in phar-macological amounts. This has resulted in attempts at optimizing the cellular and/ or molecular environment of wounds. Most data exist for chronic wounds because of their known impairments in healing. Two recent reviews of the clinical experience of topical application of growth factors to chronic wounds have been published (6,8). These experiences suggest that several growth factors may be used to manipulate healing of chronic wounds such as pressure ulcers, diabetic neurotropic foot ulcers, or venous stasis ulcers. The growth factors have been applied as single agents, in combination, or sequentially.

2.1. Platelet-Derived Growth Factor

Platelet-derived growth factor serves as the paradigm for the use of a topical growth factor to enhance chronic wound healing (8). It is the first recombinant cytokine growth factor to be approved by the U.S. Food and Drug Administration for topical application to wounds for the purpose to accelerate wound closure. Based on preclinical results, clinical trials were first conducted with topical application of PDGF-BB for the treatment of pressure ulcers (16–18). The initial trials were performed with PDGF-BB in a liquid carrier. To allow a more prolonged effect of the topically applied growth factor, subsequent trials have been reported using PDGF-BB in a sodium carboxymethylcellulose (NaCMC) gel. Rees et al. (19) have demonstrated efficacy with this formulation of PDGF-BB in 124 patients with chronic pressure ulcers.

The largest experience for any given topically applied growth factor to a single wound type has been the use of PDGF-BB to treat full-thickness diabetic foot ulcers with adequate circulation (8). The first study included 118 patients with neurotropic ulcers of greater than 8 weeks duration (20). The patients were debrided of all necrotic tissues and had a $TcPO_2$ of greater than 30 mmHg. Patients received topical application of PDGF-BB or placebo once daily until the ulcer healed or for a maximum of 20 weeks. The incidence of complete healing in patients treated with PDGF-BB was 48% (29/61) vs. 25% (14/57) for those treated with placebo ($p = 0.01$). The time to complete healing was 113 days for the treatment group compared to 126 for the placebo group ($p = 0.02$) (20). A total of four clinical trials to show efficacy and six clinical trials to prove safety of topical PDGF-BB for the treatment of lower extremity diabetic neuropathic ulcers have been performed. The conclusion from these studies and the FDA review is that topical PDGF-BB in a 100-µg/gm becaplermin gel is safe and efficacious to enhance wound healing of the diabetic foot ulcer (8,21). In addition to pressure ulcers and diabetic ulcers, studies are underway to assess the efficacy and safety of becaplermin gel in other types of chronic wounds such as venous stasis ulcers (6).

2.2. Basic Fibroblast Growth Factor

The fibroblast growth factor (FGF) family consists of at least nine homologous peptides of which three have been used extensively in preclinical wound healing studies (bFGF[FGF-2], aFGF[FGF-1], and KGF-2[FGF-10]) (6,8). Basic FGF which is mitogenic and chemotactic for fibroblasts and endothelial cells, and is a stimulus for angiogenesis, has the greatest reported clinical trial experience (8). Based on preclinical experience with contaminated animal models, the first randomized, blinded, placebo-controlled trials were conducted on patients with pressure ulcers. Fifty patients were treated with eight different dosage regimens of three different bFGF concentrations (1.0, 5.0, 10 µg/cm^2) (22). There was a trend toward faster healing in 6/8 groups treated with topical bFGF compared with the vehicle-treated groups. When all patients receiving bFGF at two institutional sites were combined as a group, the difference between the slopes of the treated and placebo curves was significant ($p < 0.05$). When the data were analyzed in terms of the number of patients achieving a 70% volume reduction, 21/35 patients receiving bFGF responded, vs. 4/14 patients in the placebo group. This outcome was significantly different ($p = 0.047$) (22).

2.3. Keratinocyte Growth Factor-2

Keratinocyte growth factor-2 (also know as FGF-10) is a member of the fibroblast growth factor family of mitogens. It has a highly selective action on epithelial cells.

In addition to promoting re-epithelialization by a direct effect on keratinocytes causing them to proliferate and migrate, KGF-2 may also stimulate granulation tissue formation by a direct chemotactic effect on fibroblasts (23,24). It was found to be more effective than either the vehicle control or KGF-1 at closing the interstices of human meshed skin grafts explanted to athymic "nude" rats (25).

Following a phase 1 clinical trial to demonstrate safety when applied topically to skin, a truncated form of recombinant human KGF-2 (repifermin) was used in a phase 2a clinical trial in patients with venous stasis ulcers (23). A randomized, double-blind, parallel-group, placebo-controlled multicenter study compared either placebo or repifermin (20 or $60\,\mu g/cm^2$) applied topically twice per week for 12 weeks. A significant difference ($p = 0.047$) was seen between the combined KGF-2 treated groups and the placebo group for subjects who achieved at least 75% healing. The treatment effect appeared greater for ulcers $\leq 15\,cm^2$ in size and ≤ 18 months in duration. For this subgroup, differences were statistically significant for both the 90% combined healed group ($p = 0.028$) and the 75% combined healed group (0.007) (23). This trial was only 12 weeks in duration; presently a large multicenter trial of longer duration and with a larger concentration of KGF-2 is being conducted.

2.4. Epidermal Growth Factor

The EGF family comprises four mammalian proteins: EGF, transforming growth factor alpha (TGF_α), amphiregulin, and heparin-binding EGF (6). Although EGF and TGF_α consistently stimulate the processes in vitro that are required for wound healing, topical treatment with these cytokines in acute and chronic human wounds in vivo has not been consistent (6). The first clinical trial of any recombinant cytokine growth factor to accelerate healing was the application of EGF in Silvadene cream (1% silver sulfadiazine) to split-thickness skin graft donor sites in burn patients (26). The control group received Silvadene alone. The study showed a statistical difference of 1- to 2.5-day healing acceleration which was not thought to be of clinical significance (6,8). A crossover study of nine patients with various chronic wounds treated with Silvadene followed by recombinant EGF was subsequently reported (27). The numbers were small, and the study design was not optimal. However, none of the nine patients healed while on Silvadene cream alone and 8/9 healed on the Silvadene–EGF regimens (8). This study has been difficult to interpret because of the multiple etiologies of the wounds and the various healing processes involved (6).

2.5. Transforming Growth Factor Beta

Transforming growth factor beta exists in at least three isoforms ($TGF_{\beta 1}$, $TGF_{\beta 2}$, and $TGF_{\beta 3}$). The three have many similarities in stimulating collagen synthesis (8). Animal studies suggest that $TGF_{\beta 3}$ may have greater anti-inflammatory properties and may inhibit scarring (28). Two studies have been reported utilizing $TGF_{\beta 2}$ in a collagen sponge vehicle for the treatment of chronic venous stasis ulcers (29). A preliminary open label trial using $0.5\,\mu g/cm^2$ of $TGF_{\beta 2}$ applied three times a week for 6 weeks showed the open area of the ulcers treated with $TGF_{\beta 2}$ had decreased by 73% while the area of the placebo-treated ulcers had increased 9%.

This trial was followed by a prospectively randomized, blinded, placebo-controlled three arm trial comparing $2.5\,\mu g/cm^2$ $TGF_{\beta 2}$ in a lyophilized collagen sponge, the collagen sponge alone, and a standardized care dressing (29). Again, the $TGF_{\beta2}$-treated ulcers responded better, decreasing by 57% compared to 30% for collagen sponge alone, and 9% for the standard dressing.

$TGF_{\beta2}$ has also been used to treat diabetic neuropathic ulcers. In a blinded study using three doses of $TGF_{\beta2}$ (0.05, 0.5, and 5.0 µg/cm^2), each demonstrated a higher rate of healing than did the vehicle control (30).

2.6. Granulocyte-Macrophage Colony-Stimulating Factor

Granulocyte-macrophage colony-stimulating factor (GM-CSF) is a hematopoietic growth factor that can stimulate leukocyte, macrophage, keratinocyte, and fibroblast activity (6,8). It has been used topically for nonhealing abdominal wounds following cancer surgery (31), and injected perilesionally in two clinical trials by DaCosta et al. (32,33) to accelerate the healing of venous stasis ulcers.

In the first trial of 25 patients, ulcers received either 400 µg of GM-CSF in four perilesional sites as a one-time injection or similar placebo injections. Fifty percent of the GM-CSF-treated patients healed vs. 11% of the placebo-treated patients (32). A follow-up dose-ranging trial compared 200–400 µg GM-CSF administered weekly for 4 weeks in 60 patients. The complete healing responses were 57% and 61% for the 200 and 400 µg groups compared to a 19% response for the placebo group ($p = 0.014$) (33). Other trials have found a significant complication rate when GM-CSF was injected perilesionally.

2.7. Insulin-Like Growth Factors

This family of proteins includes IGF-I and IGF-II that have been studied in vitro and in preclinical studies of wound healing. Also known as somatomedins, they show significant amino acid homology with insulin (8). IGF-I is very important in promoting protein synthesis and increases the proliferation of many cell types, including fibroblasts (6). Although there have been several preclinical studies suggesting that IGF-1 and IGF-II might enhance wound healing processes, to date no clinical trials have been reported. However, the action of growth hormone may be through the activation of IGF-I, and recombinant human growth hormone (rHGH) has been used in a double blind placebo-controlled trial of 37 patients with chronic leg ulcers (34). The patients were randomized to receive either 1 IU/cm^2 ulcer area of topical rHGH or placebo, in addition to "standard" treatment (compression and hydrocolloid dressing). The healing rate was 16% per week in patients receiving rHGH compared with 3% per week in the placebo group (34). With 18/37 patients failing to complete the study, it is difficult to draw conclusions about this trial. Since it is postulated that the effect of rHGH might be due to a rise in IGF-I, possibly a trial with topical IGF-I would be more successful (8).

2.8. Interleukin-1 Beta

Recombinant interleukin-1 beta (IL-1β) has several actions that contribute to wound healing including chemoattraction of cells (predominately neutrophils and macrophages) to the wound site, proliferation and fibroblast-induced release of collagenase-like activity, and stimulation of capillary endothelial cell proliferation (6,8). It also has the ability to stimulate monocytes and granulocytes and stimulate macrophages to produce other growth factors (35). A prospective randomized double-blind, placebo-controlled trial including 26 patients with pressure ulcers who were treated with either 0.01, 0.10, or 1.0 μg/cm² of rhuIL-1β or a placebo vehicle demonstrated no statistical differences among the four groups (35). However, patients receiving the highest dose of IL-1β showed different in vitro fibroblast characteristics than patients in the other groups. Fibroblast "senescence" seemed to be overcome after 28 days of treatment with IL-1β at 1.0 μg/cm²/day. Despite preclinical studies suggesting that exogenous IL-1β might shift the wound trajectory to the left, the attempt in pressure ulcers was possibly ill conceived since increased levels of proinflammatory cytokines are thought to be part of the pathobiology of wound chronicity (8,36).

2.9. Combination of Cytokine Growth Factors

If a single cytokine growth factor does not establish efficacy in manipulating healing in the chronic wound, the possibility of combinations or sequences of growth factors exists. The possibilities of combinations and sequences are nearly endless (8). Several preclinical examples of this exist (6). A small multicenter clinical trial of combined topical PDGF and IGF-1 for enhancement of diabetic foot ulcer healing did not show clinical efficacy (8). The idea of combining growth factors for topical application to wounds is the concept behind the autologous platelet releasate platelet-derived wound healing formula (PDWHF). This releasate from autologous platelets contains PDGF, TGF$_\beta$, PDAF, PDEGF, platelet factor-4, and other unknown factors (8). A controlled, double-blinded, crossover trial of 32 patients has been reported in which 81% of patients treated with PDWHF had 100% epithelization after 8 weeks of treatment compared to only 15% in the control group (37).

At least five other trials have been reported using PDWHF on lower extremity ulcers (6). Most were destined to fail by a lack of homogeneous subgroups and various etiologies of leg ulcer giving contradictory results (8). However, when only diabetic neutrophic ulcers were carefully stratified and entered into a double-blind multicenter trial, it was found that all three concentrations of PDWHF tested outperformed the saline placebo over a 20-week period (38). Only 29% of the neurotropic diabetic ulcers achieved complete healing in the placebo group compared to 80%, 62%, and 52% in the 0.01, 0.033, and 0.1 PDWHF dilution-treated groups ($p = 0.02$) (38).

2.10. Sequential Applications of Growth Factors

The availability and function of the various growth factors in normal wound healing appears to be sequential (8). Platelet and/or inflammatory cell-released factors are present in the wound at an earlier time in the healing trajectory than are fibroblast-secreted factors. Based on animal experiments of wound contraction models, a large trial investigating the sequential topical application of GM-CSF followed by bFGF in pressure ulcers was conducted (39). This demonstrated that sequential therapy was successful in shifting the healing trajectory to the left, but this particular sequence choice was not as effective as bFGF alone (39).

The most interesting part of this study was the results of long-term follow-up of these patients (40). Of the patients healing ≥85% during treatment, 84.6% were 100% healed after 1 year compared with 61% of those that healed <85% during treatment ($p < 0.05$). Since only patients receiving exogenously applied growth factors achieved >85% closure during the treatment phase of the trial, the excellent long-term outcome appears attributable to the cytokine therapy (40). Long-term outcome was better in this growth factor trial than with surgical or standard nonoperative treatment of pressure ulcers (40,41).

2.11. Combinations of Growth Factors and Antiproteases

If a single growth factor, a combination of growth factors, or a sequence of growth factors topically applied do not eventually prove successful in enhancing healing of the chronic wound, it may be due to the pathobiology of these wounds with an imbalance of the synthetic-degradation equilibrium of the extracellular matrix (1,8). There is an excess of MMPs in chronic wounds and a decrease in their natural inhibitors, TIMP-1 and TIMP-2. Not only are the degradative MMP enzymes elevated but also cathepsin G, elastase, and urokinase (42). Since all of these could theoretically degrade exogenously applied growth factors, it has been suggested that one could treat the chronic wound with natural or synthetic exogenous protease inhibitors, induce expression of endogenous antiproteases, or attack the excess neutrophil accumulation responsible for much of the protease excess (42). To re-establish the wound healing trajectory uniformly in chronic wounds, it is possible that cytokines and protease inhibitors will require simultaneous administration (1,3,8,42). Although this approach has not yet been reported in clinical trials, ointment containing EGF and a serine protease inhibitor has been tested in open rat wounds and showed improved healing (8).

3. ATTEMPTS TO MANIPULATE HEALING OF ACUTE WOUNDS WITH GROWTH FACTORS

Even when tissue repair is efficiently activated following injury and reliably passes through the tightly orchestrated cellular and molecular healing pathways of the wound healing scheme, the resultant "normal" healing trajectory requires a significant amount of time (8). Patient morbidity occurs with what is labeled "normal" healing. Acute burns are an obvious example, but all soft tissue injuries are similarly debilitating. When acute healing is delayed or incomplete, a surgical complication is the result (8). When acute wounds fail, they result in dehiscences, incisional hernia formation, gastroenteric fistulae, vascular anastomotic leaks, bronchopleural fistulae, and luminal stricture formation (8). Because of these problems, newer data are emerging using these cytokines for acute wounds that are healing with a "normal" trajectory. These attempts are to change the timing of cytokine action to shift the normal trajectory farther to the left towards "ideal" healing.

3.1. Acute Burns

Thermal burn injuries are examples of wounds whose acute healing time course can be prolonged. If the burn is deep, the wound is excised and a skin graft immediately applied. The healing is then timely and orderly resulting in a sustained anatomical and functional result. This fulfills the definition of acute wound healing (43). However, when the burn wound is more superficial, the time to epithelialization is prolonged.

Application of a growth factor to accelerate burn wound healing has recently been attempted. A clinical trial encompassing 600 patients from 32 hospitals across

China investigated the efficacy of topical bFGF to enhance the healing of partial-thickness second-degree burns (44). This study used the gold standard of histological diagnosis of depth of burn and divided the patients into superficial and deep partial-thickness burns. Superficial and deep second-degree burns treated with rbFGF healing in a mean of 9.9 ± 2.5 days and 17.0 ± 4.6 days, respectively compared with 12.4 ± 2.7 days and 21.2 ± 4.9 days for the placebo groups. The significance was $p = 0.0008$ for the superficial partial thickness burns and $p = 0.0003$ for the deep partial-thickness burns (44). Another attempt to accelerate wound healing in burns has been the application of growth factors to accelerate closure of interstices of meshed split-thickness skin grafts. This has been successful in an animal model for KGF-2, bFGF, and $TGF_{\beta 2}$ (45).

3.2. Surgical Incisions

Realizing the sigmoid-shaped curve of gain in breaking strength or tensile strength is a compromise, attempts have been made to shorten the inflammatory or lag phase of healing, accelerate the proliferative phase of healing, and modulate the remodeling phase of healing (8). One approach for accelerating the inflammatory/lag phase of wound healing is to therapeutically activate the target tissue prior to wounding. "Priming" early acute wound healing using classic wound repair cytokine growth factors such as PDGF, GM-CSF, and IL-1β has been shown to preactivate the humoral and cellular elements of acute tissue repair and to accelerate the recovery of tissue breaking strength following incision (46). The priming approach induces chemotaxis of regulatory cells important to tissue repair into the planned incision site (8). Because activated cells such as macrophages and fibroblasts are capable of synthesizing and releasing additional cytokines and are under the feedback regulation of the acute wound milieu, an in situ approach such as priming is theoretically appealing (8).

A second strategy for inducing an acceleration of the acute wound healing trajectory is to stimulate the proliferative phase of acute tissue repair molecularly. Transforming growth factor beta was the first tissue cytokine growth factor used to shift the proliferative phase of incisional healing to the left successfully and accelerate the recovery of wound tensile strength (47). Other tissue repair growth factors such as PDGF, bFGF, and $TGF_{\beta 2}$ have since shown similar promise following acute injury (46,48). In all of these preclinical studies, dermal wounds were treated at the time of incision and an acceleration of the acute healing curve again was observed.

The majority of preclinical and clinical studies of acute tissue repair have focused on the dermis. This is true despite the fact that the complications of acute wound failure clearly cross the boundary of dermal wound failure and are focused on the fascia (8). To compare fascial healing to the information available for dermal healing, a novel animal model has been developed to compare simultaneous ventral abdominal wall dermal and midline fascial (linea alba) incisions (8). By isolating the healing dermal and fascial incisions, it was possible to observe that the fascial wound regains breaking and tensile strength significantly faster than the dermis (8,15). Isolated fascial fibroblasts were also more active than dermal fibroblasts in vitro as measured by fibroblast proliferation and fibroblast-populated collagen lattice contraction (FPCL) (15). It was then hypothesized that the steeper slope of the fascial healing trajectory may be more susceptible to an acute wound healing insult and possibly susceptible to growth factor manipulation. This hypothesis has proven to be true. Major extirpative surgery such as a partial hepatectomy decreases the fascial gain of tensile strength in the surgical incision. This could be reversed by application of $TGF_{\beta2}$ at the time of fascial wound closure (49). Similarly, in an animal model of incisional hernia, both bFGF and $TGF_{\beta2}$ were able to restore defects in fascial healing (50,51). In fact, $TGF_{\beta2}$ injected into the fascia at the time of incision could totally prevent hernia formation (51).

None of these approaches have been attempted clinically. Remaining unanswered questions before clinical usage include the determination of appropriate doses to induce optimal acute tissue repair, and whether a specific combination and or sequence of acute tissue growth factor therapy will result in improved outcomes. A reliable manner for growth factor delivery to acute wounds also remains a problem, as does the effect of cytokine therapy on nondermal wounds (8). However, once all of these things are understood, earlier induction of the components of acute tissue repair may shorten the time required along the healing continuum (8).

4. EXPLANATION FOR LIMITED SUCCESS OF WOUND MANIPULATION BY GROWTH FACTORS

To date, a single growth factor, PDGF-BB, has been approved by the USFDA for topical use to enhance wound healing, and this approval has been limited to a single wound type. Although overall this appears discouraging, many individual clinical trials have been encouraging (14). How does one reconcile this apparent contradiction? First, attention must be paid to the caveats published for the design of clinical trials (14). These include not adequately controlling factors such as bacteria, ischemia, and hypoxia that are known to inhibit the various wound healing processes (6,14). Also, since various growth factors affect different processes of wound healing and the degree to which any single process plays a part in the repair of a given wound is variable, it is clear that individual growth factors should be targeted at those specific processes that a given wound uses to heal (8,14). If all of the caveats had been considered and included in growth factor clinical trial design, it is possible that more dramatic outcomes would have been achieved for wound healing enhancement (8). However, they have not always been considered in the trials reported to date. However, when trials have attempted to be careful in enrolling homogeneous subgroups by restricting etiology, transcutaneous partial pressure oxygen levels, and bacterial loads, results have often been much more favorable (6,8).

The number of growth factors that affect the various processes in the wound healing cascade is considerable. Since animal models have not been particularly helpful in predicting effective human doses, the attempts to find the correct factor, administered at the correct time, at the correct dosage has been, and will continue to be, very difficult (6). It may be that attempting to manipulate the wound with growth factors by applying them topically as discussed in this chapter will prove not to be the most effective approach. Gene therapy may prove to be a more targeted approach to using cytokines. Gene therapy uses DNA as a superpharmaceutical agent to alter cell function for an extended period of time in relation to more established direct delivery systems (52). Although gene therapy for wound healing is not yet a reality for true utility, recent preclinical experiments suggest it may prove to be effective (53,54).

5. CONCLUSION

In the past, optimization of wound healing focused on minimizing contamination, accurate tissue approximation, and providing protection. With the advent of recombinant technology, optimization can now include manipulation of the molecular and cellular wound environment with compounds such as growth factors. Although the exact manipulative scheme has not yet evolved, it is clear from the multiple attempts reported in this chapter, understanding and progress is being made.

REFERENCES

1. Nwomeh BC, Yager DR, Cohen IK. Physiology of the chronic wound. Clin Plast Surg 1998; 25:341–356.
2. Lyle WG, Phillips LG. Growth factor applications. Adv Plast Reconstr Surg 1997; 13: 89–106.
3. Bennett NT, Schultz GS. Growth factors and wound healing. Part II. Role in normal and chronic wound healing. Am J Surg 1993; 166:74–81.
4. Robson MC. Growth factors as wound healing agents. Curr Opin Biotechnol 1991; 2: 863–867.
5. Kiritsky CP, Lynch AB, Lynch SE. Role of growth factors in cutaneous wound healing: a review. Critic Rev Oral Biol Med 1993; 4:729–760.
6. Robson MC, Smith PD. Topical use of growth factors to enhance healing. In: Falanga V, ed. Cutaneous Wound Healing. London: Martin Dunitz Limited, 2001:379–398.
7. LeGrand EK. Preclinical promise of becaplermin (rhPDGF-BB) in wound healing. Am J Surg 1998; 176(suppl 2A):485–545.
8. Robson MC, Steed DL, Franz MG. Wound healing: biologic features and approaches to maximize healing trajectories. Curr Prob Surg 2001; 38:61–140.
9. Cooper DM, Yu EZ, Hennessey P, Ko F, Robson MC. Determination of endogenous cytokines in chronic wounds. Ann Surg 1994; 219:688–692.
10. Falanga V, Eaglstein WH. The trap hypothesis of venous ulceration. Lancet 1993; 341: 1006–1008.
11. Robson MC, Stenberg BD, Heggers JP. Wound healing alterations caused by infection. Clin Plast Surg 1990; 17:485–492.
12. Robson MC. Wound infection: a failure of wound healing caused by an imbalance of bacteria. Surg Clin N Am 1997; 77:637–650.
13. Ko F, Wright TE, Payne WG, Wang X, Robson MC. Bacterial degradation of growth factors. Wound Rep Regen 2001; 9:A152.
14. Robson MC, Mustoe TA, Hunt TK. The future of recombinant growth factors in wound healing. Am J Surg 1998; 176(suppl 2A):80S–82S.
15. Franz MG, Smith PD, Kirk S, Wright TE, Robson MC. Fascial healing exceeds skin. A novel model of abdominal wall repair. Surg Forum 1999; 50:604–606.
16. Robson MC, Phillips LG, Thomason A, Robson LE, Pierce GF. Platelet-derived growth factor-BB for the treatment of chronic pressure ulcers. Lancet 1992; 339:23–25.
17. Robson MC, Phillips LG, Thomason A, Altrock BW, Pence PC, Heggers JP, Johnston AF, McHugh TP, Anthony MS, Robson LE, Odom LL, Yanagihara D, Pirece GF. Recombinant human platelet-derived growth factor-BB in the treatment of pressure ulcers. Ann Plast Surg 1992; 29:193–201.
18. Mustoe TA, Cutler NR, Allman RM, Goode PS, Deuel TF, Prause JA, Bear M, Serdar CM, Pierce GF. Phase II study to evaluate recombinant PDGF-BB in the treatment of pressure sores. Arch Surg 1994; 129:213–219.
19. Rees RS, Robson MC, Smiell SM, Perry BH. Becaplermin gel in the treatment of pressure ulcers: a randomized, double-blinded, placebo-controlled study. Wound Rep Regen 1999; 7:141–147.

20. Steed D. Diabetic Ulcer Study Group: clinical evaluation of recombinant human platelet derived growth factor (rhPDGF-BB) for the treatment of lower extremity diabetic ulcers. J Vasc Surg 1995; 21:71–81.

21. Steed DL. Platelet-derived growth factor in the treatment of diabetic foot ulcers. Wounds 2000; 12:95B–98B.

22. Robson MC, Phillips LG, Lawrence WT, Bishop JB, Youngerman JS, Hayward PG, Broemeling LD, Heggers JP. The safety and effect of topically applied recombinant basic fibroblastic growth factor on healing of chronic pressure sores. Ann Surg 1992; 216: 401–408.

23. Robson MC, Phillips TJ, Falanga V, Odenheimer DJ, Parish LC, Jensen JL, Steed DL. Randomized trial of topically applied repifermin (rh-KGF-2) to accelerate wound healing in venous ulcers. Wound Rep Regen 2001; 9:347–352.

24. Tagashira S, Harada H, Katsumata T, Itoh N, Nakatsuka M. Cloning of mouse FGF-10 and upregulation of its gene expression during wound healing. Gene 1997; 197:399–404.

25. Soler PM, Wright TE, Smith PD, Maggi SP, Hill DP, Ko F, Jimenez PA, Robson MC. In vivo characterization of keratinocyte growth factor-2 as a potential wound healing agent. Wound Rep Regen 1999; 7:172–178.

26. Brown GL, Nanney LB, Griffen J, Cramer AB, Yancey JM, Curtsinger LJ, Holtzin L, Schultz GS, Jurkiewicz MJ, Lynch JB. Enhancement of wound healing by topical treatment with epidermal growth factor. N Engl J Med 1989; 321:76–79.

27. Brown GL, Curtsinger L, Jurkiewicz MJ, Nahai F, Schultz G. Stimulation of healing of chronic wounds by epidermal growth factor. Plast Reconstr Surg 1991; 88:189–196.

28. Shah M, Foreman DM, Ferguson MW. Neutralization of TGF-beta-1 and TGF-beta-2 or exogenous addition of TGF-beta-3 to cutaneous rat wounds reduces scarring. J Cell Sci 1995; 108:985–1002.

29. Robson MC, Phillips LG, Cooper DM, Lyle WG, Robson LE, Odom L, Hill DP, Hanham AF, Ksander GA. The study and effect of transforming growth factor beta-2 for the treatment of venous stasis ulcers. Wound Rep Regen 1995; 3:157–167.

30. Robson MC, Steed DL, McPherson JM, Pratt BM. Use of transforming growth factor beta-2 (TGF-beta-2) in treatment of chronic foot ulcers in diabetic patients. Wound Rep Regen 1999; 7:A266.

31. Raderer M, Kornek G, Hejna M, Koperna K, Scheithauer W, Base W. Topical granulocyte-macrophage colony stimulation factor in patients with cancer and impaired wound healing. J Nat Cancer Inst 1997; 89:263.

32. DaCosta RM, Aniceto C, Mendes MA. Double-blinded randomized placebo controlled trial of the use of granulocyte macrophage colony stimulating factor in chronic leg ulcers. Am J Surg 1997; 173:165–168.

33. DaCosta RM, Riberiro JF, Jesus FM, Aniceto C, Mendes MA. Randomized, double-blind, placebo-controlled, dose-ranging study of granulocyte-macrophage colony stimulation factor in patients with chronic leg ulcers. Wound Rep Regen 1999; 7:17–25.

34. Rasmussen LH, Karlsmark T, Aunstrop C, Avnstorp C, Peters K, Jorgensen M, Jensen LT. Topical human growth hormone treatment of chronic leg ulcers. Phlebology 1991; 6: 23–30.

35. Robson MC, Abdullah A, Burns BF, Phillips LG, Garrison L, Cowan W, Hill D, Vande-Berg J, Robson LE, Schuler S. Safety and effect of topical interleukin-1B in the management of pressure sores. Wound Rep Regen 1994; 2:177–181.

36. Mast BA, Schultz GS. Interactions of cytokines, growth factors, and proteases in acute and chronic wounds. Wound Rep Regen 1996; 4:411–420.

37. Knighton DR, Ciresi KF, Fiegel VD, Schumerth S, Butler E, Cerra F. Stimulation of repair in chronic, nonhealing, cutaneous ulcers using platelet-derived wound healing formula. Surg Gynecol Obstetr 1990; 170:56–60.

38. Holloway GA, Steed DL, DeMarco MJ, Masumoto T, Moosa HH, Webster MW, Bunt TJ, Polansky MA. A randomized, controlled, multicenter, dose response trial of activated

platelet supernatant, topical CT-102 in chronic, nonhealing, diabetic wounds. Wounds 1993; 5:198–206.

39. Robson MC, Hill DP, Smith PD, Wang X, Meyer-Seigler K, Ko F, VandeBerg JS, Payne WG, Ochs D, Robson LE. Sequential cytokine therapy for pressure ulcers: clinical and mechanistic response. Ann Surg 2002:600–611.

40. Payne WG, Ochs DE, Meltzer DD, Hill DP, Mannari RJ, Robson LE, Robson MC. Longterm outcome study of growth factor-treated pressure ulcers. Am J Surg 2001; 181: 81–86.

41. Disa JJ, Carlton JM, Goldberg NH. Efficacy of operative cure in pressure sore patients. Plast Reconstr Surg 1992; 89:272–278.

42. Yager DR, Nwometh BC. The proteolytic environment of chronic wounds. Wound Rep Regen 1999; 7:433–441.

43. Lazurus GS, Cooper DM, Knighton DR, Margolis DJ, Pecoraro RE, Rodeheaver G, Robson MC. Definitions and guidelines for assessment of wounds and evaluation of healing. Arch Dermatol 1994; 130:489–493.

44. Fu X, Shen Z, Chen Y, Xie J, Guo Z, Zhang M, Sheng Z. Randomized placebo-controlled trial of use of topical recombinant bovine basic fibroblast growth factor for second degree burns. Lancet 1998; 352:1661–1664.

45. Smith PD, Polo M, Soler PM, McClintock JS, Maggi SP, Kim YJ, Ko F, Robson MC. Efficacy of growth factors in the accelerated closure of interstices in explanted meshed human skin grafts. J Burn Care Rehab 2000; 21:5–9.

46. Smith PD, Kuhn MA, Franz MG, Wachtel TL, Wright TE, Robson MC. Initiating the inflammatory phase of incisional healing prior to tissue injury. J Surg Res 2000; 92: 11–17.

47. Mustoe TA, Pierce GF, Thomason A, Gramates P, Sporn MB, Deuel TF. Accelerated healing of incisional wounds in rats induced by transforming growth factor-beta. Science 1987; 237:1333–1336.

48. Wright TE, Hill DP, Ko F, Soler PM, Smith PD, Franz MG, Nichols EH, Robson MC. The effect of TGF-beta-2 in various vehicles on incisional wound healing. Int J Surg Invest 2000; 2:133–143.

49. Kuhn MA, Smith PD, Nguyen K, Ko F, Wang X, Wachtel TL, Robson MC, Franz MG. Abdominal wall repair is delayed during hepatic regeneration. J Surg Res 2001; 95:54–60.

50. Franz MG, Kuhn MA, Nguyen K, Wang X, Ko F, Wright TE, Robson MC. A biological approach to prevention and treatment of incisional hernias. Surg Forum 2000; 51:585–587.

51. Franz MG, Kuhn MA, Nguyen K, Wang X, Ko F, Wright TE, Robson MC. Transforming growth factor beta-2 lowers the incidence of incisional hernias. J Surg Res 2001; 97: 109–116.

52. Shea LD, Smiley E, Bonadio J, Mooney DJ. DNA delivery from polymer matrices for tissue engineering. Nat Biotechnol 1999; 17:551–554.

53. Slama J, Andree C, Winkler T, Swain WF, Eriksson E. Gene transfer. Ann Plast Surg 1995; 35:429–439.

54. Davidson JM, Whitsitt JS, Pennington B, Ballas CB, Eming S, Benn SI. Gene therapy of wounds with growth factors. Curr Top Pathol 1999; 93:111–121.

38

Vacuum-Assisted Closure of Wounds

Michael J. Morykwas
Department of Plastic and Reconstructive Surgery, Wake Forest University School of Medicine, Winston-Salem, North Carolina, U.S.A.

1. INTRODUCTION

With the concurrent advances in medical care, both patients with more severe wounds and patients with a greater degree of debilitation are surviving longer than in the past. These wounds and patients present those who provide care challenges of ever-increasing difficulty. This in turn has led to increased research and understanding of the basic mechanisms of wound healing, both for normally healing wounds and also for wounds with impaired healing. The increased knowledge of the healing mechanisms has also led to the development of additional treatment modalities, including the vacuum-assisted closure system (The V.A.C., KCI, San Antonio, TX). Since being certified by the U.S. Food and Drug Administration in 1995, the use of the V.A.C. system has exponentially increased for the treatment of a wide variety of wounds. While originally designed for the treatment of nonhealing or impaired healing wounds, its use has expanded to include virtually all types of wounds.

The components include an open cell foam dressing, an evacuation tube, and a thin film dressing to cover the wound site and create an airtight seal, a fluid collection container, and a microprocessor-controlled vacuum pump. The foam dressing is trimmed to the size of the wound, the site sealed with the thin film dressing and then the desired level of vacuum applied in the desired manner (continuous vs. intermittent application). Dressings are normally changed at 48-hr intervals.

This chapter will review some of the original studies performed that form the basis for the clinical protocols, discuss the potential mechanisms of action, and then review several types of clinical applications.

2. ANIMAL STUDIES

Swine are frequently used in wound healing studies, and were used for our studies. This is based upon the similarities of their skin to human skin (1–3). Among the desirable properties is the fact that swine are a tight-skinned animal similar to humans. Thus, the formation of granulation tissue plays a much more significant role in the healing process that in loose-skinned animals where contraction appears to be the more significant factor.

2.1. Blood Flow Studies

Three basic studies, two of which form the basis for the treatment regiment, are described. The initial study was a basic dose–response experiment that examined the local vascular response to increasing levels of applied vacuum. Full thickness defects were created on the dorsal midline of anesthetized animals, and needle probes from a laser Doppler were inserted into the tissues. The foam dressing was placed into the defect and the site sealed with a thin film dressing. After establishing the baseline flux, vacuum was applied in a stepwise manner using 25 mm mercury (Hg) increments, returning to atmospheric pressure (0 mm Hg vacuum) between each step. The response was a bell-shaped curve with the maximum increase in flux occurred at 125 mm Hg-applied vacuum, with flux increasing approximately 400× over baseline levels (4). The flux then decreased and actually was less than baseline with applied vacuum levels greater than 300 mm Hg. The decrease may be due to one of two mechanisms: stretching of the small vessels when the tissue is deformed from the applied vacuum, thus decreasing the diameter of the vessels; or the physical compression of the small vessels due to bulk movement of the tissue.

With continuous application of the vacuum, the increase in flux in the periwound tissues gradually decayed back to baseline levels through unknown mechanisms. Flux had decayed to approximately 75–80% of maximum after 5 min. In an attempt to maximize flux, and also to "reset" whatever the mechanisms are that caused the initial increase in flux, the vacuum was turned off for increasing lengths of time. With "off" times less than 2 min, there was no effect on the decay of the flux. With "off" times of 2 min or greater, the flux did return to the maximal levels with each subsequent application of 125 mm Hg vacuum. Thus to maximize local flux in the periwound tissues over an extended period of time, a 5 min "on"/2 min "off" regiment is optimal (4).

The response of periwound tissue to increasing levels of vacuum was also confirmed in paraplegic humans who had wounds in the insensate area, with the same results.

2.2. Granulation Tissue Formation

Once the level of vacuum was determined, a second set of animals was obtained and the effect of the applied vacuum on the rate of granulation tissue was performed. Three sets of 5-cm diameter wounds were created on the dorsal midline of anesthetized animals. The wounds were treated either with saline wet-to-moist dressing, continuous vacuum application, or cycled vacuum applied in a 5 min on/2 min off regiment. The animals were sedated daily and the volume of the wounds measured using an alginate impression material. The molds of the wounds were placed into a graduated cylinder and the volume of water displaced measured. Wounds were treated until the newly formed granulation tissue was flush with surrounding tissue. The diameter of each wound was measured daily to make sure the wounds were healing by new granulation tissue formation and not by contraction. The wounds did not contract during the course of the study. Each animal acted as its own control. Wounds treated with 125 mm Hg continuous vacuum filled with granulation tissue 63% faster than the saline wet-to-moist gauze-treated wounds, while the intermittent treated wounds filled with granulation tissue 103% faster (twice as fast) as the saline wet-to-moist gauze wounds (4).

2.3. Colonized Tissue/Bacterial Response

A third study examined the effects of topically applied vacuum on the tissue bacterial loads in deliberately infected wounds. Full thickness wounds were again created on the dorsum of anesthetized animals and were exposed to 10^8 organisms of either *Staphylococcus hominis* or *Staphylococcus aureus*. Wounds were either treated with saline wet-to-moist gauze dressings or with continuous vacuum at 125 mm Hg. Punch biopsies were harvested daily and the number of organisms per gram of tissue determined, with 10^5 organisms per gram of tissue as the demarcation level for infected tissue. Bacteria levels in vacuum-treated wounds went below 10^5 organisms per gram tissue between days 4 and 5. Bacterial levels in the saline wet-to-moist-treated wounds went below 10^5 organisms per gram of tissue between days 11 and 12 (4).

3. MECHANISMS OF ACTION

Upon application of the vacuum, two broad events happen: removal of fluid from the wound tissues; and movement of the periwound tissues toward the geometric center of the wound. The vacuum applied through the system increases the diffusion gradient, with fluid in the tissues flowing into the foam dressing. The vacuum also causes the foam dressing to collapse, applying tensile forces to the surrounding tissues as the tissues try to fill the defect (Fig. 1). Cells are normally anchorage-dependent, and as the tissues are drawn into the defect, the cells bound to the matrix molecules are deformed by default.

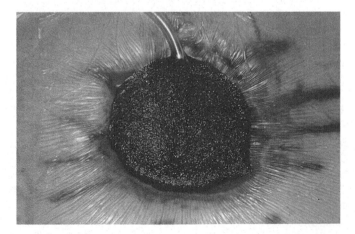

Figure 1 Collapsed foam dressing in abdominal defect from infected TRAM flap donor site. Ridges in drape and underlying tissue are representative of tensile forces placed upon periwound tissue.

3.1. Edema Control and Removal of Soluble Factors

According to Fick's law, fluid and any soluble components should flow from the tissue into the dressing due to differences in the pressure gradient between the tissue "compartment" and the dressing "compartment" (5–7). The removal of excess interstitial fluid helps restore local blood flow to more normal levels by decompressing capillaries and small venules. As is evident from earlier chapters, an extremely well-orchestrated sequence of events and biochemical mediators is required for the healing process to proceed normally. Minor disruptions in the events, whether timing or concentration-dependent, may result in a nonhealing wound or an overhealed wound. Removal of fluid from the periwound tissue also may aid in healing by removal of soluble mediators and other molecules found in the fluid. In in vitro studies, fluid removed from chronic wounds suppressed the proliferation of fibroblasts, keratinocytes, and vascular endothelial cells (8,9). Additionally, chronic wounds contain elevated levels of a variety of proteolytic molecules, which should be removed with the wound fluid (10–13). Removal of these inhibitory or suppression factors from tissues surrounding chronic wounds may allow the normal process to continue to completion.

On a practical note, removal of fluid from injured extremities should allow reapproximation of the wound edges, thus allowing for primary closure of the wound. Additionally, in situations where there is the potential for abdominal or muscle-related compartment syndromes, the removal of the fluid should decompress the tissues and help maintain normal blood flow. In this situation, the V.A.C. system does not replace the need for surgical release, but it is an adjunct used after surgical release.

3.2. Mechanical Stimulation

The direct effects of mechanical forces on tissue and cell growth and deposition have been known and postulated about for well over a century. Probably, the most famous description is Wolff's law, which simplistically paraphrased is "form follows function," e.g., bone is deposited in areas of high forces and is resorbed from areas of low forces. Similar theories for soft tissue were postulated by Thoma in 1911 (14). The gross application of forces to induce tissue growth is widely used clinically, including external osteogenic distraction (the Ilizarov technique) and soft tissue expansion (15–18). Today, the field is known as mechanical transduction, in which mechanical and physical forces applied to a cell produce a physiological or biochemical response. This is a sophisticated series of events involving the extracellular matrix, transmembrane and cytoskeletal structures, and a series of intracellular kinases (19–24). In vitro investigations of mechanical deformation of a variety of cells have shown molecular responses (calcium release) with a single stretch (25). A wide variety of molecular and genetic responses additionally occur in response to mechanical deformation, including second messenger release, stimulation of a variety of kinase-mediated pathways, upregulation of immediate early protocol-oncogenes, increased mitosis, etc (24–31). The powerful tool of gene microarray analysis has also recently been used to determine the effects of mechanical stress on vascular endothelial cell response (32).

While much of the research examining the effects of mechanical deformation and the cellular responses to the deformation is occurring in diverse fields, the knowledge from the various cell types is inter-related and should shed light on the mechanisms by which the V.A.C. technique promotes new tissue formation.

4. CHRONIC WOUNDS

A loose definition of a chronic wound is one that is not progressing in a normal orderly manner to a resolved wound. The V.A.C. system was originally developed to treat chronic and slowly healing wounds (33). A wide variety of chronic wounds respond favorably to treatment with the V.A.C. system (34–36). Prior to the start of any wound care, any necrotic tissue present in the wound must be removed; necrotic tissue can become a nidus for infection and no treatment will bring it back to life. There are several considerations when treating chronic wounds with the V.A.C. system based upon our observations during treatment of such wounds. In general, it appears that the longer a wound has been in a nonhealing stage, the slower the initial response to the applied vacuum. During the treatment of chronic wounds, particularly pressure sores, the response may reach a "plateau," a time period of a week or two in which there may not be any gross signs of healing. The wounds then restart the healing process with visible progress. The cause of this plateau is not known. Once the wound is closed, patient education is a major component to prevent recurrence of the pressure sore.

The periwound tissues of chronic wounds located on the trunk are frequently edematous and woody. The typical treatment regiment at our institution is to use continuous vacuum to withdraw this excess fluid from the periwound tissues, and cycled vacuum applied once the fluid volume decreases. It is not unusual to withdraw up to several liters of fluid from a large, old pressure sore in the first day of treatment.

Venous stasis ulcers are very painful, and a low level of vacuum should be applied continuously. Patients usually feel increased pain for a short period of time after application of the vacuum, which usually subsides. If the wound is painful during dressing changes with other modalities, it will be painful with V.A.C. dressing changes and may require prior medication. Clamping off the evacuation tube and introducing a lidocaine solution (sans epinephrine) into the foam dressing prior to the dressing change are usually effective in controlling the pain during dressing changes. However, there is a small subset of patients who will find even the lowest level of vacuum with a continuous application too painful to continue the treatment. For those patients whose wounds are successfully closed, the patient must be compliant and use preventative measures so that the ulcer does not reoccur.

Arterial insufficiency ulcers as a whole are difficult to treat and exhibit a moderate response to treatment with the V.A.C. system. While the V.A.C. system does increase local blood flow, if there is not an adequate inflow, the wound will not respond well. The long-term prognosis of these wounds is dependent upon re-establishing an adequate inflow into the extremity. Similar to the moderate response shown by arterial insufficiency ulcers, radiation ulcers and wounds in irradiated tissue respond very slowly to the V.A.C. system. Wounds which have been traditionally considered to develop into chronic wounds include envenomation and extravasation wounds. These wounds respond very well to the V.A.C. system (37,38).

Pressure sores also respond favorably to treatment with the V.A.C. system (33–35). Pressure sores in paraplegic patients in general respond more quickly and heal more rapidly than pressure sores in older, debilitated patients. This is both a function of age and usually nutritional status. In the acute setting, it is also possible to control the use of drugs and alcohol, which frequently confounds treatment of the younger spinal cord-injured patients. Care must be taken in this patient population as the patient may lie on the evacuation tubing and/or the associated tube clamp, resulting in an additional pressure sore.

A final note about patients with nonhealing wounds. Patients with iatrogenic wounds routinely will refuse treatment with the V.A.C. system, as it is a controlled, closed system and any tampering of the wound is quickly evident from the disrupted drape.

5. SUBACUTE WOUNDS

Subacute wounds are wounds such as dehisced incisions, necrotizing fasciitis, and other wound breakdowns. With dehisced incision, no new tissue is necessary to close the wound. Usually, the edges of these wounds are edematous and woody and the extra volume prevents the edges of the wound from being opposed to allow for fibrovascular growth across the gap. The constant application of vacuum with the V.A.C. system removes this excess edema, allowing for the opposing edges to drawn into contact and held in place until new tissue can bridge the gap. Unlike closure with sutures, there is not a change for the suture to break or for the suture to pull through the friable tissue at the edges of the wound. The V.A.C. system has shown to be particularly effective for the treatment of sternal wound dehiscences (39–41) (Fig. 2). When used for treatment of sternal dehiscences, care should be used when the heart is exposed.

Patients with necrotizing fasciitis should be debrided and examined daily to ensure that the infected areas have not progressed (42). The V.A.C. system promotes granulation tissue and allows for earlier coverage with split thickness skin grafts. The V.A.C. system also may be applied circumferentially on extremities without creation of a tourniquet effect (Fig. 3). With application of the vacuum, the foam dressing is

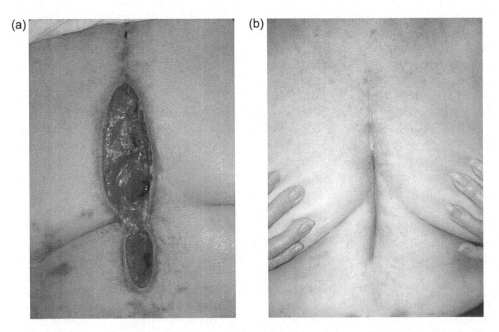

Figure 2 Dehisced sternal wound in 57-year-old female patient post-CABG. Due to the size and weight of the patient's breasts, the wound dehisced. The V.A.C. system was used at 125 mm Hg continuous vacuum for 6 weeks until the wound was totally healed. (a) Pretreatment; (b) post-treatment.

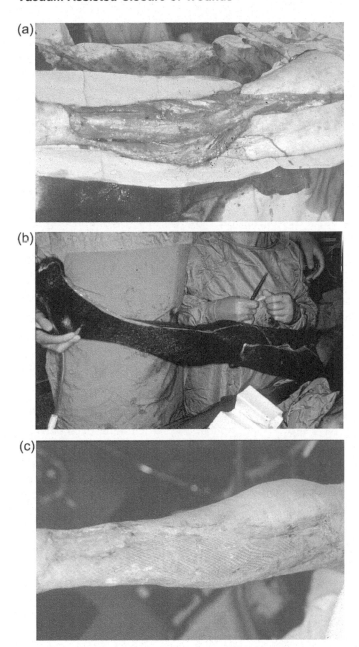

Figure 3 Necrotizing fasciitis wound on posterior of right leg of 84-year-old female patient. (a) The calf and popliteal were debrided and the posterior thigh filleted open. (b) The V.A.C. was placed circumferentially on the extremity. (c) The wound was treated for 3 weeks, at which time the posterior calf and popliteal area were covered with a split thickness skin graft and the thigh incision was closed primarily.

pulled down to the dressing/wound interface while the underlying tissues are pulled up to the dressing/tissue interface with the net effect on the tissues being zero force. This may be adversely affected by the tubing, connectors, or the tubing clamp, all of which may cause pressure problems if they are in weight-dependent positions.

6. ACUTE WOUNDS

Acute wounds respond extremely well to the V.A.C. system. These patients generally are younger and in better health than the patients with chronic wounds. Wounds such as large tissue avulsions and gunshot injuries are surrounded by a "shock zone," which is similar to the zones surrounding a burn injury. It is not unusual to remove several liters of fluid a day during the first few days of treatment with the V.A.C. system. The system is very effective in promoting granulation tissue, which can rapidly cover exposed hard structures, such as bone and tendon, and also orthopedic hardware (Fig. 4). It also reduces the edema in extremities, and may allow for earlier approximation of wound edges than otherwise possible (Fig. 5). Pediatric trauma patients produce granulation tissue at an extremely rapid rate, with the dressing usually requiring daily changes even with the use of a nonadherent intervening layer (43). Failure to change the foam dressing at appropriately short intervals may result in granulation tissue growth into the foam dressing. If ingrowth occurs, removal of the dressing is painful, disrupts the capillary buds, and can cause significant loss of blood due to oozing.

The V.A.C. system can be used for two different reasons for the treatment of burns. The first is to prevent progression of the burn injury in the hours immediately postburning. Animal studies have shown that application of vacuum to deep partial thickness burn wounds within 6 hr of injury prevented the burn from progressing as measured by depth of cell death (44). The effectiveness in the applied vacuum to prevent progression of the injury decreased at the time interval between injury and application increased. The V.A.C. system also is effective in promotion of

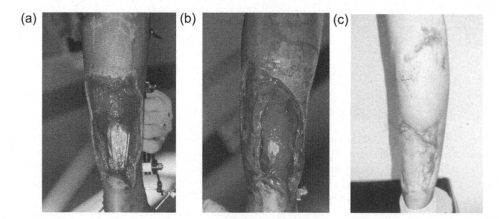

(a)   (b)   (c)

Figure 4 Avulsion injury with exposed Achilles' tendon in 27-year-old female patient who was thrown from the motor vehicle in an accident. No local donor site was acceptable for flap rotation. (a) Pretreatment. (b) After 3-week treatment with V.A.C. system immediately prior to coverage with a split thickness skin graft. The Achilles' tendon is 90% covered with granulation tissue. (c) Six-month follow-up.

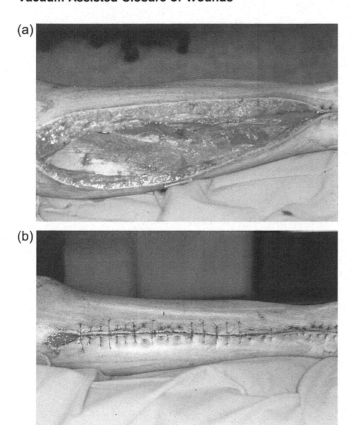

Figure 5 A 14-year-old male patient was shot in the hip region and developed a compartment syndrome in the lower part of the extremity. (a) Releasing incisions were made medial and lateral to relieve pressure. (b) Wound was closed primarily 1 week after creation of releasing incisions.

granulation tissue formation postescharotomy in preparing the wound bed to accept a split thickness skin graft.

The V.A.C. is routinely used as a bolster over both full thickness and partial thickness skin grafts at our institution (45–48) (Fig. 6). The graft is meshed or fenestrated to allow fluid egress. An intervening nonadherent layer is usually placed over the graft, then the V.A.C. dressing is sealed in place. Continuous vacuum is applied at the same pressure that was used to prepare the wound for grafting for 4 days. The common reasons for loss of skin grafts are fluid collection, shear forces, and infection. The V.A.C. system removes the fluid, is mechanically stable when under vacuum, and increases blood flow, thus decreasing bacterial load.

7. SUMMARY

The V.A.C. is an effective addition to the armamentarium for treatment of wounds. As with all wound care, wounds must be debrided of necrotic tissue. The foam

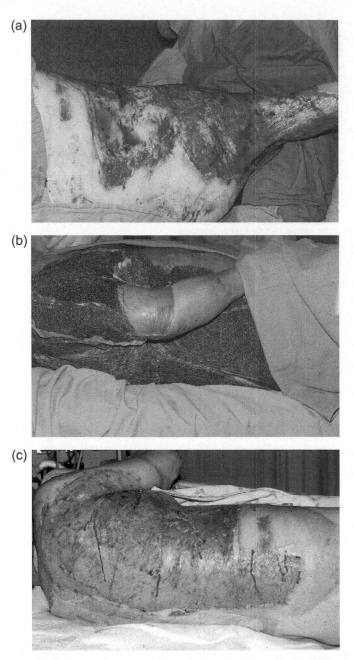

Figure 6 Fifty-eight-year-old female patients suffered from a burn injury of right trunk, axilla, and shoulder region. The wound was debrided and treated with the V.A.C. system prior to placement of split thickness skin grafts. The V.A.C. system was used for 5 days to hold skin grafts in place. (a) Prior to excision; (b) collapsed V.A.C. dressing in place over split thickness skin grafts; (c) appearance of grafts immediately after V.A.C. dressing removal. Some blood is present from disturbed staples.

dressing trimmed to the size of the wound. The site is sealed with a thin film dressing and a controlled vacuum applied. The dressing is normally changed at 48-hr intervals. A significant amount of fluid may be removed, and the mechanical deformation of the cells anchored in the surrounding tissues stimulates proliferation. While no technique will heal all wounds, the V.A.C. system has shown the ability to successfully treat a wide variety of chronic, subacute, and acute wounds.

REFERENCES

1. Montagna W, Yun JS. The skin of the domestic pig. J Invest Dermatol 1963; 41:11–21.
2. Meyer W, Schwartz R, Neurand K. The skin of the domestic animals as a model for the human skin with special reference to the domestic pig. Curr Prob Dermatol 1979; 7: 39–52.
3. Bartek MJ, LaBudde JA, Maibach HI. Skin permeability in vivo: comparison of rat, rabbit, pig and man. J Invest Dermatol 1972; 58:114–123.
4. Morykwas MJ, Argenta LC, Shelton-Brown EI, McGuirt W. Vacuum assisted closure: a new method for wound control and treatment—animal studies and basic foundation. Ann Plast Surg 1997; 38:553–562.
5. Lightfoot EN. The roles of mass transfer in tissue function. In: Bronzino JD, ed. The Biomedical Engineering Handbook. Boca Raton: CRC Press, 1995:1656–1670.
6. Nachtrieb NH. Diffusion in liquids. In: Besancon RM, ed. The Encyclopedia of Physics. New York: Reinhold Publishing Corp, 1996:168–709.
7. Wilke CR. Diffusion in gases and liquids. In: McGraw-Hill Encyclopedia of Science and Technology. 6th ed. New York: McGraw-Hill Book Company, 1987:222–226.
8. Falanga V. Growth factors and chronic wounds: the need to understand the microenvironment. J Dermatol 1992; 19:667–672.
9. Bucalo B, Eaglstein WH, Falanga V. Inhibition of cell proliferation by chronic wound fluid. Wound Repair Regen 1993; 1:181–186.
10. Wysocki AB, Staiano-Coico L, Grinnell F. Wound fluid from chronic leg ulcers contains elevated levels of metalloproteinases MMP-2 and MMP-9. J Invest Dermatol 1993; 101:64–68.
11. Wysocki AB, Grinnell F. Fibronectin profiles in normal and chronic wound fluid. Lab Invest 1990; 63:825–831.
12. Grinnell F, Ho CH, Wysocki A. Degradation of fibronectin and vitronectin in chronic wound fluid: analysis by cell blotting, immunoblotting, and cell adhesion assays. J Invest Dermatol 1992; 98:410–416.
13. Yager DR, Nwomeh BC. The proteolytic environment of chronic wounds. Wound Repair Regen 1999; 7:433–441.
14. Thoma R. Ueber die histomechanik des gefassystems und die pathogenese der angiosklerose. Virchow Arch f Path Anat 1911; 204:1–74.
15. Ilizarov GA. The tension–stress effect on the genesis and growth of tissues. Part I. The influence of stability of fixation and soft-tissue preservation. Clin Orthop Related Res 1989; 238:249–281.
16. Ilizarov GA. The tension–stress effect on the genesis and growth of tissues. Part 2. The influence of the rate and frequency of distraction. Clin Orthop Related Res 1989; 239:263–285.
17. Argenta LC, Marks MW. Tissue expansion. In: Georgiade N, ed. Essentials of Plastic, Masillofacial and Reconstructive Surgery. 2nd ed. Baltimore: Williams and Wilkins, 1990:103–113.
18. Urschel JD, Scott PG, Williams HTG. The effect of mechanical stress on soft and hard tissue repair: a review. Br J Plast Surg 1988; 41:182–186.
19. Gumbiner BM. Cell adhesion: the molecular basis of tissue architecture and morphogenesis. Cell 1996; 84:345–357.

20. Huang S, Ingber DE. The structural and mechanical complexity of cell-growth control. Nat Cell Biol 1999; 1:E131–E138.
21. Ingber DE, Dike L, Hansen L, Karp S, Liley H, Maniotis A, McNamee H, Mooney D, Plopper G, Sims J, Wang N. Cellular tensegrity: exploring how mechanical changes in the cytoskeleton regulate cell growth, migration, and tissue pattern during morphogenesis [rev]. Int Rev Cytol 1994; 150:173–224.
22. Ruoslahti E. Stretching is good for a cell. Science 1997; 276:1345–1346.
23. Takei T, Han O, Ikeda M, Male P, Mills I, Sumpio BE. Cyclic strain stimulates isoform-specific PKC activation and translocation in cultured human keratinocytes. J Cell Biochem 1997; 67:327–337.
24. Vandenburgh HH. Mechanical forces and their second messengers in stimulating cell growth in vitro. Am J Physiol 1992; 262(3 Part 2):R350–R355.
25. Wirtz HRW, Dobbs LG. Calcium mobilization and exocytosis after one mechanical stretch of lung epithelial cells. Science 1990; 250:1266–1269.
26. Sumpio BE, Banes AJ, Letton RL, Levin LG, Johnson G. Mechanical stress stimulates aortic endothelial cells to proliferate. J Vasc Surg 1987; 6:252–256.
27. Sadoshima J, Izumo S. Mechanical stretch rapidly activates multiple signal transduction pathways in cardiac myocytes: potential involvement of an autocrine/paracrine mechanism. EMBO 1993; 12:1681–1692.
28. Sadoshima J, Takahashi T, Jahn L, Izumo S. Roles of mechano-sensitive ion channels, cytoskeleton, and contractile activity in stretch induced immediate–early gene expression and hypertrophy of cardiac myocytes. PNASUSA 1992; 89:9905–9909.
29. Baudouin-Legros M, Paquet J, Brunelle G, Meyer P. Role of nuclear proto-oncogenes in the proliferation of aortic smooth muscle cells in spontaneously hypertensive rats. J Hypertens 1989; 7:S14–S15.
30. Chen KD, Li YS, Kim M, Li S, Yuan S, Chien S, Shyy JYL. Mechanitransduction in response to shear stress—roles of receptor tyrosine kinases, integrins, and Shc. J Biol Chem 1999; 26:18393–18400.
31. Jalali S, del Pozo MA, Chen K, Miao H, Li Y, Schwartz MA, Shyy JY, Chien S. Integrin-mediated mechanotransduction requires its dynamic interaction with specific extracellular matrix (ECM) ligands. PNASUSA 2001; 98:1042–1046.
32. Chen BPC, Li Y, Zhao Y, Chen K, Li S, Lao J, Yuan S, Shyy JY, Chien S. DNA microarray analysis of gene expression in endothelial cells in response to 24-hr shear stress. Physiol Genomics 2001; 7:55–63.
33. Argenta LC, Morykwas MJ. Vacuum assisted closure: a new method for wound control and treatment—clinical experience. Ann Plast Surg 1997; 38:563–577.
34. Joseph E, Hamori CA, Bergman S, Roaf E, Swann NF, Anastasi GW. A prospective randomized trail of vacuum-assisted closure versus standard therapy of chronic nonhealing wounds. Wounds 2000; 12:60–67.
35. Mendez-Eastman S. When wounds won't heal. RN 1998; 61:20–24.
36. Armstrong DG, Lavery LA, Abu-Rumman P, Espensen EH, Vazquez JR, Nixon BP, Boulton AJM. Outcomes of subatmospheric pressure dressing therapy on wounds of the diabetic foot. Ostomy/Wound Manage 2002; 48:64–68.
37. Morykwas MJ, Kennedy AC, Argenta JP, Argenta LC. Use of subatmospheric pressure to prevent doxorubicin extravasation ulcers in a swine model. J Surg Oncol 1999; 72: 14–17.
38. von Gros CME, Horch RE. Rapid aggressive soft-tissue necrosis after beetle bite can be treated by radical necrectomy and vacuum suction-assisted closure. J Cutan Med Surg 2000; 4:219–233.
39. Obdeijn MC, de Lange MY, Lichtendahl DHE, de Boer WJ. Vacuum-assisted closure in the treatment of poststernotomy mediastinitis. Ann Thorac Surg 1999; 68:2358–2360.
40. Hersh RE, Jack JM, Dahman MI, Morgan RF, Drake DB. The vacuum-assisted closure device as a bridge to sternal wound closure. Ann Plast Surg 2001; 46:250–254.

41. Gustafsson R, Johnsson P, Algotsson L, Blomquist S, Ingemansson R. Vacuum assisted closure therapy guided by C-reactive protein levels in patients with deep sternal infection. J Throc Cardiovasc Surg 2002; 123:895–900.

42. Kovacs LH, Kloeppel M, Papadapulos NA, Reeker W, Biemer E. Necrotizing fasciitis. Ann Plast Surg 2001; 47:680–681.

43. Mooney JF, Argenta LC, Marks MW, Morykwas MJ, DeFranzo AJ. Treatment of soft tissue defects in pediatric patients using the V.A.C. system. Clin Orthop Rel Res 2000; 376:26–31.

44. Morykwas MJ, David LR, Schneider AM, Whang C, Jennings DA, Canty C, Parker D, White WL, Argenta LC. Use of the V.A.C. to prevent progression of partial thickness burns in a swine model. J Burn Care Rehabil 1999; 20:15–21.

45. Genecov DG, Schneider AM, Morykwas MJ, Parker D, White WL, Argenta LC. A controlled sub-atmospheric pressure dressing increases the rate of skin graft donor site reepithelialization. Ann Plast Surg 1998; 40:219–225.

46. Schneider AM, Morykwas MJ, Argenta LC. A new and reliable method of securing skin grafts to the difficult recipient bed. Plast Reconst Surg 1998; 102:1195–1198.

47. Scherer LA, Shiver S, Chang M, Meredith JW, Owings JT. The vacuum assisted closure device: a method of securing skin grafts and improving graft survival. Arch Surg 2002; 137:930–933. Discussion 933–934.

48. Molnar JA, DeFranzo AJ, Marks MW. Single-stage approach to skin grafting the exposed skull. Plast Reconstr Surg 2000; 105:174–177.

39

Pressure Off-Loading Devices in the Treatment of Pressure Ulcers

Cathy Thomas Hess
Clinical Operations, Wound Care Strategies, Inc., Harrisburg, Pennsylvania, U.S.A.

1. INTRODUCTION

The number of people in the United States with pressure ulcers is unclear. A monograph on pressure ulcer incidence and prevalence from the National Pressure Ulcer Advisory Panel (1) found a wide range of reported rates, often varying by practice site: incidence, 0.4–38% in general acute care; 2.2–23.9% in long-term care; and 0–17% in home health care; prevalence, 10–18% in general acute care; 2.3–28% in long-term care; and 0–29% in home health care. These data should be viewed with caution, however, as variations in staging definitions, data sources used, and methodologies make it difficult to compare studies. The best estimates suggest that 2.5 million pressure ulcers are treated annually among hospitalized patients, with total annual costs of hospital-acquired pressure ulcers estimated at $ 2.2 billion to $ 3.6 billion (2).

These figures only tell part of a story. Additional dollars are spent on adjunctive therapies and products to manage the patient with a pressure ulcer. Also, after decades of published data, best practice guidelines, risk assessment tools, research and monies spent for wound care, patients continue to develop pressure ulcers and one has to ask "why."

Understanding how pressure ulcers develop has been well documented in the literature over the decades (3,4). Localized sites of cell death, pressure ulcers occur most commonly in areas of compromised circulation secondary to pressure. They may be superficial, caused by local skin irritation with subsequent surface maceration, or deep, originating in underlying tissue. Deep ulcers may go undetected until they penetrate the skin.

Most pressure ulcers develop when soft tissue is compressed between a bony prominence (such as the sacrum) and an external surface (such as a mattress or the seat of a chair) for a prolonged period. Pressure—applied with great force for a short period or with less force over a longer period—disrupts blood supply to the capillary network, impeding blood flow to the surrounding tissues and depriving tissues of oxygen and nutrients. This leads to local ischemia, hypoxia, edema, inflammation and, ultimately, cell death. The result is a pressure ulcer, also known as a bedsore, decubitus ulcer, or pressure sore.

Shear, which separates the skin from underlying tissues, and friction, which abrades the top layer of skin, also contribute to pressure ulcer development. Contributing systemic factors include infection, malnutrition, edema, obesity, emaciation, multisystem trauma, and certain circulatory and endocrine disorders.

The pathophysiology of pressure ulcer development is documented clearly. Successful pressure ulcer management requires a comprehensive approach that includes prevention, relieving pressure, restoring circulation, managing the wound, and minimizing related disorders. This chapter will focus on the off-loading devices in the management of pressure ulcers, namely support surfaces.

2. MANAGING TISSUE LOADS

Support surfaces (or tissue load management surfaces) are a major therapeutic means to managing pressure, friction, and shear on tissues. In addition, many support surfaces control moisture and inhibit bacterial growth. Support surfaces are available in various sizes and shapes for use on beds, chairs, examination tables, and operating room tables. Used with proper topical skin and wound care, turning, and repositioning, the correct support surface enhances healing of pressure ulcers and helps prevent new ones.

However, the support surface is not the only intervention that should be employed to prevent pressure ulcers from occurring. As exemplified in the Agency for Health Care Research and Quality (AHRQ) [formerly the Agency for Health Care Policy and Research (AHCPR)], effective turning and positioning schedules are the best way to offset pressure in the immobile patient (3). Any individual in bed who is assessed to be at risk for developing pressure ulcers should be repositioned at least every 2 hr if consistent with overall patient goals. A written schedule for systematically turning and repositioning the individual should be implemented. The guidelines also point out that immobile patients who are placed in a sitting position in a chair or wheelchair should be repositioned, shifting the points under pressure at least every hour or be put back to bed if consistent with overall patient management goals. Individuals who are able should be taught to shift weight every 15 min. Other strategies based on published clinical practice guidelines include the following.

- *Positioning Devices.* For individuals in bed, positioning devices such as pillows or foam wedges should be used to keep bony prominences (for example, knees or ankles) from direct contact with one another, according to a written plan.
- *Pressure Relief for the Heels.* Individuals in bed who are completely immobile should have a care plan that includes the use of devices that totally relieve pressure on the heels, most commonly by raising the heels off the bed. Do not use donut-type devices.
- *Side-Lying Positions.* When the side-lying position is used in bed, avoid positioning directly on the trochanter.
- *Bed Positioning.* Maintain the head of the bed at the lowest degree of elevation consistent with medical conditions and other restrictions. Limit the amount of time the head of the bed is elevated.
- *Lifting Devices.* Use lifting devices such as a trapeze or bed linen to move (rather than drag) individuals in bed who cannot assist during transfers and position changes.

Employing these strategies into a comprehensive plan of care addresses the first line of defense for patients at risk for skin breakdown.

The Wound, Ostomy, and Continence Nurses Society (WOCN) (4) have recently published additional strategies.

3. TYPES OF SUPPORT SURFACES

Support surfaces can be divided into two categories: pressure-reducing devices and pressure-relieving devices. A pressure-reducing device for the trochanter or hip lowers pressures below that exerted by a standard hospital mattress or chair surface. A pressure-relieving device relieves pressure at the trochanter or hip below capillary closing pressure (26–32 mmHg). Supportive devices for the heel or special positioning may be needed to eliminate pressure directly on the heel.

Support surfaces can be dynamic, with alternating inflation and deflation, or static, with the pressure load spread over a large area. An algorithm developed by AHRQ can assist the clinician in clinical decisions on the management of tissue loads (Fig. 1) (5).

4. DESCRIPTION OF TISSUE LOAD MANAGEMENT

Understanding the goals for the patient at risk or with actual skin breakdown is the first step to a successful plan. Providing a support surface environment that enhances soft-tissue viability and promotes healing of any pressure ulcers is the first line of defense (5). When the patient is placed on the appropriate support surface, the "tissue load" adequately allocates the distribution of pressure, friction, and shear on the tissues. Further, when the tissue load is distributed evenly, capillary closure pressures (accepted value at 32 mm Hg) are reduced (6). Generally if unrelieved pressures are greater than capillary closure pressure, pressure ulcers develop.

Support surfaces can be divided into two main categories: pressure-reducing and pressure-relieving devices. A pressure-reducing device is defined by the AHRQ guidelines as reduction of interface pressure, not necessarily below the level required to close capillaries. The pressure-reducing device lowers pressure compared to the standard hospital mattress or chair surface. However, it does not consistently reduce pressures below capillary closure pressures. A pressure-relieving device is defined as reduction of interface closing pressure below capillary closing pressures. On most devices, heel pressures are never reduced below capillary closure pressure (7). Supporting the heel from the ankle or calf with foam padding or special positioning or the adjustment of the patient on the support surface eliminates pressure directly on the heel. Unfortunately, patients can develop heel ulcers in any care setting (8) and on the most sophisticated support surfaces. Therefore, frequent turning and repositioning and additional off-loading devices should be implemented with any support surface intervention.

5. TISSUE LOAD MANAGEMENT SURFACES

The support surfaces categories can be broken down into mattress overlays, mattress replacements, and total bed replacements. Each product has features and benefits as well as considerations for its use.

Management of Tissue Loads (5)

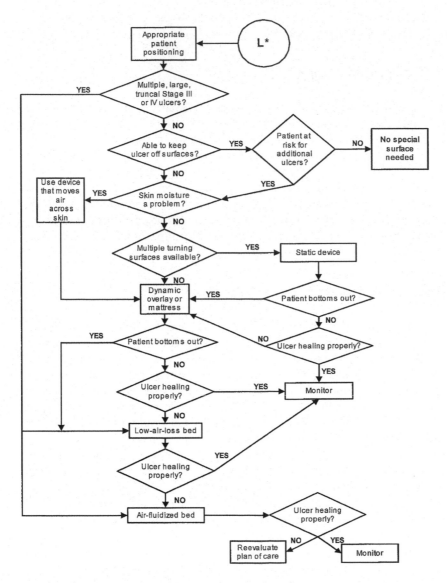

Figure 1 Algorithm for management of tissue loads.

5.1. Foam Mattress Overlays or Mattress Replacements

Many different types of foam products are available on the market today. These products vary by four parameters: density, thickness or base height, indentation load deflection, and modulus (9). Density refers to the amount of foam in the product and its ability to support the patient's weight. Thickness or base height refers to the height of the overlay from the base to where the convolution begins. Indentation load deflection (ILD) indicates the firmness of the foam and modulus is the ratio of 60% ILD to 25% ILD. The support surface should have enough compression resistance to support the weight (or load) of the patient.

The height of a two-inch convoluted foam mattress overlay does not significantly reduce pressures below the standard hospital mattress level and should be used only as a comfort measure. As opposed to two-inch convoluted foam, three-inch and four-inch foam may be an effective device to reduce pressures. These products should be evaluated for effectiveness on an individual basis. This can be accomplished by observing the patient for signs of improvement or deterioration, or by measuring the tissue interface pressures (TIP) if the equipment is available. TIP can be defined as the pressure between the patient's body and the support surface and can be measured using an electropneumatic sensor (10). Considerations for this product include the need to monitor moisture as it is not always controlled on a foam surface and there is no therapeutic benefit when used in conjunction with overlays.

5.2. Static Air Mattress Overlays and Mattress Replacements

The static air mattress overlays are filled with air using an inflating device, such as a hand-held pump. It is critical that the mattress overlay be monitored for inflation using a hand check. To perform this task, the practitioner places a hand (palm up) under the overlay and directly below the patient's bony prominence. In accordance with the AHRQ guidelines, if the practitioner feels less than an inch of support material, the patient has bottomed out and the support surface is inadequate. The air mattress replacements reduce interface pressure and replace the standard hospital mattress. These products can be manufactured in combination with other materials, such as foam. They may have removable shapes with the mattress. The recommended height is not less than 5 in. The products generally have a waterproof cover to reduce shear and friction. Considerations include proper inflation for optimal effectiveness, slippery surface may cause a patient to slide down or out of the bed, and sharp objects may damage the surface.

5.3. Alternating Air Mattress Overlays and Mattress Replacements

Dynamic motion of an alternating air mattress overlay and mattress, alternating inflation and deflation of the tubules, is used to prevent constant pressure against skin and enhance blood flow. These interconnected cells or tubules are inflated with an electric pump. Configuration of the system's chambers allows for cyclical changes in pressure within different chamber, creating a low- and high-pressure area. The cell depth of the overlay is recommended more than 3 in. Alternating air pressure mattresses recommended depth is not less than 5 in. The considerations for both products are its dependence on electricity. Proper inflation is also necessary for optimal effectiveness. Additionally, sharp objects may damage the product and the sensation of inflation and deflation may bother the patient.

5.4. Gel and Water Products as Overlays and Mattress Replacements

These products are either filled with gel or water. Though heavy in weight, they require little maintenance and are easy to clean. Gel products provide flotation with pressure reduction and may be manufactured in combination with foam. The recommended depth is no less than 2 in. The considerations of gel mattresses are that some surfaces may be slippery and proper inflation is necessary for optimal effectiveness. Additionally, limited clinical research has been done to evaluate their effectiveness.

Water products provide lower interface pressure than standard hospital mattresses and the recommended depth is not less than 3 in. The disadvantages of water mattresses are that fluid motions can make procedures and patient transfers difficult, precautions are needed to prevent microorganism growth and a water heater is required to maintain a comfortable temperature for the patient. Both products are prone to damage in the presence of sharp objects.

5.5. Low-Air-Loss Mattress Overlays and Mattress Replacements

Scales (11) first reported clinical studies of low-air-loss therapy in the early 1970s. These products prevent capillary occlusion by even distribution of weight over a number of cells or pillows, which are usually grouped by zones. Each zone of pillows is inflated with air, based primarily on the patient's height, weight, and body distribution. The flotation depth of each pillow should have a minimum depth of 5 in. This allows patient to float or immerse their bodies in any position on the product and maintain pressure relief. These products provide a generous amount of dry airflow between the patient and the support surface that controls moisture and heat buildup defraying maceration and friction. Low-air-loss settings are adjustable. Low-air-loss mattress replacements are manufactured with interconnected air cells with a minimum depth of at least 5 in. They provide the same benefits as the mattress overlay although some products have adjuvant therapies incorporated in the product. These features include percussion, pulsation, and kinetic therapy. The considerations of either product include a slippery surface that may cause a patient to slide down or out of the bed. Additionally, the motor may be noisy. The low-air-loss product with adjuvant therapy is not recommended for patients who have cervical or skeletal traction. Both products need proper inflation for optimal effectiveness; electricity to maintain inflation and sharp objects may damage the products.

5.6. Total Bed Replacement: Low-Air-Loss Therapy

These products are integrated support surfaces attached to a bed frame. They distribute the patient's body weight evenly over a sequence of pillows inflated with air by a motor. They have interconnected air cells that have a minimum depth of 5 in. Low-air-loss therapy provides a generous amount of dry airflow between the patient and the surface, which controls moisture and heat buildup and prevents maceration and friction. These systems have a dedicated power supply unit. The low-air-loss beds with adjvant features combine other therapies such as pulsation, percussion, and kinetic therapy. The considerations of these products are their slippery surface that may make patient transfers difficult. The slippery surface may also make the patient slide down in bed. The low-air-loss therapy with adjuvant features is not recommended for patients who have cervical or skeletal traction.

5.7. Total Bed Replacement: Air-Fluidized or High-Air-Loss Therapy

Air-fluidized therapy products, originally developed for burn patients in the 1960s, are an integrated system of a support surface attached to a bed frame. This therapy provides a medium that is more dense than water for patients to float on by pumping air through silicon-coated microspheres separated from the patient by a monofilament sheet. Patients float on this surface with capillary readings less than capillary closure. Air-fluidized therapy also has the capability to control large amounts bodily fluids, exudates, or drainage from the wound and is an excellent product for post-op flap and burn patients. This product, like all other support surfaces, has considerations for use. They are not recommended for mobile patients, patients with pulmonary disease, or patients with an unstable spine. The continuous circulation of warm, dry air may dehydrate the patient or desiccate the wound bed. The head of the bed cannot be raised. Finally, the weight of the product needs to be taken into consideration when placed in any site of service.

5.8. Seating Devices

If a patient is deemed at risk for skin breakdown (12,13), and the patient will be transferred to a chair or wheelchair during their course of care, the patient should be evaluated for a seating device to prevent skin breakdown or assist in off-loading pressures to a wound(s). These products are generally used in conjunction with a pressure-reducing or pressure-relieving device for the bed. The products may be static or dynamic, powered or non-powered, and constructed of air, a fluid medium, foam, or gel. Considerations for use of these products include evaluation of each patient for correct product choice based on the patient's clinical presentation and reevaluating these products routinely for effectiveness.

5.9. Selecting the Right Surface

There are many factors to consider when selecting a support surface for a patient. The first course of action is to work with a multidisciplinary team to review the patient's status and special needs. Determine if the product considered is pressure-reducing for prevention of pressure ulcers or pressure-relieving for pressure ulcer therapy. Determine the cost parameters based on the patients payer source. Review each product's benefits and considerations. Investigate the rental agreement for the facility as well as the patient's reimbursement source(s). If the patient is Medicare Part B, review the medical policy coverage and payment rules for the specific support surface (14).

   Carefully document the medical necessity for the product ongoing. The documented details are paramount and become the facts for a medical record. Now, words like consents, release of information, compliance with standards, and patient confidentiality are second nature and common in the workplace (15). The clinician understands that the medical record serves as the vehicle for demonstrating the clinician's planning, evaluating, coordination of patient care, and justification for payment.

6. CONCLUSION

Pressure ulcers can be found in all health care settings. Proper procedures and support surfaces need to be implemented upon admission to prevent and treat existing pressure ulcers. But, not all products meet the particular criteria for each individual patient. Therefore, choices must be made carefully. Off-loading devices, such as support surfaces, are not a substitution for nursing and medical care. Effective interventions demand a multidisciplinary team approach that coordinates the needs of the patient.

REFERENCES

1.   Pressure ulcers in America: prevalence, incidence, and implications for the future. An executive summary of the National Pressure Ulcer Advisory Panel monograph. Adv Skin Wound Care 2001; 14:208–215.
2.   Beckrich K, Aronovitch SA. Hospital-acquired pressure ulcers: a comparison on costs in medical vs surgical patients. Nurs Econ 1999; 17:263–271.
3.   Agency for Health Care Policy and Research (AHCPR). Pressure Ulcers in Adults: Prediction and Prevention. Rockville, MD: U.S. Department of Health and Human Services, Public Health Service, AHCPR, 1992 May. Clinical practice guideline; no. 3.
4.   Wound, Ostomy, and Continence Nurses Society (WOCN). Guideline for Prevention and Management of Pressure Ulcers. Glenview, IL: Wound, Ostomy, and Continence Nurses Society (WOCN), 2003.
5.   Bergstrom N, et al. Pressure Ulcer Treatment, Clinical Practice Guideline No. 15, AHCPR Publication No. 95–0652. Rockville, MD: U.S. Department of Health and Human Services, Public Health Service, Agency for Health Care Policy and Research, December 1994.
6.   Landis EM. Micro-injection studies of capillary blood pressure in human skin. Heart 1930; 15:209–228.
7.   Brienza DM, Geyer MJ, Sprigle S. Seating, position and support surfaces. In: Baranoski S, Ayello EA, eds. Wound Care Essentials. Philadelphia, Lippincott: Williams and Wilkens, 2004:184–216.
8.   Wong VK, Stotts NA. Physiology and prevention of heel ulcers: the Ssate of science. J WOCN 2003; 30(4):191–198.
9.   Krouskop T. Scientific aspects of pressure relief. IAET Annual Conference, Washington, DC, 1989.
10. Weaver V, Jester J. A clinical tool: updated readings on tissue interface pressure. Ostomy Wound Manage 1994; 40(5):34–43.
11. Scales JT. Pressure on the patient. In: Kenedi RM, Cowden JM, eds. Bedsore Biomechanics. London: University Park Press, 1976.
12. Braden BJ, Bergstrom N. Clinical utility of the Braden scale for predicting pressure sore risk. Decubitus 1989; 2(3):44–6,50–1.
13. Norton D. Norton scale for decubitus prevention. Krankenpflege (German periodical). 1980; 34(1):16.
14. CMS's Coverage issues manual can be found on the following website: http://cms.hhs.gov/manuals.
15. Hess CT. Clinical Guide to Wound Care 5th ed. Philadelphia, Lippincott: Williams and Wilkens, 2005.

40

Pressure Off-Loading in the Treatment of Diabetic Foot Ulcers

George Tye Liu and John S. Steinberg
Department of Orthopedics, Podiatry Division, The University of Texas Health Science Center, San Antonio, Texas, U.S.A.

From 1990 to 1998, the prevalence of diabetes mellitus has increased from 4.9% to 6.5%—a total increase of 33% (1). Accordingly, the rate of nontraumatic lower extremity amputations, one of the most serious and devastating consequences of chronic diabetes mellitus, has increased proportionately. In 2001, a report of the national hospital discharge surveys from 1997 estimated 87,720 nontraumatic lower extremity amputations related to diabetes (2). Ulceration of the diabetic foot has been recognized as the pivotal event of limb loss primarily through infection or nonhealing (3). Approximately 85% of lower extremity amputations are preceded by a plantar ulceration of the foot, most of which are reported preventable (4,5). A patient with diabetes mellitus has a 15% lifetime risk of developing a foot ulceration (6). Recently, the presence of foot ulceration has been recognized as a marker of disease progression of diabetes associated with increased mortality rates (7).

Several clinical risk factors have been attributed to the development of neuropathic lesions of the diabetic foot. Clinical reports have demonstrated the presence of sensory neuropathy in greater than 80% of diabetic subjects with foot ulcerations (5,8). Additionally, the presence of sensory neuropathy has been associated with an 8- to 15-fold risk of developing a plantar ulcerations in patients with diabetes (3,9). Component aspects of neuropathy contribute to increased ulcer risk. Lack of protective sensation from either singular high grade or repetitive low-grade trauma is attributed to advanced sensory neuropathy. Foot deformity secondary to intrinsic and extrinsic muscular atrophy and imbalance are common manifestations of motor neuropathy. Abnormal focal plantar pressure primarily about the forefoot often ensues since the weightbearing distribution function of the foot has been impaired. Lastly, autonomic neuropathy clinically manifests with dishydrosis and severe xerosis predisposing plantar skin to fissures.

Elevated plantar pressure of the foot has been identified as a significant independent risk factor for plantar ulcerations in a multivariant model (3). Factors surrounding the critical level of plantar foot pressure required to create foot lesions have not been clearly identified (10). Altered focal pressures beneath bony prominences may be attributed to structural abnormalities of the foot due to inherent foot deformities. In addition, muscular imbalance due to neuropathy as described above or charcot neuroarthropathy are noted contributors. Mueller et al. (11) reported ulcerations of submetatarsals two, three, or four with compensated forefoot varus deformities, submetatarsal five ulcerations with uncompensated forefoot varus deformities, and submetatarsal one ulcerations with uncompensated forefoot valgus deformities. Midfoot ulcerations were commonly seen with charcot midfoot collapse (12). Additionally, limited joint mobility secondary to nonenzymatic glycosylation of soft tissues including tendons has been associated with altered gait and elevated focal plantar pressures (13). Biomechanical deformities such as hammertoes and hallux abductovalgus formation in patients with neuropathy often serve as a source for repetitive pressure in tight shoes. Prominent submetatarsal heads due to retrograde force from the proximal phalanx and anterior migration of the fat pad are predisposed to increased pressure and subsequent ulceration. Other factors that are commonly overlooked are the presence of thick mycotic nails and calluses. With tight-fitting shoegear, mycotic nails may serve as a source of pressure against the nail bed creating a subungual lesion. The presence of plantar or dorsal hyperkeratosis may indicate areas of the foot exposed to increased repetitive pressure or shear. Routine plantar callus debridement has been shown to reduce peak plantar pressures between 26% and 30% (14,15).

A history of pathology, including prior amputation or ulceration, contributes to the risk of developing a new ulcer or re-ulceration of previously healed site. The risk is in part due to altered gait patterns and redistribution of plantar pressures commonly encountered after minor amputations of the foot (16–18). Speculatively, a history of pathology may represent the presence of predisposing factors necessary for developing an ulceration. Various reports have indicated that new or recurrent ulceration will occur in 20–58% of patients with previous history (19,20). Subsequent, re-amputation at the foot will occur in approximately in 40% of patients with previous history of foot amputations (21).

Combinations of individual factors have been found to contribute to cumulative risk (3). Patients with only clinical neuropathy were 1.7 times more likely to develop a plantar ulceration. With both neuropathy and deformity, patients were 12.1 times more likely to develop ulceration. Patients with neuropathy, deformity, and history of pathology were 36.4 times more likely to develop a plantar ulceration.

Though clinical studies have shown that abnormal plantar pressure is an independent risk factor for the development of plantar ulcerations, abnormal foot pressures alone may not cause ulcerations (22). Sensory neuropathy has been identified as the permissive factor for plantar ulceration in a deformed foot distributing altered loads.

Mechanical stresses at the level of skin-to-interface contact are ultimately responsible for the creation of neuropathic lesions of the foot. Vertical loads and horizontal shear forces are two component ground reactive forces encountered at the foot surface in normal ambulation. Horizontal shearing forces of the foot comprise approximately 73–80% of the stance phase pressure. This is encountered as a result of both acceleration and deceleration as the lower extremity progresses though the gait cycle (23). Ctercteko et al. (24), in 1981, demonstrated that neuropathic plantar ulcerations occurred at sites of maximal vertical loading. In 1983 Pollard and Le Quesne (25) utilized a shear transducer to show that the site of healed ulcerations corresponded with areas of maximal longitudinal shear force and as well as vertical load.

In addition to mechanical destruction of the skin with exposure to mechanical stresses, vertical and horizontal loading of the foot also has been shown to cause local tissue ischemia. Fromy et al. (26) demonstrated that skin blood flow response to locally applied pressure was significantly delayed in diabetic patients with neuropathy compared to control subjects and diabetic patients without neuropathy. The role of shear forces on ischemic skin breakdown has been identified to have a cumulative effect with vertical loading. Animal studies have shown that vertical pressures of 290 mmHg were required to create ulceration in skin but only 45 mmHg was required to create an ulceration when both pressure and horizontal shear were applied (27). Bennett et al. (28) also demonstrated that the vertical forces required to cause complete occlusion of superficial capillaries of the palm are reduced by 50% when approximately $100 \, g/cm^2$ of force is introduced.

Another factor that can influence tissue breakdown is nonenzymatic glycosylation of keratin, an important structural protein of skin (29). This intermolecular crosslinking of collagen has been purported to produce rigidity and stiffness in skin and subcutaneous tissues. Crossed-linked collagen has been reported to be resistant to normal methods of metabolic degradation by collagenases (30). Clinical studies have demonstrated association between diabetic patients with neuropathy and elevated durometer of plantar skin (31). Loss of resilient properties may compromise plantar skin ability to attenuate horizontal shearing forces encountered during gait leaving it susceptible to breakdown.

The cumulative effect of vertical and shear stresses on the insensate foot is the mechanical factors associated with soft tissue destruction. Propagation of ulcer size is mitigated by the premise coined "edge effect" (32). Ulcers produce a discontinuity of stress through the plantar skin during ambulation thereby causing increased focus stress fields around the periphery of the wound. These destructive shear and vertical forces are heightened at the edges of the ulcer propagating further tissue damage. This prevents the normative reparative process from occurring to achieve successful wound healing. This process was clinically noted by Brand (33) demonstrating that maximal soft tissue damage occurred at the edges of wounds and not the center.

The concept of pressure off-loading may be characterized by the modern adage that it is not what is placed on the wound, but what is taken off that effects successful healing. Clearly, a multitude of treatments may address specific aspects of wound healing; however, if mechanical factors are not addressed, healing of neuropathic wounds may be delayed or halted altogether. Pressure off-loading of ulcers addresses several mechanical etiologies of ulcer formation. Increasing surface area contact of the weightbearing surface of the foot, focal contact pressures may be relieved as they are more evenly distributed to other areas of the foot. By relieving pressure, shear forces are also alleviated as the relationship of the two variables are linear. Material protection of ulcerations from vertical and shear forces may allow a sufficient relief for ulcer healing in the absence of destructive forces and frequent episodes of local ischemia.

The primary and most fundamental aspect of pressure off-loading of the diabetic foot ulceration is debridement. Debridement of diabetic wounds has been shown to improve ulcer healing by removal of chronic fibrotic and necrotic tissues thus converting a problem chronic wound into an acute wound (34,35). However, the unforeseen secondary benefit of debridement is the removal of thick callused tissues of which stiffness contributes to the mechanical destructive stresses across the neuropathic wound. Neuropathic foot ulcerations often present with a peripheral undermined margins of hyperkeratotic tissue representing the wound edge's reaction to repetitive shear stresses by a process known as the "edge effect" (32). Proliferation of this thick and stiff hyperkeratotic wound edge increases the destructive forces causing recurrent and repetitive inflammatory autolysis of the peripheral edge of the ulceration and thus impeding closure. With debridement of this undermined portion of the wound, contributory damaging stresses about the wound are removed allowing granulation and subsequent epithelialization to occur. The hallmark of an adequately debrided and offloaded wound is the absence of peripheral undermining at the wound edges (36). Several studies have specifically evaluated the role of pressure and shear reduction of neuropathic ulcers after debridement, while other clinical studies have demonstrated decreased vertical pressures and shear stresses with debridement at sites of hyperkeratotic callused tissues on the sole of the foot (14,15).

Alteration of biomechanics of the lower extremity has been the focus of design of pressure off-loading devices. However, the second highly important factor of off-loading neuropathic foot ulcers is the insole material selection. The direct absorption of destructive vertical and shear forces is known to occur at the foot–material interface. With abnormal focal pressure distribution secondary to motor neuropathy, foot deformity, and sensory neuropathy, the role of an insole is to be soft enough to maximize the surface area of foot contact, yet stiff and resilient enough to resist material failure and breakdown. In the diabetic neuropathic foot, the role of insole materials is to maximize surface area of contact by conforming to the contours of the sole thus effectively distributing weightbearing forces and diminishing focal pressure concentrations around the ulceration. Traditionally, material selection has been largely subjective and based upon anecdotal evidence. There is little evidence in the literature regarding material selection in the treatment of diabetic neuropathic ulcerations. However, some experimental and clinical studies have attempted to substantiate the utilization of some widely used materials by quantitating their material characteristics. Plastazote is expanded closed-cell polyethylene foam that is available in three densities (#1 medium, #2 firm, #3 rigid) of increasing durometer. PPT is open-cell urethane foam. Pelite is closed-cell, expanded crossed-linked, thermoplastic polyethylene foam also available in graded densities. Sorbothane is a viscoelastic polymer. Spenco is closed-cell neoprene foam with nylon top covering. Ideal materials should maximize surface area of contact to effectively diminish focal areas of vertical pressure and attenuate destructive horizontal shear forces. Laboratory studies evaluating material behavior under cyclic vertical and shear compression tests have shown that the greatest loss in thickness is medium-grade plastazote, second greatest being firm-grade plastazote. However, medium-grade plastazote was also shown to have better force distribution characteristics by dissipating transmitted force better than Spenco, PPT, and Sorbothane. Both findings are consistent with the clinically observed phenomenon of "bottoming out." Softer materials dissipate force but are subjected to rapid material fatigue and failure. PPT was shown as the most durable material resisting permanent deformation in both vertical and shear compression testing and accordingly having a lower force dissipation profile. This characteristic may be advantageous to the lifespan of the material. The inability of a material to conform to the sole of the foot substantially decreases the capacity to attenuate abnormal ground reactive forces (37). Statistically significant reduction in bare forefoot pressures was shown in nondiabetic subjects ambulating on sheets of medium and firm-grade plastazote, Spenco, and PPT (38,39). Clinical studies have demonstrated the effectiveness of accommodative insole materials in the statistical reduction of mean peak plantar pressures in diabetic neuropathic feet (40–42). Lavery et al. (42) reported a statistical reduction of mean peak plantar pressures with a plastazote/urethane insole in various shoes compared to their noninsoled counterparts. The role of combination bi- or tri-laminar materials is unknown; however, utilizing a softer top layer maximizing surface area of contact supported beneath with a firmer material for attenuation of vertical forces has been shown in clinical observations to improve durability of insole lifespan while deforming enough to absorb the abnormal ground reactive forces.

Still the gold standard, the total contact cast (TCC) has been the consensus initial off-loading device for plantar diabetic foot ulcerations. This casting method, which recommends minimal padding to allow the cast to conform to the contours of the foot and leg, was introduced by Paul Brand at the Hansen's Disease Center for the treatment of neuropathic plantar ulcers in patients with leprosy (43). Anatomic molding of casting material against the foot and leg has been shown to increase surface area of contact effectively reducing the focal reactive ground forces (both vertical and shear) at the ulcer site. The mechanism of unloading is attributed to increased proportion of plantar load transferred to the rearfoot, one-third of total load received by the cast walls, and metatarsal off-loading by cavity of soft foam in the forefoot (44). Various studies have demonstrated consistent reduction in plantar pressures and subsequent decrease in healing times with the TCC. Approximately 86% reduction in forefoot pressures was shown in a TCC compared to a cast shoe (44). In a randomized prospective clinical trial, the percentage of diabetic ulcer healing in patients over a 12 week period was 89.5% for the TCC followed by the removable cast walker (RCW) and half-shoe which were shown to be 65.0% and 58.3%, respectively. Accordingly, the average healing time in the TCC, RCW and half-shoe was 33.5, 50.4, and 61.0 days, respectively (45). Success of the TCC in this study was not only attributed to the off-loading capacity but also a significant reduction in the patients' weightbearing activity compared to a below-ankle device.

1. STUDY SHOWING DECREASE IN PRESSURE

Additional benefits of TCC include a reduction of mechanical stress against the ulcerated tissues, edema control through compression, protection from external trauma, forced compliance with the device, and retaining ambulatory functional status. Successful application of the TCC is skill-dependent. Adequate padding must be applied to avoid local skin irritation along bony prominences but excessive padding may lead to poor fit and pistoning within the cast and possibly causing new ulcer formation. Routine changing of the TCC is necessary to inspect the progression of wound healing, to provide local wound care and to ensure continued anatomic fit. The initial application of the TCC is often removed after 3 days and the subsequent casts are removed every 7–10 days. The use of TCCs has been reported in the off-loading of plantar neuropathic ulcerations which are noninfected and nonischemic. Healing rates ranging from 72% to 90% have been reported.

With total contact casting, the inability of physicians to monitor the casted extremity for formation of iatrogenic ulcerations from cast irritation and development of wound infections was a concern of some physicians. In addition, cast technicians or physicians with specific expertise in the application of a TCC are rare. Due to these limitations, other alternative means and devices to off-loading neuropathic ulcerations have been investigated. Removable cast walkers (RCW), a below-knee device like the TCC, have been found to have similar off-loading characteristics in providing the neuropathic ulceration relief from plantar destructive forces. Advantages of this device have been the convenience for routine wound care, access to continue monitoring of the wound, and ease of application. Unna boots or ancillary compression devices to control edema may be used concomitantly with the RCW.

Additionally, its re-usability has made the RCW cost effective when compared to the TCC. Each application of a TCC averages 60–80 dollars in material costs alone, while the average cost of one RCW ranges from 150 to 200 dollars. With an average of five to seven weeks of weekly cast changes and wound care required to heal a neuropathic ulcer, RCW may be considered an expense saving investment. However, it is the removability of this device which has been attributed to patient compliance issues and subsequent delayed healing times of neuropathic ulcerations. Therefore, patient education of their disease process and the fundamental role of these off-loading devices in the treatment of the neuropathic wound are necessary to address potential compliance issues. Lavery et al. determined that there was little difference between the DH Walker (Royce Medical) and TCC in reducing peak plantar pressures for ulcers beneath the hallux, first metatarsal, and lesser metatarsal heads. The study also demonstrated that not all commercially available RCWs have the consistent effectiveness in off-loading neuropathic wounds. The level of pressure reduction in forefoot ulcers with the DH Walker and TCC was shown to be significantly more effective than the 3D Walker, Aircast Walker, and CAM Walker. However, all RCWs were statistically found to reduce forefoot pressures beneath ulcerations better than a therapeutic extra depth shoe. Also, many of the above companies and others have now developed and refined diabetic ulcer off-loading RCWs and these are yet to be tested in the comparison off-loading trial. It is the belief of the authors that many of these refined diabetic RCWs offload more effectively and would compare more favorably to the DH Walker. In a randomized clinical trial, Armstrong et al. was able to achieve 65% healing in a 12 week period with the use of pneumatic RCW. With the reported off-loading effectiveness, cost saving potential and ease of application, RCWs may be considered a practical treatment alternative for primary care providers in addressing neuropathic wounds of the high-risk diabetic patient.

Rocker bottom soles have been shown to alter distribution of plantar pedal pressures. Bauman et al. (46) were one of the first groups to investigate the effect of different rocker sole designs on plantar pressure reduction in the neuropathic foot of leprosy patients. Nawoczenski et al. (47) later demonstrated that curved and pivot rocker soled shoes reduced forefoot pressures in normal subjects. The rocker bottom modifications on standard shoes, healing sandal, and postoperative shoe have been shown to decrease plantar pressures specifically in the forefoot region. The limitation of dorsiflexion at the level of the metatarsophalangeal joint has been shown to limit the progression of weight transfer through the metatarsal head during the toe-off phase of the gait cycle. Thus, the pressure distribution is shared by the forefoot region at a shorter pressure–time integral. Clinical studies in both neuropathic and non-neuropathic patients without ulcers have demonstrated a statistically significant reduction of peak plantar forefoot pressures ranging from 23% to 34% in a rocker bottom sole compared to a standard post-operative flat soled shoe (48,49). Shoe designs with various degrees of forefoot rocker sole designs demonstrated a pressure reduction average of 35–65% beneath the heel and central forefoot. The most effective design possessed a rocking angle of 23 degrees and a rocking point at 65% of the length of the sole reducing forefoot peak pressures by an average of 31% compared to a standard shoe but only the 43% peak pressure reduction in the central forefoot being statistically significant (50). This pressure reduction finding coincided with analysis of gait measures which showed that the maximal reduction of metatarsal head pressure occurred with axis location placed 55–60% of the shoe length (51). In one experimental study, peak pressures in the medial and central forefoot as well as the digital area displayed a reduction by 30% compared to a standard extra-depth shoe, but the pressures were found to be elevated in the heel, midfoot, and lateral forefoot areas (52). This finding coincides with studies which have demonstrated less effective off-loading in the medial and lateral forefoot which clinically may be clinically ineffective for 1st and 5th ray ulcerations commonly seen in cavovarus foot deformities (50,53). In general, indication of use is primarily restricted for forefoot ulcerations only and may be considered an alternative in patients who have severe gait instability with risk of injury from falling with a below-knee off-loading device. However, the authors recommend that shoe type devices be reserved for long-term off-loading of the extremity once ulcer healing has been achieved. Acute ulceration on the plantar surface of the foot will be most effectively off-loaded in a device such as a TCC or RCW which extends above the ankle and onto the leg. It is this characteristic of redistributing the pressure directly from the ground onto the leg which seems to have the most impact in ulcer off-loading/healing.

Many other devices are commercially available for off-loading of the plantar diabetic foot ulceration. These include wedge type shoes, post-operative shoes, custom molded insoles, custom molded sandals, and padding directly applied to the skin surrounding the ulceration. In addition, attempts at using traditional devices such as crutches, walkers, and wheelchairs are common. While many of these devices do reduce pressure at the ulcer site, they are generally not as effective or consistent as the use of a TCC or RCW. Many patients with diabetes do not have the strength, coordination, or balance to utilize crutches and walkers safely. By placing a device such as a TCC or RCW on the affected extremity, the therapeutic benefit will be achieved with every step the patient makes rather than dependent on the patient's compliance to an easily removable device such as a wedge shoe. Patient education and compliance are paramount to a successful treatment plan. Recent data from Armstrong reveal that patients with ulceration take majority of their steps within the home, yet it is common for patients to only wear their off-loading device when ambulating outside the home.

Identification of the cause of pressure has a role in prevention of recurrence. Deformity has been identified as a cumulative risk factor increasing the probability of ulcer development in the diabetic neuropathic foot. In the neuropathic forefoot, deformities such as hammertoes, bunions, and prominent metatarsal heads are subject to contact irritation and subsequent ulcer formation within an ill-fitting shoe. In the Charcot midfoot rockerbottom deformity, central plantar osseous prominence serves as a focal point of pressure. If healing fails with traditional off-loading devices, surgical resection of the osseous prominence or foot reconstruction to alleviate the present deformity may be necessary to relieve the focus of stress. Additionally, recent literature has directed increased importance to the soft tissue balancing that can often be achieved by a simple surgical procedure in the face of a chronic ulceration or increased forefoot pressure. This can include a percutaneous tendo-achilles lengthening or other tendon procedures to address functional gait deformity such as equinus.

The selection of the appropriate off-loading device in the treatment of the diabetic neuropathic ulcer is multifactorial. Concerns that guide this process should include location of ulceration, presence of infection or ischemia, gait stability of the patient, and lifestyle issues. With ulcerations recalcitrant to appropriate off-loading modalities, surgical intervention may be indicated to correct the underlying osseous deformity creating the area of focal tissue destruction.

REFERENCES

1. Mokdad A, Ford ES, Bowman BA, et al. Diabetes Trends in the U.S. 1990–1998. Diabetes Care 2000; 23:1278–1283.
2. Anonymous. Hospital discharge rates for nontraumatic lower extremity amputation by diabetes status—United States, 1997. MMWR—Morbidity & Mortality Weekly Report. 2001; 50:954–958.
3. Lavery LA, Armstrong DG, Vela SA, et al. Practical criteria for screening patients at high risk for diabetic foot ulceration. Arch Intern Med 1998; 158:157–162.
4. Apelqvist J, Ragnarson-Tennval G, Persson U, et al. Diabetic foot ulcers in a multidisciplinary setting: an economic analysis of primary healing and healing with amputation. J Intern Med 1994; 235:463–471.
5. Pecoraro RE, Reiber GE, EM, B. Pathways to diabetic limb amputation: basis for prevention. Diabetes Care 1990; 13:513–521.
6. Palumbo PJ, LJ, M. Peripheral vascular disease and diabetes. Diabetes in America: Diabetes Data Compiled 1984. Washington, DC: U.S. Govt Printing Office, 1985.
7. Boyko EJ, Ahroni JH, Smith DG, et al. Increased mortality associated with diabetic foot ulcer. Diabet Med 1996; 13:967–972.
8. Boulton AJ. Lawrence lecture. The diabetic foot: neuropathic in aetiology? Diabet Med 1990; 7:852–858.
9. Young MJ, Breddy JL, Veves A, et al. The prediction of diabetic neuropathic foot ulceration using vibration perception thresholds. A prospective study. Diabetes Care 1994; 17:557–560.
10. Armstrong DG, Peters EJG, Athanasiou KA, et al. Is there a critical level of plantar foot pressure to identify patients at risk for neuropathic foot ulcerations? J Foot Ankle Surg 1998; 37:303–307.
11. Mueller MJ, Minor SD, Diamond JE, et al. Relationship of foot deformity to ulcer location in patients with diabetes mellitus. Phys Ther 1990; 70:356–362.
12. Armstrong DG, LA, L. Elevated peak plantar pressures in patients who have Charcot arthropathy. J Bone Joint Surg Am 1998; 80:365–369.
13. Fernando DJ, Masson EA, Veves A, et al. Relationship of limited joint mobility to abnormal foot pressures and diabetic foot ulceration. Diabetes Care 1991; 14:8–11.
14. Pitei DL, Foster A, Edmonds M. The effect of regular callus removal on foot pressures. J Foot Ankle Surg 1999; 38:251–255; discussion 306.
15. Young MJ, Cavanagh PR, Thomas G, et al. The effect of callus removal on dynamic plantar foot pressures in diabetic patients. Diabet Med 1992; 9:55–57.
16. Armstrong DG, LA, L. Plantar pressures are higher in diabetic patients following partial foot amputation. Ostomy Wound Manage 1998; 44:30–32, 34, 36.
17. Garbalosa CJ, Cavanagh PR, Wu G, et al. Foot function in diabetic patients after partial amputation. Foot Ankle Int 1996; 17:43–48.
18. Lavery LA, Lavery DC, TL, Q-F. Increased foot pressures after great toe amputation in diabetes. Diabetes Care 1995; 18:1460–1462.
19. Helm PA, Walker SC, GF, P. Recurrence of neuropathic ulceration following healing in a total contact cast. Arch Phys Med Rehab 1991; 72: 967–970.
20. Uccioli L, Faglia E, Monticone G, et al. Manufactured shoes in the prevention of diabetic foot ulcers. Diabetes Care 1995; 18:1376–1378.
21. Armstrong DG, Lavery LA, Harkless LB, et al. Amputation and reamputation of the diabetic foot. J Am Podiatr Med Assoc 1997; 87:255–259.
22. Masson EA, Hay EM, Stockley I, et al. Abnormal foot pressures alone may not cause ulceration. Diabet Med 1989; 6:426–428.
23. Tappin JW, KP, R. Study of the relative timing of shearing forces on the sole of the forefoot during walking. J Biomed Eng 1991; 13:39–42.
24. Ctercteko GC, Dhanendran M, Hutton WC, et al. Vertical forces acting on the feet of diabetic patients with neuropathic ulceration. Br J Surg 1981; 68:608–614.

25. Pollard JP, Quesne LP. Method of healing diabetic forefoot ulcers. Br Med J 1983; 286:436–437.
26. Fromy B, Abraham P, Bouvet C, et al. Early decrease of skin blood flow in response to locally applied pressure in diabetic subjects. Diabetes 2002; 51:1214–1217.
27. Dinsdale SM. Debubitus ulcers: role of pressure and friction in causation. Arch Phys Med Rehab 1974; 55:147–152.
28. Bennett L, Kavner D, Lee BK, et al. Shear vs pressure as causative factors in skin blood flow occlusion. Arch Phys Med Rehab 1979; 60:309–314.
29. Delbridge L, Ellis CS, Robertson K, et al. Nonenzymatic glycosylation of keratin from stratum corneum of the diabetic foot. Br J Dermatol 1985; 112:547–554.
30. Hamlin CR, Kohn RR, JH, L. Apparent accelerated aging of human collagen in diabetes mellitus. Diabetes 1975; 24:902–904.
31. Piaggesi A, Romanelli M, Schipani E, et al. Hardness of plantar skin in diabetic neuropathic feet. J Diabetes Complications 1999; 13:129–134.
32. Armstrong DG, KA, A. The edge effect: how and why wounds grow in size and depth. Clin Podiatr Med Surg 1998; 15:105–108.
33. Brand PW. Other insensitive foot types similar to diabetes. Management of the diabetic foot. Baltimore: Williams and Wilkins, 1987.
34. Attinger CE, Bulan E, Blume PA. Surgical debridement. The key to successful wound healing and reconstruction. Clin Podiatr Med Surg 2000; 17:599–630.
35. Steed DL, Donohoe D, Webster MW, et al. Effect of extensive debridement and treatment on the healing of diabetic foot ulcers. Diabetic Ulcer Study Group. J Am Coll Surg 1996; 183:61–64.
36. Armstrong DG, Lavery LA, Vazquez JR, et al. How and why to surgically debride neuropathic diabetic foot wounds. J Am Podiatr Med Assoc 2002; 92:402–404.
37. Brodsky JW, Kourosh S, Stills M, et al. Objective evaluation of insert material for diabetic and athletic footwear. Foot Ankle 1988; 9:111–116.
38. Leber C, Evanski PM. A comparison of shoe insole materials in plantar pressure relief. Prosthet Orthot Int 1986; 10:135–138.
39. Sanfilippo PB II, Stess RM, Moss KM. Dynamic plantar pressure analysis. Comparing common insole materials. J Am Podiatr Med Assoc 1992; 82:507–513.
40. Ashry HR, Lavery LA, Murdoch DP, et al. Effectiveness of diabetic insoles to reduce foot pressures. J Foot Ankle Surg 1997; 36:268–271; discussion 328–269.
41. Boulton AJ, Franks CI, Betts RP, et al. Reduction of abnormal foot pressures in diabetic neuropathy using a new polymer insole material. Diabetes Care 1984; 7:42–46.
42. Lavery LA, Vela SA, Fleischli JG, et al. Reducing plantar pressure in the neuropathic foot. A comparison of footwear. Diabetes Care 1997; 20:1706–1710.
43. Coleman WC, Brand PW, JA, B. The total contact cast: a therapy for plantar ulceration on insensitive feet. J Am Podiatr Med Assoc 1984; 74:548–552.
44. Shaw JE, Hsi WL, Ulbrecht JS, et al. The mechanism of plantar unloading in total contact casts: implications for design and clinical use. Foot Ankle Int 1997; 18:809–817.
45. Armstrong DG, Nguyen HC, Lavery LA, et al. Off-loading the diabetic foot wound: a randomized clinical trial. Diabetes Care 2001; 24:1019–1022.
46. Bauman J, Girling J, PW, B. Plantar pressures and trophic ulcerations: an evaluation of footwear. J Bone Joint Surg Br 1963; 45:652–673.
47. Nawoczenski DA, Birke JA, Coleman WC. Effect of rocker sole design on plantar forefoot pressures. J Am Podiatr Med Assoc 1988; 78:455–460.
48. Fuller E, Schroeder S, Edwards J. Reduction of peak pressure on the forefoot with a rigid rocker-bottom postoperative shoe. J Am Podiatr Med Assoc 2001; 91:501–507.
49. Giacalone VF, Armstrong DG, Ashry HR, et al. A quantitative assessment of healing sandals and postoperative shoes in off-loading the neuropathic diabetic foot. J Foot Ankle Surg 1997; 36:28–30.
50. Praet SF, Louwerens JW. The influence of shoe design on plantar pressures in neuropathic feet. Diabetes Care 2003; 26:441–445.

51. van Schie C, Ulbrecht JS, Becker MB, et al. Design criteria for rigid rocker shoes. Foot Ankle Int 2000; 21:833–844.
52. Schaff PS, Cavanagh PR. Shoes for the insensitive foot: the effect of a "rocker bottom" shoe modification on plantar pressure distribution. Foot Ankle 1990; 11:129–140.
53. Boyko EJ, Ahroni JH, Stensel V, et al. A prospective study of risk factors for diabetic foot ulcer. The Seattle Diabetic Foot Study. Diabetes Care 1999; 22:1036–1042.

41

Skin Grafting: Surgical Techniques

Yuji Yamaguchi, Satoshi Itami, and Kunihiko Yoshikawa
Department of Dermatology, Osaka University Graduate School of Medicine,
Suita, Osaka-fu, Japan

1. INTRODUCTION

Current surgical alternatives to wound healing by secondary intention include free skin grafts, local flaps, free flaps, tissue expansion, or bioengineered skin equivalents. Among these surgical techniques, free skin grafts are still by far the most reliable method, especially to repair defects caused by skin cancers. Some clinicians may insist that free skin grafts are underused when compared with flaps in plastic and reconstructive surgery, and skin grafts are regarded as old-fashioned procedures. Many cutaneous surgeons, however, choose them to treat skin defects caused by cancers and major trauma because of their ability to act as a window for detecting recurrence of high-risk lesions and their simplicity of use in covering large lesions. Skin grafting has also become a popular method for treating chronic ulcers including venous ulcers, pressure sores, ischemic ulcers, diabetic ulcers, radiation induced ulcers, and wounds caused by collagen diseases. All skin surgeons have their own techniques; however, there are principles that every surgeon must follow. This chapter briefly describes skin grafting in respect to its history, classification, indications, mechanism of take, and individual procedures. We also intend this chapter to be helpful for residents who are about to learn surgical techniques.

2. HISTORY

Skin graft procedures are supposed to have been originated by the Hindu Tilemaker caste approximately 3000 years ago, but Western medicine remained exclusively ignorant of reconstructive surgery until the beginning of the 19th century (1–4), when Baronio, Cooper, Dieffenbach, Leroux, and Buenger were successful with their skin grafts. After Bert's article on animal skin grafting was published in 1863, Reverdin, who published his remarkable and much-cited article on pinch grafts in 1869, Ollier, who reported thin split-thickness skin graft (STSG) in 1872, and Wolfe, who reported on full-thickness skin grafts (FTSGs) in 1875, followed. Thiersch and Krause also reported on the use of thin STSG in 1886 and FTSGs in 1893, respectively. More than 100 years have passed since the great discoveries of these pioneers. Our understanding of skin grafting has progressed along with the rapid development of molecular and cellular biology techniques.

3. CLASSIFICATION AND INDICATIONS

Skin grafts can be classified into three types: full-thickness skin grafts (FTSGs), split-thickness skin grafts (STSGs), and others (Table 1). The FTSGs consist of epidermis and the entire dermis including adnexal structures such as hair follicles, sebaceous glands, and sweat glands. Also, FTSGs contain slight adipose tissue because dermo-subcutaneous fat interface is undulated, similar to epidermo-dermal interface. The STSGs consist of epidermis and a part of dermis. Also, STSGs are subdivided into thin (0.125–0.275 mm), medium (0.275–0.4 mm), and thick (0.4–0.75 mm) depending on the amount of dermis. Others include artificial skin grafts (5,6), which are discussed in Chapter 47, pure epidermal sheet grafts (7–10), and composite grafts, which consist of at least two tissue components such as skin [either pure epidermis, dermis (11), partial-thickness skin, or full-thickness skin], fat, cartilage, muscle, fascia, and bone. Pure epidermal sheet grafts are useful to treat palmoplantar wounds through epithelial–mesenchymal interactions (10) and to treat vitiligo (7,8). Composite grafts are sometimes useful to reconstruct nasal alar rim defects. Composite grafts can be narrowly defined as the combination of full-thickness skin with adipose tissue or cartilage. Such grafts do not take easily because these tissues cannot transport tissue fluid to the grafted dermis and also act as obstacles to revascularization of the graft. Dermal grafts, dermal fat grafts, mucous grafts are also occasionally used for the special component augmentations.

In addition to covering deep skin defects down to the fascia on every site of the body, FTSGs can be used to repair facial defects caused by skin cancers (Table 2). They may be especially useful for covering defects of the nasal tip, nasal dorsum, nasal ala, lateral nasal sidewall, lower eyelid, and ear if there is a suitable recipient site. In general, avascular tissue such as exposed bone, cartilage, tendon, or nerve

Table 1 Classification and Characteristics of Various Skin Grafts

	Composition	Take	Cosmesis	Strength	Donor sites
FTSG	E + D + pF	F	M	M	Nearby site, inguinal
STSG					
Thick	E + pD	F	M	M	Thigh, buttock, etc.
Medium	E + pD	M	F	F	
Thin	E + pD	G	F	F	
Others					
PESG	E	G	M[a]	M[a]	Thigh, buttock, etc.
ASG	E, D, E + D	F	M[a]	M[a]	Inguinal, foreskin
CG	S + F, S + C, etc.	P	M[a]	G	Ear cartilage, etc.
DG	D	M	M[a]	M	Abdomen, etc.
FG	F	F	M[a]	M	Abdomen, etc.
MG	M	M	M[a]	M	Buccal mucosa

FTSG, full-thickness skin graft; STSG, split-thickness skin graft: PESG, pure epidermal sheet graft; ASG, artifical skin graft; CG, composite graft; DG, dermal graft: FG, dermal fat graft: MG, mucus graft; E, epidermis; D, dermis; pD, partial dermis; F, fat; pF, partial fat; S, full-thickness skin: C, cartilage; M, mucosa; P, poor; F, fair, M, moderate; G, good.
[a] The results vary because of limited use.

Table 2 Choice of Treatment for Various Skin Defects

	Skin defect				
	Small shallow	Small deep	Large shallow	Large deep	Larger ($>3\%$) deep
Choice					
2nd Intention	+++	++	++		
Direct closure	++	++			
Local flap	++	+++		+	
PESG	+		+		
STSG	+		++		++ (expand[a])
FTSG		++		++	+ (expand[a])
ASG	+	+	+	+	++
Free flap				+	+
Others				Tissue expansion[b] Cadaver skin graft	Xenograft

2nd Intention, wound healing by second intention; PESG, pure epidermal sheet graft; STSG, split-thickness skin graft; FTSG, full-thickness skin graft: ASG, artificial skin graft.
+, possible; ++, suggested; +++, strongly suggested
[a] Mesh grafting or patch grafting is necessary.
[b] This can be only used when benign tumor resections including scars are planned in advance.

devoid of periosteum, perichondrium, peritenon, or perineurium, respectively, cannot support FTSGs, although small areas may be grafted with the bridging phenomenon. Also, FTSGs can provide relatively good color, texture, and thickness matches for properly selected defects under the proper circumstances. Wound contraction is minimized when skin is grafted to the recipient site where no adipose tissue remains (12).

Although precise mechanistic differences are poorly understood in the survival of STSGs and FTSGs (13,14), STSGs are considered to be effective for the treatment of chronic lower extremity ulcerations because their thinner nature requires less vascular supply (15–17). Skouge (18) has discussed the indications for STSGs in detail. They can cover large skin defects that cannot be repaired by a local flap or would heal too slowly by secondary intention. When the recipient sites are still too large to be covered with autologous STSGs, mesh grafting (19,20) or patch grafting (21) techniques are conventionally used to expand the graft skin. Instead of autologous STSGs, cultured autografts, cultured allografts, allogeneic cadaver skin grafts, or xenografts are also alternatives to treat patients with wounds of large surface area, which generally lack adequate donor tissue for autografts. Although FTSGs are also useful to cover surgical defects in areas at high risk for tumor recurrence as compared with flaps, STSGs are more ideal than FTSGs for detecting recurrent tumors through the grafted skin. The main disadvantages of STSGs over FTSGs are: (a) less optimal cosmetic appearance, (b) the presence of a donor site wound requiring postoperative care, (c) greater contraction when grafted on a deep wound down to fascia, and (d) requirement of the special instrument and equipment to harvest large donor skin.

4. MECHANISM OF TAKE

The mechanism of graft healing can be divided into three phases on the basis of the vascular supply in dermal components: the plasmatic imbibition phase, the inosculatory phase, and the revascularization phase (3,4). During the plasmatic imbibition phase, the transplanted tissues imbibe the wound fluid, gaining up to 40% in weight during the first 24 hr (22). The inosculatory phase marks the occurrence of anastomoses between the vessels of the donor skin and the recipient sites in the dermis, usually at 2 or 3 days postgrafting (3). The revascularization phase is the stage of vascular proliferation with sprouting and budding of vessels in both donor and recipient sites. The mechanism of graft healing thus involves angiogenesis; however, it is difficult to explain the healing mechanism of epidermal grafts including cultured epithelial sheet grafts and pure epidermal sheet grafts obtained by suction blisters or enzymatic treatments. Yamaguchi et al. (12) proposed a fourth phase, keratinocyte activation phase, in the healing process of pure epidermal sheet grafts and STSGs but not FTSGs on the basis of the fact that the epidermis in the grafted thin skin but not full-thickness skin possesses the enhanced expression of β1-integrin, which is one of the adhesion molecules and is associated with cell–matrix adhesion. Furthermore, keratinocytes in the grafted thin skin produce growth factors and cytokines, such as transforming growth factor (TGF)-α, TGF-β, platelet-derived growth factor (PDGF), vascular endothelial growth factor (VEGF), activin, interleukin (IL) -6, and heparin-binding EGF-like growth factor, which may play a role in stimulating wound healing through their pharmacologic properties (23,24). This newly described phase may begin as part of the inosculatory phase and may persist into early revascularization. The enhanced keratinocyte activity in STSG may help explain why STSGs take better than FTSGs in chronic leg ulcers (16) and why prewounding of the donor site augments the stimulatory properties of the donor skin by initiating the healing process prior to grafting (25).

The raw surface areas that grafts cannot cover (this occurs in mesh grafting, patch grafting, or fissures between grafts and surrounding areas) heal by secondary intention, which is divided into three phases: the inflammatory phase, the proliferation phase, and the remodeling phase (26–28). The inflammatory cells, including macrophages, produce various cytokines and lead to the induction of granulation tissue formation, reepithelialization, and wound contraction. Granulation tissue consists of new vessels that migrate into the wound (called angiogenesis or neovascularization) and the accumulation of fibroblasts and dermal matrix (called fibroplasias). Reepithelialization occurs as a consequence of keratinocyte migration and proliferation.

5. PROCEDURES

5.1. FTSGs

Careful preoperative evaluations, meticulous intraoperative techniques, and postoperative care are required for successful FTSGs. Technique is explained in detail showing a typical operative record of a case for FTSGs.

1. Systemic anesthesia was given to treat a 32-year-old man with dermatofibrosarcoma protuberans on the right anterior chest (systemic or local anesthesia can be selected by the size and the location of the wound, the general condition, etc.).
2. Tumor resection caused a skin defect down to fascia approximately 10 cm in diameter. Right cephalic vein was ligated with the use of 4-0 silk. Other miscellaneous vessels were also well coagulated with an electrical coagulator or 4-0 silk ligation because inadequate coagulation causes hematoma.

3. A template of the defect was made by pressing a filter paper. (Any other flexible material will do.) The template was then placed on the donor site, the left inguinal area, devoid of pubic hair. (When the patient is preadolescent, it is very important to presume the hair-bearing area in advance.) Although some articles (3,29) suggest the donor site size must be approximately 3–5% larger than the defect presuming shrinkage, the donor size we took was exactly the same as the recipient size to minimize donor site sacrifice.

4. The donor skin was cut along with the designed outline, using a No. 15 blade scalpel. Defatting of the graft, which is essential for adequate revascularization, was done at the same time excising the donor skin. (Most textbooks say that defatting is performed after the donor skin is excised, but the defatting can be performed while excising the donor skin.) Using a skin hook, the graft was placed on the ring or little finger, dermal side up. Almost all fat was trimmed with sharp iris scissors or with a No. 15 blade scalpel during the harvest of the donor skin. This step prevents unnecessary adipose tissue loss of the donor site.

5. The donor site was closed in a linear-layered fashion. Occasionally, trimming is necessary to remove a dog ear, which can be covered with a triangular local flap.

6. The donor skin was then grafted dermis side down to the recipient bed and was trimmed to provide a perfect fit.

7. 4-0 silk sutures (60 cm) were placed around the periphery at opposite edges of the graft to tie over the dressing. Running 5–0 nylon sutures were then placed between the silk sutures. Several bolster-type anchoring sutures were placed centrally to enhance fixation. The narrow space between the graft and recipient site was washed with isotonic saline solution using a 30-mL plastic syringe connected with an elastic needle to prevent hematoma or seroma, after which Adaptic gauze (Johnson & Johnson, New Brunswick, NJ) with antibiotic ointment was applied. Finally, the rolled gauze was placed and tie-over bolster dressings were placed to immobilize the graft.

8. Because postoperative care is extremely important for the perfect FTSG take, right arm motion including adduction, abduction, flexion, and extension was prohibited for 5 days by using a chest band.

Short-term problems that cause graft failure include hematoma, seroma, infection, and shearing force between the graft and the wound bed. Meticulous hemostasis, pressure dressing, and postoperative care are the keys to avoid hematoma and seroma formation. Oral antibiotics are helpful to prevent infection. Extreme caution is needed to treat patients with diabetes mellitus and severe vasculitis because normal wound healing is retarded in these patients (28). Postoperative care was uneventful in this patient. Half of the sutures were removed at 7 days postgrafting and the remaining half at 14 days postgrafting.

Long-term complications include cosmetic and functional problems. Generally speaking, skin grafts are depressed during their first 2–4 weeks and gradually correct themselves after a couple of months. Hypertrophic scars and keloids sometimes occur especially in Black and Asian individuals, who would need further treatment (30). Functional complications occur as a result of wound contracture, which is especially severe when the graft is placed on a deep skin defect down to fascia of the neck,

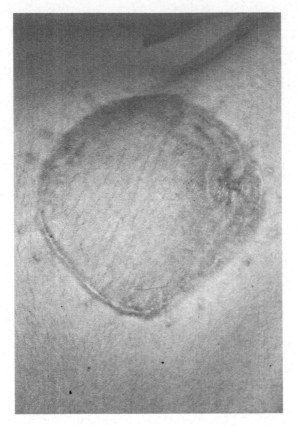

Figure 1 FTSG used to treat a skin defect down to pectoralis major caused by dermatofibro-sarcoma protuberans on the right anterior chest. (Photograph was taken 1 year postgrafting.)

the dorsal hand, the axilla, and the dorsal foot. No recurrence has been seen for 1 year in this patient (Fig. 1).

Figure 2 shows another example of FTSG used to treat a deep skin defect down to fascia caused by malignant eccrine poroma on the right dorsal hand. Post-operative care included immobilization by casting for 1 week after grafting. Similar techniques for FTSGs have been described elsewhere (3,29,31,32).

5.2. STSGs

The technique is similar to that of FTSGs except for the method to obtain the graft (3,16,33). There are generally two types of skin-harvesting methods: a freehand tech-nique using scalpels, razor blades, double edged razor blades (the Weck blade), and knives (the Humby knife and the Blair knife) and a technique using a special device such as a nonelectrical dermatome (e.g., Padgett) or an electrical dermatome (e.g., Brown, Padgett, Zimmer, Davol-Simon). When using the nonelectrical dermatome, it is important to attach the donor skin firmly and evenly to the concave surface of the equipment with glue and to lift the dermatome slightly upward during the oscilla-tion of the dermatome blade so as not to cut the intact skin after applying downward pressure to the donor skin. To use an electrical dermatome, it is important for the surgeon to place tension at the end of the donor site with one hand and to apply firm

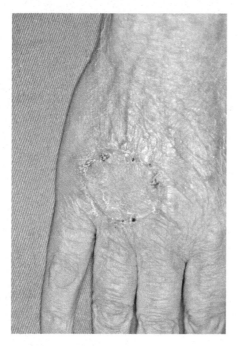

Figure 2 An example of FTSG to treat a skin defect down to fascia caused by malignant eccrine poroma on the right dorsal hand. (Photograph was taken 3 weeks postgrafting.)

downward pressure in an even manner with the other hand. The donor wound can be covered with occlusive dressing therapy (Chapter 50), as it is shallow and heals within a week or two. Mesh grafting (16,19,20) and patch grafting (21) are useful for grafting lower extremity chronic wounds because the raw surface area between the grafts allows fluid and discharge to escape from the underlying wound bed.

Figure 3 shows an example of STSG used to treat a deep skin defect down to buccal muscle caused by basal cell epithelioma that occurred on the left cheek. Compared with FTSG, wound contraction was slightly severe; however, with STSG, the detection of the tumor recurrence is easier because the thin skin acts as a window. In addition, the immobilization of the grafted skin is generally less strict than that of FTSG, with regard to healing time and method of fixation.

5.3. PESGs

The technique is also similar to that of STSGs and FTSGs except for the method of obtaining the graft. There are generally two types of skin-harvesting techniques: an enzymatic treatment (10,12,34,35) and a suction blister roof method (7,8,36). The epidermal sheets can be obtained by incubating split-thickness skin with dispase, the enzyme that separates epidermis from dermis, at 37°C for 30 min. Again, the donor wound can be covered with an occlusive dressing. Details are discussed elsewhere, but the application of this method by us is restricted to the palmoplantar wounds so far (10). Suction blister roof technique is quite commonly used to surgically treat stable vitiligo since Falabella reported it in 1971 (7). A current alternative to a large suction device (or equipment) for harvesting epidermal sheets (36) is a simple device made of two plastic injection syringes and a three-way tap (37). At

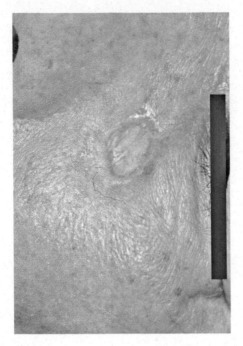

Figure 3 An example of STSG used to a skin defect down to buccal muscle caused by basal cell carcinoma on the cheek.

first, local anesthesia is administered to the donor skin, usually at the abdomen or anterior thigh, to reduce the blister formation time. A piston-removed syringe connected to a three-way tab, then to a larger size syringe, is placed on the donor skin. The larger syringe should have two to three times the suction capacity of the syringe. Negative pressure is created by the connected larger syringe, then the three-way tab is closed immediately to keep inside pressure of the skin-applied syringe negative, and the larger syringe is removed. Continuous negative pressure causes a suction blister to form within an hour, and the blister roof is harvested and grafted as mentioned previously. Quick healing and no scar formation of the doner site are other advantages of this method.

REFERENCES

1.　Davis JS. The history of plastic surgery. Ann Surg 1941; 113:641–656.
2.　Hauben DJ, Baruchin A, Mahler A. On the history of the free skin graft. Ann Plast Surg 1982; 9:242–245.
3.　Johnson TM, Ratner D, Nelson BR. Soft tissue reconstruction with skin grafting. J Am Acad Dermatol 1992; 27:151–165.
4.　Ratner D. Skin grafting. From here to there. Dermatol Clin 1998; 16:75–90.
5.　Phillips TJ. New skin for old: developments in biological skin substitutes. Arch Dermatol 1998; 134:344–349.
6.　Falanga V, Margolis D, Alvarez O, et al. for the Human Skin Equivalent Investigators Group. Rapid healing of venous ulcers and lack of clinical rejection with an allogeneic cultured human skin equivalent. Arch Dermatol 1998; 134:293–300.

7. Falabella R. Epidermal grafting. An original technique and its application in achromic and granulating areas. Arch Dermatol 1971; 104:592–600.

8. Njoo MD, Westerhof W, Bos JD, Bossuyt PM. A systematic review of autologous transplantation methods in vitiligo. Arch Dermatol 1998; 134:1543–1549.

9. Yamaguchi Y, Hosokawa K, Sumikawa Y, Kakibuchi M, Yoshikawa K. The use of autologous and bioengineered epidermis to control fibrosis and improve cosmesis. Wounds 2000; 12:68–75.

10. Yamaguchi Y, Kubo T, Tarutani M, Sano S, Asada H, Kakibuchi M, Hosokawa K, Itami S, Yoshikawa K. Epithelial–mesenchymal interactions in wounds: treatment of palmoplantar wounds by non-palmoplantar pure epidermal sheet grafts. Arch Dermatol 2001; 137:621–628.

11. Schiozer WA, Hartinger A, von Donnersmarck GH, Muhlbauer W. Composite grafts of autogenic cultured epidermis and glycerol-preserved allogeneic dermis for definitive coverage of full thickness burn wounds: case reports. Burns 1994; 20:503–507.

12. Yamaguchi Y, Hosokawa K, Kawai K, Inoue K, Mizuno K, Takagi S, Ohyama T, Haramoto U, Yoshikawa K, Itami S. Involvement of keratinocyte activation phase in cutaneous graft healing: comparison of full-thickness and split-thickness skin grafts. Dermatol Surg 2000; 26:463–469.

13. Gingrass P, Grabb WC, Gingrass RP. Skin graft survival on avascular defects. Plast Reconstr Surg 1975; 55:65–70.

14. Wolfort S, Rohrich RJ, Handren J, May JW. The effect of epinephrine in local anesthesia on the survival of full- and split-thickness skin grafts: an experimental study. Plast Reconstr Surg 1990; 86:535–540.

15. Kirsner RS, Falanga V, Eaglstein WH. The biology of skin grafts. Skin grafts as pharamcologic agents.. Arch Dermatol 1993; 129:481–483.

16. Kirsner RS, Falanga V. Techniques of split-thickness skin grafting for lower extremity ulcerations. J Dermatol Surg Oncol 1993; 19:779–783.

17. Kirsner RS, Eaglstein WH, Kerdel FA. Split-thickness skin grafting for lower extremity ulcerations. Dermatol Surg 1997; 23:85–91.

18. Skouge JW. Techniques for split-thickness skin grafting. J Dermatol Surg Oncol 1987; 13:841–849.

19. MacMillan BG. The use of mesh grafting in treating burns. Surg Clin North Am 1970; 50:1347–1359.

20. Golden GT, Power CG Jr, Skinner JR, Fox JW, Hiebert JM, Edgerton MT, Edlich RF. A technic of lower extremity mesh grafting with early ambulation. Am J Surg 1977; 133:646–647.

21. Gang RK, Arturson G, Hakelius L. The effect of split skin allografts on wound epithelialization from autologous patch grafts. An experimental study in rabbits. Scand J Plast Reconstr Surg 1981; 15:1–4.

22. Converse JM, Uhlschmid GK, Ballantyne DL. "Plasmatic circulation" in skin grafts. The phase of serum imbibition. Plast Reconstr Surg 1969; 43:495–499.

23. Martin P. Wound healing—aiming for perfect skin regeneration. Science 1997; 276: 75–81.

24. Regauer S, Compton CC. Cultured keratinocyte sheets enhance spontaneous re-epithelialization in a dermal explant model of partial-thickness wound healing. J Invest Dermatol 1990; 95:341–346.

25. Kirsner RS, Falanga V, Kerdel FA, Katz MH, Eaglestein WH. Skin grafts as pharmacological agents: pre-wounding of the donor site. Br J Dermatol 1996; 135:292–296.

26. Kirsner RS, Eaglstein WH. The wound healing process. Dermatol Clin 1993; 11:629–640.

27. Singer AJ, Clark RAF. Cutaneous wound healing. N Engl J Med 1999; 341:738–746.

28. Yamaguchi Y, Yoshikawa K. Cutaneous wound healing: an update. J Dermatol 2001; 28:521–528.

29. Branham GH, Thomas JR. Skin grafts. Otolaryngol Clin North Am 1990; 23:889–897.

30. Munro KJ. Treatment of hypertrophic and keloid scars. J Wound Care 1995; 4:243–245.

31. Petruzzelli GJ, Johnson JT. Skin grafts. Otolaryngol Clin North Am 1994; 27:25–37.
32. Ablove RH, Howell RM. The physiology and technique of skin grafting. Hand Clin 1997; 13:163–173.
33. Valencia IC, Falabella AF, Eaglstein WH. Skin grafting. Dermatol Clin 2000; 18:521–532.
34. Hosokawa K, Hata Y, Yano K, Matsuka K, Ito O. Treatment of tattoos with pure epidermal sheet grafting. Ann Plast Surg 1990; 24:53–60.
35. Yamaguchi Y, Itami S, Tarutani M, Hosokawa K, Miura H, Yoshikawa K. Regulation of keratin 9 in nonpalmoplantar keratinocytes by palmoplantar fibroblasts through epithelial–mesenchymal interactions. J Invest Dermatol 1999; 112:483–488.
36. Kiistala U, Mustakallio KK. In-vivo separation of epidermis by production of suction blisters. Lancet 1964; 1:1444–1445.
37. Gupta S, Kumar B. Suction blister induction time: 15 minutes or 150 minutes? Dermatol Surg 2000; 26:754–756.

42

Cultured Skin Substitutes

Markéta Límová
Department of Dermatology, University of California San Francisco, San Francisco, California, U.S.A.

1. INTRODUCTION

Loss of skin coverage is a significant challenge for the clinician as well as a major medical problem in our society and the western world. Whether it is acute wounds due to surgery or a burn, chronic wounds such as venous, diabetic or decubitus ulcers, or from other causes, these all have a tremendous impact on the cost of medical care (1,2).

Significant progress has been made in our understanding of wound healing (3–6). Various synthetic occlusive dressings have been developed over the last several decades which are based upon the concept of moist wound healing and can be broadly divided into several categories by their chemical composition and physical properties (7–10). However, even with these materials being widely available, there are still wounds that for one reason or another do not heal no matter how hard one tries to optimize the wound environment. Also, these dressings do not provide the permanent coverage and protection from the environment in instances when the wound is simply too large to epithelialize from the periphery and where the depth of injury has eliminated all appendigeal structures.

With our increased understanding of wound healing pathophysiology, efforts have been dedicated to improving and stimulating wound healing with biologically active materials. These include various individual growth factors or a mixture of growth factors that could be used as a pharmacological agent, animal derived skin-type coverings as well as artificially produced living human tissue. These biosynthetic skin substitutes have allowed clinicians to treat patients with large body surface area defects, difficult to treat ulcerations and other chronic wounds without rejection, creation of a secondary donor site wound, as well as help reduce scarring of the wound bed. A variety of epidermal, dermal, and composite skin substitutes are beginning to be available on the market today and a number are still in the process of development (11–13). In this chapter, we will focus on the various bioengineered human skin substitutes and their role in healing acute and chronic wounds.

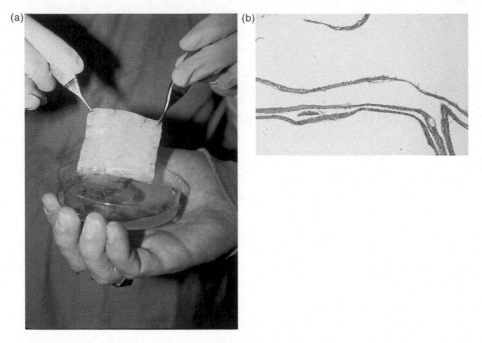

Figure 1 Cultured keratinocyte autograft. (Courtesy of the author.) (a) Thin sheet of cells mounted onto petrolatum impregnated gauze. (b) Microscopic appearance; sheets are only a few cell layers thick.

2. CULTURED EPIDERMAL GRAFTS

For many years, the "gold standard" of wound closure has been the autologous skin graft. Unfortunately, in patients with massive burns, the availability of donor sites is limited. Also, harvesting skin grafts creates secondary wounds which can lead to additional complications and scarring. Scientists have attempted to culture human and other mammalian tissues, including human keratinocytes, since the 1950s. Unfortunately, the initial attempts produced only small colonies of cells and it was not until 1975 when Rheinwald and Green (14) described a new way of culturing human keratinocytes, which allowed rapid expansion of the original sample several thousand fold; in essence from two to three square centimeters of skin one could grow between one and two square meters of human epidermis.

The technique involves taking a small skin biopsy which is processed to yield a single cell keratinocyte suspension. This is then inoculated onto a layer of irradiated 3T3 mouse fibroblasts, incubated in a growth medium with various supplements until the cells reach confluence and the process is repeated several times. The final cultured sheets are enzymatically released from the support surface, attached to a petrolatum impregnated gauze and are ready to be placed on the wound as shown in Figure 1. Since the original report, variations on the technique have been developed in order to improve efficiency (15,16). Cultured epithelial autografts (CEAs) are commercially available in the United States under the name Epicel (Genzyme Biosurgery, Cambridge, MA).

The first attempt to use CEAs in clinical practice was in 1980 in an adult burn patient (17). This technique was shown to be life saving in 1981 when these grafts were used to treat 97–98% body surface burns in two pediatric patients, a condition which, without this skin substitute, would have been uniformly fatal (18).

Since that time, hundreds of patients have been treated with CEAs in burn units in this country and around the world (19–21). These grafts not only have been shown to stimulate wound healing, but can provide permanent epidermal coverage in wounds where no other source of intrinsic keratinocytes exists such as full thickness burns below the level of epidermal appendages. In patients with large total body surface area burns, CEAs have improved their survival to over 85% even in instances where previously they would have had a uniformly fatal outcome (Genzyme Biosurgery data on file). Many clinicians will agree that ultimately the cosmetic appearance of these grafts is equal or better than split-thickness skin grafts, even though initially they are quite fragile and susceptible to shear injury and infection. The "take" of these grafts has been reported to be anywhere from less than 20% to 100% and is dependent on the condition of the wound bed, postoperative care and clinician's technique. Also, graft placement may have to be repeated several times to achieve complete coverage and healing.

Importantly, CEAs need to be applied to a clean and well-vascularized wound bed. While the tissue culture is in process, the burn eschar is excised and the wound is covered with a cryopreserved dermal substitute or a bioengineered dressing that functions as a temporary skin covering (22–27). These materials not only protect the wound while the CEAs are being grown, but help also provide some permanent dermal replacement, which improves the final graft take and functional results. The CEAs are relatively simple to use; they are placed onto the wound along with the supporting petrolatum gauze as close together as possible and secured in place with sutures or staples. The wound is then dressed with a nylon mesh and absorbent gauze dressings which are changed as necessary. During the postoperative period, it is important to avoid mechanical trauma and friction as well as various antiseptic agents which can be toxic to the graft (28). The gauze backings are removed after 7–10 days and the site is dressed according to the appropriate protocol.

Though the CEAs can clinically have quite impressive results, they do pose several problems in addition to the cost, fragility, and handling issues. The grafts need to be used within several hours once they are prepared in order to maintain maximum viability of the cells. Since there are only a few laboratories around the country that can produce these autografts and in their fresh state they have to be hand delivered to the clinician, transportation becomes a significant issue. For this reason, several centers have been experimenting with different cryopreservation techniques so that the grafts may be grown and harvested at the optimum time and preserved in individual pouches for future use. These can be shipped frozen to the clinician or medical center where they are thawed, rinsed, and are ready to use. This process does not seem to significantly affect the graft viability (29). Another issue with the production of CEAs is the time it takes to grow the sheets. From the time the skin sample is harvested from the patient, it takes approximately three weeks to go through all the steps of the tissue culture process to produce the grafts. This, of course, presents a delay in the treatment and the subsequent increase in morbidity and mortality.

In order to have an immediate skin replacement available and to eliminate creating donor sites, researchers have looked at the possibility of using allogeneically derived tissue, that is, using cells from an unrelated donor. Initially it was thought that these cultured epithelial grafts could survive indefinitely since cultured human epithelial sheets do not synthesize HLA-DR markers, are generally free of Langerhans cells, melanocytes other immunologically recognized markers and do not stimulate allograft rejection in vivo (30,31). The first clinical trials evaluating cultured keratinocyte allografts have been done in the 1980s and have indeed shown that these grafts will stimulate wound healing by release of a variety of growth factors and are seemingly retained in the wound (32–36). It is now perceived that cultured epithelial allografts do not persist in the wound indefinitely, though it is not clear how long these grafts do remain in the wound bed. By DNA analysis or Y-chromosome probe in sex mismatched patients, it has been shown that allografts are entirely replaced by host epidermal cells. The time in various studies has been anywhere from a few weeks to several months, but over time allografts are slowly replaced with the hosts own cells (37).

The usefulness of cultured epithelium is not limited only to burn victims. Clinicians have used cultured epithelial grafts on a variety of other conditions including large surgical defects from excision of cancers or congenital nevi, lining of mastoid cavity for postoperative otorrhea, ulcers of epidermolysis bullosa, pyoderma gangrenosum as well as leg ulcers of various etiologies (38–44). Keratinocytes from various other stratified squamous epithelia can be cultured as well and have been used for urethral reconstruction, grafting of oral mucosal defects, and other uses (45,46).

In 1986, Hefton et al. first reported using cultured epithelial autografts on leg ulcers and a year later, Leigh et al. demonstrated the usefulness of CEAs in similar clinical studies (47,48). Since then, a number of groups have reported using cultured epithelium, autologous or allogeneic, fresh or cryopreserved, on leg ulcers of various etiologies (49–55). These grafts are relatively easy to use and require minimal equipment, though as in burn patients, one must pay particular attention to the preparation of the wound bed and handling of the grafts. In relatively small wounds, such as leg ulcers, cultured epithelial grafts seem to work by releasing a variety of growth factors and extracellular matrix molecules (56). This in turn stimulates the granulation tissue of the wound bed and proliferation of keratinocytes in the wound periphery; the so called "edge effect." Even with patients own keratinocyte sheets, the actual graft take would be seen in only 20–30% of the time (personal observation). Treatment with cultured epithelial grafts was most effective in patients with venous insufficiency ulcers with healing rates of 70–80% in 4–9 weeks, though a majority of the wounds showed at least some improvement. The treatment protocol is described elsewhere (54). A clinical case to illustrate the point is shown in Figure 2.

There have been few long-term follow-up studies of sites treated with cultured epithelial grafts. Within 1–2 weeks after grafting, the healed sites develop fully stratified epithelium and within 6 weeks repopulate with recipient Langerhans cells and melanocytes (57). Weeks and months after healing, the sites closed with cultured epithelial grafts exhibited skin fragility and spontaneous blistering similar to that seen in STSG donor and recipient sites. This has been shown to be due to abnormal reconstruction of the baseline membrane zone and a delay in formation of anchoring fibrils and the lack of rete ridges (58,59).

The best long-term study of sites treated with CEAs was done by Compton et al. (60) who evaluated biopsy specimens of healed sites of burn wounds excised to fascia and grafted with CEAs over a 5-year period. These were compared to healed interstices of STSG healed sites. Their initial findings were similar to previously reported observations regarding appearance of the epidermis, Langerhans cells, melanocytes, and basement membrane zone. However, one year or more later sites regenerated a normal rete ridge pattern, anchoring fibrils, regenerated elastin and remodeled to resemble true dermis. The control sites did not show these changes, except for anchoring fibril maturation in the 5-year period.

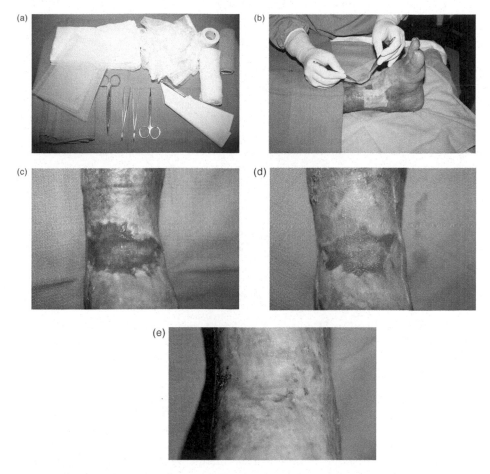

Figure 2 Clinical use of cultured keratinocyte autografts. (Courtesy of the author.) (a) Surgical tray used for grafting. (b) The individual grafts are placed on the wound in overlapping fashion. (c) Ulcer of 27 years duration prior to grafting. (d) Appearance of the ulcer 1 week later—note decrease in size and central island of graft "take." (e) Ulcer healed in 6 weeks.

Another type of cultured autologous epidermal graft available only in Europe at this time is EpiDex (Modex Therapeutics Ltd, Laussane, Switzerland). These grafts are cultured from outer root sheet cells of antigen hair follicles plucked from the patient's scalp. The outer root sheet contains the precursor cells for epidermal keratinocytes that are recruited in the natural wound healing process. These cells retain a high proliferative capacity irrespective of the age of the hair follicle donor. Under tissue culture conditions, the cells proliferate and differentiate resulting in an epidermal equivalent that closely resembles human epidermis within a 2–3-week time period.

After harvesting the hair follicles, the cells are processed in a series of steps that allow the creation of cryopreserved cell suspension that is used to create the final product. The grafts are produced as one centimeter diameter discs that are mounted onto a silicone membrane to facilitate handling. The individual autograft discs are placed in a nonoverlapping fashion into the wound bed. They are then secured in

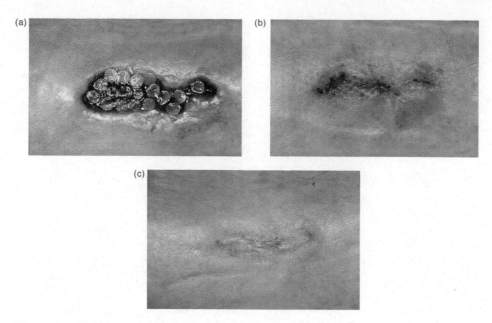

Figure 3 Clinical use of EpiDex. (Courtesy of Modex Therapeutics Ltd.) (a) Individual discs are placed into the debrided wound. (b) Appearance of the wound after 16 days showing significant decrease in size. (c) Healed wound at 42 days after application.

place with a sterile dressing. Figure 3 shows EpiDex placed into a wound and the subsequent healing. In the clinical trials of EpiDex and chronic recalcitrant ulcers that have failed other treatment methods, these grafts showed a greater than 40% area decrease in 8 weeks in 86% of the wounds with approximately 34% of the ulcers healed at the 8-week time point. Overall, the technique has several advantages. It is an easy, noninvasive procedure that does not require obtaining a skin biopsy, the source of cells and the quality of the cell material are independent of the patient's age and it does allow for permanent graft take in some instances. Also, one has a relatively unlimited supply of cells for the final cultures so multiple grafting sessions can be performed with only one harvesting of hair cells. Clinical trials evaluating EpiDex in a variety of clinical situations are ongoing in Europe and soon will begin in this country as well.

3. DERMAL SKIN SUBSTITUTES

Though skin barrier function depends on the epidermis, dermal tissue is needed for the optimal functional and cosmetic results when grafting with cultured epithelial grafts (61). Extra-cellular matrix is important for cultured epithelial autograft "take" in the postoperative period. While fibroblasts play a role in remodeling, keratinocyte differentiation, and matrix synthesis, it may take years to regenerate actual dermis-like tissue.

Cryopreserved allogeneic skin has been considered the "gold standard" on full thickness burns. It is specially processed to provide an acellular three-dimensional dermal tissue and is commercially available as AlloDerm (LifeCell Corporation, Branchburg, NJ). It is placed on the wound after eschar excision and its epidermis is removed prior to meshed split-thickness graft or cultured epithelial autograft placement (23,26). Though this technique produces good results, more widely available dermal substitute was desirable and has lead to the development of synthetic dermal substitutes.

Integra Dermal Regeneration Template (Integra LifeSciences, Plainsboro, NJ) is a nonliving dermal substitute made from bovine collagen and glycosaminoglycans covered with a synthetic silicone membrane. A similar material, TransCyte (Advanced Tissue Sciences, La Jolla CA), consists of porcine collagen coated nylon mesh bonded to a silicone membrane. During the manufacturing process, allogeneic fibroblasts cultured on the mesh produce matrix proteins and growth factors. These are retained after the material is frozen, which destroys all cellular activity. Both of these materials are FDA approved and have been used in burn patients to provide coverage of excised partial and full thickness burns until split thickness skin grafts or cultured keratinocyte autografts become available (62). TransCyte has recently been shown to decrease pain, healing time, and cost of care compared to standard care in patients with partial thickness burn wounds (63). We have used TransCyte at our clinic following CO_2 laser resurfacing with similar results.

The only commercially available "living" dermal replacement is Dermagraft (Advanced Tissue Sciences, La Jolla, CA). It is a cryopreserved human fibroblast derived dermal substitute, which has been approved by the FDA in October 2001 for the treatment of full thickness diabetic foot ulcers of greater than 6-week duration. Dermagraft is manufactured by culturing human neonatal fibroblasts onto a bioabsorbable polyglactin mesh. The proliferating cells secrete growth factors, cytokines, collagen, and matrix proteins to create a three-dimensional dermal substitute that contains metabolically active living cells. The final product sheet ($2'' \times 3''$) is cryopreserved and can be delivered to the clinician. The therapeutic properties are

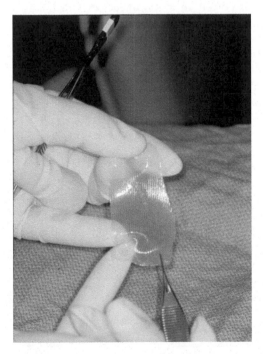

Figure 4 Appearance of Dermagraft prior to placement into the wound. (Courtesy of the author.)

dependent on the cell viability through cryopreservation, which is approximately 60% (64). Prior to use, Dermagraft undergoes a simple thawing and rinsing procedure, is cut to size and secured in the wound bed with dressings as shown in Figure 4. The success of this product, as with all cultured tissues depends on its use in a clear, noninfected, viable wound bed that has been debrided and the treatment is done in conjunction with pressure-relieving footwear (65–67). The fibroblasts used in the cell culture have been extensively tested and have not been shown to transmit any infectious agents.

A variety of other synthetic "living" dermal substitutes have also been described, including collagen-based implants, fibroblasts plated onto spongy collagen, collagen–glycosaminoglycan membranes with fibroblasts or hyaluronic acid dressing or polyglactin mesh seeded with fibroblasts (68–71). All of these materials improve graft take, increase collagen synthesis and dermal remodeling. Unfortunately, none of these materials are available commercially at this time.

4. FULL THICKNESS SKIN SUBSTITUTES

The most technologically advanced full thickness skin substitutes that are currently available on the market are essentially full thickness replacements of human skin. These materials are a composite of cultured human fibroblasts grown on a collagen sponge and on one side covered with a sheet of cultured human keratinocytes. The cells mature in a normal pattern so the resulting material histologically resembles normal skin although it is without appendigeal structures and the undulations of the rete ridges, which are characteristic of intact skin.

The first such material to be approved by the FDA for clinical use was Apligraf (Organogenesis Inc., Canton, MA). It is produced in a modified petri dish and shipped in a refrigerated container to the clinician as shown in Fig. 5. The material can be easily peeled off the supporting mesh and carrier medium, is resilient, relatively easy to handle and has a shelf life of several days.

Apligraf is currently approved for the treatment of chronic ulcers due to venous insufficiency that have not responded to standard care, though it has also been used in a variety of other clinical settings such as acute surgical defects following Mohs micrographic surgery, blistering disorders, ulcerations due to inflammatory conditions such as pyoderma gangrenosum, on split thickness donor sites, pressure ulcers, and a number of other skin defects.

Eaglstein et al. (72) found that Apligraf produced excellent healing in 58 patients with surgical incision sites with no toxicity. A comparison of Apligraf, autograft, and standard polyurethane film dressing in 20 patients with acute surgical wounds showed that pain relief, healing time, and cosmetic outcomes were similar in sites treated with Apligraf as with split thickness autograft, while sites treated with a polyurethane film took two days longer to heal and had a worse cosmetic outcome (73). This is consistent with other studies in surgical wound patients. Apligraf has been used successfully in patients with epidermolysis bullosa to close the erosions (74,75). A small randomized control trial of Apligraf in diabetic foot ulcers showed improved wound closure in the treatment group compared to the standard care control group (76).

In a large multicenter clinical trial of 287 patients with nonhealing venous ulcers, Falanga et al. (77) showed that Apligraf was significantly more effective than multilayered compression therapy (63% vs. 49%, respectively) and median time to

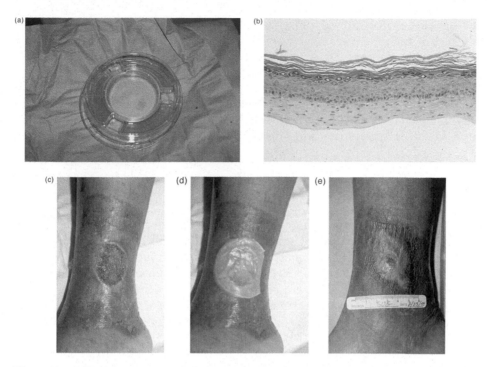

Figure 5 Apligraf. (Courtesy of the author.) (a) Cultured skin substitute is grown and delivered in a modified petri dish. (b) Microscopic appearance is similar to normal skin. (c) Appearance of ulcer prior to Apligraf placement—lesion was present for 2 years and failed a multitude of treatments. (d) Apligraf is placed into the wound a secured in place. (e) The wound completely epithelialized in 5 weeks.

wound closure was also significantly less in Apligraf patients compared to the control group (61 days vs. 181 days). Overall, treatment with Apligraf was found to be superior to standard compression therapy in healing larger and deeper longstanding ulcers. A review of this trial suggested that the material should be used before more invasive therapy, such as traditional skin grafting is undertaken. As with other bioengineered tissue materials, a clean debrided wound base that is relatively free of necrotic, fibrinous, or infected tissue is needed for it to be effective. Generally, several applications over a few weeks are used in the wound healing process. The material itself is absorbed into the wound base and over time stimulates wound healing or it is assimilated into the wound and clinically appears to engraft itself without inflammation or rejection. However, as with other allogeneic skin substitutes, it is ultimately replaced by the host's epithelial and dermal cells (78).

A similar material available on the market is OrCel (Ortec International, Inc., New York, NY). It received FDA approval in March 2001 for the treatment of ulcers due to epidermolysis bullosa and in September 2001, approved for the treatment of split thickness skin graft donor sites. It is currently in the last stage of a large multicenter trial for the treatment of venous insufficiency ulcerations and pilot trials for the treatment of ulcers due to diabetes. It is shipped frozen in a sealed pouch to the clinician; after a brief thawing and rinsing procedure, it can be placed onto the wound and secured with a nonadherent dressing of choice. In clinical trials, the earlier nonfrozen version of OrCel as well as the currently commercially available cryopreserved material showed 100% wound closure in three months in approximately 70% of the patients compared to the control group, which achieved closure in 26–37% of the patients. DNA analysis performed on OrCel treated donor site patient tissue samples showed no trace of allogeneic cell DNA after two or three weeks (Ortec International data on file).

Composite grafts with autologous keratinocytes and fibrils have been used recently in a pediatric burn patient. Though this is not available commercially, such material would be the ultimate skin substitute (79).

5. FUTURE DIRECTIONS

Since it appears that wound healing with bioengineered living skin substitutes is at least in part due to the release of growth factors, the next logical step has been the development of genetically modified cells which secrete various growth factors. Though this is at its earliest stages, retrovirally transduced fibroblasts and keratinocytes that produce platelet derived growth factor or vascular endothelial growth factor have been successful in clinical models (80,81). These techniques seem to be promising. However, the issues regarding disease transmission and cell transformation still need to be addressed (82,83).

Since culturing keratinocytes to confluence changes them from a hyperproliferative state to irreversible terminal differentiation, research has shifted from differentiated sheets to single cell suspensions or subconfluent sheets. As a cell suspension, the cells could proliferate in the wound and reform an epidermis directly in the wound (84). This in turn could lead to decreased scar formation in addition to decreased morbidity in burns and other wounds. Here the technical difficulty lies in holding the cells on the wound surface and this has been done using a xenograft or fibrin gel (85,86). These techniques still require enzymatic release of cells from the culture surface, which may damage anchoring fibrils. To avoid this step, cells have been cultured on collagen coated dextran beads and transplanted into wounds successfully (87). Another method described is the growth of cells to preconfluence on polymer membranes and inserting them into the wound (88,89).

Though these techniques are in their earliest stages of development, it is likely that in the not too distant future, we will have improved our understanding of wound healing and developed a skin replacement that optimizes the closure of any wound. Not only will these bioengineered grafts provide permanent wound coverage, but could also deliver gene therapy for local or systemic conditions. Traditional split-thickness skin grafts may very well become a thing of the past.

REFERENCES

1. Waldorf H, Fewkes J. Wound healing. Adv Dermatol 1995; 10:77–96.
2. Limova M. New therapeutic options for chronic wounds. Dermatol Clin 2002; 20: 357–363.
3. Hunt TK, Mueller RV, Goodson WH III. Wound healing. Current Surgical Diagnosis and Treatment. Norwalk: Lange, 1994:89–90.
4. Eaglstein WH, Falanga V. Chronic wounds. In: Barbul A, ed. The Surgical Clinics of North America: Wound Healing. Vol. 77. Number 3. Philadelphia: WB Saunders, 1997:689.

5. Trengrove NJ, Stacey MC, MacAuley S, Bennett N, Gibson J, Burslem F, Murphy G, Schultz G. Analysis of the acute and chronic wound environment: the role of proteases and their inhibitors. Wound Repair Regen 1999; 7:442–452.

6. Loots MA, Lamme EN, Zeegelaar J, Mekkes JR, Bos JD, Middelkoop E. Differences in cellular infiltrate and extracellular matrix of chronic diabetic and venous ulcers versus acute wounds. J Invest Dermatol 1998; 111:850–857.

7. Eaglstein WH. Occlusive dressings. J Dermatol Surg Oncol 1993; 19:716–720.

8. Motta GJ. Dressed for success: how moisture-retentive dressings promote healing. Nursing 1993; 23:26–33.

9. Nickerson D, Freiberg A. Moisture-retentive dressings: a review of the current literature. Can J Plast Surg 1995; 3:35–38.

10. Kannon GA, Garrett AB. Moist wound healing with occlusive dressings. A clinical review. Dermatol Surg 1995; 21:583–590.

11. Bello YM, Phillips TJ. Recent advances in wound healing. JAMA 2000; 283:71–78.

12. Bello YM, Falabella AF, Eaglstein WH. Tissue-engineered skin. Current status in wound repair. Am J Clin Dermatol 2001; 2:305–313.

13. Mulder GT. The role of tissue engineering in wound care. An update on the most recent developments and treatments in tissue engineering and recommendations and considerations for practice. J Wound Care 1999; 8:21–24.

14. Rheinwald JG, Green H. Serial cultivation of strains of human epidermal keratinocytes: the formation of keratinizing colonies from single cells. Cell 1975; 6:331–343.

15. Pittlekow MR, Scott RE. New techniques for the in vitro culture of human skin keratinocytes and perspectives on their use for grafting of patients with extensive burns. Mayo Clin Proc 1986; 61:771–777.

16. Grimwood RE. Keratinocyte culture techniques: methods leading to the successful grafting of cultured epidermal cells. J Assoc Mil Dermatol 1988; 14:4–7.

17. O'Connor NE, Mulliken JB, Banks-Schlegel A, Kehinde O, Green H. Grafting of burns with cultured epithelium prepared from autologous epidermal cells. Lancet 1981; 1: 75–78.

18. Gallico GG III, O'Connor NE, Compton CC, Kehinde O, Green H. Permanent coverage of large burn wounds with autologous cultured human keratinocytes. N Engl J Med 1984; 311:448–451.

19. Eldad A, Burt A, Clarke JA, Gusterson B. Cultured epithelium as a skin substitute. Burns Incl Therm Inj 1987; 13:173–180.

20. Kumagai N, Nishima H, Tanabe H, Hosaka T, Ishida H, Ogino Y. Clinical application of autologous cultured epithelia for the treatment of burn wounds and burn scars. Plast Reconstr Surg 1988; 82:99–108.

21. Herzog SR, Meyer A, Woodley D, Peterson HD. Wound coverage with cultured autologous keratinocytes. J Trauma 1988; 28:195–198.

22. Heck EL, Bergstrasser PR, Baxter CR. Composite skin grafts: frozen dermal allografts support the engraftment and expansion of autologous epidermis. J Trauma 1985; 25: 106–112.

23. Cuono C, Langdon R, McGuire J. Use of cultured epidermal autografts and dermal allografts as skin replacement after burn surgery. Lancet 1986; 1:1123–1124.

24. Langdon RC, Cuono CB, Birchall N, Madri JA, Kuklinska E, McGuire J, Moellmann GE. Reconstruction of structure and cell function in human skin grafts derived from cryopreserved allogeneic dermis and autologous cultured keratinocytes. J Invest Dermatol 1988; 91:478–485.

25. Hansbrough JF, Boyce ST, Cooper MI, Foreman TJ. Burn wound closure with cultured autologous keratinocytes and fibroblasts attached to a collagen–glycosaminoglycan substrate. JAMA 1989; 262:2125–2130.

26. Teepe RG, Kreis RW, Koebrugge EJ, Kempenaar JA, Vloemans AF, Hermans RP, Boxma H, Dokter J, Hermans J, Ponec M, et al. The use of cultured autologous epidermis in the treatment of extensive burn wounds. J Trauma 1990; 30;269–275.

27. Gao ZR, Hao ZQ, Nie LJ, Liu GF. Coverage of full skin thickness burns with allograft inoculated with autogenous epithelial cells. Burns Incl Therm Inj 1986; 12:220–224.

28. Tatnall FM, Leigh IM, Gibson JR. Comparative toxicity of antimicrobial agents on transformed human keratinocytes. J Invest Dermatol 1987; 89:316.

29. Pye RJ. Cultured keratinocytes as biological wound dressings. Eye 1988; 2:172–178.

30. Morhenn VB, Benike CJ, Cox AJ, Charron DJ, Engleman EG. Cultured human epidermal cells do not synthesize HLA-DR. J Invest Dermatol 1982; 78:32–37.

31. Hefton JM, Amberson JB, Biozes DG, Weksler ME. Loss of HLA-DR expression by human epidermal cells after growth in culture. J Invest Dermatol 1984; 83:48–50.

32. Hefton JM, Madden MR, Finkelstein JL, Shires GT. Grafting of burn patients with allografts of cultured epidermal cells. Lancet 1983; 2:428–430.

33. Thivolet J, Faure M, Demidem A, Mauduit G. Long-term survival and immunological tolerance of human epidermal allografts produced in culture. Transplantation 1986; 42:274–280.

34. Madden MR, Finkelstein JL, Staiano-Coico L, Goodwin CW, Shires GT, Nolan EE, Hefton JM. Grafting of cultured allogeneic epidermis on second- and third-degree burn wounds on 26 patients. J Trauma 1986; 26:955–962.

35. Gilchrest BA, Karassik RL, Wilkins LM, Vrabel MA, Maciag T. Autocrine and paracrine growth stimulation of cells derived from human skin. J Cell Physiol 1983; 117:235–240.

36. Thivolet J, Faure M, Demidem A. Cultured human epidermal allografts are not rejected for a long period. Arch Dermatol Res 1986; 278:252–254.

37. Arons JA, Wainwright DJ, Jordan RE. The surgical applications and implications of cultured human epidermis: a comprehensive review. Surgery 1992; 111:4–11.

38. Gallico GG III, O'Connor NE, Compton CC, Remensnyder JP, Kehinde O, Green H. Cultured epithelial autografts for giant congenital nevi. Plast Reconstr Surg 1989; 84:1–9.

39. Premachandra DJ, Woodward BM, Milton CM, Sergeant RJ, Fabre JW. Treatment of postoperative otorrhoea by grafting of mastoid cavities with cultured autologous epidermal cells. Lancet 1990; 335:365–367.

40. McGuire J, Birchall N, Cuono C, Moellmann G, Kuklinska E, Langdon R. Successful engraftment of allogeneic keratinocyte cultures in recessive dystrophic epidermolysis bullosa. Clin Res 1987; 35:702A.

41. Carter DM, Lin AN, Varghese MC, Caldwell D, Pratt LA, Eisinger M. Treatment of junctional epidermolysis bullosa with epidermal autografts. J Am Acad Dermatol 1987; 17:246–250.

42. Cony M, Donatien PH, Beylot C, Geniaux M, Maleville J, Bezian JH, Taieb A. Treatment of leg ulcers with an allogeneic cultured-keratinocyte-collagen dressing. Clin Exp Dermatol 1990; 15:410–414.

43. Limova M, Mauro T. Treatment of pyoderma gangrenosum with cultured epithelial autografts. J Dermatol Surg Oncol 1994; 20:833–836.

44. Beldon P. Management of chronic venous leg ulcers using a new autologous skin graft system. J Wound Care 1999; 8:380–382.

45. Romagnoli G, De Luca M, Faranda F, Bandelloni R, Franzi AT, Cataliotti F, Cancedda R. Treatment of posterior hypospadias by the autologous graft of cultured urethral epithelium. N Engl J Med 1990; 323:527–530.

46. De Luca M, Albanese E, Megna M, Cancedda R, Mangiante PE, Cadoni A, Franzi AT. Evidence that human oral epithelium reconstituted in vitro and transplanted onto patients with defects in the oral mucosa retains properties of the original donor site. Transplantation 1990; 50:454–459.

47. Hefton JM, Caldwell D, Biozes DG, Balin AK, Carter DM. Grafting of skin ulcers with cultured autologous epidermal cells. J Am Acad Dermatol 1986; 14:399–405.

48. Leigh IM, Purkis PE, Navsaria HA, Phillips TJ. Treatment of chronic venous ulcers with sheets of cultured allogenic keratinocytes. Br J Dermatol 1987; 117:591–597.

49. Phillips TJ, Kehinde O, Green H, Gilchrest BA. Treatment of skin ulcers with epidermal allografts. J Am Acad Dermatol 1989; 21:191–199.
50. Phillips TJ, Gilchrest BA. Cultured epidermal grafts in the treatment of leg ulcers. Adv Dermatol 1990; 5:33–48.
51. Marcusson JA, Lindgren C, Berghard A, Toftgård R. Allogeneic cultured keratinocytes in the treatment of leg ulcers. Acta Derm Venereol (Stockholm) 1992; 72:61–64.
52. De Luca M, Albanese E, Cancedda R, Viacava A, Faggioni A, Zambruno G, Giannetti A. Treatment of leg ulcers with cryopreserved allogeneic cultured epithelium: a multicenter study. Arch Dermatol 1992; 128:633–638.
53. Teepe RGC, Roseeuw DI, Hermans J, Koebrugge EJ, Altena T, de Coninck A, Ponec M, Vermeer BJ. Randomized trial comparing cryopreserved cultured epidermal allografts with hydrocolloid dressings in healing chronic venous ulcers. J Am Acad Dermatol 1993; 29:982–988.
54. Limova M, Mauro T. Treatment of leg ulcers with cultured epithelial autografts: treatment protocol and five year experience. Wounds 1995; 7:170–180.
55. Phillips TJ. Cultured epidermal allografts—A temporary or permanent solution? Transplantation 1991; 51:937–941.
56. Carver N, Leigh IM. Keratinocyte grafts and skin replacements. Int J Dermatol 1991; 30:540–551.
57. Aihara M. Ultrastructural study of grafted autologous cultured human epithelium. Br J Plast Surg 1989; 42:35–42.
58. Woodley DT, Peterson HD, Herzog SR, Stricklin GP, Burgeson RE, Briggaman RA, Cronce DJ, O'Keefe EJ. Burn wounds resurfaced by cultured epidermal autografts show abnormal reconstruction of anchoring fibrils. JAMA 1988; 259:2566–2571.
59. Petersen MJ, Lessane B, Woodley DT. Characterization of cellular elements in healed cultured keratinocyte autografts used to cover burn wounds. Arch Dermatol 1990; 126:175–180.
60. Compton CC, Gill JM, Bradford DA, Regauer S, Gallico GG, O'Connor NE. Skin regeneration from cultured epithelial autografts on full-thickness burn wounds from 6 days to 5 years after grafting: a light, electron microscopic, and immunohistochemical study. Lab Invest 1989; 60:600–611.
61. Coulcomb B, Dubertret L. Skin cell culture and wound healing. Wound Repair Regen 2002; 10:109–112.
62. Loss M, Wedler V, Kunzi W, Meuli-Simmen C, Meyer VE. Artificial skin, split-thickness autograft and cultured autologous keratinocytes combined to treat a severe burn injury of 93% of TBSA. Burns 2000; 26:644–652.
63. Demling RH, DeSanti L. Closure of partial-thickness facial burns with a bioactive skin substitute in the major burn population decreases the cost of care and improves outcome. Wounds 2002; 14:230–234.
64. Mansbridge J, Liu K, Patch R, Symons K, Pinney E. Three-dimensional fibroblast culture implant for the treatment of diabetic foot ulcers: metabolic activity and therapeutic range. Tissue Eng 1998; 4:403–414.
65. Gentzkow GD, Iwasaki S, Hershon K, Mengel M, Prendergast JJ, Ricotta J, Steed D, Lipkin S. Use of Dermagraft, a cultured human dermis, to treat diabetic foot ulcers. Diabetes Care 1996; 19:350–354.
66. Gentzkow GD, Jensen J, Pollak R, Kroeker R, Lerner J, Lerner M, Iwasaki S. Improved healing of diabetic foot ulcers after grafting with Dermagraft, a living human dermal replacement. Wounds 1999; 11:77–84.
67. Finch PM, Hyder E. Treatment of diabetic ulceration using Dermagraft. The Foot : 1999; September:156–163.
68. Kuroyanagi Y, Yamada N, Yamashita R, Uchinuma E. Tissue-engineered product: allogeneic cultured dermal substitute composed of spongy collagen with fibroblasts. Artif Organs 2001; 25:180–186.

69. Tanaka M, Nakakita N, Kuroyanagi Y. Allogeneic cultured dermal substitute composed of spongy collagen containing fibroblasts: evaluation in animal test. J Biomater Sci Polym Ed 1999; 10:433–453.

70. Harris PA, di Francesco F, Barisoni D, Leigh IM, Navsaria HA. Use of hyaluronic acid and cultured autologous keratinocytes and fibroblasts in extensive burns. Lancet 1999; 353:35–36.

71. Cooper ML, Hansbrough JF, Spielvogel RL, Cohen R, Bartel RL, Naughton G. In vivo optimization of a living dermal substitute employing cultured human fibroblasts on a biodegradable polyglycolic acid or polyglactin mesh. Biomaterials 1991; 12:243–248.

72. Eaglstein WH, Alvarez OM Auletta M, Leffel D, Rogers GS, Zitelli JA, Norris JE, Thomas I, Irondo M, Fewkes J, Hardin-Young J, Duff RG, Sabolinski ML. Acute excisional wounds treated with a tissue-engineered skin (Apligraf). Dermatol Surg 1999; 25: 195–201.

73. Muhart M, McFalls S, Kirsner RS, Elgart GW, Kerdel F, Sabolinski ML, Hardin-Young J, Eaglstein WH. Behavior of tissue-engineered skin: a comparison of a living skin equivalent, autograft, and occlusive dressing in human donor sites. Arch Dermatol 1999; 135:913–918.

74. Falabella AF, Schachner LA, Valencia IC, Eaglstein WH. The use of tissue-engineered skin (Apligraf) to treat a newborn with epidermolysis bullosa. Arch Dermatol 1999; 135:1219–1222.

75. Falabella AF, Valencia IC, Eaglstein WH, Schachner LA. Tissue-engineered skin (Apligraf) in the healing of patients with epidermolysis bullosa wounds. Arch Dermatol 2000; 136:1225–1230.

76. Brem H, Balledux J, Bloom T, Kerstein MD, Hollier L. Healing of diabetic foot ulcers and pressure ulcers with human skin equivalent: a new paradigm in wound healing. Arch Surg 2000; 135:627–634.

77. Falanga V, Margolis D, Alvarez O, Auletta M, Maggiacomo F, Altman M, Jensen J, Sabolinski M, Hardin-Young J. Rapid healing of venous ulcers and lack of clinical rejection with an allogeneic cultured human skin equivalent. Arch Dermatol 1998; 134: 293–300.

78. Phillips TJ, Manzoor J, Rojas A, Isaacs C, Carson P, Sabolinski M, Young J, Falanga V. The longevity of a bilayered skin substitute after application to venous ulcers. Arch Dermatol 2002; 138:1079–1081.

79. Caruso DM, Schuh WH, Al-Kasspooles MF, Chen MC, Schiller WR. Cultured composite autografts as coverage for an extensive body surface area burn: case report and review of the technology. Burns 1999; 25:771–779.

80. Breitbart AS, Grande DA, Laser J, Barcia M, Porti D, Malhotra S, Kogon A, Grant RT, Mason JM. Treatment of ischemic wounds using cultured dermal fibroblasts transduced retrovirally with PDGF-B and VEGF121 genes. Ann Plast Surg 2001; 46:555–561.

81. Supp DM, Bell SM, Morgan JR, Boyce ST. Genetic modification of cultured skin substitutes by transduction of human keratinocytes and fibroblasts with platelet-derived growth factor-A. Wound Repair Regen 2000; 8:26–35.

82. Beele H. Artificial skin: past, present and future. Int J Artif Organs 2002; 25:163–173.

83. Boyce ST. Design principles for composition and performance of cultured skin substitutes. Burns 2001; 27:523–533.

84. Harris PA, Leigh IM, Navsaria HA. Pre-confluent keratinocyte grafting: the future for cultured skin replacements? Burns 1998; 24:591–593.

85. Kaiser HW, Stark GB, Kopp J, Balcerkiewicz A, Spilker G, Kreysel HW. Cultured autologous keratinocytes in fibrin blue suspension, exclusively and combined with STS-allograft (preliminary clinical and histological report of a new technique). Burns 1994; 20:23–29.

86. Horch RE, Bannasch H, Stark GB. Transplantation of cultured autologous keratinocytes in fibrin sealant biomatrix to resurface chronic wounds. Transplant Proc 2001; 33:642–644.

87. Voigt M, Schauer M, Schaefer DJ, Andree C, Horch R, Stark GB. Cultured epidermal keratinocytes on a microspherical transport system are feasible to reconstitute the epidermis in full-thickness wounds. Tissue Eng 1999; 5:563–572.
88. Barlow Y, Burt A, Clarke JA, McGrouther DA, Lang SM. The use of a polymetric film for the culture and transfer of subconfluent autologous cultured keratinocytes to patients. J Tissue Viability 1992; 2:33–36.
89. Dvorankova B, Smetana K Jr, Konigova R, Singerova H, Vacik J, Jelinkova M, Kapounkova Z, Zahradnik M. Cultivation and grafting of human keratinocytes on a poly(hydroxyethyl methacrylate) support to the wound bed: a clinical study. Biomaterials 1998; 19:141–146.

43
Oxygen and Wound Healing

Noah A. Rosen
Department of Surgery, Boston University Medical Center, Boston, Massachusetts, U.S.A.

Harriet W. Hopf and Thomas K. Hunt
Departments of Anesthesia and Surgery, University of California San Francisco, Wound Healing Laboratory, San Francisco, California, U.S.A.

1. INTRODUCTION

Wounding disrupts the microvasculature, rendering tissue ischemic. Platelets aggregate to prevent exsanguination, but widen the area of impaired circulation. Silver studied the oxygen microclimate in wounds using Clark microelectrodes in a rabbit ear chamber wound model.* He found that the oxygen tensions of the dead-space of the wound, at distances of more than 120–140 mcm beyond the nearest capillary, were less than 3 mmHg (1). The delivery of oxygen to this dead-space is dependent on the diffusion of oxygen from the surrounding capillaries (2). The higher the capillary oxygen tension, the greater the driving force for diffusion.

The oxygen tension at the capillary level can be increased by increasing arterial oxygen tension (increasing inspired oxygen concentration) or by increasing blood flow to the tissue surrounding a wound (Fig. 1) (3). Silver demonstrated that in rabbits breathing room air, the oxygen gradient from capillary to dead-space went from 90 mmHg to zero in 150 mcm. When the animals inspired 100% oxygen, the capillary oxygen tension increased to 450 mmHg, but the gradient in the wound went to zero in approximately the same distance (1). This implies that in rabbits breathing room air, the inflammatory cells (neutrophils first, then macrophages in 24–48 hr) recruited into the wound exist in a relatively hypoxic state. When oxygen diffusion into the dead-space is increased, oxygen utilization by the inflammatory cells also increases. Normal skin cells consume relatively little oxygen; about 0.7 mL/100 mL of blood flow at normal perfusion (3,4). Wound cells consume only a little more oxygen, producing energy largely via the hexose-monophosphate shunt (glucose + oxygen → lactate + superoxide). The increased oxygen is not

---

*Wounds were created in rabbit ears and chambers were inserted that allowed two-dimensional healing to be studied under direct vision.

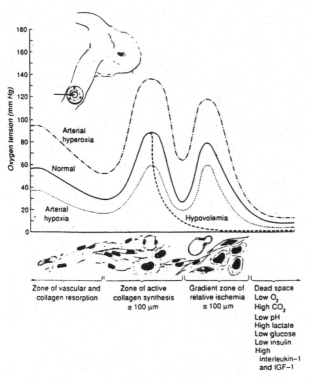

Figure 1 Oxygen tissue measurements across a healing wound measured in a rabbit ear wound healing chamber. Tissue oxygen tension increases at each capillary. The effect of hyperoxia, hypoxia, and hypovolemia on the oxygen gradient driving diffusion into the dead space of the wound is demonstrated. (From Ref. 21.)

used for cellular metabolism, but rather is consumed by the inflammatory cells to accelerate repair and fight infection. Inflammatory cells largely use oxygen to produce oxidants. Oxygen has been shown to be vitally important for collagen synthesis, epithelization, angiogenesis, and bacterial killing. Oxygen is required at relatively high concentrations for some part of each of these processes, and oxidants are a primary signal for the growth factors that direct the wound healing process (5).

2. WOUND INFECTION

Resistance to bacterial infection in wounds depends on neutrophils. One component of phagocyte bacterial killing is oxidative killing. Molecular oxygen is converted by the neutrophil to high-energy radicals, such as superoxide, hydroxyl, peroxide, aldehydes, hypochlorite, hypoiodite, and others, all of which are toxic in varying degrees to bacteria (6, Fig. 2). The rate of production of these toxic radicals is directly proportional to oxygen tension (7). Allen et al. showed that superoxide production in neutrophils is half-maximal for oxygen tensions from 45 to 80 mmHg and maximal at oxygen tensions greater that 300 mmHg. They found that bactericidal activity would rise 3- to 4-fold if mean oxygen tension in a wound increased from 15 to 100 mmHg (8). *Staphylococcus aureus, Escherichia coli, Proteus* spp, *Salmonella*

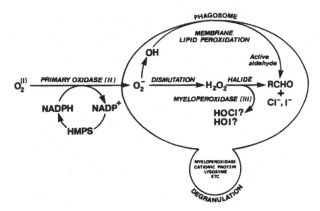

Figure 2 Schema of neutrophil oxidative killing mechanisms. (From Ref. 6.)

spp, and *Klebsiella* spp are killed at rates proportional to local oxygen tension (7,9). Hohn et al. measured in vitro leukocyte killing of *S. aureus* 502A from 0 to 150 mmHg. They found a 50% loss of bacterial killing when oxygen tension was reduced to 0 mmHg, with the major loss of killing capacity for oxygen tensions below 30 mmHg (6,17, Fig. 3).

Hohn et al. studied the clearance of *S. aureus* from subcutaneous wound cylinders implanted in rabbits. They showed that clearance of bacteria was retarded in the hypoxic group and accelerated in the hyperoxic group (10, Fig. 4). Knighton et al. studied the effect of increased environmental oxygen (45%) on *E. coli* wound

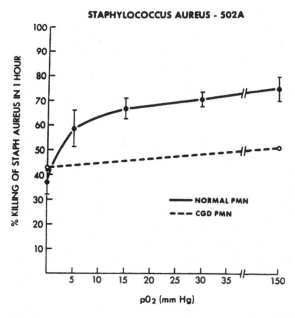

Figure 3 CGD PMN = leukocytes from chronic granulomatous disease patients that lack the oxidase enzyme. Lack of the enzyme is equivalent to lack of the substrate (oxygen) for the enzyme. (From Ref. 6.)

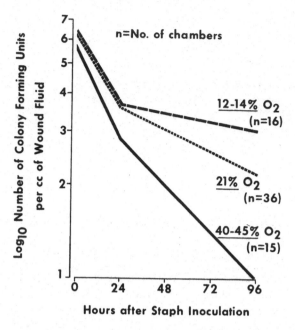

Figure 4 Clearance of bacteria from wound cylinders in relation to inspired oxygen concentration. (From Ref. 10.)

infections in an intradermal injection model in guinea pigs.* They found that supplemental oxygen significantly decreased the size and number of necrotic lesions (6,11), (Fig. 5) and enhanced bacterial clearance from the wound (12). Hopf et al. (13) demonstrated in postsurgical patients that subcutaneous tissue oxygen tension was inversely proportional to the rate of wound infection (Fig. 6).

3. COLLAGEN SYNTHESIS

During collagen formation, the transcribed polypeptide chains (procollagen) require post-translational modification to allow formation of the triple helix that provides the strength of collagen and allows it to be exported from fibroblasts. The hydroxylation of prolyl and lysyl residues by the enzymes prolyl and lysyl hydroxylase requires molecular oxygen as a cofactor (14). The K_m value for the hydroxylation of proline in vitro is approximately 25 mmHg (15). Thus, the V_{max} of this enzyme occurs at or above 200 mmHg. As tissue oxygen falls from about 50 mmHg, there is a steep decline in collagen production. Without oxygen, collagen intramolecular cross bonding and final assembly cannot proceed.

Using a wound cylinder model in rabbits,[†] Hunt and Pai (16) showed that collagen accumulation increased with increasing arterial oxygen tension, (Fig. 7). Similar results were found in postoperative surgical patients (17,18, Fig. 8), where collage deposition is proportional to tissue PO_2. Shandall et al. studied oxygen ten-

---

*Bacteria was injected intradermally and induration and necrosis were measured at 24 and 48 h
[†]Dead-space wounds were created by placing wire mesh cylinders subcutaneously along the dorsum of rabbits.

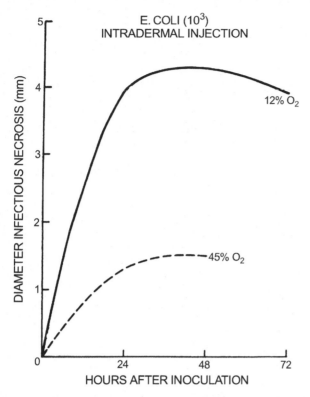

Figure 5 Mean lesion diameter was greater in animals breathing hypoxic mixtures. (From Ref. 6.)

sion and colonic anastomotic healing in rabbits. They found that perianastomotic oxygen tension correlated with hydroxyproline content and breaking strength. The leakage rate for anastomoses constructed with a perianastomotic oxygen tension of above 55 mmHg was 10%, compared to a 100% leakage rate for oxygen tensions less than 25 mmHg (Fig. 9) (19).

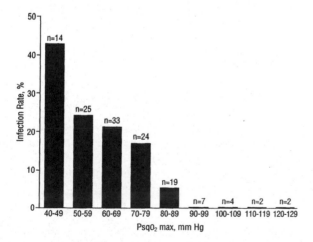

Figure 6 Infection rate is inversely proportional to maximal subcutaneous wound oxygen tension. (From Ref. 13.)

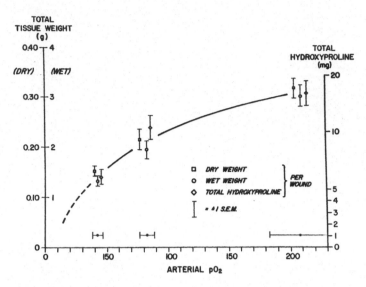

Figure 7 Wound tissue collagen as a function of arterial oxygen tension. Hydroxyproline was assayed by removing the wound cylinders 25 days after placement and assaying the contents. (From Ref. 16.)

4. ANGIOGENESIS

The goal of angiogenesis is to re-establish blood flow to wounds, thus decreasing the diffusion distance from capillary to dead-space. Silver showed that capillary ingrowth increases the oxygen tension of the wound dead-space (1). The hypoxia present in the dead-space initiates angiogenesis, but this process simultaneously requires oxygen to proceed (20). This environment exists with a steep gradient present between the surrounding capillaries and wound dead-space. Knighton et al. (21) showed in rabbit ear chamber wounds that if this gradient was abolished, by allowing the central dead-space to equilibrate with atmospheric oxygen, angiogenesis ceased (21, Fig. 10). Oxygen drives collagen formation in the basement membrane of the new blood vessels. Without oxygen, new vessels are fragile and leaky. Gibson et al. (22) demonstrated that increased environmental oxygen (including hyperbaric oxygen) increases angiogenesis in a mouse matrigel model* (Fig. 11).

5. EPITHELIZATION

Medawar demonstrated in tissue culture without oxygen, epidermal movement and cell division are brought to a standstill. He further found that the rate of epithelial cell division increases with increasing oxygen tension (23,24). In open rat wounds, Pai et al. demonstrated that hyperoxia increases the rate of epithelization and hypoxia decreases this rate. The oxygen effect was slight, however, with an accelerated closure of about 15% (Fig. 12) (25). Uhl et al. (26) showed that in mouse ear

---

*Matrigel, a reconstituted basement membrane complex, was injected subcutaneously in mice and then harvested and examined microscopically for neovascularization.

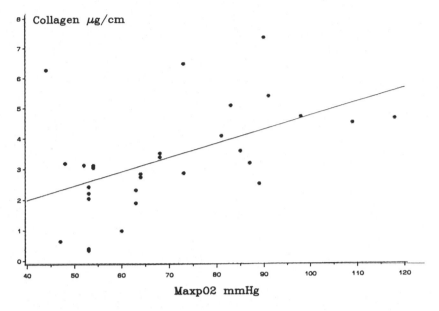

Figure 8 The regression line reflects the relation between collagen accumulation in postsurgical patients on day 5 and maximal tissue oxygen tension. (From Ref. 17.)

wounds, treatment with hyperbaric oxygen reduced the time for complete epithelization by 2 days.

6. CLINICAL IMPLICATIONS

Prevention of wound hypoxia is critical to avoid wound infections and wound healing failure. In practice, this requires maximizing tissue perfusion and arterial oxygen tension. Blood flow to subcutaneous tissue and skin is approximately 20% of cardiac output, although metabolic oxygen demands of subcutaneous tissue require only a

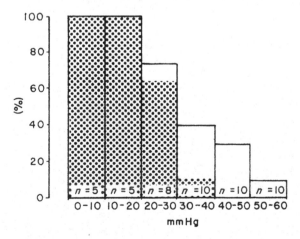

Figure 9 Leakage rate and tissue oxygen tension: stippled = major leaks (death); clear = minor leak (localized collection at day 10). (From Ref. 19.)

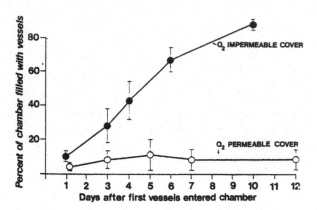

Figure 10 Raising the central dead space oxygen concentration, by use of a permeable ear chamber cover allowing equilibration with room air, completely abolished normal vessel growth. (From Ref. 21.)

fraction of this perfusion. Subcutaneous tissue serves as: (1) a reservoir of blood volume providing volume to the central circulation in cases of hypovolemia (for example, due to hemorrhage or dehydration) and (2) the major site of thermoregulation. Subcutaneous perfusion is almost entirely controlled by the sympathetic nervous system. Local warming is the only input known to be able to overcome sympathetically induced vasoconstriction.

Maintenance of high wound oxygen levels has been shown to improve acute wound healing outcomes. The keys to maintaining a high oxygen tension in wounds are prevention of vasoconstriction (euvolemia, treating pain, warming) and maintenance of high arterial oxygen tension (increasing inspired oxygen concentration). Arkilic et al. (27) showed that an aggressive intraoperative fluid

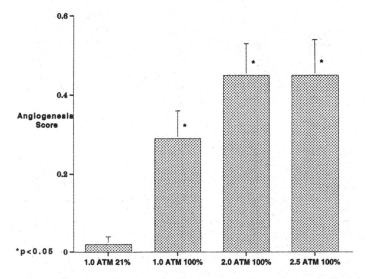

Figure 11 Angiogenesis score in implanted matrigel on day 7 after placement as a function of increasing oxygen tension. Sections of matrigel are microscopically graded: $0 =$ no vessels; $0.5 =$ scattered vessels; and $1 =$ maximal vessels in all quadrants. (From Ref. 22.)

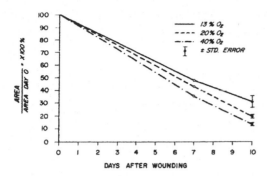

Figure 12 Healing of open wounds in rats at different inspired oxygen concentrations. (From Ref. 25.)

resuscitation protocol (16–18 mL/kg/hr) for colorectal surgical patients increased tissue oxygen tension compared to a conservative protocol (8 mL/kg/hr). Hartmann et al. (28) demonstrated that the patients who received more fluid on the day of operation had increased accumulation of collagen in healing wounds. Kurz et al. (29) showed that maintaining core normothermia (36.6°C) intraoperatively in colorectal surgery patients decreased the rate of wound infections from 19% to 6%, and increased collagen deposition, compared with hypothermic patients (34.7°C). Greif et al. (30) showed that the administration of 80% oxygen to colorectal surgical patients intraoperatively and 2 hours postoperatively decreased the incidence of wound infections by more than 50% compared to patients who received 30% oxygen (5.2 % vs. 11.2%).

7. SUMMARY

A high partial pressure of oxygen is required for collagen synthesis, epithelization, angiogenesis, and bacterial killing. The rate constants for oxygen for these components of wound repair all fall within the range of 25–100 mmHg. The measured wound tissue oxygen tension in surgical patients breathing room air is in this range (13,30). These processes are maximized only for tissue oxygen tensions greater than 250 mmHg. Any impairment of blood flow to the surrounding wound capillaries or decreased arterial oxygen tension will impair wound repair and immunity.

REFERENCES

1. Silver IA. The measurement of oxygen tension in healing tissue. Progr Resp Res 1969; 3:124–135.
2. Silver IA. The physiology of wound healing. In: Hunt TK, ed. Wound Healing and Wound Infection: Theory and Surgical Practice. New York: Appleton-Century-Crofts, 1980:11–31.
3. Hopf HW, Jensen JA, Hunt TK. Calculation of subcutaneous tissue blood flow. Surg Forum 1988; 39:33–36.
4. Evans NT, Naylor PF. Steady states of oxygen tension in human dermis. Respiration Physiol 1966; 2:46–60.
5. Sen CK, Khanna S, Babior BM, Hunt TK, Ellison, EC, Roy S. Oxidant induced vascular endothelial growth factor expression in human keratinocytes and cutaneous wound healing. J Biol Chem 2002; 277:33284–33290.

6. Hunt TK, Knighton DR, Price DC, Mathes SJ, Halliday B, Gottrup F, Hohn DC, Jonsson K. Oxygen in the prevention and treatment of infection. In: Root RK, Trunkey DD, Sande MA, eds. New Surgical and Medical Approaches in Infectious Diseases. New York: Churchill Livingstone, 1987:1–16.

7. Hohn DC, Mackay RD, Halliday B, Hunt TK. Effect of O_2 tension on microbicidal function of leukocytes in wounds and in vitro. Surg Forum 1976; 27:18–20.

8. Allen DB, Maguire JJ, Mahdavian M, Wicke C, Marcocci L, Scheuenstuhl H, Chang M, Le AX, Hopf HW, Hunt TK. Wound hypoxia and acidosis limit neutrophil bacterial killing mechanisms. Arch Surg 1997; 132:991–996.

9. Mandell GL. Bactericidal activity of aerobic and anaerobic polymorphonuclear neutrophils. Infect Immun 1974; 9:337–341.

10. Hohn DC. Host resistance to infection: established and emerging concepts. In: Hunt TK, ed. Wound Healing and Wound Infection: Theory and Surgical Practice. New York: Appleton-Century-Crofts, 1980:264–279.

11. Knighton DR, Halliday B, Hunt TK. Oxygen as an antibiotic: the effect of inspired oxygen on infection. Arch Surg 1984; 119:199–204.

12. Knighton DR, Fiegel VD, Halverson T, Schneider S, Brown T, Wells CL. Oxygen as an antibiotic: the effect of inspired oxygen on bacterial clearance. Arch Surg 1990; 125: 97–100.

13. Hopf HW, Hunt TK, West JW, Blomquist P, Goodson WH, Jensen AJ, Jonsson K, Pary PB, Rabkin JM, Upton RA, von Smitten K, Whitney JD. Wound tissue oxygen tension predicts the risk of wound infection in surgical patients. Arch Surg 1997; 132:997–1004.

14. Kivirkko KI, Risteli L. Biosynthesis of collagen and its alterations in pathological states. Med Biol 1976; 54:159–186.

15. Hutton JJ, Tappel Al, Undenfriend S. Cofactor and substrate requirements of collagen proline hydroxylase. Arch Biochem 1967; 118:231–236.

16. Hunt TK, Pai MP. The effect of varying ambient oxygen tensions on wound metabolism and collagen synthesis. Surg Gynecol Obstet 1972; 135:561–567.

17. Jonsson K, Jensen JA, Goodson WH, Scheuenstuhl H, West J, Hopf HW, Hunt TK. Tissue oxygenation, anemia, and perfusion in relation to wound healing in surgical patients. Ann Surg 1991; 214:605–613.

18. Hartmann M, Jonsson K, Zederfeldt B. Effect of tissue perfusion and oxygenation on accumulation of collagen in healing wounds. Eur J Surg 1992; 158:521–526.

19. Shandall A, Lowndes R, Young HL. Colonic anastomotic healing and oxygen tension. Br J Surg 1985; 72:606–609.

20. Feng JJ, Hussain MZ, Constant J, Hunt TK. Angiogenesis in wound healing. J Surg Path 1998; 3:1–7.

21. Knighton DR, Silver IA, Hunt TK. Regulation of wound-healing angiogenesis: effect of oxygen gradients and inspired oxygen concentration. Surgery 1981; 2:262–270.

22. Gibson JJ, Angeles AP, Hunt TK. Increased oxygen tension potentiates angiogenesis. Surg Forum 1997; 48:696–699.

23. Medawar PB. The behaviour of mammalian skin epithelium under strictly anaerobic conditions. Q J Micr Sci 1947; 88:27–37.

24. Medawar PB. The cultivation of adult mammalian skin epithelium. Q J Micr Sci 1948; 89:187–196.

25. Pai MP, Hunt TK. Effect of varying oxygen tension on healing of open wounds. Surg Gynecol Obstet 1972; 135:756–758.

26. Uhl E, Sisjo A, Haapaniemi T, Nilsson G, Nylander G. Hyperbaric oxygen improves wound healing in normal and ischemic tissue. Plas Recon Surg 1994; 93:835–841.

27. Arkilic CF, Taguchi A, Sharma N, Ratnaraj J, Sessler DI, Read TE, Fleshman JW, Kurz A. Supplemental perioperative fluid administration increases tissue oxygen pressure. Surgery 2003; 133:49–55.

28. Hartmann M, Jonsson K, Zederfeldt B. Effect of tissue perfusion and oxygenation on accumulation of collagen in healing wounds. Randomized study in patients after major abdominal operations. Eur J Surg 1992; 158:521–526.
29. Kurz A, Sessler DI, Lenhardt R. Perioperative normothermia to reduce the incidence of surgical wound infections and shorten hospitalization. Study of wound infection and temperature group. N Eng J Med 1996; 334:1209–1215.
30. Greif R, Akca O, Horn E, Kurz A, Sessler DI. Supplemental perioperative oxygen to reduce the incidence of surgical-wound infection. N Eng J Med 2000; 342:161–167.

44

Hyperbaric Oxygen Therapy

Caroline E. Fife
Department of Anesthesiology, University of Texas Health Science Center, and Memorial Hermann Center for Wound Healing, Houston, Texas, U.S.A.

1. INTRODUCTION

In hypoxic wounds, as Hunt has observed, the question is not *whether* increased tissue oxygen is of benefit to healing, but how much. The mechanism by which oxygen is supplied to the tissues is via respiration of oxygen and subsequent delivery by the vasculature. If any additional oxygen is going to be delivered to hypoxic tissues, it must be breathed. Hyperbaric oxygen therapy (HBO$_2$T) is a treatment in which a patient breathes 100% oxygen while inside a pressure vessel (chamber) at an atmospheric pressure greater than sea level. Monoplace chambers accommodate a single patient and the entire chamber is usually pressurized with 100% oxygen that the patient breathes directly (Fig. 1). Multiplace chambers accommodate two or more patients (and usually an attendant) and the chamber is pressurized with compressed air while the patients breathe 100% oxygen via masks, head hoods, or endotracheal tubes (Fig. 2). According to the U.S. Food and Drug Administration, topical oxygen, in which isolated parts of the body are exposed to 100% oxygen, does not constitute HBO$_2$T. Topical oxygen should not be equated with HBO$_2$T and is not reimbursable by Medicare.

This chapter briefly reviews the physiology of HBO$_2$T, its effects on the healing process, and the clinical data to support its use as part of the continuum of wound management.

2. HOW HBO$_2$T INCREASES TISSUE OXYGEN LEVELS

Under normal circumstances, breathing air at sea level, the arterial partial pressure of oxygen (PO$_2$) is about 100 mmHg. In healthy individuals, the hemoglobin is about 97% saturated under those conditions. Increasing inspired oxygen concentration at sea level has little effect on the *hemoglobin* because it is already nearly saturated. A gram of fully saturated hemoglobin carries 1.35 cc of oxygen, bound chemically to the hemoglobin molecule. Note on the graph in Figure 3 (1), assuming a healthy person with a normal amount of hemoglobin (15 g), and 100% saturation of hemoglobin, the oxygen carrying capacity will be 20 cc of oxygen for every 100 cc

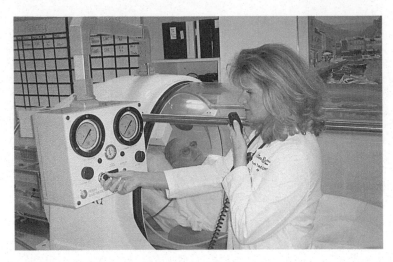

Figure 1 Monoplace hyperbaric chambers are usually compressed with oxygen. (Photo courtesy of the Texas Wound and Lymphedema Center, Tomball Regional Hospital.)

of blood, otherwise defined as 20 volumes percentage (vol.%) (Fig. 3). In contrast, blood plasma carries only 0.3 cc of oxygen for every 100 cc of blood (0.3 vol.%), so blood plasma makes no real contribution to oxygen carrying capacity when one breathes air at sea level. However, once hemoglobin is fully saturated, the only way to increase oxygen carrying capacity is to increase *plasma-dissolved* oxygen. Breathing pure oxygen at sea level increases the plasma-dissolved oxygen only 2 vol.%, because oxygen is not particularly soluble in plasma. However, as atmospheric pressure increases, an increasing amount of oxygen is dissolved in blood

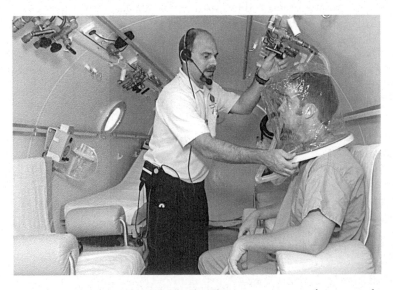

Figure 2 Multiplace hyperbaric chambers can accommodate more than one patient and an attendant. They are usually compressed with air and patients breath oxygen from a hood, mask, or endotracheal tube. (Photo by Richard Cunningham; courtesy of the Memorial Hermann Hyperbaric Center, Houston, Texas.)

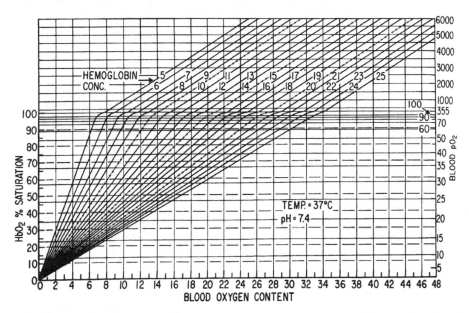

Figure 3 Hemoglobin oxygen saturation is displayed on the left vertical axis; blood oxygen tension from 0 to 6000 mmHg on the right. The lower horizontal axis depicts blood oxygen content in volumes per cent from 0 to 48. Various hemoglobin concentrations are plotted diagonally across the graph. Note that, assuming hemoglobin is constant, the only way to significantly increase oxygen carrying capacity (vol.%) is to dramatically increase blood PO_2. (From Ref. 1.)

plasma. Breathing oxygen at two times sea level atmospheric pressure, referred to as 2 atmospheres absolute (ATA), will result in an arterial PO_2 of about 1400 mmHg, a 10-fold increase in arterial oxygen tension. Under hyperbaric conditions, enough oxygen can be dissolved in plasma to keep tissues alive in the total absence of hemoglobin. Boerma et al. (2) demonstrated the potential importance of plasma dissolved oxygen in his historic study, "Life Without Blood," in which unanesthetized pigs with an average hemoglobin of 0.45 g/dL behaved normally when kept on pure oxygen at an atmospheric pressure of 3 ATA. Although the appropriate treatment for life-threatening anemia continues to be transfusion, there are many case reports in which HBO_2T was successfully used to prolong life in Jehovah's Witness patients who refused transfusion (3). Blood oxygen carrying capacity will have increased from 20 vol.% to about 24 vol.%, almost entirely due to an increase in *plasma* oxygen carrying capacity. Following the graph in Figure 3, with a hemoglobin of 5 g and a PO_2 of 100 mmHg, the oxygen carrying capacity is only about 7 vol.%. However, under hyperbaric conditions, at a depth of about 3 ATA, an arterial PO_2 of 2000 mmHg can be achieved so that even with a hemoglobin of 5 mg, the oxygen carrying capacity can be raised to approximately 14 vol.%. In general, the blood oxygen carrying capacity increases approximately 2 vol.% for every atmosphere of pressure increase.

In patients without life-threatening anemia who undergo HBO_2T, the dramatic increase in arterial oxygen levels during treatment also increases the driving force for oxygen diffusion. For example, at 3 ATA, the diffusion radius of oxygen into the extravascular compartment is estimated to increase from about 64 to 247 μm at the precapillary arteriole (Fig. 4) (3). This may allow a small number of capillaries

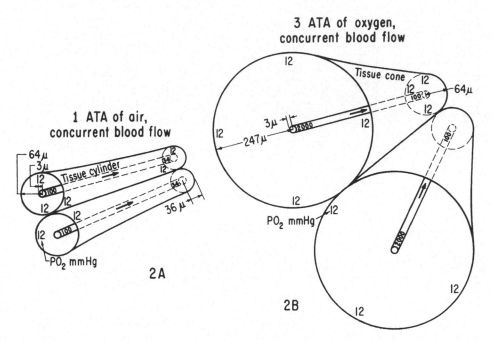

Figure 4 Oxygen diffusion into tissues: the diffusion of oxygen from a capillary into surrounding tissues using the Krogh–Erlang equation. During exposure to 1 ATA of oxygen of air (2A), the diffusion distance for oxygen at the arterial end is about 64 μm. With the blood PO₂ falling from 100 to 34 mmHg within the capillary during transit, the radius of oxygenated tissue at the venous end is relatively small. At 3 ATA, a larger cone of oxygenated tissue is depicted around the capillary, about 240 μm at the arterial end, and perhaps 64 μm at the venous end, assuming concurrent blood flow (2B). (Modified from Ref. 3.)

to supply a larger volume of tissue, an effect that might be important in crush injury or threatened flaps.

Oxygen, like any drug, has overdose and side effects. Pressure itself can cause barotrauma to gas spaces in the body, most commonly the middle ear. Approximately 1–10% of patients experience ear pain from difficulty equalizing the middle ear through the Eustachian tubes. Rupture of the tympanic membrane is uncommon but possible. Occasionally, tympanostomy tubes are necessary for patients to undergo HBO₂T. At the termination of treatment, as the atmospheric pressure of the chamber decreases and gas expands, air must be able to exit the lungs freely. Rare cases of pneumothorax have been described, and this could lead to arterial gas embolization and death. Patients with severe obstructive lung disease are not candidates for HBO₂T. Central nervous system oxygen toxicity is reported at a rate of 1:2000–1:10,000, manifested as grand mal seizures, with the risk possibly enhanced by hypoglycemia. This is an effect of hyperbaric oxygen on brain neurotransmitters, but there are no long-term negative effects. Pulmonary oxygen toxicity is not an issue with the short duration treatments given for wound healing problems. However, critically ill patients with necrotizing infections who may be maintained on high oxygen partial pressures in the intensive care unit require special consideration. Hyperbaric oxygen also has an effect on the lens of the eye which, in some patients, causes a transient myopia after a course of therapy. This effect seems to resolve after 3–6 months and does not appear to be linked to cataract development. The hyperbaric physician must evaluate the patient with regard to the safety and the appropriateness of HBO$_2$T. Patients with chronic obstructive lung disease must be assessed carefully. Seizure disorders must be controlled, and a variety of other underlying disease processes can affect patients in the hyperbaric environment, which is why hyperbaric physicians receive specialized training. Patients must then be frequently assessed as to their response to treatment and whether continued HBO$_2$T is warranted.

3. THE PHYSIOLOGICAL EFFECTS OF OXYGEN IN WOUND HEALING

Hyperbaric oxygen therapy improves host immune response by increasing leukocyte bactericidal activity (4,5), enhancing the neutrophil oxidative burst, and promoting leukocyte killing of aerobic gram-positive organisms, including *Staphylococcus aureus*, and aerobic gram-negative organisms (6). It is cytotoxic to anaerobes. It may therefore decrease morbidity, mortality, and the need for operative intervention in various necrotizing infections. It has proved effective as adjunctive therapy in animal models of chronic *S. aureus* and *Pseudomonas aeruginosa* osteomyelitis (7). In addition to enhanced bacterial killing, HBO$_2$T also raises decreased oxygen tensions found in infected bone to normal or even above normal levels. Hyperbaric oxygen therapy enhances the transport of aminoglycoside antibiotics across the cell wall (gentamicin, tobramycin, amikacin and perhaps others) increasing the efficacy of these drugs which may be inhibited *in vivo* by the local tissue hypoxia common in many patients with severe wounds (8).

Hyperbaric oxygen therapy reduces local tissue edema by arterial vasoconstriction while maintaining higher than normal local oxygen delivery to wounded tissue. In addition to the biochemical effects discussed above, oxygen has direct vascular effects. It causes vasoconstriction in both arterial and venous vessels. Hyperbaric oxygen therapy has been shown to reduce edema and congestion, effects that contribute to its adjunctive use in threatened replantations (9). While vasoconstriction induced by HBO$_2$T may reduce blood "in-flow" by 20%, the amount of oxygen supplied by the plasma is increased, as described above, so oxygen delivery is maintained (10,11). Hyperbaric oxygen therapy prevents leukocyte mediated postischemia reperfusion (IR) injury (12). The most intriguing aspect of HBO$_2$T is its now well-described ability to mitigate ischemia reperfusion injury, both in musculoskeletal tissue and in the brain. The mechanism is by preventing the adhesion of leukocytes to the venule wall and thus limiting the production of oxygen-free radicals which cause arteriolar vasoconstriction.

Hyperbaric oxygen therapy has long been known to enhance collagen deposition in hypoxic tissues as well as increasing angiogenesis (13,14). At the cellular level, these benefits of HBO$_2$T must be mediated by cytokines. Recent data by Mustoe have demonstrated that HBO$_2$T modulates the signal transduction pathway that regulates the gene expression for platelet-derived growth factor (PDGF) -beta receptor. Not only does this suggest a possible synergistic effect between HBO$_2$T and PDGF administration, but may also explain one of the mechanisms by which HBO$_2$T enhances angiogenesis. Hyperbaric oxygen therapy also stimulates osteoclast and osteoblast function which is impaired under hypoxic conditions. Marx et al. (15) have demonstrated that HBO$_2$T enhances angiogenesis in ischemic irradiated tissues. Histopathological studies have shown that the etiology of delayed radiation injury is endarteritis with tissue hypoxia and secondary fibrosis (16).

Dental extractions or surgical reconstructions performed in previously irradiated
tissue have high rates of complication and failure unless preoperative HBO_2T is
performed (17–20).

4. AN EVIDENCE-BASED REVIEW OF THE EFFECTS OF HBO_2T IN WOUND HEALING

Hyperbaric oxygen therapy is considered the primary treatment for decompression
illness, arterial gas embolism, and carbon monoxide poisoning (21). The following
indications are accepted by the Undersea and Hyperbaric Medical Society (UHMS)
as adjunctive uses of HBO_2T in various wound healing problems: acute thermal
burns, clostridial myonecrosis, other necrotizing soft tissue infections, compromised
skin grafts and flaps, crush injury, compartment syndrome, other acute traumatic
ischemias, osteoradionecrosis, soft tissue radionecrosis, refractory osteomyelitis,
and other wounds with demonstrated periwound hypoxia. The 2003 Hyperbaric
Oxygen Committee Report, available from the UHMS, provides an evidence-based
review of the literature for each indication (22). Several exhaustive evidence-based
reviews of world literature have been conducted by the following organizations or
entities: BlueCross/BlueShield (BCBS) Technology Assessment 1999, American
Diabetes Association Foot Council 1999, British Journal of Medicine 2000, 2001,
and the Medical Services Advisory Committee, Australia. Independently, they concluded that the data for acute ischemia, acute infection, diabetic ulcers, and radiation
supported the utility of HBO_2T (23–26).

In 2001, the AHRQ made an extensive literature review in preparing a report
to CMS. They reviewed 13 published, peer-reviewed studies, of which 7 were randomized, controlled trials (27–29). All diabetic wounds were Wagner III–IV. There
were a total of 606 patients in the HBO_2T groups with a 71% bipedal limb salvage
rate. In the combined control groups, there were a total of 463 patients with a
53% bipedal limb salvage rate. Compare this to the Regranex (becalpermin) clinical
trials of diabetic foot ulcer healing. In 922 patients over four trials, 478 patients
received Regranex, with healing rates of 43%, compared to control healing rates
of 29%. However, these involved only Wager II, well vascularized ulcers (30). It
would seem that the hyperbaric data compare very favorably in the area of efficacy
and limb salvage with much more limb threatening wounds.

The Faglia study was a randomized, controlled trial of 70 diabetic ulcer
patients consecutively admitted and randomized to receive HBO_2T vs. standardized
conventional care. The HBO_2T treatment protocol was 2.5 ATA for 90 min initially
then 2.4 ATA for subsequent treatments. In the HBO_2T-treated group (mean treatment number 38 ± 8), 3 patients (8.6%) underwent major amputations, 2 below the
knee (BKA), 1 above the knee, (AKA). In the non-HBO_2T-treated group, 11 patients
(33%) underwent major amputations, 7 BKA and 4 AKA ($P = 0.016$). Multivariate
analysis of major amputation on all the considered variables confirmed the protective role of HBO_2T in diabetic foot ulcers.

5. HYPERBARIC TREATMENT PROTOCOLS

Treatment protocols vary depending on the diagnosis and the severity of the wound.
The "dose" of oxygen is determined by the atmospheric pressure and the duration of

treatment. The number of treatments should be determined by patient response. Treatments for wound healing problems are usually delivered at 2.0–2.4 ATA. Outcome data failed to show a statistical difference in diabetic wound healing when analyzed by treatment pressure (2.0 vs. 2.4 ATA) (31). This is probably because after some minimum threshold is reached, increasing treatment pressure will not confer additional benefit. Usual wound healing protocols are between 90 and 120 min.

Treatments may be once or twice per day depending on the severity and type of wound. Necrotizing infections are usually treated twice per day at least initially. Outcome data in diabetic foot ulcerations show that the average number of treatments in patients who benefited was 35 and diminishing returns are reached at approximately 40 treatments (31). Appropriate use of HBO_2T requires the direct and frequent input of a trained hyperbaric physician.

6. PATIENT SELECTION FOR HYPERBARIC OXYGEN THERAPY

To use HBO_2T cost effectively, patients who are going to heal spontaneously should be screened out, as well as those patients who are destined to fail. Transcutaneous oximetry (TCOM) represents a simple, noninvasive method for assessing the likelihood of spontaneous healing and as a screening tool for vascular disease. Generally, values less than 30–40 mmHg are considered inadequate for spontaneous healing. If TCOMs are adequate, the wound may be followed with conservative management. If TCOMs suggest ischemia, further vascular testing can be performed, and after revascularization, TCOMs can be rechecked again. Patients with low TCOMs can be referred for HBO_2T. This process is depicted in Figure 5.

We evaluated the outcome of a series of 29 consecutive diabetic patients with limb threatening lesions who underwent angioplasty for revascularization. After a mean follow-up period of 12 months, 23 patients (79%) experienced progressive healing with 15 (65%) being discharged from hyperbarics by the end of the follow-up period. Mean time to wound healing was 3 months. Six patients (21%) had poor outcomes, 2 requiring BKA due to osteomyelitis despite technically successful angioplasties, 1 was amputated due to a worsening wound, and 3 could not be revascularized. Transcutaneous oximetry improved in all the patients who were successfully revascularized from 27.8 ± 9.9 to 54.5 ± 14.7 mmHg ($P < 0.0001$). Patients whose post procedure TCOMs remained below 40 received HBO_2T to assist with wound healing. Transcutaneous oximetry performed better than Doppler ABI in predicting the technical success of angioplasty as well as in screening the patients who were referred for angioplasty, and in determining which patients would get HBO_2T afterward (32).

Transcutaneous oximetry, which uses a modified Clark electrode in a heated thermistor, is in common usage at many wound-healing centers. It has the disadvantage of requiring intact skin for measurement, and thus may be used only in the peri-wound area. Since this technique relies on the diffusion of oxygen to the heated electrode, highly calloused, edematous or infected skin decreases the reliability of measurements. The accuracy of TCOM was evaluated in a retrospective analysis of over 1000 patients with diabetic foot ulcers all of whom underwent treatment with HBO_2T, with an overall success rate of 75.6% (31). Forty-eight percent of the hyperbaric patients had a baseline TCOM below 20 mmHg, yet the failure rate was only 35% (31). This may suggest the effectiveness of HBO_2T. For this reason, while baseline sea level air TCOM levels are used to determine whether the wound

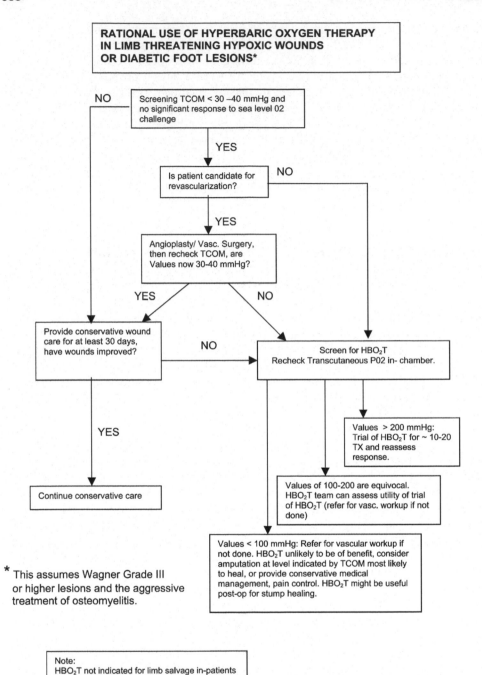

Figure 5 Rational use of hyperbaric oxygen therapy in limb threatening hypoxic wounds or diabetic foot lesions: patients can be screened for tissue hypoxia with transcutaneous oximetry. Revascularization must be a priority. In-chamber TCOM is the most accurate way to determine the likelihood of benefit from HBO_2T.

might heal spontaneously, they are of no value in determining whether HBO_2T will be of benefit. An increase in periwound TCOM while breathing oxygen at sea level was useful in selecting patients likely to benefit from HBO_2T. If oxygen-breathing TCOM values increased to above 35 mmHg at sea level, the likelihood of benefiting from subsequent HBO_2T was 77% and the test was 69% accurate. The absolute increase (in mmHg) with oxygen breathing was better than the percentage increase (or ratio) over baseline, because many patients with a baseline near zero were not healed if their HBO_2T doubled or tripled (e.g., going from 2 to 6 mmHg). However, the most reliable test for benefit from HBO_2T was the increase in periwound TCOM while breathing oxygen in the hyperbaric chamber. If in-chamber TCOM increased to 200 mmHg or better, the likelihood of benefiting from HBO_2T was 94%, and this test was 75% accurate. These data did not directly demonstrate the effectiveness of HBO_2T because there was no control group of similar patients who did not receive the therapy. However, for many of these patients with modified Wagner III or IV lesions, HBO_2T was the only alternative to amputation. In light of the overall success rate of 75.6% in this large series of patients, the benefit of HBO_2T is encouraging. These data confirm those previously reported by Wattel et al. that patients with transcutaneous oxygen values of about 450 mmHg in the vicinity of the wound while breathing pure oxygen at 2.5 atm abs are predictive of healing, whereas patients with values of 100 mmHg are likely to require amputation (33).

Two case studies illustrate this process. Patient A is a 62-year-old African-American male with noninsulin dependent diabetes mellitus and severe peripheral vascular disease. The tissue over the dorsal right foot spontaneously necrosed and after debridement exposed all anterior tendons (Fig. 6). Transcutaneous oximetry revealed a value of 10 mmHg with no significant response to sea level oxygen breathing. Magnetic resonance angiography demonstrated complete occlusion of the right superficial femoral artery (SFA), peroneal and anterior tibial arteries (AT), with severe disease of the posterior tibial (PT) and dorsalis pedis. The SFA was successfully stented, and the AT and PT were dilated via angioplasty. Postprocedure TCOMs were improved but still borderline for spontaneous healing (39 mmHg). In-chamber TCOM was 410 mmHg, suggesting that HBO_2T was likely to be beneficial, and was initiated. The patient received a total of 36 treatments, with improved

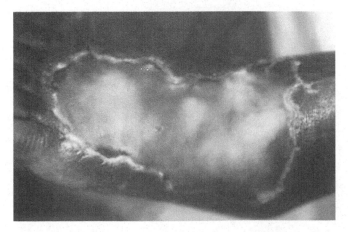

Figure 6 Patient A: 62-year-old male with NIDDM and vascular disease, baseline TCOM of 10 mmHg.

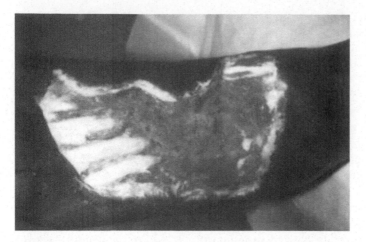

Figure 7 Postangioplasty and 28 of an eventual 36 HBO_2T with granulation tissue beginning to form.

granulation tissue (Fig. 7), so HBO_2T was discontinued while conservative treatment with moist dressings continued. Complete wound healing was achieved in a patient who would otherwise likely have required amputation (Fig. 8). Patient B is a 68-year-old Hispanic male with noninsulin dependent diabetes and severe peripheral vascular disease, status post an aortobifemoral bypass and an axillobifemoral bypass on the right. Nevertheless, he required an above the knee amputation on the right for ischemia, and presented with a dehisced surgical wound (Fig. 9). Transcutaneous oximetry revealed values adjacent to the wound of only 1 and 9 mmHg, with no significant response to sea level oxygen breathing (e.g., 16 and 32 mmHg, respectively), confirming severe ischemia. The patient had no other revascularization options.

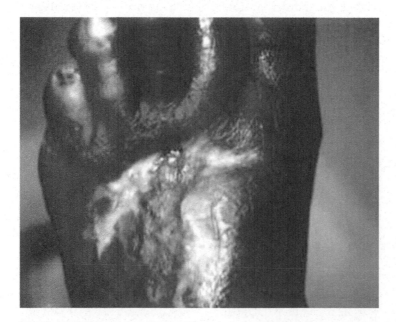

Figure 8 Healed wound after 20 weeks of further conservative wound care.

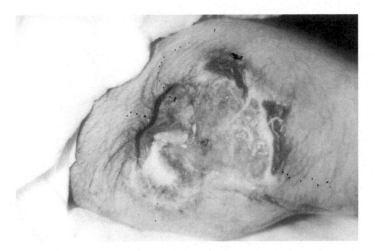

Figure 9 Patient B: 68-year-old male with NIDDM and severe vascular disease status post-numerous bypass procedures, nonhealing AKA stump. TCOM: 1 and 9 mmHg adjacent to wound.

However, in-chamber TCOM was 365 mmHg adjacent to the wound, so a course of HBO_2T was initiated. After 15 treatments, a confluent granulation bed was apparent (Fig. 10). In addition, the patient was begun on V.A.C. (KCI, Inc.). Hyperbaric oxygen therapy was then discontinued, and the patient continued to receive treatment with the V.A.C. He went on to complete closure with conservative wound care (Fig. 11).

Hyperbaric oxygen therapy treatments usually last only 1–2 hr, raising the question as to whether this time period is sufficient to affect biological processes. Data confirm that oxygen tension values may remain elevated for up to 3 hr after the cessation of hyperbaric therapy (34). Faglia et al. (29) documented a highly

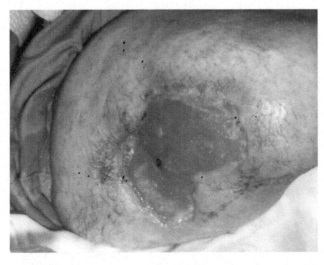

Figure 10 Confluent granulation tissue after 15 HBO_2T and treatment with the V.A.C. (KCI Inc.). HBO_2T is discontinued.

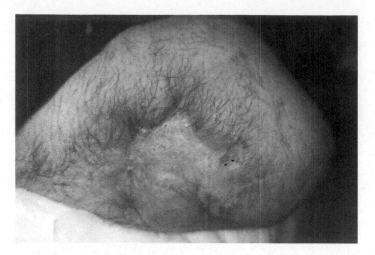

Figure 11 Healed wound 16 weeks from initiation of treatment.

significant and long-lasting increase in transcutaneous oxygen values in diabetic patients who benefited from HBO_2T. Marx et al. have demonstrated the same changes in ischemic irradiated tissues.

A sea level TCOM assessment has an accuracy of about 70%, while the accuracy of in-chamber TCOM approaches 75%. Even with these effective screening tools, prediction would still be incorrect in one out of four cases and patients who might benefit from HBO_2T would be deprived of the therapy. Therefore, these "cut-off" scores must serve as guides to therapy. A rational approach might be to provide a trial of therapy and then reassess the patient on the basis of clinical progress or improved TCOM values after a reasonable trial of therapy (e.g., 15–20 treatments).

7. MEDICARE COVERAGE GUIDELINES

In a coverage memorandum published December 27, 2002, CMS stated, "The evidence is adequate to conclude that HBO therapy is clinically effective and thus reasonable and necessary in the treatment of certain patients with limb threatening diabetic wounds of the lower extremity" (Transmittal AB-01-183). To qualify for HBO_2T in the treatment of a diabetic foot ulcer, patients must meet each of the following three criteria: (1) Type I or Type II diabetes with a lower extremity wound *due to diabetes* (2) Wagner Grade III or higher wound, and the (3) patient must have failed a 30-day course of adequate, standard wound therapy. "Standard wound therapy," is defined as: (1) assessment of vascular status and correction, if possible, of vascular problems in the affected limb, (2) optimization of glucose control, (3) debridement of necrotic tissue, (4) maintenance of moist wound bed, (4) appropriate off-loading, (5) and treatment of infection. "Measurable signs of healing," is defined as a decrease in wound volume or size, a decrease in exudate, or a decrease in necrotic tissue. Once HBO_2T is begun, CMS requires that the wound be re-evaluated every 30 days during the HBO_2T course and continued HBO_2T will not be covered if there are no measurable signs of healing.

Hyperbaric oxygen therapy is a treatment provided by a physician with specific expertise and training. CMS expanded coverage of HBO_2T for diabetic foot ulcers based on a careful review of the data. The cost of a primary amputation in 1986 was reported to be in excess of $ 40,000 (35). The cost of a course of HBO_2T to save a limb (assuming an average of 35 treatments) is approximately $ 18,000. When patients are carefully selected, appropriately followed, and HBO_2T is discontinued at maximal benefit, HBO_2T can reduce amputation rate and save health care dollars.

REFERENCES

1. Fuson RL, Saltzman HA, Starmer CF, Smith WW. Normogram for oxygen content, saturation and pressure at hyperbaric conditions. Anesthesiology 1966; 27(2):176–179.
2. Boerma I, Meijne NG, Brummelkamp WK, Bouma S, Mensch MH, Kamermans F, Stern Hanf M, Van Aalderen W. Life without blood. A study of the influence of high atmospheric pressure and hypothermia on dilution of the blood. J Cardiovasc Surg 1960; 1:133–146.
3. Saltzman HA. Rational normobaric and hyperbaric oxygen therapy. Ann Intern Med 1967; 67(4):843–852.
4. Hohn DC. Oxygen and leukocyte microbial killing. In: Davis JC, Hunt TK, eds. Hyperbaric Oxygen Therapy. Bethesda, Maryland: Undersea Medical Society Inc., 1977: 101–110.
5. Knighton DR, Fiegel VD. Oxygen as an antibiotic: the effect of inspired oxygen on infection. Arch Surg 1990; 125:97–100.
6. Mader JT, Adams KR, Wallace WR, Calhoun JH. Hyperbaric oxygen as adjunctive therapy for osteomyelitis. Infect Dis Clin N Am 1990; 4:433–444.
7. Mader JT, Brown GL, Guckian JC, Wells CH, Reinarz JA. A mechanism for the amelioration by hyperbaric oxygen of experimental staphylococcal osteomyelitis in rabbits. J Infect Dis 1980; 142:915–922.
8. Mader JT, Adams KR, Couch LA, Sutton TE. Potentiation of tobramycin by hyperbaric oxygen in experimental *Pseudomonas aeruginosa* osteomyelitis. Presented at the 27th Interscience Conference on Antimicrobial Agents and Chemotherapy, 1987.
9. Chang N, Goodson WH III, Gottrup F, Hunt TK. Direct measurement of wound and tissue oxygen tension in postoperative patients. Ann Surg 1983; 197:470–478.
10. Robson MC, Stenberg BD, Heggers JP. Wound healing alterations caused by infection. Clin Plast Surg 1990; 17(3):485–492.
11. Hunt TK. The physiology of wound healing. Ann Emerg Med 1988; 17:1265–1273.
12. Zamboni WA. Applications of hyperbaric oxygen therapy in plastic surgery. In: Oriani G, Marroni A, Wattel F, eds. Handbook on Hyperbaric Oxygen Therapy. New York: Springer-Verlag, 1996.
13. Davis JC, Hunt TK, eds. Problem Wounds: The Role of Oxygen. New York: Elsevier, 1988.
14. Davis JC, Hunt TK. Hyperbaric Oxygen Therapy. Bethesda, Maryland: Undersea Medical Society, 1977.
15. Marx RE, Ehler WJ, Tayapongsak P, Pierce LW. Relationship of oxygen dose to angiogenesis induction in irradiated tissue. Am J Surg 1990; 160:519–524.
16. Rubin P. Late effects of chemotherapy and radiation therapy: a new hypothesis. Int J Radiat Oncol Biol Phys 1984; 10:5–34.
17. Marx RE, Ames JR. The use of hyperbaric oxygen in bony reconstruction of the irradiated and tissue-deficient patient. J Oral Maxillofac Surg 1982; 40:412–420.
18. Marx RE. A new concept in the treatment of osteoradionecrosis. J Oral Maxillofac Surg 1983; 41:351–357.

19. Marx RE, Johnson RP. Problem wounds in oral and maxillofacial surgery: the role of hyperbaric oxygen. In: Davis JC, Hunt TK, eds. Problem Wounds: The Role of Oxygen. New York: Elsevier, 1988:65–123.

20. Marx RE, Johnson RP, Kline SN. Prevention of osteoradionecrosis: a randomized prospective clinical trial of hyperbaric oxygen versus penicillin. J Am Dent Assoc 1985; 11:49–54.

21. Tibbles PM, Edelsberg JS. Hyperbaric-oxygen therapy. New Engl J Med 1996; 334: 1642–1648.

22. Feldmeier J, ed. Hyperbaric oxygen therapy: 2003 Committee Report. Kensington, MD: Undersea and Hyperbaric Medical Society, 2003.

23. Hyperbaric Oxygen Therapy for Wound Healing—Parts I, II, III. BlueCross BlueShield Association Assessment Program August 1999; 14(2), December 1999; 14(15), December 1999; 14(16). Blue Cross Blue Shield Association Technology Evaluation Center.

24. Medical Services Advisory Committee (MSAC), Department of Health and Aged Care, Australia, Hyperbaric Oxygen Therapy, November 2000, MSAC Applications 1018–1020 Assessment Report.

25. American Diabetes Association (April 7–8, 1999). Consensus Development Conference on Diabetic Foot Wound Care. Diabetes Care 1999; 22(8):1354–1360.

26. ADA Consensus Development Conference on Diabetic Foot Wound Care. Diabetes Care 1999; 22(8):1354, Consensus Panel: Cavanagh, Buse, Frykberg, Gibbons, Lipsky, Pogach, Reiber, Sheehan.

27. Baroni G, Porro T, Faglia E, Pizzi G, Mastropasqua A, Oriani G, Pedesini G, Favales F. Hyperbaric oxygen in diabetic gangrene treatment. Diabetes Care 1987; 10:81–86.

28. Doctor N, Pandya S, Supe A. Hyperbaric oxygen therapy in diabetic foot. J Postgrad Med 1992; 38(3):112–114.

29. Faglia E, Favales F, Aldeghi A, Calia P, Quarantiello A, Oriani G, Michael M, Campagnoli P, Morabito A. Adjunctive systemic hyperbaric oxygen therapy in treatment of severe diabetic foot ulcer. A randomized study. Diabetes Care 1996; 19:1338–1343.

30. Embil JM, Papp K, Sibbald G, et al. Recombinant human platelet-derived growth factor-BB (becaplermin) for healing chronic lower extremity diabetic ulcers: an open label clinical evaluation of efficacy. Wound Rep Reg 2000; 8:162–168.

31. Fife CE, Buyukcakir C, Otto GH, Sheffield PJ, Warriner RA, Love TL, Mader J. The predictive value of transcutaneous oxygen tension measurement in diabetic lower extremity ulcers treated with hyperbaric oxygen therapy; a retrospective analysis of 1144 patients. Wound Rep Reg 2002; 10:198–207.

32. Hanna GP, Fujise K, Kjellgren O, Field S, Fife CE, Schroth G, Clanton T, Anderson V, Smalling RW. Infrapopliteal transcatheter interventions for limb salvage in diabetic patients: importance of aggressive interventional approach and role of transcutaneous oximetry. Am J Cardiol 1997; 30:664–669.

33. Wattel FE, Mathieu MD, Fossati P, Neviere RR, Coget JM. Hyperbaric oxygen in the treatment of diabetic foot lesions. Search for healing predictive factors. J Hyperb Med 1991; 6(4):263–268.

34. Sheffield PJ, Workman WT. Noninvasive tissue oxygen measurements in patients administered normobaric and hyperbaric oxygen by mask. Hyperb Oxyg Rev 1985; 6(1):47–62.

35. Mackey WC, McCullough JL, Conlon TP, Shepard AD, Deterlin RA, Callow AD, O'Donnel TF. The cost of surgery for limb-threatening ischemia. Surgery 1986; 99:26–35.

45

The Art and Science of Wound Dressings in the Twenty-First Century

Liza Ovington
Ovington & Associates, Inc., Allentown, Pennsylvania, U.S.A.

1. A BRIEF HISTORY OF WOUND DRESSINGS

Mankind has described the art of dressing a wound since our earliest written records. Sumerian cuneiform tablets dated prior to 2000 B.C. contain lists of different types of wounds and injuries along with passages detailing how best to treat them (1,2). Topical treatments included applications of poultices incorporating ingredients such as plant matter, mud, milk, wine, and oil. The Edwin Smith surgical papyrus, an Egyptian document dated 1650 B.C. but believed to be a copy of a much older document, describes 48 cases of wounds and details their treatment. A later Egyptian document, the Ebers Papyrus, discusses the preparation of various topical concoctions for dressing wounds. The basic recipe for an Egyptian wound dressing appears to have consisted of lint, grease, and honey applied to strips of cotton or linen, which were then placed into and over the wound. Lint refers to vegetable fibers that likely served an absorbent role. Grease consisted of animal fats that may have served as a barrier to external contamination. Honey is the most often cited ingredient in a number of Egyptian wound preparations (1) and was perhaps used empirically for its antibacterial properties. Today, we have evidence that unprocessed honey contains natural antibacterial constituents and also exerts an osmotic effect that dehydrates bacteria and reduces tissue edema (3,4). In addition to any antibacterial effects, honey as well as the grease probably prevented the cotton or linen bandages used by the Egyptians from adhering to the wound surface. Interestingly, these features of absorption, acting as a physical barrier, and preventing infection and adherence to the wound are still desirable characteristics of a wound dressing.

Moving forward in time, a pertinent figure in Greek medicine with relevance to wound healing was Galen of Pergamum. Galen was a second century physician who wrote of his medical observations and beliefs in a series of 83 volumes of text that influenced the European practice of medicine until the Renaissance. Galen gained experience in wound management when he acted a perhaps the first "sports medicine physician" and cared for injured gladiators. Gladiatorial games generated many wounds and Galen had opportunities to experiment with a variety of ways of dressing them. He observed that wounds healed optimally when the topical dressing maintained a continuously moist environment at the wound surface. He described creating such an environment with cotton cloth and a sponge and refers to the difficulty of keeping dressing moist during the heat of the summer in the following passage (4):

> ...as I have previously explained, it is necessary to keep the wound continuously moist, because if the dressings dry out, the ulcer becomes inflamed. This is true especially in summer, at which time when the pontifices of Pergamum were celebrating the appointed gladiatorial games, I cured the most seriously injured by covering the wounds by a cloth wet with astringent wine and kept moist both day and night by a superimposed sponge...

Galen was perhaps the first physician to recognize the clinical benefit of moist wound healing and the inherent challenges in creating and maintaining that environment with appropriate wound dressings. However, his observations did little to change the art of dressing wounds and the materials used in preparing dressings did not vary significantly through the course of Greek and Roman civilization, the Middle Ages and the Renaissance.

The history of wound dressings finally took a major turn in the 20th century when clinical researchers rediscovered and scientifically documented what Galen had observed empirically centuries earlier—that wounds in a continuously moist environment heal more rapidly than those allowed to dry out. Early modern evidence of improved healing rates that can be achieved by keeping a wound in a moist environment is found in the 1948 dissertation of a Swedish doctoral student, Oscar Gilje (5). Gilje noted that venous ulcers treated with occlusion by adhesive tape exhibited dramatic healing results compared to those that were not occluded. However, while tape could occlude a wound and keep it moist, it was not a practical wound dressing because it lacked absorbency and existing absorbent dressing materials (gauze) were not effective at maintaining a continuously moist environment. Consequently, Gilje's findings also had little effect on changing clinical practice until more advanced dressing materials became available. Luckily, in the 1950s, the textile industry was producing synthetic fibers and fabrics from polymers including nylon, polyethylene, polypropylene, polyesters, polyvinyl alcohols, acrylics, and olefins (6). It was not long before scientists began investigating the use of these polymeric materials in wound management.

Perhaps the most referenced evidence of the positive effects of a continuously moist environment on healing is the work published by George Winter in Nature in 1962 (7). In his landmark study, in a swine model of wound healing, he described an almost 50% increase in the epithelialization rate for partial thickness wounds occluded with polyethylene film when compared to wounds left exposed to the air. Winter also tested polyester and polypropylene films (8). In 1963, Howard Maibach repeated Winter's study in human volunteers and found a similar increase in the epithelialization rate for occluded wounds (9). Potential mechanisms for the increased healing rates were suggested when histological studies of wounds healing in an moist environment vs. wounds healing in a dry environment demonstrated that the dry environment results in further tissue death beyond the original cause of the wound or "dehydration necrosis" (8,10). Studies have also been shown that resurfacing epithelial cells move farther and faster in a moist environment whereas a dry environment can effectively retard their progress (8). Further studies of wounds healing in a moist environment have shown that the fluid that is retained at the wound surface occlusion contains proteolytic enzymes and functional growth factors that facilitate an optimal and expedient healing process (11). In dry wounds, these enzymes and proteins may be presented only deeper in the tissue and in lower concentrations.

Results from studies such as these eventually led to the widespread commercial development of polymeric dressings for wound management in the late 1970s and that development continues today. Polymers can essentially be custom made to meet specific performance parameters such as gas permeability, absorbency, and physical format. Due to this possible customization of polymers, the range of materials suitable for use as wound dressings has grown exponentially beyond natural plant fibers. Manmade polymeric products such as films, foams, hydrogels, alginates, and hydrocolloids are now available for wound management. Even more recently, wound dressings are incorporating biomaterials and active ingredients with unique functions.

2. WOUND DRESSING CHOICES IN THE 21ST CENTURY

2.1. Functions: Passive vs. Active Wound Dressings

Wound dressings in the 21st century are still evolving—both in terms of new material developments as well as new performance parameters or functions. Many dressings that may differ widely in their physical composition can be divided into two broad functional categories—those that are *passive* and those that are *active*.

Passive wound dressings may be characterized as those that function in terms of affecting local moisture levels in the damaged tissues but do not cause a significant change in any other local chemical or cellular constituents. These dressings have traditionally been referred to as moisture retentive or semiocclusive dressings or described as promoting the continuously moist wound environment recommended by Galen and Winter. Their composition is variable; however, they are almost always composed of ingredients that are "foreign" to the local tissue environment. Most of the polymeric dressings mentioned earlier fall into this category. Depending on their specific ingredients, passive wound dressings may balance local tissue moisture levels by different means (to be discussed in greater detail in the next section).

Active dressings, on the other hand, may be characterized as those that function primarily by changing some specific chemical (other than water) or cellular parameter in the local wound tissues. These dressings may also influence the local moisture levels but this is not their primary mechanism of action. Their materials of composition are often ingredients that are native to tissue—such as collagen or other matrix proteins—and that are effectively "recognized" by local cells. They may also contain ingredients that interact in some ways with local wound cells or chemicals. Active wound dressings can be thought of as increasing or decreasing some specific chemical or cellular parameter of the local tissues.

3. PASSIVE DRESSING CATEGORIES

Passive dressings function primarily by affecting tissue moisture levels. It is important to remember that the desirable continuously moist local tissue environment does not mean that the wound should be covered in fluid. Wound tissues should be physiologically moist, not too dry but not too wet. In the early inflammatory phase of healing, the wound tissues may be overly moist and not only lose fluid through

Table 1 Examples of Passive Wound Dressings

Dressing category	Sample brands (manufacturer)	Dressing function
Foams	Tielle (Johnson & Johnson)	Absorb wound exudate
	Allevyn (Smith & Nephew)	
	Mepilex (Molnlycke)	
Alginates	Kaltostat (ConvaTec)	Absorb wound exudate
	Tegagen (3M)	
	NuDerm (Johnson & Johnson)	
Hydrocolloids	Duoderm (ConvaTec)	Maintain moisture
	Comfeel (Coloplast)	
	Restore (Hollister)	
Transparent films	OpSite (Smith & Nephew)	Maintain moisture
	Bioclusive (Johnson & Johnson)	
	Tegaderm (3M)	
Hydrogels—amorphous	Intrasite (Smith & Nephew)	Supply moisture
	NuGel (Johnson & Johnson)	
	Curasol (HealthPoint)	
Hydrogels—sheets	Vigilon (Bard)	Supply moisture
	NuGel (Johnson & Johnson)	
	Elastogel (Southwest Technologies)	

evaporation, but also through exudate production. Chronic or nonhealing wounds are often stalled in the inflammatory phase and therefore exude fluid continuously. Excessive wound exudate must be managed to prevent maceration or "water logging" of the tissues as well as potential soiling of clothes and linens. Also, certain wound etiologies may be associated with very high exudate levels such as venous leg ulcers or wounds in a setting of lymphedema. In these cases, a dressing must be able to manage the exudate by absorption in order to maintain optimal tissue moisture levels. Alternatively, if tissue moisture levels are already depleted due to evaporative moisture loss, the wound dressing must be able to restore moisture.

Passive wound dressings usually fall into one of these three categories with regard to their effects on tissue moisture levels—dressings that absorb excessive wound exudate, dressings that maintain existing levels of tissue moisture, and those which supply moisture to the tissues (Table 1).

3.1. Passive Dressings That Absorb Exudate

In any situation where a wound is producing moderate to high levels of exudate, an absorbent dressing is needed. Absorbent dressings are those types that have a high capacity for capturing and holding fluid. They will require fewer dressing changes within a set period of time as opposed to dressings that are not as absorbent (e.g., gauze) and therefore enable undisturbed wound healing and less labor time on the part of the clinician or caregiver. Foam and alginate dressings are both excellent passive dressing choices when absorbency is needed.

Foam dressing are most often polyurethane in composition but may be composed of other polymers as well. The polymer solution has been "foamed"—which is to say that air bubbles have been introduced to create tiny, open cells that are capable of filling with and holding fluids. Foams will actively take up fluids into their structure, removing it from the wound surface and holding it in the open cells—the same operating principle as a kitchen sponge. The absorbed fluid in the foam also maintains humidity at the wound surface, preventing tissue dehydration. Foam dressings are one of the most variable categories of passive dressings (from brand to brand) and may differ from one another in several aspects. They may be of varying thicknesses—which will, of course, impact their overall absorbent capacity. Foam dressings may also have adhesive borders that enable them to adhere directly to the skin surrounding the wound—or not, requiring that some other means of securement to the patient be used (e.g., tapes). Also, foams may have a waterproof coating on one side—or they may not. If there is a waterproof coating, the side containing that coating is often colored (e.g., pink or blue) to indicate the difference between the sides. This visual cue is to ensure that the dressing is not placed on the wound with the waterproof side down—which would, of course, defeat the absorbency function.

A potential shortcoming of foam dressings occurs when the wound to be dressed is a deep cavity or has undermining or sinus tracts. A general principle of wound management is that the dressing used should gently fill all open spaces of the wound to prevent the premature closure of the proximal portion of the wound, thereby creating an abscess. Most foams are resilient and do not conform well to depth or cavities (e.g., if you take a foam and fold it in half then let go of it; it usually unfolds quickly to become flat again). While there are a few foams designed especially for cavities, if the wound has significant depth and needs absorbency, a different type of absorbent dressing may be called for.

Alginate dressings are a more conformable type of absorbent passive dressing that may be particularly useful in the management of exuding cavity wounds. Alginates are composed of a polymer derived from brown seaweed and present visually as a soft, beige fiber. The fibers are compressed and entangled to form a flat sheet or simply bunched together in a rope form. Alginate fibers have a very high absorbent capacity and upon absorption of wound fluid they swell and gel to create a moist mass on top of the wound. It is important to secure an alginate dressing with secondary dressing that will keep it in place on the patient and also prevent the gelled fibers from drying out over time. The use of alginates should be limited to wounds with moderate-to-heavy exudate as they may dehydrate a wound with minimal exudate.

3.2. Passive Dressings That Maintain Moisture

As wounds progress in healing and begin to granulate, their exudate production lessens and dressing absorbency becomes less important. Indeed, when the exudate levels decrease, continued use of an absorbent dressing may actually dehydrate the wound tissues. At this phase of healing, what is needed is a passive dressing that can maintain the natural moisture level of the newly forming tissues. Two types of passive dressings that provide this function are hydrocolloid dressings and transparent film dressings.

Hydrocolloid dressings are composed of a homogeneous mixture of adhesive, absorptive, and elastomeric ingredients. They present visually as a caramel colored wafer and are sticky across the entire wound contact surface. This stickiness or tack is due to their adhesive components and enables the hydrocolloid to adhere very securely to the dry, intact skin around the wound. The hydrocolloid will not stick to the moist tissues of the wound because its surface will gel upon prolonged contact with moist tissues. The upper surface of hydrocolloid dressings is usually coated with a transparent film, which renders it waterproof. They are capable of extended wear times (3–5 days or longer depending on wound status) and can be worn in the shower. Hydrocolloids do have the ability to absorb small amounts of wound exudate but they do so very slowly and are not likely to dry a wound out. Most hydrocolloids are available in both regular and extrathin formats, the latter of which are very conformable to the topography of the body. Hydrocolloid wafers are not appropriate choices for cavity wounds, but there are paste versions that can be used to fill in the cavity prior to covering with the wafer form.

Transparent film dressings are thin, transparent sheets of a polymer, which has been coated on one side with an adhesive. They are engineered to transmit less water vapor than the average wound loses and so they are capable of maintaining a moist wound environment. Film dressings are waterproof but have no ability to absorb fluids and wound exudate may accumulate beneath the film surface with highly exudative wounds. When this occurs, the pooled exudate may break the adhesive seal and leak out. This creates a potential hygiene problem for the patient as well as a portal of entry for exogenous bacteria. In addition to treating superficial wounds, these transparent film products are also used as i.v. site dressings, as secondary or retention dressings over other topical products and even prophylactically to protect against friction damage to skin in susceptible areas of bedridden patients.

3.3. Passive Dressings That Supply Moisture

When wounds are already dehydrated and therefore covered by dead or dying tissues, they need to be debrided in order to heal optimally. When the amount of dead tissue is not significant or when the patient is not a candidate for surgical debridement, the healthcare professional may opt for autolytic debridement. Autolytic debridement is the slow digestion of the dead cells by endogenous phagocytes and enzymes and a moist local wound environment facilitates it. This is a scenario in which the goal is to actively add moisture to the wound. It may also be of interest to add moisture to wounds that are just beginning to dry out, before desiccation has already set in. To effectively add moisture, a wound dressing must contain water and the dressing categories that fulfill the function of supplying moisture are the amorphous hydrogels and sheet hydrogels. These two types of hydrogels are similar in composition—containing significant portions of water and smaller amounts of polymers and thickening agents.

Amorphous hydrogels may be packaged in tubes, foil packets, or spray bottles or impregnated into a gauze pad. They are primarily water in composition and present as translucent gels of varying viscosity, which can be applied directly to the wound surface. However, in the case of a deep wound, the gel should not be used to "fill" but only to coat the surfaces of the wound cavity which should then be filled with some other material such as moistened gauze. Filling a cavity wound with a gel will provide too much moisture and may macerate the wound.

Sheet hydrogels present visually as a wafer consisting of three-dimensional networks of cross-linked hydrophilic polymers (polyethylene oxide, polyacrylamides, and polyvinylpyrrolidone), which physically entrap water. Depending on the brand, they can be up to 96% water in composition; therefore, their absorbent capacity is low. Most hydrogel sheets are nonadhesive and require the use of a secondary dressing for securement to the patient and to keep them from drying out. Some hydrogel sheets have an adhesive border of film or foam material, which enables them to be attached to the intact skin around the wound. A unique characteristic of the sheet hydrogels is their cooling effect on the skin. This cooling effect may contribute to transient pain relief for the patient. They are particularly soothing when used on excoriated skin or thermal burns.

4. ACTIVE DRESSING CATEGORIES

Passive dressings as described in the prior section have been available and in use for wound management for 20 years. Their primary function is to maintain physiologic levels of hydration in exposed tissues by absorbing excessive exudate, maintaining moisture, or donating moisture to tissues. This interaction with the physical environment of the wound has been shown to facilitate optimal healing rates. Recently, dressings have been developed which interact with the biochemical and cellular environment of the wound. These dressings are "active" in the sense that they quantitatively *change* something about the wound. Key biochemical and cellular parameters of the wound environment that are candidates for a quantitative change via dressing technology include protease levels, bacterial levels, and bacterial chemical levels.

5. REDUCING PROTEASES IN THE WOUND ENVIRONMENT

Changing something about the wound is of particular interest when the wound in question is not healing. Nonhealing wounds of multiple etiologies have been shown to exhibit similar biochemical imbalances (12). Research studies have shown consistent differences in the array and levels of chemicals found locally in the tissues and fluids of normally healing wounds are compared to those found in wounds with slow healing or no healing. Specifically, the levels of proteolytic enzymes are found to be different in healing vs. nonhealing wounds of many etiologies. A particular family of structurally related proteolytic enzymes called matrix metalloproteases (MMPs) has been found to be persistently elevated in chronic wounds that are not progressing towards closure (13). These proteolytic enzymes normally play a role in cellular migration through the extracellular matrix as well as in controlled proteolysis stimulated by cytokines in the inflammatory phase of healing. Matrix metalloproteases exist in healing wounds but their levels tend to peak during the inflammatory phase of healing and then decline as the wound fills with granulation tissue and resurfaces with new epithelial tissue. In chronic nonhealing wounds, when levels of these enzymes remain persistently high, it is believed to result in uncontrolled degradation of existing or newly deposited extracellular matrix components such as collagen, glycosaminoglycans, and proteoglycans; as well as degradation of the various growth factor proteins necessary to co-ordinate healing. The net result of this uncontrolled local proteolysis in the wound is that granulation tissue is not deposited and the healing process appears to arrest in the inflammatory phase. Excessive levels of MMPs have been demonstrated in nonhealing wounds of many etiologies and are thought to develop due to multiple causes including high levels of bacteria in the wound, the presence of nonviable tissues, and repetitive mechanical trauma to the wound.

5.1. Collagen Dressings to Reduce Proteases in Nonhealing Wounds

An active dressing specifically targeted towards reducing local levels of MMPs in nonhealing wounds is comprised of a homogeneous mixture of 55% bovine collagen and 45% oxidized regenerated cellulose. When placed in the wound bed, this collagen-based dressing chemically binds to members of the MMP family of enzymes and renders them inactive, bringing their active levels back down into the ranges found in healing wounds, which may then allow healing to progress (Table 2) (14). It has also been further shown that the collagen-oxidized regenerated cellulose material protects local growth factor proteins from being degraded by the MMPs. Growth factors are small molecular weight proteins that essentially transmit messages between cells that result in increased cell proliferation and migration as well as in the production and deposition of extracellular matrix proteins. Therefore, the collagen-oxidized regenerated cellulose dressing may facilitate the wound healing process in complimentary ways—by directly reducing elevated protease levels and indirectly increasing local growth factor levels by protecting them from proteolytic degradation.

5.2. Collagen Dressings

Other collagen dressings have been available in the market; however, they do not contain oxidized regenerated cellulose, so they do not reduce MMP levels in non-healing wounds to the same extent as the one previously described. However, pure collagen dressings are thought to be active products in their own right. The collagen in these dressings may be derived from a variety of animal sources including cow-hide, cow or chicken tendon, and pig intestine. Because collagen is an evolutionarily conserved protein, the origin of the protein makes little difference in terms of its function. These collagen dressings are available in multiple physical formats such as gels or pastes, powders or granules, and sheets or sponges. The exogenous collagen in these dressings is thought to have the same effects on cells in the wound as endogenous collagen. It is known, for example, that exogenous bovine collagen is hemostatic—as is endogenous collagen. It is also known from tissue culture studies that exogenous collagen is chemotactic for fibroblasts and macrophages (15). Finally, exogenous collagen implants in animal models have been shown to act as a three-dimensional scaffold to guide the ingrowth of tissue. It is therefore believed that exogenous collagen dressings may have the same effects in the wound

Table 2 Collagen-Based Dressings

Dressing name	Active ingredient	Dressing format	Manufacturer
Promogran wound matrix	55% Bovine collagen and 45% oxidized regenerated cellulose	Sheet	Johnson & Johnson
Fibracol plus collagen dressing with alginate	90% Bovine collagen and 10% alginate	Sheet	Johnson & Johnson
Medifill	100% Bovine collagen	Powder	Biocore
Oasis	100% Porcine collagen	Sheet	HealthPoint

environment as endogenous collagen—it recruits cells into the local wound environment and stimulates their proliferation to facilitate healing progress.

6. REDUCING BACTERIA AND BACTERIAL CHEMICALS IN THE WOUND ENVIRONMENT

The presence of bacteria in and on the superficial soft tissues to the extent that healing progress is delayed or blocked has been described as "critical colonization" (16–18). Traditionally, colonization of a wound has referred to the presence of proliferating bacteria on superficial tissues without injury to or reaction from the host. "Critical colonization" is differentiated from "noncritical" colonization, because it does involve injury to the host. Sibbald et al. (17) have defined critical colonization as a transition point of increased bacterial burden, which occurs when a wound is progressing from superficial colonization towards more invasive local infection.

Critical colonization has been described as clinically indistinct; however, there is a growing consensus about potential local indicators of this condition (17–20). These local indicators are subtle signs of an increased superficial bacterial burden and are thought to precede classic signs of invasive clinical infection. Increasing levels of pain, serous exudates, and odor, changes in the color and texture of granulation tissue, rapid onset or return of slough tissue, wound deterioration, or simply failure to heal are all potential signs that a wound may be critically colonized.

Critical colonization and its clinical effects are not due simply to the quantity of bacteria in and on the superficial soft tissues but more specifically to the quality of the bacteria in terms of their virulence factors—or biochemical products and metabolites. These bacterial virulence factors mediate local injury to the host through specific effects on the cells and extracellular matrix components in the local wound environment and ultimately impede healing progress. Two common classes of bacterial virulence factors include toxins that are produced and secreted into the host environment directly from viable, proliferating bacteria (exotoxins), and toxins that are released from bacterial cell walls upon lysis or death (endotoxins).

Bacterial exotoxins and endotoxins are known to stimulate inflammation and the increased production of inflammatory mediators and proteolytic enzymes by macrophages and neutrophils, which can result in wound deterioration (21,22). Robson et al. (21,23) demonstrated a quantitative correlation between bacterial counts and abnormal (e.g., fragile, edematous, and hemorrhagic) granulation tissue in inoculated animal wounds. Bacterial growth in the wound environment was also been shown to promote collagen lysis and tissue damage mediated not only by the action of bacterial collagenases, but also by the action of macrophage-derived collagenases. Additionally, it is known that the presence of bacterial toxins and metabolites can inhibit the migration of new epithelium across the wound bed, further delaying wound closure (21).

Endotoxins are associated only with gram-negative bacteria; however, endotoxin concentrations in the local environment of most chronic wounds can be very high since these wounds are often heavily colonized with gram-negative species. Data have shown that up to 38% of bacterial species in noninfected wounds are gram-negatives increasing to up to 48% in infected wounds (24).

7. ACTIVE ANTIMICROBIAL DRESSINGS

Recently, dressings that contain and release antimicrobial agents at the wound surface have entered the market. The objective of these dressings is to provide a sustained release of the antiseptic agent at the wound surface to provide a long-lasting antimicrobial action in combination with maintenance of physiologically moist environment for healing (Table 3).

Iodine has been complexed with a polymeric cadexomer starch vehicle to form a topical gel or paste. The cadexomer moiety provides exudate absorption from the wound, which results in a concomitant slow release of low concentrations of free iodine from the vehicle. The wound healing effects of this particular iodophor have been studied in nine randomized controlled trials. The majority of the studies targeted venous leg ulcers (25–28); however; diabetic foot ulcers and pressure ulcers were addressed in two of the trials (29,30). Overall, these clinical studies in chronic wounds have consistently shown that the is not only effective at reducing bacterial counts in the wound, it also appears to positively affect the healing process when compared to standard treatments (usually gauze and saline) and to the cadexomer starch vehicle alone.

Silver has also been recently incorporated into a wide variety of semiocclusive dressing formats such as foams, hydrocolloids, alginates, and hydrofibers. All of these products release silver cations into the wound as they absorb or come in contact with wound exudate. No comparative clinical trials of these products in the management of infected chronic wounds are yet available.

One particular silver-containing dressing has been evaluated in the management of infected chronic wounds. This dressing consists of silver, which has been impregnated into an activated charcoal cloth, and finally encased, in nylon sleeve. The silver in the product is not freely released at the wound surface, but kills bacteria that have been adsorbed onto the activated charcoal component. Activated charcoal has been shown to adsorb not only bacteria, but also their toxins that increase inflammatory mediators and promote tissue damage (31–33). This cloth format of

Table 3 Antimicrobial Dressings

Dressing name	Antimicrobial ingredient	Dressing format	Manufacturer
Acticoat	Ionic silver	Wound contact layer	Smith & Nephew
Acticoat absorbent	Ionic silver	Calcium alginate	Smith & Nephew
Actisorb silver 220	Ionic silver and activated charcoal	Silver-impregnated activated charcoal cloth	Johnson & Johnson Wound Management
Arglaes	Ionic silver	Transparent film or powder	Medline Industries
Aquacel AG	Ionic silver	Hydrofiber	Convatec
Contreet H	Ionic silver	Hydrocolloid	Coloplast
Contreet F	Ionic silver	Foam	Coloplast
Iodosorb	Molecular iodine	Gel or paste	HealthPoint Ltd.
Silvasorb	Ionic silver	Hydrogel sheet or amorphous gel	Medline Industries
Silverlon	Ionic silver	Silver coated nylon cloth	Argentum, LLC

activated charcoal has demonstrated the ability to adsorb bacteria from solution (34) and has been associated with in vitro reductions in colony forming units of common wound pathogens as well as with in vivo improvements in wound size and epithelialization.

8. SUMMARY

Wound dressings are continually evolving in their material forms and performance parameters or functions to address the local needs of healing tissues. Balancing local tissue moisture levels is an important performance parameter for many types of wound dressings. Moisture-balancing dressings may be generally referred to as passive in the sense that they do not change any other chemical or cellular aspect of the wound environment. Dressings that balance moisture fall into three main categories—absorbent dressings, dressings that maintain moisture, and dressings that supply moisture. Selection of a particular type of passive dressing may depend on the type of wound being treated or the healing phase.

Dressings that change something in the local wound environment other than or in addition to moisture may be referred to as active dressings. Active dressings either increase or decrease some biochemical or cellular characteristics of a nonhealing wound. Currently, the local characteristics that may be addressed by active dressings include levels of local proteolytic enzymes, bacteria, and bacterial toxins.

REFERENCES

1. Majno G. The Healing Hand: Man and Wound in the Ancient World. Cambridge, MA: Harvard University Press, 1975.
2. Oxford Clinical Communications, Inc. A Brief History of Wound Healing. Philadelphia, PA: Oxford Clinical Communications, 1998.
3. Subrahmanyam M. A prospective randomised clinical and histological study of superficial burn wound healing with honey and silver sulfadiazine. Burns 1998; 24(2):157–161.
4. Subrahmanyam M. Topical application of honey in the treatment of burns. Br J Surg 1991; 78(4):497–498.
5. Gilje O. Ulcus Cruris in venous circulation disturbances: investigations of etiology, pathogenesis and therapy of leg ulcers. Acta Dermatol Venereol 1948; 28:454–467.
6. Grun B. The Timetables of History. New York, NY: Simon and Schuster, 1982.
7. Winter GD. Formation of scab and the rate of epithelialization of superficial wounds in the skin of the young domestic pig. Nature 1962; 193:293–294.
8. Winter GD. Epidermal regeneration studied in the domestic pig. In: Rovee DT, Maibach HI, eds. Epidermal Wound Healing. Chicago: Year Book Medical Publishers, 1972: 71–112.
9. Hinnman CD, Maibach HI. Effect of air exposure and occlusion on experimental human skin wounds. Nature 1963; 200:377–378.
10. Rovee DT, Kurowsky CA, Labun J, Downes AM. Effect of local wound environment. In: Rovee DT, Maibach HI, eds. Epidermal Wound Healing. Chicago: Year Book Medical Publishers, 1972:159–181.
11. Chen WY, Rogers AA, Lydon MJ. Characterization of biologic properties of wound fluid collected during the early stages of wound healing. J Invest Dermatol 1992; 99(5):559–564.
12. Trengove NJ, Stacey MC, MacAuley S, et al. Analysis of the acute and chronic wound environments: the role of proteases and their inhibitors. Wound Repair Regen 1999; 7(6):442–452.

13. Ovington LG. Overview of matrix metalloprotease modulation and growth factor protection in wound healing. Part 1. Ostomy Wound Manage 2002; 48(6 suppl):3–7.

14. Cullen B, Watt PW, Lundqvist C, Silcock D, Schmidt RJ, Bogan D, Light ND. The role of oxidised regenerated cellulose/collagen in chronic wound repair and its potential mechanism of action. Int J Biochem Cell Biol 2002; 34(12):1544–1556.

15. Mian M, Beghe F, Mian E. Collagen as a pharmacological approach in wound healing. Int J Tissue React 1992; 14(suppl):1–9.

16. Dow G, Browne A, Sibbald RG. Infection in chronic wounds: controversies in diagnosis and treatment. Ostomy Wound Manage 1999; 45(8):23–27, 29–40.

17. Sibbald RG, Williamson D, Orsted HL, Campbell K, Keast D, Krasner D, Sibbald D. Preparing the wound bed—debridement, bacterial balance, and moisture balance. Ostomy Wound Manage 2000; 45(11):14–35.

18. Cooper R, Kingsley A, White R. . Wound Infection and Microbiology. Highbury House, Whitstone, Holsworthy: Medical Communications UK Ltd., 2002.

19. Cutting KF, Harding KGH. Criteria for identifying wound infection. J Wound Care 1994; 3(4):198–201.

20. Schultz GS, Sibbald RG, Falanga V, Ayello EA, Dowsett C, Harding K, Romanelli M, Stacey MC, Teot L, Vanscheidt W. Wound bed preparation: a systematic approach to wound management. Wound Repair Regen 2003; 11(suppl 1):S1–S28.

21. Robson MC, Stenberg BD, Heggers JP. Wound healing alterations caused by infection. Clin Plastic Surg 1990; 17(3):485–492.

22. Smalley JW. Pathogenic mechanisms in periodontal disease. Adv Dental Res 1994; 8(2):320–328.

23. Robson, MC. Wound infection: a failure of wound healing caused by an imbalance of bacteria. Surg Clin N Am 1997; 77(3):637–650.

24. Bowler PG. Wound pathophysiology, infection and therapeutic options. Ann Med 2002; 34(6):419–427.

25. Steele K, Irwin G, Dowde N. Cadexomer iodine in the management of venous leg ulcers in general practice. Practitioner 1986; 230(1411):63–68.

26. Harcup JW, Saul PA. A study of the effect of cadexomer iodine in the treatment of venous leg ulcers. Br J Clin Pract 1986; 40(9):360–364.

27. Ormiston MC, et al. Controlled trial of iodosorb in chronic venous ulcers. Br Med J (Clin Res Ed) 1985; 291(6491):308–310.

28. Skog E, et al. A randomized trial comparing cadexomer iodine and standard treatment in the outpatient management of chronic venous ulcers. Br J Dermatol 1983; 109(1):77–83.

29. Apelqvist J, Ragnarson Tennvall G. Cavity foot ulcers in diabetic patients: a comparative study of cadexomer iodine ointment and standard treatment. An economic analysis alongside a clinical trial. Acta Derm Venereol 1996; 76(3):231–235.

30. Moberg S, Hoffman L, Grennart ML, Holst A. A randomized trial of cadexomer iodine in decubitus ulcers. J Am Geriatr Soc 1983; 31(8):462–465.

31. Pegues AS, Sofer SS, McCallum RE, Hinshaw LB. The removal of 14C labeled endotoxin by activated charcoal. Int J Artif Organs 1979; 2(3):153–158.

32. Du XN, Niu Z, Zhou GZ, Li ZM. Effect of activated charcoal on endotoxin adsorption. Part 1. An in vitro study. Biomater Artif Cells Artif Organs 1987; 15(1):229–235.

33. Naka K, Watarai S, Tana, Inoue K, Kodama Y, Oguma K, Yasuda T, Kodama H. Adsorption effect of activated charcoal on enterohemorrhagic *Escherichia coli*. J Vet Med Sci 2001; 63(3):281–285.

34. Thomas S, Fisher B, Fram P, Waring M. Odour absorbing dressings: a comparative study. Available at: World Wide Wounds on Line Journal April 1998: http://www.worldwidewounds.com/1998/march/Odour-Absorbing-Dressings/odour-absorbing-dressings.html. Accessed June 5, 2003.

46
Topical Treatment of Wound Infection

Heather Orsted
Skin and Wound Management, Calgary Home Care, Calgary, Alberta, Canada

R. Gary Sibbald
Dermatology Daycare and Wound Healing Clinic, Sunnybrook and Women's College Health Sciences Centre, Toronto, Ontario, Canada

1. CASE STUDY

An 80-year-old woman presents with a shallow leg ulcer (2×3) on her (l) medial lower leg. The patient has been diagnosed with a venous leg ulcer and, in spite of a best practice approach using high-compression therapy previously, was not healing at the expected rate. In fact, recently it is more painful, a clear exudate has developed and is larger in size.

2. INTRODUCTION

Wound-care clinicians are faced with dilemma of assessing the relationship of bacteria in chronic wounds. We must develop an approach to determine if we are to use antimicrobials and when to choose topical, systemic, or both.

Some experts estimate that there may be a million different bacteria with only 1% (10,000) identified. Of that 1%, only a fraction has been shown to be associated with human diseases (1). Medical science has countered with the development of ~5000 antibiotics, including 1000 have been carefully investigated and about another 100 that are used clinically to treat infections (2).

The Healthcare Cost and Utilization Project (HCUP) (3) in 1996 revealed that complications of acute surgical procedures [surgical site infections (SSIs)] and chronic skin and subcutaneous tissue infections were diagnosis no. 27 and no. 28 identified in the United States. The Centers for Disease Control (CDC) (4) reported SSIs were the third most common nosocomial infection accounting for 14–16% of all nosocomial infections in hospitalized patients. Stotts and Hunt (5) reported the statistics on prevalence and incidence of pressure ulcers as high in all healthcare settings with a reported 50% mortality rate when both pressure ulcers and bacteremia were present. The statistics for both acute (SSIs) and chronic wounds (e.g., pressure ulcers) indicates that wound infection is a significant health problem.

Bacteria are always present and are held in balance (bacterial balance) by the healthy host (host resistance) (6). Bacterial imbalance and frank infection are always

599

potential complications for any wound if bacteria are allowed to over-run host resistance (6,7). Many bacteria commonly found in wounds are potentially pathogenic and may be detrimental to wound healing despite the fact that they usually exist as commensals in their natural human habitats. Bacteria only compete with normal cells for oxygen and nutrients, but their byproducts are toxic to normal cells (8). As bacterial balance is explored, it is important to remember that it is only one of several key components in the wound-healing paradigm (Fig. 1) and correction of it alone will not ensure wound healing.

A holistic approach needs to be taken when managing bacteria in a wound.

Topical treatment of a wound infection requires assessment and care related to three concepts:

1. Host resistance and wound bioburden (patient risk):
   a. Maximize host response to minimize bioburden.
2. Wound bed preparation (product/treatment selection):
   a. Cleansing and debridement to reduce the bacterial load.
   b. Appropriate use of products based on the needs of the wound and condition of the patient:
      i. Consider the characteristics and properties of the wound-care products and antimicrobials.
3. Wound-care outcomes (Protocol efficacy):
   a. Assess and monitor progress of healing.

3. WOUND BIOBURDEN ASSESSMENT

3.1. Host Resistance

Healing is a complex series of biological interactions that are affected by host resistance and the local wound environment. One of the best ways to support bioburden

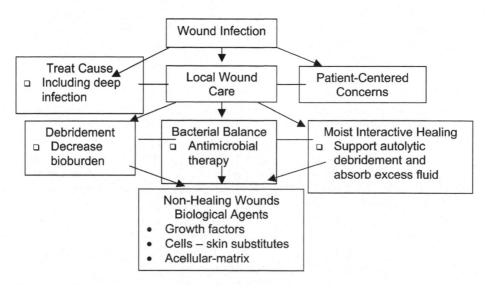

Figure 1   Preparing the wound bed. (Modified from Ref. 9.)

management is through the identification and support of the host resistance. Health is not a static state, and individuals with wounds frequently experience other infections and illnesses that put wound healing at a disadvantage (10). Host resistance may be influenced by many factors such as age, poor tissue O_2 perfusion, excess pressure, bacterial imbalance, stress, concomitant conditions, adverse effects from treatments, and malnutrition. Wound-care practice should be based on the recommendation of a holistic patient assessment for the risk of infection combined with wound assessment (11–14). It is not uncommon to see a wound deteriorate during concomitant illness (an acute flu or chronic diagnosis of diabetes) related to host susceptibility leading to bacterial imbalance. Early identification of these risks may be linked to the initiation of antimicrobial prophylaxis. The quality and chronicity of the wound may also predict an increased risk infection. Chronic wounds do not react to bacteria in the same way that acute wounds do (10,15). In chronic wounds, the wound healing vigor has altered (16).

3.2. Bioburden Load

All wounds contain bacteria; however, a balance or equilibrium usually exists between the bacteria and the host. Bacteria, in low concentrations, according to Tonge (12) may even aide in desloughing, stimulate inflammation, and assist in the healing of a wound. If the bacterial balance is upset in favor of the bacteria, colonization will occur with the risk of infection (10). Wound infection is a result of the complex interaction between the number of organisms, the virulence of the organisms involved, and the resistance of the host, *with host resistance being the most important* (17,18). The challenge for healthcare professionals is to distinguish the infected wound from the colonized wound, to identify the offending organism, and to initiate a treatment plan and evaluate the outcome (19).

The bacterial burden of a wound can be assessed by a variety of methods: clinical observations, laboratory (wound and blood cultures), and occasionally, radiological assessment. The diagnosis of infection is a clinical decision based with supporting evidence gathered from laboratory and radiological assessments. Traditional signs of local infection (superficial/deep infection) are described as rubor (vasodilation), dolor (cytokine mediated stimulation of nociceptive/neuropathic nerve fibers), callor (increased temperature due to enhanced metabolic activity and blood flow), and tumor (increased vessel permeability leading to edema) (17). Signs of systemic infection (systemic infection) include fever, leukocytosis, and a sudden high glucose in individuals with diabetes (20). Cooper, in an article by Gillen (21), describes the role of the nurse as the "wound tender" when the nurse refers to the meticulous assessment required to make appropriate therapeutic choices. Nurses (and other clinicians) should see wound healing at a rate of ∼5 mm/week (22). However, in chronic wounds, healing does not occur in a timely fashion. The signs of infection may be less obvious than in acute wounds. Several papers have demonstrated variable signs and symptoms of bacterial imbalance or infection in chronic wounds: increased wound size, dormancy, delay in healing, increased pain, increased exudate, foul odor, discoloration, friable tissue, bridging or pocketing of the wound (12,18,22–24). Davis, in an article by Tonge (12), describes these characteristics when refers to a new stage termed "critical colonization" (Table 1).

By dividing the signs and symptoms into superficial, deep, and systemic compartments, the clinician can determine when to use a topical approach vs. a systemic

Table 1 Clinical Signs of Wound Infection

Superficial increased bacterial burden	Deep wound infection	Systemic infection
Nonhealing	Pain	Fever
Bright red granulation tissue	Swelling, induration	Rigors
Friable and exuberant granulation	Erythema	Chills
New areas of breakdown or necrosis on the wound surface (slough)	Increased temperature	Hypotension
	Wound breakdown	Multiple organ failure
	Increased size or satellite areas	
Increased exudate that may be translucent or clear before becoming purulent	Undermining	
	Probing to bone	
Foul odor		

Source: From Sibbald (2003).

approach to bacterial management. To further complicate the assessment of increased bacterial burden, increasing bacterial numbers may be silent only becoming recognizable with the advent of sepsis (12,14). This extreme is demonstrated as necrotizing fasciitis is initially recognized as a local infection (cellulitis); however, it rapidly spreads and without intervention can result in a systemic infection leading to the loss of a limb or life within 24–96 hr (21). Gardner et al. (25) focus on the importance of a complete assessment when they report on a study of the use of a clinical sign and symptom checklist (CSSC) tool. Their tool was used at the bedside to assist the clinician in the detailed assessment required to accurately incorporate all the pertinent data into a wound assessment.

In integrating the micro-organism (load × virulence) with host resistance, Bowler (6) asks that we put wounds on a microbial continuum and explore what happens as either/or the host weakens or the micro-organism gains strength.

Bacteria are known to react to the hostile environment they often encounter by creating biofilms. Biofilms, according to the CDC, are involved in 65% of human bacterial infections (26). The National Institute for Health (NIH) has described biofilms as an accumulation of micro-organisms (colony) in a polysaccharide matrix that is adherent to a biological or nonbiological surface (27). Rather than behaving as a primitive, planktonic (free floating), unicellular organism struggling for survival, biofilms represent microbial colonies, affixed to solid surfaces like catheters or medical implants and have their own defense and communication system (28–30). In chronic wounds, the presence of debris or two surfaces of different viscosities will often favor the development of biofilm or biofilm-like structures. Biofilms grow slowly in one or more locations and are often slow to produce overt symptoms, usually from releasing single planktonic cells that seed local infection. They have been linked to mortalities in Legionnaire's disease and fatal lung infections in cystic fibrosis. Traditionally, bacterial cells release antigens and stimulate the production of antibodies causing a host response that fights the bacteria. When biofilms are present, antibodies are not effective in killing the bacteria and may cause immune complex damage to surrounding tissues. Biofilms have three known characteristics that may provide additional protection for the bacteria against antibiotic therapy.

1. Biofilms secrete a protective glycocalyx that surrounds the affixed colony and differs from the traditional individual, planktonic, and bacterial cell walls.
2. Some biofilms can survive without dividing by reverting to a resting state or living off nutrients from their neighbors.
3. Biofilms intermittently release planktonic cells that can reseed the bacteria and may lead to recurrent infection.

Therefore, the antibiotic therapy may reverse the symptoms of infection but fails to penetrate the full depth of the biofilm and kills the biofilm-associated bacteria. After cycles of antibiotic therapy, symptoms recur with the release of planktonic cells (29). Science has discovered the biofilm-organism adaptation but is still struggling with ways to effectively treat and prevent biofilm formation.

Wound cultures are another method of assessing the microbiology of the wound. The most common culture technique is obtaining a semiquantitative swab from the wound surface and culture plating. Reports of >100,000 bacteria/g or the presence of beta-hemolytic streptococci, associated with clinical signs and symptoms, indicate an infection (10,31,32). The culture can be used to confirm the diagnosis, identify the number and specific organisms involved, and identify antibiotic resistances and sensitivities. Healthcare professionals should perform cultures on wounds *suspected* to be out of bacterial balance. However, the problem of distinguishing between an infected wound and a colonized wound continues to be a challenge.

4. BIOBURDEN MANAGEMENT

4.1. Wound Bed Preparation (Debridement)

Dead tissue is the food source for bacteria and one of the biggest causes for increased bacterial burden in the chronic wound. The reduction of the bacterial load through wound bed preparation should be of primary importance to the healthcare professional (9). According to Rodeheaver (34), wound cleansing in the broadest sense includes aggressive debridement of all devitalized tissue, extensive use of fluids for cleansing, and selective use of topical antimicrobial agents to control bacterial contamination.

Wound debridement is the single most important action to reduce the level of bacterial contamination in the chronic wound. Bacteria thrive in devitalized tissue and exudate (34). Debridement choices should match the needs of the wound/patient, skill and practice parameters of the clinician, and availability of resources.

Cleansing choices can be categorized into cleansing by mechanical force or cleansing by solutions. Solutions should not be toxic to healthy tissue and should be used with enough mechanical force to remove the necrotic tissue, exudate, metabolic waste, and dressing residue from the wound surface but not enough to traumatize (35). The strength of the cleanser is directly proportionate to their cleansing capacity and toxicity to the cells; therefore, the cleansing capacity needs to be balanced against toxicity to wound-healing cells (34). Depending on wound characteristics and patient risk factors, saline or water is usually the cleanser of choice. The use of antiseptics as wound cleansers remains very controversial (36).

4.2. Antimicrobials

There remains much controversy over which antimicrobials are safe and effective to use in wounds, and with the emergence of resistance to systemic antimicrobials, selection of a specific topical therapy becomes more of a clinical decision.

There are two ways to obtain chemical control of micro-organisms in a wound: using a chemical that causes a lethal event, *cidal* or using a chemical that prevents microbial growth without causing death, *static* (37). Antimicrobials may either be categorized as a sterilant, disinfectant, antiseptic, chemotherapeutic, or antibiotic. Disinfectants (for inanimate objects) and antiseptics (for living tissue) do not necessarily destroy all living organisms. Chemotherapeutics and antibiotics inhibit specific organisms in a precise way (selective toxicity), without unduly harming the host. Antiseptics and antibiotics are often used and misused with the hope of reducing or eliminating bacteria from a wound (Table 2) (37).

Traditionally, antiseptics have not just been used as wound cleansers and irrigations but they are also used as a dressing through their application in wound packing. Unlike antibiotics, they do not selectively kill bacteria without harming other tissue. However, new therapeutic options have been made less toxic to living tissue. Much of the data used to support the use of these products have been obtained either in vitro or without an appropriate control. Many of the studies demonstrate the benefit of an antiseptic-soaked gauze dressing at reducing bacterial numbers in a wound, and when compared with a normal saline-soaked dressing as a control, the normal saline dressing actually shows lower numbers of bacteria (34). The debriding action of the normal saline gauze provides for the reduction of bacteria rather than a nonselective kill action related to the antiseptic. Dilution of antiseptics to reduce toxicity lacks the studies to prove efficacy. In vitro studies have not significantly demonstrated that these agents are *doing no harm*. For more indepth reading on the subject Drousou et al. (38) have attempted to provide the clinician with an exhaustive review of the literature surrounding the use of antiseptics on wounds. Antiseptics, however, have the advantage of rarely selecting for resistant microbial strains and being topical do not rely on the bloodstream for access to the wound. This is particularly important in ischemic or nonhealable wounds where reducing bacterial burden is more important than living tissue toxicity (33). Table 3 reviews potentially harmful and harmful antiseptics commonly used in wound care.

Two new forms of well-known topical synthetic antimicrobial therapies (antiseptics) have recently emerged as a front-line treatment of critically colonized wounds and local wound infections, such as cadexomer iodine and nanocrystalline silver.

Cadexomer iodine has a slow-release delivery system in the form of a starch-based material known as cadexomer (40). These starch molecules are absorbent and as they absorb fluid they expand and release the iodine into the wound. This free iodine is responsible for the documented antibacterial effects of the product (40). The effects of the product are multiple as in what follows.

1. The cadexomer formulation absorbs exudates forming a hydrogel that also supports autolytic debridement.
2. Free iodine is released in low concentrations to kill bacteria but is less toxic to living cells.
3. Repeated studies have demonstrated that the effects of cadexomer iodine not only reduce bacterial numbers, but also positively affect the healing process.
4. In some patients, cadexomer iodine may trigger the inflammatory response

Table 2 Definition of Terms

Antibiotic: A chemical substance produced by micro-organisms that has the capacity in dilute solutions to selectively inhibit the growth (static) or to kill (cidal) other micro-organisms. Inhibit specific organisms in a precise way (selective toxicity) without harming the host (i.e., Bactroban)

Antiseptic: A disinfectant substance produced synthetically that can be used on either skin or wounds, which either kills (cidal) or prevents the multiplication (static) of potentially pathogenic micro-organisms. Antiseptics can be dilute disinfectants and are not selective; therefore, it can be toxic to host particularly in high concentrations (sodium hypochlorite in lower concentrations, silver, iodine)

Bioburden: The microbial loading of the skin and/or wounds with normal commensals and potential pathogens

Biofilm: A colony of micro-organisms surrounded a polysaccharide matrix (glycocalyx) that is adherent to a biological or nonbiological surface. Biofilms affix to solid surfaces like catheters or medical implants and have their own defense and communication systems. Antibiotic therapy may reverse the symptoms of infection but fails to penetrate the full depth of the biofilm and kill the bacteria

Contaminated: Presence of nonreplicating micro-organisms on the wound surface that have not attached to the tissue

Colonized: The presence of replicating micro-organisms attached to tissue with no overt host immunological reaction or clinical symptoms

Critically colonized: A situation where host defenses cannot maintain the balance of micro-organisms in a wound, signs of critical colonization may be subtle

Disinfectant: A nonselective synthetic agent that disinfects by killing or removing micro-organisms from inert surfaces. It is too toxic to be used on living, viable tissue (i.e., sodium hypochlorite in higher concentrations, glutaraldehyde)
  High-level disinfection kills all organisms, except high levels of bacterial spores
  Intermediate-level disinfection kills mycobacteria, most viruses, and bacteria with
  a chemical germicide
  Low-level disinfection kills some viruses and bacteria with a chemical germicide

Infection: The presence of multiplying micro-organisms in body tissues resulting in spreading cellular injury due to competitive metabolism, toxins, intracellular replication, or antigen-antibody response. May demonstrate classic signs of inflammation such as erythema, heat, swelling, pain, or the more subtle signs such as delayed healing, friable, bleeding granulation tissue, unexpected pain, abnormal smell, bridging and pocketing at the base of wound.

Sterilant: A substance that achieves complete destruction of all micro-organisms, including highly resistant endospores. The major sterilizing agents used in hospitals are (a) moist heat by steam autoclaving, (b) ethylene oxide gas, and (c) dry heat. There are a variety of chemical germicides (sterilants) that have been used for purposes of reprocessing reusable heat-sensitive medical devices and appear to be effective when used appropriately. These chemicals are rarely used for sterilization but appear to be effective for high-level disinfection of medical devices that come into contact with mucous membranes during use

Source: Modified from Ref. 33.

Silver is another well-known topical antimicrobial. One of the key difficulties has been the effective delivery of the silver to the tissues (40). The active agent in the silver compounds is the positively charged silver atom (cation). In the wound environment, the positively charged silver atom binds to serum proteins or reacts with chloride anions, which makes it unavailable for antibacterial activity and may actually delay healing. To facilitate continuous silver release, silver is present in high

Table 3 Potentially Harmful and Harmful Antiseptics Used in Wound Care

Antiseptics	Agent	Mode of action	Comments
Use with caution or avoid use	Hypochlorite, e.g., Hygeol, Eusol, Dakins	Lysing cell walls, acts as a chemical debrider, and should be discontinued with healing tissue	Concerns regarding cytotoxicity dependent on dilution. Short term as a debrider. Rapidly deactivated in the presence of pus, may be painful, and delays healing by damaging cells and capillaries
	Povidine iodine, e.g., Betadine	Method of use makes it a debrider rather than antimicrobial	Concerns regarding cytotoxicity dependent on dilution. Potential toxicity in vivo related to concentration and exposure
	Hydrogen peroxide	Very little antimicrobial activity but acts as an effective debrider in dissolving blood clots	Concerns regarding cytotoxicity. Safety concerns about use in open wounds due to reports of tissue embolism
	Chlorhexidine	Highly effective as hand washing agent and for surgical scrub. Binds to stratum corneum and has persisting activity	Toxicity in wounds has not yet been established, may be a therapeutic agent
	Acetic acid	Provides an acetic wound environment which is unsuitable to pseudomonas	Concerns regarding cytotoxicity regarding to dilution. Short-term approach
Do not use	Gentian violet	Kills gram positive and some yeasts such as *Candida*, more effective at higher pH but can select out overgrowth of gram negative	Carcinogenic and cytotoxic. May cause erosions, ulcers, or areas of necrosis especially on mucous membranes
	Isopropyl alcohol	Used as a disinfectant on intact skin for bactericidal and viricidal effects	Cytotoxic and may cause dryness and irritation on intact skin
	Mecurochrome	A very weak antiseptic with action inhibited in the presence of organic debris	Epidermal cell toxicity, dermatitis, systemic toxicity and death through topical application, possible aplastic anemia

Source: From Refs. 33, 34, 39.

concentration (SSD) or released over a prolonged period (silver foam, alginate, and hydrocolloid dressings). A new technology, which creates small particles of silver known as nanocrystalline silver, allows the silver to be soluble in water. Nanocrystalline silver has demonstrated to reduce the number of viable bacteria to below detection levels and has shown no detrimental effects on wound healing (41) (Table 4).

Topical antibiotic therapy may be considered in wounds that have a covert or mild infection with no signs of tissue invasion (47). It would be reasonable for the clinician to consider a 2-week trial of topical antimicrobials if superficial signs are present. Owing to the development of antibiotic resistance, the avoidance of any topical treatment that is also used systemic is strongly encouraged. Topical antibiotics have been shown to provoke delayed hypersensitivity reactions, superinfections by resistant organisms, and select for resistant bacteria if used indiscriminately or for long periods of time (33). Resistance to antibiotics has been described as a crisis in the United States; therefore, topical antibiotics that also can be used systemically should be avoided (e.g., gentamycin) (33). Many of the new antimicrobials also have fungus and yeast as a target. Table 5 reviews topical antimicrobials commonly used in wound care.

The advantage of the newer antiseptic bacterial dressings (cadexomer iodine and ionized silver dressings) is the combination of bacterial balance with moisture balance. Traditional antimicrobials, such as silver sulfadiazine cream, have no wound exudate absorbing properties and may leave behind a residual eschar of debris that needs to be removed. These preparations are used for the superficial compartment increased bacterial burden with reassessment frequently recommended at biweekly intervals. The antibacterial spectrum of these agents is covered in the chart (Table 5), but resistance can emerge in individual cases.

When MRSA is found in a chronic wound, we can often consider stopping all antibiotic or antiseptic formulations or using topical therapy to attempt decolonization. Topical agents effective for MRSA on the surface of the wounds include silver and cadexomer dressings along with silver sulfadiazine cream, combinations of polysporin and gramicidin cream, and fusidic acid cream. To avoid the emergence of resistance, mupirocin is reserved in some centers for the treatment of MRSA.

Pseudomonas is often a problem on the wound surface. Our topical options include dilute acetic acid compresses or soaked dressings. Five percent acetic acid is white vinegar and this is diluted one in five or one in 10 to achieve 0.5–1% concentration to apply to chronic wounds. The acetic acid decreases the pH on the wound surface, which inhibits the growth of *Pseudomonas* organisms. Side effects include local burning and stinging, as well as some cytotoxicity. Topical antimicrobial choices for *Pseudomonas* include the cadexomer iodine and silver dressings along with silver sulfadiazine and the combination of polymyxin and gramicidin. An odor in chronic wounds often suggests that anaerobic organisms are present and metronidazole may be effective topically to kill anaerobes on the surface and decrease odor.

Topical antimicrobials should ideally have three key characteristics:

1. They should have low tissue toxicity
2. They are not used systemically (topical use selects resistant organisms)
3. They are not common sensitizers

Low tissue toxicity prevents topical agents from inhibiting healing. The more toxic topical antiseptics in Table 3 should be reserved for nonhealable wounds where the decrease in local bacteria and the need to dry the wound surface are more important than cytotoxicity. At the debridement stage of wounds with the ability to heal,

Table 4 Silver Preparations Used in Wound Management

Preparation	Current use	Product	Benefits	Disadvantages
Silver salts				
Silver nitrate	0.5% solutions in burn wounds	Silver nitrate solution	Easy to use; Host cytotoxicity (42–44)	Staining; May lead to electrolyte imbalance
Silver sulfadiazine	1% in carrier cream–chronic wounds	Flamazine, Silvadene, SD cream	Low cytotoxicity (in vivo) (45)	Cytotoxic (in vitro) (46)
Silver–calcium–sodium phosphates	Coextruded in polymer matrix—for superficial wounds with limited exudate	Arglades	Residual antimicrobial activity lasts from 24 hr to 4 days	Limited absorption of fluid
Silver–sodium carboxy-methylcellulose dressing	Dressing containing 1.2% ionic silver released via ion exchange	Aquacel-AG	Provides fluid lock to prevent excess wound fluid from macerating surrounding skin	Low concentration of silver released; Fluid lock may trap bacteria
Silver-coated foam	Highly exudating chronic wounds	Contreet Foam	Provides bacterial balance in a foam dressing	Low concentration of silver released with high absorption
Silver combined with hydrocolloid	Chronic wounds with increased bacterial burden	Contreet-HC	Provides odor control under hydrocolloid dressing	Moderate fluid absorption and low concentration of silver release
Adsorbed silver				
Silver charcoal	Silver adsorbed onto charcoal for odor control	Actisorb	Silver kills organisms that are adsorbed onto the charcoal	No release of silver into the wound

Nanocrystalline silver				
Silver coating and absorptive core	Burns / Chronic wounds	Acticoat Burn	Equivalent to silver nitrate in burns with less frequent dressing changes	Release of high concentration of ionized silver
Silver coating—three layers with two absorptive cores	Leg ulcers and other chronic wounds for upto 7 days wear time	Acticoat 7	Sustained release of bactericidal concentrations of silver over 7 days	Useful for weekly compression therapy in venous ulcers
Silver-coated foam	Heavily exudating chronic wounds	Acticoat Moisture Control	Provides a fluid equilibrium between dressing and wound fluid	Controls bioburden in dressing and wound fluid
Silver-coated calcium alginate	Moderately exudating chronic wounds	Acticoat Absorbent	Provides absorption and hemostasis	Bioabsorbable controlling bacteria, fluid, and hemorrhage

Source: From RG Sibbald, with permission.

Table 5 Antimicrobials (Antiseptics and Antibiotics) Frequently Used in Wound Care

	Agent	Spectrum					Comments
		Staph	MRSA	Strep	Pseud	Anaer	
Safe and effective	Cadexomer iodine[a]	✓	✓	✓	✓	✓	Broad spectrum including viral and fungal
	Ionized silver[a] (for other agents, see Table 4)	✓	✓	✓	✓	✓	Useful in sloughy wounds
	Silver sulfadiazine	✓	✓	✓	✓		Limited potential for resistance
	Polymyxin B sulfate–gramicidin	✓	✓	✓	✓	✓	Cream combination does not contain bacitracin in paste/ointment formulations
Selective use	Mupuricin	✓	✓	✓			Reserve for MRSA
	Metronidazole					✓	Reserve for anaerobes and odor control
	Benzyl peroxide	✓					Frequently causes sensitization when used for leg/other ulcers
Use with caution	Gentamycin	✓		✓	✓		Reserve for oral and IV
	Fucidic acid	✓	✓	✓			Sensitizer
	Polymyxin B sulfate	✓	✓	✓	✓		Sensitizers including both neomycin and Bacitracin that is in combined ointment formulations
	Bacitracin zinc–Neomycin						

[a] Antiseptics
Source: From Ref. 9.

Table 6 Bacterial Assessment and Management in Chronic Wounds

Bacterial burden	Contaminated or colonized	Critically colonized	Infection		
			Superficial	Deep	Systemic
	Adhere to principles of good wound care (cleansing, debridement, and moisture balance). Assess/monitor host and wound (address cause and patient-centered concerns)				
	Wound is progressing host stable No C&S	Subtle S&S and change in host C&S	S&S of superficial infection C&S	S&S of deep infection C&S	Constitutional S&S C&S
Monitor change in lab values and possible x-ray					
Antiseptics/antibiotics					
Topical	–	+	+	+	+
Systemic	–	Possible	Possible	+	+

Source: Adapted from Ref. 9.

there may be a role for topical antiseptic agents when increased bacterial burden needs to be controlled before promoting moist interactive healing. Agents such as the aminoglycoside gentamicin, when applied topically, will select out resistant organisms on the wound surface. Resistance is cross acquired to all of the aminoglycosides and when the resistant organisms invade the deep bacterial compartment, a very useful first line system class of antibiotics will be ineffective.

The skin is a dynamic organ that is very well equipped to process antigens applied externally and mount an immune response (48). Topical agents are more likely to cause allergic reactions, and leg ulcers with a defect in the cutaneous barrier will absorb these agents more efficiently than any other skin disorder. With this high sensitization potential, clinicians need to avoid common sensitizers when treating cutaneous increased bacterial burden. Neomycin is a very common sensitizer and it can cross sensitize to the aminogycoside antibiotics because it contains the same backbone. Bacitracin is a part of most combination topical antibiotic ointments and has now reached the top 10 sensitization list for North America. Lanolin, a derivative of wool, is in many tulle dressings and fusidic-acid ointment. It is a rare allergen on intact skin, uncommon allergen in persons with atopic dermatitis, and a strong allergen in persons with leg ulcers. It is also found in many moisturizers along with unwanted perfume sensitizers. Benzoyl peroxides are also useful antimicrobial agents but their sensitization potential should limit their use.

5. CONCLUSION

Wound infections occur when there is an imbalance between the host resistance and the invading organism favoring organism proliferation and tissue destruction. The outcome of the impact of the bacteria in the wound bed remains dependent on the interaction of the host and microbial factors. With the recognition of the bacterial biofilm defense mechanism, the challenge of infection control continues to present itself to healthcare professionals. We must be vigilant, especially in the chronic wound (Table 6) where signs of infection may be subtle. The identification of subclinical bacterial damage, known as critical colonization, emphasizes the need for early recognition and antibacterial treatment. There are now safe and effective topical antimicrobial choices combined with moisture balance dressings available to support bacterial balance in the wound. The selective yet appropriate use of these topical antimicrobials will not reduce the risk of invasive deep tissue infection in normal or compromised hosts.

REFERENCES

1. Office of Technology Assessment, Congress of the United States. Impacts of Antibiotic Resistant Bacteria. (www.wws.princton.edu/cgibin/byteserv.prl).
2. Hoel D, Williams DN. Antibiotics: past, present, and future. Unearthing nature's majic bullets. Postgrad Med 1997; 101(1):114–123.
3. Health Care Cost and Utilization Project (http://www.hcup-us.ahrq.gov/home.jsp).
4. Centers for Disease Control and Prevention Management. NNIS—National Nosocomial Infections Surveillance System. About NNIS Antimicrobial Resistance ICU Surveillance Report, 1999 (www.cdc.gov/ncidod/hip/surveill/nnis.htm).
5. Stotts NA, Hunt TK. Managing bacterial colonization and infection. Clin Geriatr Med 1997; 13(3):565–573.

6. Bowler P. The 10^5 bacterial growth guideline: reassessing its clinical relevance in wound healing. Ostomy Wound Manag 2003; 49(1):44–53.

7. Neil J, Munro C. A comparison of two culturing methods for chronic wounds. Ostomy Wound Manag 1997; 43(3):20–30.

8. Bowler P. The anaerobic and aerobic microbiology of wounds: a review. Wounds 1998; 10(6):170–178.

9. Sibbald RG, Williamson D, Orsted H, Campbell K, Keast D, Krasner D, Sibbald D. Preparing the wound bed—debridement, bacterial balance, and moisture balance. Ostomy Wound Manag 2000; 40(11):14–35.

10. Robson MC. Wound infection: a failure of wound healing caused by an imbalance of bacteria. Surg Clin North Am 1997; 77(3):637–650.

11. Fowler E. Wound infection: a nurse's perspective. Ostomy Wound Manag 1998; 44(8):44–53.

12. Tonge H. The management of infected wounds. Nurs Stand 1997; 12(12):49–53.

13. Stotts NA, Wipke-Tevis D. Co-factors in impaired wound healing. Ostomy Wound Manag 1996; 42(2):44–54.

14. Krasner D. Minimizing factors that impair wound healing: a nursing approach. Ostomy Wound Manag 1995; 41(1):22–30.

15. Tarnuzzer R, Schultz G. Biochemical analysis of acute and chronic wound environments. Wound Repair Regen 1996; 4(3):321–325.

16. Hunt TK, Hopf HW. Wound healing and wound infection. Surg Clin North Am 1997; 77(3):587–605.

17. Dow G, Browne A, Sibbald RG. Infection in chronic wounds: controversies in diagnosis and treatment. Ostomy Wound Manag 1999; 45(8):23–40.

18. van Rijswijk L. To culture, or not...and if yes, how? Ostomy Wound Manag 1997; 43(3):21.

19. Cuzzell J. The right way to culture a wound. Am J Nurs 1993; 93(5):48–50.

20. Benbow M, Burg G, Matinez FC, Eriksson E, Flour M, Meaume S, Moffatt CJ, Neumann HAM, Rodeheaver GT, Romanelli M, Stark GB, Téot L, Werner KG, Wolff K. Guidelines for the Outpatient Treatment of Chronic Wounds and Burns. Oxford: Blackwell Science Ltd, 1999.

21. Gillen PB. Necrotizing fasciitis: early recognition and aggressive treatment remain important. J Wound Ostomy Continence Nurs 1995; 22(5):219–222.

22. Cutting K. Wounds and evidence of infection. Nurs Stand 1997; 11(25):49–51.

23. Cutting K, Harding KG. Criteria for identifying wound infection. J Wound Care 1994; 3(4):198–202.

24. Gardner SE, Frantz RA, Doebbeling BN. The validity of the clinical signs and symptoms used to identify localized wound infections. Wound Repair Regen 2001; 9(3):178–186.

25. Gardner SE, Frantz RA, Troia C, Eastman S, MacDonald M, Buresh K, Healy D. A tool to assess clinical signs and symptoms of localized infection in chronic wound: development and reliability. Ostomy Wound Manag 2001; 47(1):40–47.

26. Potera C. Forging a link between biofilms and disease. Science 1999; 283(5409): 1837–1839.

27. NIH Guide: Research on Microbial Biofilms Research on Microbial Biofilms, May 14, 1998. PA NUMBER: PA-98–070 (grants.nih.gov/grants/guide/pa-files/PA-98–070.html).

28. Serralta VW, Harrison-Balestra C, Cassaniga AL, Davis SC, Mertz PM. Lifestyles of bacteria in wounds: presence of biofilms? Wounds 2001; 13(1):29–34.

29. Costerton JW, Stewart PS, Greenberg EP. Bacterial biofilms: a common cause of persistent infections. Science 1999; 248(5418):1318–1322.

30. Kolter R, Losick R. One for all and all for one. Science 1998; 280(5361):226–227.

31. Brown DL, Smith DJ. Bacterial colonization/infection and the surgical management of pressure ulcers. Ostomy Wound Manag 1999; 45(1A):109s–118s.

32. Lookingbill DP, Miller SH, Knowles RC. Bacteriology of chronic leg ulcers. Arch Dermatol 1978; 114:1765–1768.
33. White RJ, Cooper R, Kingsley A. Wound colonization and infection: the role of topical antimicrobials. Br J Nurs 2001; 10(9):563–576.
34. Rodeheaver G. Wound cleansing, wound irrigation, wound disinfection. In: Chronic Wound Care. 3rd ed. Wayne, Pennsylvania: Health Management Publications 2001.
35. Campton-Johnston S, Wilson J. Infected wound management: advanced technologies, moisture-retentive dressings, and die-hard methods. Crit Care Nurse Quarterly 2001; 24(2):64–77.
36. Hall Angeras M, Brandberg A, Falk A, Seeman T. Comparison between sterile saline and tap water for the acute traumatic soft tissue wounds. Eur J Surg 1992; 158:147–150.
37. Cooper R, Lawrence JC. The role of antimicrobial agents in wound care. J Wound Care 1996; 5(8):374–380.
38. Drousou A, Falabella A, Kirsner R. Antiseptics on wounds: an area of controversy. Wounds 2003; 15(5):149–166.
39. Lineweaver W, Howard R, Soucy D, et al. Topical antimicrobial toxicity. Arch Surg 1985; 120:367–370.
40. Ovington LG. Battling bacteria in wound care. Home Healthc Nurs 2001; 19(10): 622–631.
41. Wright JB, Lam K, Burrell RE. Wound management in an era of increasing bacterial antibiotic resistance: a role for topical silver treatment. Am J Infect Control 1998; 26(6):572–577.
42. Hall RE, Bender G, Marquis RE. In vitro effects of low intensity direct current generated silver on eukaryotic cells. J Oral Maxillofac Surg 1988; 46:128.
43. Bador K. Organ deposition of silver following silver nitrate therapy for burns. Plast Reconstr Surg 1966; 37:550.
44. Cooms C, Wan A. Do burn patients have a silver burning? Burns 1992; 18:180.
45. Paddock HN, Schultz GS, Perrin KJ, Moldawer LL, Wright B, Burrell RE, Mozingo DW. Clinical assessment of silver-coated antimicrobial dressing on MMPs and cytokine levels in non-healing wounds. Ann Mtg Pres Wound Healing Society, Baltimore, MD, 28th May–1st June, 2002.
46. McCauley RL, Linares HA, Pelligrini V, Herndon DN, Robson MC, Haggers JP. In vitro toxicity of topical antimicrobial agents to human fibroblasts. J Surg Res 1989; 46:267.
47. Dow G. Infection in chronic wounds. In: Chronic Wound Care. 3rd ed. Wayne, Pennsylvania: Health Management Publications 2001.
48. Sibbald RG, Cameron J. Dermatological aspects of wound care. In: Chronic Wound Care. 3rd ed. Wayne, Pennsylvania: Health Management Publications, 2001.

SUGGESTED READING

1. Armstrong DG. The Use of Silver as an Antimicrobial. Alpha and Omega Worldwide LLC, 2000.
2. Barrett T. Recognition and treatment of surgical wound infections. Today's OR Nurse 1992 October:11–14.
3. Bennett LL, Rosenblum RS, Perlov C, Davidson JM, Barton RM, Nanney LB. An in vivo comparison of topical agents on wound repair. Plast Reconstr Surg 2000; 108:675–685.
4. Bowler P, Davies BJ. The microbiology of infected and non-infected leg ulcers. Int J Dermatol 1999; 38(8):573–578.
5. Cruse PJE, Foord R. The epidemiology of wound infection. Surg Clin North Am 1980; 60(1):27–39.

6. Davis SC, Mertz PM, Eaglestein WH. The wound environment: implications from research studies for healing and infection. In: Chronic Wound Care. 3rd ed Wayne, Pennsylvania: Health Management Publications 2001.

7. Gilchrist B. Infection and culturing. In: Krasner D, Kane D, eds. Chronic Wound Care. 2nd ed. Wayne, Pennsylvania: Health Management Publications, 1997:109–114.

8. Heggers JP. Defining infection in chronic wounds: methodology. J Wound Care 1998; 7(9):452–456.

9. Hirshberg J, Rees RS, Marchant B, Dean S. Osteomyelitis related to pressure ulcers: the cost of neglect. Adv Skin Wound Care 2000; 13(1):25–29.

10. Holzapfel L, Jacquet-Francillon T, Rahmani J, Achard P, Marcellin E, Joffre T, Lallement PY, Bousquet A, Devaux S, Coupry A. Microbiological evaluation of infected wounds in 214 adults. J Accid Emerg Med 1999; 16:32–34.

11. Kramer SA. Effect of povidone–iodine on wound healing: a review. J Vasc Nurs 1999; 17(1):17–23.

12. Lawrence JC, Ameen H. Swabs and other sampling techniques. J Wound Care 1998; 7(5):232–233.

13. Lazarus GS, Cooper DM, Knighton DR, Margolis DJ, Percoraro RE, Rodeheaver G, Robson MC. Definitions and guidelines for assessment of wounds and evaluation of healing. Wound Rep Regen 1994; 2(3):165–170.

14. Leaper DJ. Antiseptic toxicity in open wounds. Nurs Times 1988; 84(25):77–79.

15. Mertz PM, Davis SC, Oliveira-Gandia M, Eaglstein WH. The wound environment: implication from research studies for healing and infection. Wounds 1996; 8(1):1–8.

16. Oliveria-Gandia M, Davis SC, Mertz PM. Can occulsive dressing composition influence proliferation of bacterial wound pathogens? Wound Compend Clin Res Pract 1998; 10(1):4–11.

17. O'Meara SM, Cullum NA, Najid M, Sheldon TA. Systematic review of antimicrobial agents used for chronic wounds. Br J Surg 2001 January:4–21.

18. Papasain CJ, Kragel PJ. The microbiology laboratory's role in life-threatening infectons. Crit Care Nurs Quarter 1997; 20(3):44–59.

19. Scott Ward R, Saffle JR. Topical agents in burn wound care. Phys Ther 1995; 75(6): 526–538.

20. Stotts NA. Determination of bacterial burden in wounds. Advances in Wound Care 1995; 8(4):28–46–28–52.

21. Stotts NA, Cavanaugh CE. Assessing the patient with a wound. Home Healthc Nurs 1999; 17(1):27–35.

22. Stotts NA, Whitney JD. Identifying and evaluating wound infection. Home Healthc Nurs 1999; 17(3):159–165.

23. Thomson PD, Taddonio TE. Wound infection. In: Krasner D, Kane D, eds. Chronic Wound Care. 2nd ed. Wayne, Pennsylvania: Health Management Publications, 1997:90–96.

24. van Rijswijk L. The fundamentals of wound assessment. Ostomy Wound Manag 1996; 42(7):40–52.

25. Young T. Managing MRSA wound infection and colonization. Nurs Times Plus 2000; 96(14):14–16.

26. Zhou LH, Nahm WK, Badiavas E. Yufit T, Falanga V. Slow release iodine preparation and wound healing: in vitro effects consistent with lack of in vivo toxicity in human chronic wounds. Br J Dermatol 2002; 146:365–374.

47

Systemic Therapies in Wound Healing

Ysabel M. Bello and Anna F. Falabella
Department of Dermatology and Cutaneous Surgery, University of Miami School of Medicine, Miami, Florida, U.S.A.

1. INTRODUCTION

Wound healing is a dynamic process that includes three overlapping phases: inflammation, tissue formation, and tissue remodeling. It involves soluble mediators, blood cells, extracellular matrix, and parenchymal cells (1). Several systemic therapies such as pentoxifylline, cilostazol, stanozolol, oxandrolone, prednisone and methylprednisolone, infliximab, antimicrobials, horse chestnut seed extract, growth factors, and aspirin have been suggested to speed or augment the healing of certain types of wounds.

2. PENTOXIFYLLINE

Pentoxifylline is a substituted methylxanthine structurally similar to theophylline and caffeine, which significantly increases cerebral and peripheral blood flow and increases tissue oxygen tension. The mechanism of action includes increased red blood cell and white cell deformability, decreased whole blood viscosity, decreased platelet aggregation and adhesion, and decreased fibrinogen concentration. It has been used in peripheral vascular disease (claudication), cerebrovascular disease, hearing disorders, retinal vein thrombosis, ulcers due to thalassemia, livedo vasculitis, and diabetic foot ulcers. Oral pentoxifylline was reported in a review of nine randomized trials involving 572 patients to be a helpful therapy in addition to compression bandaging for the treatment of venous ulcers at a dose of 400 mg three times a day (2). A prospective, randomized, double-blind, parallel, placebo-controlled, multicenter study in 131 patients, receiving pentoxifylline 400-, 800 mg or placebo tablets three times a day for up to 24 weeks, found that patients who received higher dose of pentoxifylline had greater and earlier healing than the lower dose or compression alone (3). A dose-dependent rate of ulcer healing was reported in the same study. Pentoxifylline does have some gastrointestinal effects including dyspepsia, nausea, vomiting, or diarrhea, as well as dizziness, which act as limiting factor for its use in some patients.

Several other agents, not currently available in the United States, have been studied in Europe. Daflon, which is a Pentoxifylline-like medication, Sulodexide, which is a heparin-like molecule and a proteoglycan called mesoglycan, all given systemically have sped healing of venous ulcers in combination with compression therapy.

Daflon, a micronized purified flavonoid fraction, has been studied in Europe in addition to compression therapy and standardized local care in a double-blind randomized placebo-controlled study (4). This study reported that a two-month course of Daflon 500 mg twice a day significantly accelerates complete healing patients with ulcers $\leq$10 cm.

Sulodexide, a highly purified glycosaminoglycan with profibrinolytic and anti thrombin action, has been reported to heal more venous ulcers. In a randomized-controlled trial in 94 patients, sulodexide (daily intramuscular injection for 30 days and then orally for 30 days) in addition to compression therapy showed that 58% of the patients in the treatment group healed compared to 36% in the compression alone or control group (5).

Mesoglycan, a sulphated polysaccharide compound, resulted in a significantly faster and more frequent ulcer healing when given (30 mg/day intramuscular for 3 weeks followed by 100 mg orally) as an adjunct to compression therapy and appropriate wound care (6).

3. CILOSTAZOL

Cilostazol is a type III phosphodiesterase inhibitor that has been approved for use in intermittent claudication with significant improvement in pain and walking distance at a dose of 100 mg twice daily. It is metabolized by the cytochrome P-450 system and caution is required regarding possible drug interactions. Adverse effects include headache, diarrhea, and dizziness. This antiplatelet and antithrombotic pharmacological agent has been reported to promote wound healing in a small case series of five patients with chronic limb ischemia (7). A pharmacological approach may be an alternative when revascularization is not an option.

4. STANOZOLOL

Stanozolol, a synthetic anabolic steroid derived from testosterone, with one of the largest anabolic/androgenic ratio and fibrinolytic properties (8). It is capable of improving the skin induration and hyperpigmentation of the legs that occurs in patients with venous insufficiency (lipodermatosclerosis). A prospective double-blind, placebo-controlled randomized study in 60 patients with lipodermatosclerosis receiving stanozolol 5 mg or placebo twice daily for 6 months plus compression stocking have shown that Stanozolol caused reduction in the area of lipodermatosclerosis (9). Stanozolol has also been reported to be a safe and effective treatment of the cutaneous manifestations caused by cryofibrinogenemia, including that seven of the eight patient's ulcers healed, prompt reduction of pain, improvement in livedo reticularis and purpura (10). Stanozolol can induce sodium retention with edema and hypertension, as well as acne, dysmenorrhea, liver function, and lipid abnormalities, all these side effects seem to be reversible. However, the asymptomatic reversible increase of liver transaminases and temporary lowering of HDL may pose a risk for patients with coronary artery disease (11).

5. OXANDROLONE

Oxandrolone an anabolic steroid is indicated as an adjunctive therapy to promoteweight gain after weight loss following extensive surgery, chronic infections, or severe trauma. It has been studied in a prospective randomized study in the recovery phase after major burns. The effect of oxandrolone combined with a high protein diet (2 g/kg/day) significantly increased the rate of restoration of weight gain postburn (12). Oxandrolone plus amino acid supplement have shown to promote wound healing in individuals with spinal cord injury who have long-standing pressure wounds (13). Many of these patients are malnourished and elderly, and the key is to optimize their nutrition.

6. PREDNISONE AND METHYLPREDNISOLONE

The systemic administration of prednisone has been reported to reduce the inflammatory component of pyoderma gangrenosum, halting the progression of ulcers and preventing development of new lesions (14). There are no randomized double-blinded prospective trials investigating the treatment of pyoderma gangrenosum but the best clinical evidence is systemic corticosteroids in the initial phase, such as a high dose of prednisone usually 100–200 mg/day that is tapered slowly to discontinuation (15). Pulse therapy with methylprednisolone (1 g/day for 5 consecutive days) was described long time ago to halt progressive pyoderma gangrenosum (16). Combination of corticosteroids with other drugs have been used as a corticosteroid-sparing alternative treatment for pyoderma gangrenosum to avoid the unfortunatly long-term side effects of corticosteroids.

7. INFLIXIMAB

Infliximab is a chimeric immunoglobulin G monoclonal antibody that binds to tumor necrosis factor alfa (TNF-α). It binds specifically and with high affinity to free and membrane-bound TNF, neutralizing its effect in vivo. Infliximab is administered through i.v. infusion. It has been approved for human use by the FDA (Food and Drug Administration) for reduction in signs and symptoms of rheumatoid arthritis in patients who have inadequate response to methotrexate; in patients with moderately to severely active Crohn's disease who have an inadequate response to conventional therapy; and in reduction in number of draining enterocutaneous fistulae in patients with fistulizing Crohn's disease. Its efficacy has been described in patients with inflammatory bowel disease and concomitant pyoderma gangrenosum or psoriasis (17–19). Pyoderma gangrenosum ulcers began to decrease in size and healed after infusion with infliximab. Further studies are needed to demonstrate the efficacy of infliximab in the treatment of pyoderma gangrenosum, as well as the long-term risks and benefits.

8. ANTIMICROBIALS

The increase in antimicrobial resistance is related to the overuse of broad-spectrum agents. The careful use of antimicrobials and the use of sensitivities as per antibiogram should be implemented in order to reduce resistance emergence. New antimicrobials have been approved by the FDA in the United States for the treatment of resistant infections which include quinupristin-dalfopristin (Synercid), linezolid (Zyvox), gatifloxacin (Tequin), and moxifloxacin (Avelox) (20). Others such as tigecycline, daptomycin, and oritavancin are in stages of development (21). However, cases of resistance to these new antimicrobials have already been reported.

9. HORSE CHESTNUT SEED EXTRACT

Horse chestnut seed extract (*Aesculus hippocastanum*) is an herbal remedy with an active component called escin, that appears to improve symptoms in patients with chronic venous insufficiency (22). This oral drug treatment is an attractive option for discomfort and poor compliance associated with the conservative compression therapy of chronic venous insufficiency. A review of three observational studies and 13 randomized controlled trials indicated that horse chestnut seed extract is an effective and safe short-term treatment for chronic venous insufficiency; however, further studies are required to evaluate long-term effectiveness and safety (23). The recommended dose is 50 mg of escin twice daily.

10. GROWTH FACTORS

A preliminary study on the administration of intramuscular naked plasmid DNA encoding for fibroblast growth factor type 1 to patients with end-stage peripheral arterial occlusive disease reported significant increase in ankle brachial index, and reduction in pain (24). Similar trends were observed in a phase I study of direct administration of adenovirus vector containing human vascular endothelial growth factor cDNA to patients with claudication (25). Fibroblast growth factor, as well as vascular endothelial growth factor, seem promising therapeutic agents. Larger randomized controlled studies are encouraged.

11. ASPIRIN

Aspirin has been studied for the treatment of venous leg ulcer. In a small study, 20 patients were randomized to aspirin (300 mg/day enteric-coated) plus compression vs. compression alone (26). In this small study, aspirin plus compression was superior to compression alone. Something as inexpensive as aspirin may have utility for patients with venous leg ulcers.

12. ESTROGEN

Estrogen in the form of hormone replacement therapy showed in a case cohort study including elderly patients were less likely to develop a venous leg ulcer or a pressure ulcer than those who did not use hormone replacement therapy (27). However, recent randomized clinical trials suggested that estrogen plus progestin does not confer cardiac protection and may increase risk of coronary artery disease among generally healthy post-menopausal women, and this report may limit its prescription (28).

13. CONCLUSION

Many therapies have been developed and proven to be effective for the treatment of specific wounds, but etiology, character, size, amount of exudate, and presence of concomitant diseases need to be considered to make the best choice among available therapies. Compression and off-loading need to be provided simultaneously with certain systemic therapies. The need for new therapies exists, but the costs, regulatory issues, as well as reimbursement are barriers for drug development.

REFERENCES

1. Singer A, Clark R. Cutaneous wound healing. N Engl J Med 1999; 341:738–746.
2. Jull A, Walters J, Arroll B. Pentoxifylline for treating venous leg ulcers. Cochrane Database of Systematic Reviews 2002.
3. Falanga V, Fujitani RM, Diaz C, et al. Systemic treatment of venous leg ulcers with high doses of pentoxifylline: efficacy in a randomized, placebo-controlled trial. Wound Rep Reg 1999; 7:208–213.
4. Guilhou J, Dereure O, Marzin L, et al. Efficacy of Daflon 500 mg in venous leg ulcer healing: a double-blind, randomized, controlled versus placebo trial in 107 patients. Angiology 1997; 48:77–85.
5. Scondotto G, Aloisi D, Ferrari P, Martini L. Treatment of venous leg ulcers with sulodexide. Angiology 1999; 50:883–889.
6. Arosio E, Ferrari G, Santoto L, Gianese F, Coccheri S, Group TMVI. A placebo-controlled, double-blind study of mesoglycan in the treatment of chronic venous ulcers. Eur J Vasc Endovasc Surg 2001; 22:365–372.
7. Dean S, Vaccaro P. Successful pharmacologic treatment of lower extremity ulcerations in 5 patients with chronic critical limb ischemia. J Am Board Fam Pract 2002; 15:55–62.
8. Helfman T, Falanga V. Stanozolol as a novel therapeutic agent in dermatology. J Am Acad Dermatol 1995; 32:254–258.
9. McMullin G, Watkin G, Coleridge Smith P, Scurr J. Efficacy of fibrinolytic enhancement with stanozolol in the treatment of venous insufficiency. Aust NZ J Surg 1991; 61: 306–309.
10. Kirsner RS, Eaglstein WH, Katz MH, Kerdel F, Falanga V. Stanozolol causes rapid pain relief and healing of cutaneous ulcers caused by cryofibrinogenemia. J Am Acad Dermatol 1993; 28:71–74.
11. Arsenault EF, Carson P, Falanga V. Extent and reversibility of laboratory abnormalities in patients treated with stanozolol. American Academy of Dermatology 60th Annual Meeting, New Orleans, 2002.
12. Demling R, DeSanti L. Oxandrolone, an anabolic steroid, significantly increases the rate of weight gain in the recovery phase after major burns. J Trauma 1997; 43:47–51.
13. Spungen A, Koehler K, Modeste-Duncan R, Rasul M, Cytryn A, Bauman V. 9 clinical cases of nonhealing pressure ulcers in patients with spinal cord injury treated with an anabolic agent: a therapeutic trial. Adv Skin Wound Care 2001; 14:139–144.
14. Hickman J, Lazarus G. Pyoderma gangrenosum: new concepts in etiology and treatment. In: Moschella S, ed. Dermatology Update: Review for Physicians. New York: Elsevier, 1979:325.
15. Wollina U. Clinical management of pyoderma gangrenosum. Am J Clin Dermatol 2002; 3:149–158.

16. Johnson R, Lazarus G. Pulse therapy, therapeutic efficacy in the treatment of pyoderma gangrenosum. Arch Dermatol 1982; 118:76.

17. Ljung T, Staun M, Grove O, Fausa O, Vatn M, Hellstrom P. Pyoderma gangrenosum associated with crohn disease effect of TNF-alpha blockade with infliximab. Scand J Gastroenterol 2002; 37:1108–1110.

18. Botros N, Pickover L, Das K. Image of the month. Pyoderma gangrenosum caused by ulcerative colitis. Gastroenterology 2000; 118:654, 809.

19. Tan MH, Gordon M, Lebwohl O, George J, Lebwohl MG. Improvement of pyoderma gangrenosum and psoriasis associated with Crohn disease with anti-tumor necrosis factor alpha monoclonal antibody. Arch Dermatol 2001; 137:930–933.

20. Longworth DL. Microbial drug resistance and the roles of the new antibiotics. Cleve Clin J Med 2001; 68:496–497, 501–502, 504.

21. Kauffman C. Therapeutic and preventive options for the management of vancomycin-resistant enterococcal infections. J Antimicrob Chemother 2003; 51:iii23–30.

22. Pittler MH, Ernst E. Horse-chesnut seed extract for chronic venous insufficiency. Arch Dermatol 1998; 134:1356–1360.

23. Siebert U, Brach M, Sroczynski G, Berla K. Efficacy, routine effectiveness, and safety of horsechesnut seed extract in the treatment of chronic venous insufficiency. A meta-analysis of randomized controlled trials and large observational studies. Int Angiol 2002; 21:305–315.

24. Comerota A, Throm R, Miller K, et al. Naked plasmid DNA encoding fibroblast growth factor type 1 for the treatment of end-stage unreconstructible lower extremity ischemia: preliminary results of a phase I trial. J Vasc Surg 2002; 35:930–936.

25. Rajagopalan S, Trachtenberg J, Mohler E, et al. Phase I study of direct administration of a replication deficient adenovirus containing the vascular endothelial growth factor cDNA(C1-1023) to patients with claudication. Am J Cardiol 2002; 90:512.

26. Layton A, Ibbotson S, Davies J, Goodfield M. Randomised trial of oral aspirin for chronic venous leg ulcers. Lancet 1994; 344:164–165.

27. Margolis DJ, Knauss J, Bilker W. Hormone replacement therapy and prevention of pressure ulcers and venous leg ulcers. Lancet 2002; 359:675–677.

28. Manson J, Hsia J, Johnson K, Rossouw J, Assaf A, Lasser N. Estrogen plus progestin and the risk of coronary heart disease. N Engl J Med 2003; 349:523–534.

48

Keloids and Hypertrophic Scars

Adriana Villa, Varee Poochareon, and Brian Berman
Department of Dermatology and Cutaneous Surgery, University of Miami School of Medicine, Miami, Florida, U.S.A.

1. DEFINITION

Keloids and hypertrophic scars are considered to be atypical manifestations of the wound healing process following trauma to the skin. These scars consist of excessive dense fibrous tissue growing in all directions, resulting in a prominent elevation above the skin (1). First described over 3000 years ago on Egyptian papyrus, keloids were later specifically defined in 1806 by Alibert, who proposed the term *cheloide* (from the Greek *chele*, or "crab claw"), in an effort to describe the lateral growth of scar tissue into the surrounding uninvolved skin (2).

2. CLINICAL AND DIAGNOSTIC BACKGROUND

2.1. Comparison of Keloids and Hypertrophic Scars

Physically similar in appearance, keloids and hypertrophic scars are considered by some researchers to be relatively indistinguishable, despite significant differences in their behavior.

A summary of these differences can be found in Table 1.

3. PATHOGENESIS

3.1. Wound Healing and Derailments Leading to Keloid or Hypertrophic Scar Formation

It seems hypertrophic scars and keloids represent an aberration or derailment in a wide array of these fundamental processes of wound healing. It is also believed that immunologic processes, and not primarily alterations in fibroblast function alone, are important in the formation of excessive scar tissue. Current data on morphologic, immunohistochemical, and biological characteristics involved in abnormal wound healing processes for both scar types will be presented here. Normal wound healing processes are presented elsewhere in this text.

Table 1 Clinical and Diagnostic Comparison of Hypertrophic Scars and Keloids

Hypertrophic scars	Keloids
Early appearance (within 4 weeks after original injury)	May take months to years to appear after original injury
May have spontaneous regression (within 12–18 months) (3)	Tendency to persist
Surgery indicated as a treatment (Z-plasties)	Recur after surgery (50% of the time)
Located on flexor surfaces more often than extensor areas	Located on earlobes, anterior chest, cheeks, among others, and rarely involves the joints
Remain limited to the boundaries of the initial site of injury (4)	Extend beyond the original wound
Light microscopy findings[a]: large nodules containing cells and collagen within the mid-to-deep part of the scar (collagen nodule) (3)	Light microscopy findings[a]: large collagen bundles, less oriented compared with hypertrophic scars. Abundant eosinophils, mast cells, plasma cells, and lymphocytes (3,18)
Electron microscopy findings: collagen fibers are smaller, more regular, and have higher interfibrillar distance compared with keloids (2)	Electron microscopy findings: presence of large, broad bundles of pink collagen separated by an amorphous ground substance (5)
	Higher metabolic activity and less degradation of newly synthesized collagen proteins (6)
	Higher expression of proliferating cell nuclear antigen (7)
Complications: contractures and possible loss of function and restriction of movement if overlying a joint	Complications: tenderness, pain, burning, and pruritus (found to be the most common symptom in an earlier survey) (11)

[a] On a histologic basis, both keloids and hypertrophic scars are characterized by a high density of fibroblast and collagen fibrils, rich vasculature, thickened epidermal cell layer, and high mesenchymal cell density.

3.2. Cells Involved in Wound Healing Processes

3.2.1. *Fibroblasts*

During the hemostasis stage of the wound healing process, fibroblasts on abnormal scar tissue have difficulty in mediating fibrinolysis because they exhibit an intrinsically low level of plasminogen activator and a high level of the inhibitor activity. The result is a lower plasmin concentration and an inferior breakdown of fibrin (10). Fibroblasts in excessive scar tissue show normal growth parameters but produce abnormal amounts of extracellular matrix (11). In keloid-derived fibroblasts, fibronectin production is increased (12), and its activity continues at high level for months to years in hypertrophic scars and keloids (13,14). Fibronectin concentration is higher mainly in perivascular areas and in the collagen nodule of excessive scar tissue (14). Myofibroblasts, the final phenotype of the fibroblast during granulation-tissue formation, persist in hypertrophic scars after the wound is fully epithelialized (8). This may be important in the pathogenesis of scar contracture, seen exclusively in hypertrophic scars. During the transition between granulation tissue and scar formation, keloid fibroblasts may undergo apoptosis, at a rate lower than fibroblasts found in normal scars (see Sec. 3.3.4).

3.2.2. Platelets

During hemostasis, degranulation of platelets is responsible for the release and activation of an array of potent growth factors, including epidermal growth factor, insulin-like growth factor (IGF-1), platelet-derived growth factor, and transforming growth factor (TGF)-β, which function as chemotactic agents for the recruitment of inflammatory cells such as neutrophils, macrophages, mast cells, epithelial cells, endothelial cells, and fibroblasts (5).

3.2.3. Macrophages

Macrophages can possibly initiate the formation of hypertrophic scars and keloids by the release of fibroblast-activating cytokines (i.e., TGF-β and platelet-derived growth factor) and are found in abundant numbers in active hypertrophic scars (15–17). Among the cytokines macrophages produce, interleukin-1α and -1β are not only responsible for induction of inflammatory cell adhesion and migration, but also for extracellular matrix degradation via stimulation of the release of matrix metalloproteinases (18,19) and induction of collagenase activity (20,21). A decrease in wound levels of interleukin-1 was found in patients with keloidal scars, correlating with the extent of their deformity (22). This may result in extracellular matrix accumulation and scar formation at the site of the injury.

3.2.4. Mast Cells

Mast cells, found in higher numbers in hypertrophic scars (23,24), may have a role in excessive scar tissue formation. The cells can be stimulated by immunoglobulin E to expel their cytoplasmic granules containing histamine, heparin, serotonin, acid hydrolase, chymase, and several growth factors, most of them involved in dermal matrix production (29). There is a correlation between immunoglobulin E levels and the incidence of excessive scar formation for race, sex, and age (25).

3.2.5. Keratinocytes

Keratinocytes are an important source of growth factors. In hypertrophic scars, they show an increased proliferation and differentiation, a reduced epidermal interleukin expression, and an increased platelet-derived growth factor expression (26,27). An immunologic role of hypertrophic scars and keloid keratinocytes may be shown by their expression of human leukocyte antigen class 2 and intercellular adhesion molecule-1, not present on normal scar keratinocytes (4,28). It was reccently established that keratinocytes overlying the keloid lesion promote proliferation and inhibit apoptosis of the underlying fibroblasts, by increasing the expression of TGF-β1, mitogen-activated protein kinase (MAPK) family phosphorylation, and Bcl-2, via soluble factors (double paracrine action) (29).

3.2.6. Other Cells

The skin's immune surveillance system may also play an important role in the formation of excessive scar tissue. Langerhans cells, (30) activated T-lymphocytes, (17) and macrophages (31) have been found in increased number in hypertrophic scars (21,35,36). Burn patients show a higher level of interleukin-6 expression compared with control patients (32). Keloid patients show antinuclear antibodies from different immunoglobulin classes against fibroblasts, epithelial, and endothelial cells as further proof of immunologic involvement. These antibodies were not found in hypertrophic scars (33,34).

3.3. Significant Processes and Factors in Abnormal Wound Healing

3.3.1. Neovascularization

Neovascularization in hypertrophic scars and keloids is characterized by an excess of new microvessels when compared with normal scars. These microvessels, late in the granulation stage, show occlusion of the lumina because of an excess of endothelial cells (35,36).

There is reduced tissue oxygen concentration in excessive scar tissue. This may be due to the microvessel occlusion (37) or possibly because of a high tissue metabolic rate or reduced oxygen diffusion to the wound space (38). Hypoxia promotes angiogenesis and stimulates fibroblasts to proliferate and produce collagen, accounting for the bulk of the excessive scar tissue (4,35,39). Collagen deposition concentrates between the lateral branches of the new microvessels. In excessive scar tissue, the deposition results in collagen nodules of various shapes and sizes (40).

3.3.2. Remodeling

In conditions of excessive tissue fibrosis, hyaluronic acid and proteoglycans remain at supranormal levels (41). In hypertrophic scars, hyaluronic acid is found mainly as a narrow strip in the papillary dermis, whereas in keloids it is mainly found in the thickened granular or spinous layers of the epidermis (11). The role of hyaluronic acid in excessive scar tissue formation may be in creating a pericellular boundary, maintaining TGF-β1 around the cell's environment, while potentiating the bioactivities of TGF-β1 as a collagen-production stimulator. It may also stabilize the plasma protease inhibitor–collagenase complex, thereby not only increasing collagen production but also inhibiting its degradation (41).

After wounding in hypertrophic scars and keloids, the relative amount of type III collagen remains increased compared with normal scar and normal skin (42,43). The collagen synthesis in keloids can continue for several years, instead of declining at 6 months and then decreasing to a normal turnover after 2 or 3 years. One possible mechanism to explain this is an overexpression of the IGF signal transduction pathway, which has been shown to increase the expression of type I and type III procollagen. IGF-1 receptor is overexpressed in keloidal fibroblasts compared with normal fibroblasts (44).

3.3.3. Growth Factors

Transforming growth factor-β activates extracellular matrix production and seems to be the most responsible for excessive scar tissue formation. Fibroblasts on hypertrophic scars and keloids proved to be more sensitive (45) to and respond to a lower concentration of TGF-β (46,47). In vitro, TGF-β reduces the collagenase-mediated degradation of wound matrix (48,49).

In the pathogenesis of keloids, the immune response seems to be of great importance. In the normal wound healing process, interferon (IFN)-α downregulates collagen synthesis (26,53), IFN-γ reduces collagenase activity (53), and IFN-α, -β, and -γ inhibit keloidal fibroblast production of collagen I, III, and VI and reduce messenger RNA proliferation of rapidly dividing fibroblasts (51). Reductions of IFN-α, IFN-γ, and tumor necrosis factor-α concentration have been found in keloids (22,31,52). IFN-α and -β also reduce fibroblast production of glycosaminoglycans (GAGs), which form the scaf-folding for deposition of dermal collagen. IFN-γ enhances GAG production (53). Studies have shown that IFN-γ modulates a p53 apoptotic pathway by inducing apoptosis-related genes.

3.3.4. Apoptosis

Downregulation of multiple apoptosis-related genes in human keloid tissue has been demonstrated (54). Keloid fibroblasts may undergo apoptosis at a rate lower than that of a normal scar, depositing collagen and other extracellular matrix proteins and proteoglycans beyond that expected in normal wound healing. Apoptosis may participate as well in downregulation of the inflammatory cell infiltration phase. Mutations in p53, a protein synthesized following DNA damage, are believed to predispose cells to hyperproliferation, possibly resulting in keloid formation. In addition, p53 is a potent suppressor of interleukin-6, a cytokine implicated in hyper-proliferative and fibrotic conditions (57). Of the downregulated apotosis-related genes already identified, there is a group of promoters such as tumor TRADD, c-*myc*, proto-oncogene, NIP3, and HDLC1, as well as inhibitors such as DAD-1, G-S-T, G-S-T-M, and glutathione peroxidase (54).

Bcl-2, an antiapoptotic gene, was found to stain intensely in keloid tissue dermis and its level of expression was highest when cocultured with keloid derived keratinocytes (29). The existing data show a difference between apoptotic gene expression of keloids and normal scars.

4. TREATMENT

4.1. Commonly Used Treatments

No single therapeutic modality is best for all keloids. Location, size, depth of the lesion, age of the patient, and past response to treatment all may determine the type of therapy used. Standardization of the criteria involved in evaluating keloids and hypertrophic scars separately is required to determine effectiveness and indications of treatment. Suggested variables for assessment of therapeutic intervention should include epidemiology, etiology, age of the lesion, symptoms, photographic documen-tation, location, volume (linear dimensions or calcium alginate molds), induration (55), color, histology (whenever possible), and patient-satisfaction scales after treat-ment. Often it is optimal to support the modalities of occlusion, compression, and corticosteroidism as in the product Scarguard (80). Table 2 reviews current treat-ments available for keloids and hypertrophic scars.

4.2. Other Potential Therapies

Based upon in vitro data, there are antifibrotic agents that may be potentially helpful clinically. However, there are limited clinical studies to support their efficacy in the treatment of keloids and hypertrophic scars at the present time. Such agents include

Table 2 Commonly Used Treatments Available for Keloids and Hypertrophic Scars

Modality	Mechanism	Efficacy	Complications
Silicone-containing dressings	Antikeloidal effects appear to result from a combination of occlusion and hydration rather than from the effect of silicone (56)	Previous studies showed 28% had no or slight improvement, 37.5% moderate improvement, and 34% excellent improvement (56). In one of the studies on keloidal scars alone, 34% of keloidal scars showed flattening after 6 months of continuous gel use (57). Improvement has been reported in scar volume, tenderness, firmness, and pruritus. Silicone gel is favored in some cases due to the benign nature of treatment.	Benign
Compression	Reduction in the cohesiveness of collagen fibers in pressure-treated hypertrophic scars (58)	Overall, 60% of patients treated with these devices (button compression, pressure earrings, pressure-gradient devices, among others) showed 75–100% improvement (1). Water-impermeable, non-silicone-based occlusive dressing worn continuously for 2 months reduced average keloid height 35% (59). Semi-permeable, semi-occlusive non-silicone-based dressing worn for 1–2 months showed statistically significant reduction in keloid height (Fig. 3), tenderness, pruritus (60).	
Corticosteroids	May downregulate collagen gene expression within the keloid (61), alter glycosaminoglycan synthesis, and reduce production of inflammatory mediators and fibroblast proliferation during wound healing (1).	Mainstay of treatment. However, in most of the older scars and keloids, can only soften and flatten the scars and can provide symptomatic relief (Fig. 4). May be effectiveas monotherapy when given every 4–6 weeks at doses of 40 mg/mL (3). Lower doses may be used in softer keloids.	Repeated injections may lead to atrophy, telangiectasia formation, and pigmentary alteration

Radiation	Destroys fibroblasts from both normal and keloidal skin. The extracellular matrix gene expression seems to be affected by radiation as well (62).	Radiotherapy is rarely used as monotherapy today	See adjuvant radiotherapy for complications
Interferons	Suppress collagen synthesis, may reduce transforming growth-factor-β (TGF-β) (4). IFN-$\alpha 2b$ enhances keloidal collagenase activity, reduce glycosaminoglycan synthesis, and induces apoptosis (50).	When used as a monotherapy IFN-$\alpha 2b$ resulted in a 41 and 46% reduction in area after 2 injections, 4 days apart (50). Because of cost and side effects of the injections, interferons are not used as single agents for keloid treatment.	Low-grade fever, flu-like illness for 48–72 hours after injection. Pain on injection site.
Surgical excision	Removes the bulk of the keloidal scar, replaces a broad-based scar with a thin, more cosmetically acceptable scar.	Excisional surgery alone has been shown to yield a 45–100% recurrence rate (3), and should very rarely be used as a solitary modality. Excision combined with other postoperative modalities show lower recurrence rates than those previously reported for excisional surgery alone.	
Adjuvant therapies to surgery Adjuvant corticosteroids	Same mechanism as monotherapy.	Injections usually given immediately after excision, 2–3 weeks postoperatively, followed by repeat injections every 4 weeks. Majority of studies show less than 50% recurrence (63); this rate is higher in keloids in comparison with hypertrophic scars.	Same complications as monotherapy.

(Continued)

Table 2 Commonly Used Treatments Available for Keloids and Hypertrophic Scars (*Continued*)

Modality	Mechanism	Efficacy	Complications
Adjuvant radiotherapy	Same mechanism as monotherapy.	Radiation after surgical excision can prevent recurrence of keloidal scars in approximately 75% of cases at one-year follow-up (4). Most frequently used treatment was superficial x-rays of 900 cGy or greater, in fractions given within 10 days of surgery (3). adiation is mainly reserved for scars resistant to other treatment modalities.	Few case reports describe the development of malignancy after radiation therapy of keloids (64). Caution is advised when treating young children, and areas around the breasts and thyroid (65).
Adjuvant interferon therapy	Same mechanism as monotherapy.	Injected interferon into the suture line of keloid excision sites may reduce recurrences prophylactically. Statistically significant fewer keloid recurrences were found in a study of 124 keloid lesions after postoperative treatment using interferon α-2b injected into keloid excision sites (18%) versus excised alone (51%) and TAC-treated sites. When using IFN-γ2b as adjuvant therapy to laser or surgical excision, recurrences of 33% at 3 years and 19% (63) have been found	Same complications as monotherapy.
Adjuvant imiquimod	Induces local production of interferon at the site of application resulting in a negative balance on collagen prodction. Imiquimod 5% cream alters the expression of genes associated with apoptosis on keloidal tissue (66).	Postoperative application of imiquimod 5% cream starting the night of surgery, for 8 weeks , on 13 earlobe keloids excised from 12 patients showed a recurrence rate of 0% at week 24 (67).	No systemic symptoms of interferon toxicity detected. Local reactions: mild eczematous erythema and transitory hyperpigmentation (67).

| Laser therapy | Can burn, coagulate, or evaporate the keloid tissue. Wounds made by a laser beam have less tendency to show scar contraction (68). | CO_2 laser (cuts and cauterizes) was associated with 0–93% recurrence rates, and when combined with postoperative injected steroids, was associated with 16–74% recurrence rates (69). Neodymium:yttrium–aluminum–garnet (Nd:YAG) laser in practice has shown recurrences of 0–100% (70,71). The 585-nm pulsed dye laser (more vascular-specific laser) reduces subjective symptoms, color, and height in keloidal or hypertrophic scars (72) with improvement in 57–83% of the cases. | |
| Cryotherapy | Cryosurgical media, such as liquid nitrogen, affect the microvasculature and cause cell damage via intracellular crystals, leading to tissue anoxia | 1, 2, or 3 freeze-thaw cycles lasting 10–30 seconds each are used. Treatment may need to be repeated every 20–30 days. Cryosurgery led to total resolution with no recurrences in 51–74% of patients after 30 months of follow-up observation (73). | Painful. May not be appropriate in patients with darker skin because of the risk of hypopigmentation. |

β-aminopropionitrile, penicillamine, colchicine, and putrescine, all of which inhibit collagen biosynthesis and cross-linking in vitro (74). Tranilast, an antiallergic drug, decreases collagen and GAG synthesis by reducing TGF-β1 (75). Topical retinoids inhibit collagen metabolism (76). Antihistamine drugs may also be helpful, considering the role histamine possibly plays in overhealing (77). Pentoxifylline inhibits proliferation of fibroblasts and reduces the production of collagen, fibronectin, and GAGs (78). Calcium antagonists affect extracellular-matrix protein reorganization, inducing procollagenase synthesis by fibrotic cells (79).

4.3. Prevention

Various modalities of treatment of keloids and hypertrophic scars have been presented here. However, it is important to note that the first rule of treatment involves prevention and patient education. Suggestions for the prevention of these lesions include avoidance of nonessential cosmetic surgery in patients known to form keloids and closure of all surgical wounds with minimal tension. Surgeons should also avoid mid-chest incisions and those crossing joint spaces, ensuring incisions follow skin creases whenever possible. Adjuvant therapies to surgery, with the exception of radiation, may also be considered.

5. CONCLUSIONS

Keloids and hypertrophic scars are fairly common lesions that, despite their similar clinical appearances, are separate entities in behavior, morphology, and pathophysiology. The majority of studies, however, don't make clear distinction between the two. There is a need for developing studies that solely examine keloids or hypertrophic scars, with special attention to standardizing criteria for diagnosis and assessment, in order to find uniquely reliable and successful therapies for each entity. Keloids and hypertrophic scars are subjects open to further study. We have tried to present the most current concepts with respect to excessive scarring, but many recent developments have arisen that merit further study, especially in the realm of immunology, which holds a great deal of value with regard to both pathogenesis and future treatment options.

REFERENCES

1. Berman B, Kapoor S. Keloid and hypertrophic scar. eMedicine (www.emedicine.com) 2001; 2(11):1–12.
2. Berman B, Bieley HC. Keloids. J Am Acad Dermatol 1995; 33:117.
3. Shaffer JJ, Taylor SC, Cook-Bolden F. Keloidal scars: a review with a critical look at therapeutic options. J Am Acad Dermatol 2002; 46:S63.
4. Brody GS. Keloids and hypertrophic scars. Plast Reconstr Surg 1990; 86:804.
5. Ehrlich HP, Desmouliere A, Diegelmann RF, et al. Morphological and immunological differences between keloid and hypertrophic scar. Am J Pathol 1994; 145:105.
6. Ueda K, Furuya E, Yasuda Y, Oba S, Tajima S. Keloids have continuous high metabolic activity. Plast Reconst Surg 1999; 104:694–698.
7. Nakaoka H, Miyauchi S, Miki Y. Proliferating activity of dermal fibroblasts in keloids and hypertrophic scars. Acta Dermatol Venereol 1995; 75:102–104.
8. Ehrlich HP, Desmouliere A, Diegelmann RF, et al. Morphological and immunological differences between keloid and hypertrophic scar. Am J Pathol. 1994; 145:105.

9. Cosman B, Crikelair GF, Gaulin JC, Lattes R. The surgical treatment of keloidal scars. Plast Reconstr Surg 1961; 27:335.

10. Tuan TL, Zhu JY, Sun B, Nichter LS, Nimni ME, Laug WE. Elevated levels of plasminogen activator inhibitor-1 may account for the altered fibrinolysis by keloid fibroblasts. J Invest Dermatol 1996; 106:1007.

11. Bertheim U, Hellstrom S. The distribution of hyaluronan in human skin and mature, hypertrophic and keloid scars. Br J Plast Surg 1994; 47:483.

12. Oliver N, Babu M, Diegelmann R. Fibronectin gene transcription is enhanced in abnormal wound healing. J Invest Dermatol 1992; 99:579.

13. Kischer CW, Wagner HN Jr, Pindur J, et al. Increased fibronectin production by cell lines from hypertrophic scar and keloid. Connect Tissue Res 1989; 23:279.

14. Kischer CW, Hendrix MJ. Fibronectin (FN) in hypertrophic scars and keloids. Cells Tissue Res 1983; 231:219.

15. Elias JA, Rossman MD, Daniele RP. Inhibition of human lung fibroblast growth by mononuclear cells. Am Rev Respir Dis 125:701,182.

16. Wahl SM, Wahl LM, McCarthy JB. Lymphocyte-mediated activation of fibroblast proliferation and collagen production. J Immunol 1978; 121:942.

17. Castagnoli C, Trombotto C, Ondei S, et al. Characterization of T-cell subsets infiltrating post-burn hypertrophic scar tissues. Burns 1997; 28:565.

18. Postlerhwaite AE, Lachman LB, Mainardi CL, Kang AH. Interleukin 1 stimulation of collagenase production by cultured fibroblasts. J Exp Med 1983; 157:801.

19. Elias JA, Gustilo K, Baeder W, Freundlich B. Synergistic stimulation of fibroblast prostaglandin production by recombinant interleukin 1 and tumor necrosis factor. J Immunol 1987; 138:3812.

20. Meyer FA, Yaron I, Yaron M. Synergistic, additive, antagonistic effects on interleukin-1 beta, tumor necrosis factor alpha, and gamma-interferon on prostaglandin E, hyaluronic acid, and collagenase production by cultured synovial fibroblasts. Arthritis Rheum 1990; 33:1518.

21. Postlethwaite AE, Raghow R, Striclin GP, Poppleton H, Seyer JM, Kang AH. Modulation of fibroblast functions by interleukin-1: increased steady state accumulation of type I procollagen messenger RNAs and stimulation of other functions but not chemotaxis by human recombinant interleukin 1 alpha and beta. J Cell Biol 1998; 106:311.

22. McCauley RL, Chopra V, Li YY, Herdon DN, Robson MC. Altered cytokine production in black patients with keloids. J Clin Immunol 1992; 2:300.

23. Craig SS, De Blois G, Schwartz LB. Mast cells in human keloid, small intestine, and lung by an immunoperoxidase technique using a murine monoclonal antibody against tryptase. Am J Pathol 1986; 124:427.

24. Hebda PA, Collins MA, Tharp MD. Mast cell and myofibroblast in wound healing. Dermatol Clin 1993; 11:685.

25. Smith C, Smith JC, Finn MC. The possible role of mast cells (allergy) in the production of keloid and hypertrophic scarring. J Burn Care Rehabil 1987; 8:126.

26. Niessen FB, Andriessen MP, Schalkwijk J, Visser L, Timens W. Keratinocyte derived cytokines play a role in the formation of hypertrophic scars. J Pathol 2001; 194(2):207.

27. Andriessen MP, Niessen FB, Van de Kerkhof PC, Schalkwijk J. Hypertrophic scarring is associated with epidermal abnormalities: an immunohistochemical study. J Pathol 1998; 186:192.

28. Castagnoli C, Stella M, Magliacani G, Ferrone S, Richiardi PM. Similar ectopic expression of ICAM-1 and HLA class II molecules in hypertrophic scars following thermal injury. Burns 1994; 20:430.

29. Zhang LQ, Laato M, Muona P, Penttinen R, Oikarinene A, Peltonen J. A fibroblast cell line cultured from a hypertrophic scar displays selective downregulation of collagen gene expression: barely detectable messenger RNA levels of the pro alpha I (III) chain of type III collagen. Arch Dermatol Res 1995; 287:534.

30. Cracco C, Stella M, Teich Alasia S, Filogamo, G. Comparative study of Langerhans cells in normal and pathological human scars. II. Hypertrophic scars. Eur J Histochem 1992; 36:53.

31. Castagnoli C, Stella M, Berthod C, Magliacani G, Richiardi PM. TNF production and hypertrophic scarring. Cell Imunol 1993; 147:51.

32. Ueyama M, Maruyama I, Osame M, Sawada Y. Marked increase in plasma interleukin-6 in burn patients. J Lab Clin Med 1992; 120:693.

33. Janssen de Limpens AM, Cormane RH. Studies on the immunologic aspects of keloids and hypertrophic scars. Arch Dermatol Res 1982; 274:259.

34. Placik OJ, Lewis VL Jr. Immunologic associations of keloids. Surg Gynecol Obstet 1992; 175:185.

35. Kisher CW, Sheltar MR, Chvapil M. Hypertrophic Scars and Keloids: A review and new concept concerning their origin. Scan Electron Microsc 4:1699–1082.

36. Kischer CW. The microvessels in hypertrophic scars, keloids and related lesions: a review. J Submicrosc Cytol Pathol 1992; 24:281.

37. Knighton DR, Silver IA, Hunt TK. Regulation of wound-healing angiogenesis-effect of oxygen gradients and inspired oxygen concentration. Surgery 1981; 90:262.

38. Sloan DF, Brown RD, Wells CH, Hilton JG. Tissue gasses in human hypertrophic burn scars. Plast Reconstr Surg 1978; 61:431.

39. Kischer CW, Thies AC, Chvapil M. Perivascular myofibroblasts and microvascular occlusion in hypertrophic scars and keloids. Hum Pathol 1982; 13:819.

40. Kischer CW, Pindur J, Krasovitch P, Kischer E. Characteristics of granulation tissue which promote hypertrophic scarring. Scanning Microsc 1990; 4:877.

41. Alaish SM, Yager DR, Diegelmann RF, Cohe IK. Hyaluronic acid metabolism in keloid fibroblasts. J Pediatr Surg 1995; 30:949.

42. Friedman DW, Boyd CD, Mackenzie JW, et al. Regulation of collagen gene expression in keliods and hypertrophic scars. J Surg Res 1993; 55:214.

43. Di Cesare PE, Cheung DT, Perelman N, Libaw E, Peng L, Nimmi ME. Alteration of collagen composition and cross-linking in keloid tissues. Matrix 1990; 10:172.

44. Yoshimoto H, Hiroshi I, Ohtsuru A, et al. Overexpression of insulin-like growth factor-1 (IGF-1) receptor and the invasiveness of cultured keloid fibroblasts. Am J Pathol 1999; 154:883–889.

45. Tredget EE. The molecular biology of fibroproliferative disorders of the skin: potential cytokine therapeutics. Ann Plast Surg 1994; 33:152.

46. Russel SB, Trupin KM, Rodriguez Eaton S, et al. Reduced growth-factor requirement of keloid-derived fibroblasts may account for tumor growth. Proc Natl Acad Sci USA 1988; 85:587.

47. Garner WL, Karmiol S, Rodriguez JL, et al. Phenotypic differences in cytokine responsiveness of hypertrophic scar versus normal dermal fibroblasts. J Inves Dermatol 1993; 101:875.

48. Quaglino D Jr, Nanney LB, Ditesheim JA, Davison JM. Transforming growtyh factor-beta stimulates wound healing and modulates extracellular matrix gene expression in pig skin: incisional wound model. J Invest Dermatol 1991; 97:34.

49. Overall CM, Wrana JL, Sodek J. Independent regulation of collagenase, 72-kDa progelatinase, and metalloendoproteinase inhibitor expression in human fibroblasts by transforming growth factor-beta. J Biol Chem 1989; 264:1860.

50. Berman B, Duncan MR. Short-term keloid treatment in vivo with human interferon alfa-2b results in a selective and persistent normalization of keloidal fibroblast collagen, glycosaminoglycan, and collagenase production in vitro. J Am Acad Dermatol 1989; 21:694.

51. Elias JA, Jimenez SA, Freundlich B. Recombinant gamma, alpha, and beta interferon regulation of human lung fibroblast proliferation. Am Rev Respir Dis 1987; 135:62.

52. Peruccio D, Castagnoli C, Stella M, et al. Altered biosynthesis of tumour necrosis factor (TNF) alpha is involved in postburn hypertrophic scars. Burns 1994; 20:118.

53. Berman B, Flores F. Interferons. In: Wolverton SE, ed. Philadelphia: W.B. Saunders Co., 2001:339–357.

54. Sayah DN, Soo C, Shaw WW, et al. Downregulation of apoptosis-related genes in keloid tissues. J Surg Res 1999; 87:209.

55. Flores J, Berman B, Burdick A, Jonusas AM. The effectiveness of a new method for assessing induration. J Am Acad Dermatol 1998; 39:1021.

56. Chang CC, Kuo YF, Chiu HC, Lee JL, Wong TW, Jee SH. Hydration, not silicone, modulates the effects of keratinocytes on fibroblasts. J Sug Res 1995; 59:705.

57. Mercer NS. Silicone gel in the treatment of keloid scars. Br J Plast Surg 1989; 42:83.

58. Kischer CW, Shetlar MR, Shetlar CL. Alteration of hypertrophic scars induced by mechanical pressure. Arch Dermatol 1975; 111(1):60.

59. Bieley HC, Berman B. Keloids. Effects of a water-impermeable, non-silicone-based occlusive dressing on keloids. J A Acad Dermatol 1996; 35:113.

60. Young A, Tan P, Berman B, Villa A, Poochareon V. Topical application of a semipermeable, semiocclusive, non-silicone-based dressing for keloid treatment. Cosmet Dermatol In press.

61. Kauh YC, Roud S, Mondragon G, Tokarek R, diLeonardo M, et al. Major suppression of pro-alfa 1 (I) type I collagen gene expression in the dermis after keloid excision and immediate intrawound injection of triamcinolone acetonide. J Am Acad Dermatol 1997; 37:586.

62. Lee KS, Jung JB, Ro YJ, Ryoo YW, Kim OB, Song JY. Effects of x-irradiation on survival and extracellular matrix gene expression on cultured keloid fibroblasts. J Dermatol Sci 1994; 8:33.

63. Berman B, Flores F. Recurrence rates of excised keloids treated with postoperative triamcinolone acetonide injections or interferon alfa-2b injections. J Am Acad Dermatol 1997; 37:755.

64. Rockwell WB, Cohen IK, Ehrlich HP. Keloids and hypertrophic scars: a comprehensive review. Plast Reconstr Surg 1989; 84:827.

65. Botwood N, Lewanski C, Lowdell C. The risks of treating keloids with radiotherapy. Br J Radiol 1999; 72:1222.

66. Jocob SE, Berman B, Naossiri M, Vincet V. Topical application of immiguimod 5% cream to keloids alters expression genes associated with apoptosis Br J Dermatol: 149(s66) 62–65.

67. Kaufman J, Berman B. Pilot study of the effect of postoperative imiquimod 5% cream on the recurrence rate of excised keloids. J Am Acad Dermatol 2002; 46(4):S209–S211.

68. Hendrick DA, Meyers A. Wound healing after laser surgery. Otolaryngol Clin North Am 1995; 5:969.

69. Norris JE. The effect of carbon dioxide laser treatment on the recurrence of keloids. Plast Reconstr Surg 1991; 87:44.

70. Castro DJ, Abergel RP, Meeker CA, Dwyer RM, Lesavoy MA, Vitto J. Effects of the Nd:YAG laser on DNA synthesis and collagen production in human skin fibroblast cultures. Ann Plast Surg 1984; 11:214–222.

71. Sherman R, Rosenfeld H. Experience with the Nd:YAG laser in the treatment of keloid scars. Ann Plast Surg 1998; 21:231.

72. Alster TS, Williams CM. Treatment of keloid sternotomy scars with 585 nm flashlamp-pumped pulsed-dye laser. Lancet 1995; 8959:1198.

73. Zouboulis CC, Orfanos CE. (Cryosurgical treatment of hypertrophic scars keloids.) Kryochirurgische Behandlung von hypertrophen Narben and Keloiden. Hautarzi 1990; 12:683.

74. Peacock EE Jr. Pharmacologic control of surface scarring in human beings. Ann Surg 1981; 5:592.

75. Suzawa H, Kikuchi S, Arai N, Koda A. The mechanism involved in the inhibitory action of tranilast, an anti-allergic drug, on the release of cytokines on PGE2 from human monocytes–macrophages. Jpn J Pharmacol 1992; 2:85.

76. Daly TJ, Weston WL. Retinoid effects on fibroblast proliferation and collagen synthesis in vitro and on fibrotic disease in vivo. J Am Acad Dermatol 1986; 4(Pt 2):900.
77. Bairy KL, Rao CM, Ramesh KV, Kulkarni DR. Effects of antihistamines on wound healing. J Exp Biol 1991; 4:398.
78. Berman B, Duncan MR. Pentoxifylline inhibits the proliferation of human fibroblasts derived from keloid, scleroderma and morphea skin in their production of collagen, glycosaminoglycans and fibronectin. Br J Dermatol 1990; 3:339.
79. Lee RC, Ping JA. Calcium antagonists retard extracellular matrix production in connective tissue equivalent. J Surg Res 1990; 5:463.
80. Eisen D. A pilot study to evaluate the efficacy of ScarGuard in the prvention of the scars. Internat J Dermatol 2004; 5(2).

49
Pain Management

Diane L. Krasner
Rest Haven—York, York, Pennsylvania, U.S.A.

1. INTRODUCTION

The pain experienced by most chronic wound pain sufferers is typically a complex, multidimensional phenomenon (1,2). It usually involves procedural pain (such as pain from debridement, dressings, or therapies) as well as nonprocedural pain (such as body image changes, loss of function, suffering, or ache and anguish) (3,4). Only in the past decade and a half has the importance of the chronic wound pain experience been truly appreciated by wound care providers (5–8).

To date, only a handful of specialty wound centers have algologists or anesthesiologists on the interdisciplinary team. The evidence to date suggests that wound pain management in hospitals still leaves much to be desired (9,10). In an ideal world, pain specialist doctors and nurses would be part of every chronic wound care team. When that is not feasible, having a pain specialist who can be regularly consulted may be the next best thing. Another option may be to designate the member of the wound care team who has the most interest in pain management to be the watchdog, to co-ordinate pain management efforts, and to advocate for the appropriate pain plans of care for patients. Whichever approach you choose, attending to wound pain is no longer an option—pain management is essential for advanced wound caring (11).

While research has not yet conclusively demonstrated that decreasing wound pain will improve the time to healing of wounds, it seems intuitively likely to be the case. Decreasing a person's pain response is an important and quantifiable outcome measure of care that clinicians will find useful in this age of outcome imperatives. Painful wounds often frustrate both patient and caregiver. They may represent failed expectations from the patient's point of view, the providers—or both. They may be palliative wounds that will never heal. Painful wounds are much more, therefore, than mere physical damage to skin and tissue. The psychological aspects of managing chronic wound pain—addressing the suffering, the ache and anguish—are as essential as relieving the physical pain. Changes in body image, activities of daily living, productivity, and functional status are usually significant contributors to the overall wound pain experience.

During interviews for my dissertation, a phenomenological study that explored the lived experience of chronic wound pain (12), Mr. Beech (a pseudonym), a tough truck driver with a 7-year history of a nonhealing venous ulcer, said to me one day, "Do you know how much courage it takes to come back to this clinic every week, knowing I'm going to be tortured?" Would *you* go to the dentist for a root canal without an anesthetic? Of course, not! But this is the expectation for far too many wound patients. Even our language reflects our bias in common phrases such as "Bite the bullet," "No pain, no gain," and "Grin and bear it."

We *can* do better. We *must* do better. By opening our eyes and ears to the issue of wound pain (13) and employing the strategies that will be discussed in this chapter, we can reduce the pain and suffering that far too many patients with chronic wounds still experience.

> The real voyage of discovery
> consists not in seeking new landscapes,
> but in having new eyes.
>
> —*Marcel Proust*

> When wounds are painful,
> They are trying to communicate that something is wrong.
> All we have to do is listen.
>
> —*Lia van Rijswijk*

2. CHRONIC WOUND PAIN

Interest in chronic wound pain has evolved slowly in contrast to interest in burn (acute wound) pain or to the science of wound healing both of which have grown by leaps and bounds. Brief mention of the pain experienced by chronic wound suffers was occasionally mentioned in the chronic wound literature prior to the 1990s (14,15). The 1990s saw an emerging interest in the phenomenon with the publication of various descriptive studies addressing the experiences of leg ulcer patients in pain (16–18), as well as the impact of the wound pain experience on health-related quality of life (19,20). Interventional research on the subject is just reaching the research agenda. So, at the beginning of the 21st century, it is fair to say that our research base for practice related to chronic wound pain is spotty and superficial. There is certainly much more room for research into this important area for practice.

3. CLASSIFICATION OF CHRONIC WOUND PAIN

Pain has classically been categorized in several different ways: nociceptive (tissue injury) vs. neuropathic (nerve injury), procedural vs. nonprocedural, acute vs. chronic, and acute vs. chronic malignant vs. chronic nonmalignant. In every case, it is recognized that the pain experience is multidimensional and that people commonly experience more than one type of pain, either sequentially or concurrently (1). The implication of this is that frequently multiple approaches and/or polypharmacy are required for a person to achieve an acceptable level of pain relief.

In 1995, this researcher, after experiencing three surgeries each of which involved wound complications (21–24), developed a model entitled The Chronic

Wound Pain Experience Model. This model is based on empirical experience and makes a distinction between acute noncyclic wound pain, acute cyclic wound pain, and chronic wound pain (25) (Fig. 1). This author suggests that in the real world, distinguishing between one-time or very limited painful stimuli (such as one-time debridements or drain tube removals) vs. cyclic painful stimuli (such as

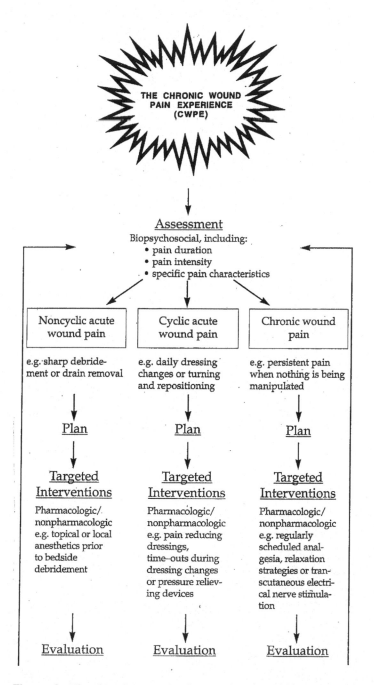

Figure 1 The chronic wound pain experience model. (©1995 Diane L. Krasner.)

daily dressing changes) vs. chronic painful stimuli (such as the continuous burning or throbbing of a wound) can help clinicians to distinguish the type of pain-reducing interventions that may be needed for a particular individual. So, for example, Mr. Beech with a chronic painful venous ulcer may need the following strategies that address all three dimensions of his chronic wound pain experience:

For acute noncyclic wound pain secondary to debridement:

- EMLA® topically under a transparent film dressing 1 hr prior to the debridement
- Oral analgesia following the procedure

For acute cyclic wound pain secondary to exudate build-up and dressing changes:

- Wound cleansing
- Pain-reducing dressings
- Reduced dressing change schedule by employing advanced wound dressings
- Periwound skin barriers

Chronic wound pain secondary to swelling and neuropathic pain:

- Compression therapy
- Antidepressant medication for neuropathic pain

4. RESOURCES

Several excellent sources for information generally on pain and specifically wound pain are worthy of mention. In 1992, the Agency for Health Care Policy and Research (AHCPR) published the first in a series of Clinical Practice Guidelines entitled Acute Pain Management: Operative or Medical Procedures and Trauma (26). In 1994, Guideline #9 was published entitled Chronic Malignant Pain (27). Both of these guidelines provide excellent starting points for clinicians interested in standards of care for pain management in general.

In 1994, the AHCPR also published a guideline addressing The Treatment of Pressure Ulcers (28). This guideline briefly mentions pressure ulcer pain, recommending:

- Assess all patients with pain related to the pressure ulcer or its treatment (*page 30*).
- Management pain by eliminating or controlling the source of pain (e.g., covering wounds, adjusting support surfaces, repositioning. Provide analgesia as needed and appropriate (*page 31*).
- Prevent or manage pain associated with debridement as needed (*page 49*).

In 2002, the European Wound Management Association (EWMA) published a position document on wound pain at wound dressing changes (29). This excellent resource consists of a series of review articles on the following topics:

- Pain at Wound Dressing Changes (CJ Moffatt)
- Understanding Wound Pain and Trauma: An International Perspective (CJ Moffatt, PJ Franks, H Hollingworth)
- The Theory of Pain (H Wulf, R Baron)
- Pain at Wound Dressing Changes: A Guide to Management (M Briggs, JE Torra, Bou)

- The EWMA position document on wound pain can be downloaded from the Internet at www.tendra.com

5. CHRONIC WOUND PAIN ASSESSMENT

Chronic wound pain comes from a variety of sources, most commonly secondary to tissue trauma, treatments, devices, swelling, infection, and nerve damage. As with all types of pain, it is a subjective phenomenon defined and experienced by the individual. McCaffery captured this important recognition in her 1972 definition of pain: "Pain is whatever the experiencing person says it is and exists whenever he [/she] says it does" (30). Many other definitions of pain exist and the reader is referred to the extensive literature on pain for further definitions.

It has been suggested that pain be viewed as the fifth vital sign. Routine assessment of pain along with temperature, pulse, respirations, and blood pressure is advocated by many. Following the pain initiative in 2001 by the Joint Commission on the Accreditation of Healthcare Organizations in the United States, many facilities added pain scores to their vital signs flow sheets.

6. PAIN TOOLS AND SCALES

The pain assessment tools in general use today range from simple visual analogue scales (VASs) to complex multidimensional instruments. All have their purpose and place. Because of the subjective nature of the pain experience, it is only appropriate for the person experiencing pain to determine his/her own score. It is never considered appropriate for a healthcare professional to rate a person's pain level for him. The AHCPR Panel on Acute Pain Management emphasized this in the strongest terms in the 1992 AHCPR Clinical Practice Guideline #1: The single most reliable indicator of the existence and intensity of acute pain—and any resultant affective discomfort or distress—is the patient's self report (26).

This mandate presents challenges for those chronic wound patients who, due to stroke or other illnesses, are unable to express themselves. In such cases, this author recommends relying on expert knowing (31) and experience and intuiting the person's level of pain form your prior experience with similar patients with the given type of wound/etiology and pain. The reader is referred to articles by Herr and Mobily (32,33) for further discussion of this topic and information about the assessment of pain in the elderly.

The gold standard for measuring pain for research and clinical purposes is the 10-mm horizontal VAS. On this scale, the left anchor marks "No pain" and the right anchor marks "Pain as bad as it can be." The person is asked to point to the place on the line representing the intensity of his pain at the current moment, known as present pain intensity (PPI). This scale can also be used to measure pain distress. Visual analogue scales may not be intuitive or easily comprehended by all people. In such situations, an alternative scale, such as a numeric scale, a descriptor scale, or the Faces pain scale (34) may be used. Dallam et al. (9) showed a good correlation between the VAS and the Faces scales in their study of hospitalized elderly patients with pressure ulcer pain.

Pain assessment should be done on a regular basis. Enlightened clinicians often routinely measure pain prior to and following procedures that are known to cause pain such as debridements or dressing changes to assure that adequate pain control has been achieved. Some clinicians advocate asking the person a second question, "Where do you want your pain level to be" and using that level as the target for treatment and level for measuring effectiveness of the interventions. For people experiencing ongoing pain, it is often helpful to have them keep a pain dairy in order to understand the fill extent and daily variation in the pain experience. In depth pain assessment can be obtained using the McGill Pain Questionnaire or the Short Form-McGill Pain Questionnaire (35). Other pain descriptors that are often assessed include pain duration (e.g., periodic, intermittent, and persistent) and pain characteristics (e.g., descriptors such as sharp, burning, etc.).

7. MANAGEMENT TACTICS AT THE TIME OF DRESSING CHANGE

Dressing change pain, which is considered procedural or acute cyclic pain, is often cited by chronic wound patients as the worst pain they experience. This may illustrate the problems caused by using antiquated dressings, such as gauze wet-to-dry dressings, that are ripped out of the wound and reinjure it with each dressing change—starting the wounding process all over again. Many strategies can be employed to minimize wound dressing change pain including:

1. Using pain-reducing dressings that cover the wound bed and exposed nerve endings, adhere as little as possible and leave minimal residue behind. Examples include hydrogels, foams, nonadherent dressings, or specialty absorptive dressings like hydrofibers or alginates. Dressings that cause pain should be avoided, such as wet-to-dry gauze and adhesive dressings on certain areas of the body,
2. Managing wound exudates properly, so that it does not pool in the wound bed causing local pressure and pain or leak out of the wound bed macerating or denuding the surrounding skin. If wound margins become macerated or denuded, cover them to prevent pain and further damage with a moisture barrier ointment (e.g., petrolatum and zinc oxide), a hydrocolloid or thin hydrocolloid dressing (that will stick to denuded skin) or a special wound barrier dressing,
3. Avoiding the use of cytotoxic agents such as full strength povidone iodine, which in and of themselves often cause pain when applied to wounds,
4. Minimizing the frequency of dressing changes by selecting advanced wound dressings that require daily or every other day changes (as opposed to twice a day or three times a day dressing changes),
5. Selecting a time of day for the dressing changes when that individual can best tolerate the dressing change (e.g., mornings for morning people and evenings of night owls),
6. Giving the person permission to call time-out if the pain gets to be too great. Burn research has demonstrated that giving people this control reduces pain scores related to dressing changes (26),
7. Allowing people who are able to change their own dressings, which often causes less pain than when someone else does it, and
8. Using diversionary tactics at dressing changes to help reduce the pain experienced, such as conversation, music, or imagery.

8. DEVICE APPLICATION AND REMOVAL

The application and removal of specialty devices, such as tubes, drains, and the vacuum-assisted closure device (the VAC®) (KCI, San Antonio, TX) can cause pain or exacerbate pre-existing pain. The planned used of anesthetics and analgesia can offer considerable relief. Preventive dosing is always more effective than addressing its pain when it is already peaking.

The application and removal of the V.A.C. on a painful wound poses special challenges for healthcare providers. Specific strategies can be implemented to reduce V.A.C.-related wound pain. There are reviewed in detail in an article published in Ostomy Wound Management 2002 by this author (36). Some of the strategies include:

1. Instilling normal saline or lidocaine solution into the V.A.C. tubing for 1 hr to 1 hr prior to sponge removal,
2. Lining the wound bed with a nonadherent impregnated gauze (e.g., adaptic), white V.A.C. foam, an amorphous hydrogel or for heavily draining wounds, an alginate dressing prior to applying the gray V.A.C. sponge,
3. Preventing periwound maceration by applying a skin sealant, a hydrocolloid or thin hydrocolloid dressing to the wound margin before applying the V.A.C. drape,
4. Premedicating the patient in sufficient time for the analgesic to have its peak effect at the time of dressing change,
5. Covering exposed tissue with normal saline moistened gauze during the procedure to minimize dehydration of the tissues,
6. Using sufficient personnel to minimize the time it takes to perform the V.A.C. dressing change, and
7. Taking the person for the V.A.C. dressing change to a special procedures room or the OR for more intense pain management if the above measures do not control the person's pain.

9. OTHER STRATEGIES FOR REDUCING PROCEDURAL PAIN

Other procedures that often elicit wound pain include routine turning and repositioning and mobilization of the person with a wound. These procedures are essential, of course, for overall well-being, maintenance of function, and prevention of pneumonia and other immobility-related disorders, and should not be eliminated due to pain unless the person is terminal and a decision for palliative care has been made. Rather, every effort should be made to reduce the pain experienced by the use of pressure-relieving or reducing devices, splints, immobilizers, abdominal binders and so on, all of which can help reduce the pain experienced. Using lift sheets to lift and move bed-bound patients, instead of draw sheets (that drag) helps to prevent painful friction and shear injuries. For many patients, splinting or immobilizing the wounded area (e.g., the use of an abdominal binder for a midline incision or wound) can offer significant comfort.

10. STRATEGIES FOR MANAGING NONPROCEDURAL PAIN

Common sources of nonprocedural pain in people with chronic wounds include swelling, inflammation, and infection. Edema can be controlled by thoughtful positioning (e.g., elevation of swollen extremities as much as possible) as well as the appropriate selection of dressings, compression therapy, and devices to reduce edema. The etiology of wound inflammation or infection should be identified and treatment initiated to address the cause(s). The reader is referred to Chapter 10, in this textbook.

Changes in body image, activities of daily living, sleep patterns, and productivity are commonly seen with chronic wound patients and contribute to the psychological suffering that many chronic wound patients experience. Depression is not uncommon and warrants referral to a trained healthcare professional.

11. SPECIAL CONSIDERATIONS

Nonhealing chronic wounds or palliative wounds occur due to malignancy, host immunocompromise, or the inability of the host to muster the energy needed for wound healing (37,38). For these types of wounds, where healing is not the goal of care, pain management and prevention of infection or wound deterioration often become the key objectives. Frequently, these patients will require extraordinarily high levels of analgesia to control their pain, especially as tumors in wounds grow and increase in size and depth. Creative dressing strategies can go a long way towards alleviating the pain and suffering associated with these types of wounds. Odor control and exudates management are usually key factors to be addressed.

12. CONCLUSION

In today's healthcare environment, where measuring outcomes have become the gold standard, the interdisciplinary team can use the reduction in wound patients' pain scores as a quantitative measure of the effectiveness of the wound care in addition to "time to healing" measures. For those patients with palliative, nonhealing wounds for whom healing is not a realistic outcome, reduction in pain may be the most realistic outcome measure. No one can argue the importance of reducing pain and suffering for improving a person's health-related quality of life. From the suffering person's perspective, wound pain and its sequelae are often the most significant problems. So, remember these words of wisdom from an ancient Greek epigrapher, as you strive to provide the best in modern wound care for your patients:

> To cure—occasionally.
> To relieve—often.
> To comfort—always.

REFERENCES

1. Wall P, Melzack R, eds. Textbook of Pain. 2d ed. Edinburgh, Scotland: Churchill Livingtone, 1994.
2. Rice A. Pain, inflammation and wound healing. J Wound Care 1994; 3(5):246–249.
3. Morris DB. The Culture of Pain. Berkeley: University of California Press, 1991.
4. Price P. Quality of life.
5. Walsche C. Living with a venous ulcer: a descriptive study of patients. In: Krasner DL, Rodeheaver GT, Sibbald RG, eds. Chronic Wound Care: A Clinical Source Book for

Healthcare Professionals. Wayne, PA: HMP Communications, 2001:91–97 experiences. J Adv Nurs 1995; 22:1092–1100.

6. Hofman D, Ryan TJ, Arnold F, Cherry GW, Lindholm C, Bjellerup M, Glynn C. Pain in venous leg ulcers. J Wound Care 1997; 6(5):222–224.

7. Krasner D. Painful venous ulcers: themes and stories about living with the pain and suffering. J Wound Ostomy Continence Nurs 1998; 25(3):158–168.

8. Krasner D. Painful venous ulcers: themes and stories about their impact on quality of life. Ostomy Wound Manage 1998; 44(9):38–49.

9. Dallam L, Smyth D, Jackson B, Krinsky R, O'Dell C, Rooney J, Breen C, Amella E, Ferrara L, Freeman K. Pressure ulcer pain: assessment and quantification. J Wound Ostomy Continence Nurs 1995; 22(5):211–218.

10. Hollinworth H. Nurses' assessment and management of pain at wound dressing changes. J Wound Ostomy Continence Nurs 1995; 4(2):77–83.

11. Krasner DL, Rodeheaver GT, Sibbald RG. Advanced wound caring for a new millennium. In: Krasner DL, Rodeheaver GT, Sibbald RG, eds. Chronic Wound Care: A Clinical Source Book for Healthcare Professionals. Wayne, PA: HMP Communications, 2001:3–6.

12. Krasner DL. Carrying on despite the pain: living with painful venous ulcers: a Heideggerian hermeneutic analysis. Doctoral Dissertation. Ann Arbor, MI: UMI, 1997.

13. van Rijswijk L. Wound pain. In: McCaffery M, Pasero C. Pain Clinical Manual. St. Louis: Mosby, 1999.

14. Thomas S. Pain and wound management. Community Outlook 1989, July 11–15.

15. Callam MJ, Harper DR, Dale JJ, Ruckley CV. Chronic leg ulceration: socio-economic aspects. Scott Med J 1988; 33:358–360.

16. Phillips T, Stanton B, Provan A, Lew R. A study of the impact of leg ulcers on quality of life: financial, social and psychologic implications. J Am Acad Dermatol 1994; 31(1):49–53.

17. Pieper B. A retrospective analysis of venous ulcer healing in current and former drug users of injected drugs. J Wound Ostomy Continence Nurs 1996; 23(6):291–296.

18. Pieper B, Rossi R, Templin T. Pain associated with venous ulcers in injecting drug users. Ostomy Wound Manage 1998; 44(11):54–66.

19. Franks P, Moffatt C, Connolly M, Mosanquet N, Oldroyd M, Greenhalgh RM, McCollum CN. Community leg ulcer clinics: effect on quality of life. Phlebology 1994; 9:83–86.

20. Hamer C, Cullum N, Roe B. Patients' perceptions of chronic leg ulceration. Proceedings of the 2nd European Conference in Advances in Wound Management. London, England: Macmillin Magazines, Ltd, 1992.

21. Krasner D. Using a hydrogel, foam and dressing retention sheet. Ostomy Wound Manage 1992; 38(3):28–33.

22. Ponder R, Krasner D. Gauzes and related dressings. Ostomy Wound Manage 1993; 39(5):48–60.

23. Krasner D. Treating postoperative wounds with an amorphous hydrogel. J Wound Care 1993; 2(3).

24. Krasner D. Caring for the person experiencing chronic wound pain. In: Krasner DL, Rodeheaver GT, Sibbald RG, eds. Chronic Wound Care: A Clinical Source Book for Healthcare Professionals. Wayne, PA: HMP Communications, 2001:79–89.

25. Krasner D. The chronic wound pain experience: a conceptual model. Ostomy Wound Manage 1995; 41(3):20–27.

26. Acute Pain Management Guideline Panel. Acute pain management: operative or medical procedures and trauma. Clinical Practice Guideline #1. AHCPR Pub. No. 92–0032. Agency for Health Care Policy and Research, Public Health Service, U.S. Department of Health and Human Services, Rockville, MD, February 1991.

27. Jacox A, Carr C, Payne R, et al. Management of cancer pain. Clinical Practice Guideline No. 9. AHCPR Publication No. 94–0592. Agency for Health Care Policy and Research,

U.S. Department of Health and Human Services, Public Health Service, Rockville, MD, March 1994.

28. Bergstrom N, Bennett M, Carlson C, et al. Treatment of pressure ulcers. Clinical Practice Guideline, No. 15. AHCPR Pub. No. 95–0622. U.S. Department of Health and Human Services, Public Health Service, Agency for Health Care Policy and Research, Rockville, MD, 1994.

29. Pain at wound dressing changes. Position Document. European Wound Management Association. London: Medical Education Partnership, 2002. Downloadable from the Internet at www.tendra.com.

30. McCaffery M. Nursing Management of the Patient with Pain. Philadelphia: Lippincott, 1972.

31. Benner P. From Novice to Expert: Excellence and Power in Clinical Nursing Practice. Menlo Park, CA: Addison Wesley, 1984.

32. Herr K, Mobily P. Pain assessment in the elderly: clinical considerations. J Gerontol Nurs 1991; 17(4):12–19.

33. Herr K, Mobily P. Comparison of selected pain assessment tools for use with the elderly. Appl Nurs Res 1993; 6(1):39–46.

34. Whaley & Wong.

35. Melzack R. The McGill Pain Questionnaire: major properties and scoring methods. Pain 1975; 1:277–299.

36. Krasner D. Managing wound pain for patients with vacuum-assisted closure devices. Ostomy Wound Manage 2002; 48(5).

37. Barton P, Parslow N. Malignant wounds: holistic assessment and management. In: Krasner DL, Rodeheaver GT, Sibbald RG, eds. Chronic Wound Care: A Clinical Source Book for Healthcare Professionals. Wayne, PA: HMP Communications, 2001:699–710.

38. Rolstad BS, Nix D. Management of wound recalcitrance and deterioration. In: Krasner DL, Rodeheaver GT, Sibbald RG, eds. Chronic Wound Care: A Clinical Source Book for Healthcare Professionals. Wayne, PA: HMP Communications, 2001:731–742.

50
Nutrition and Wound Healing

Robert H. Demling
Harvard Medical School and Burn Center, Brigham and Women's Hospital, Boston, Massachusetts, U.S.A.

1. INTRODUCTION

It has long been recognized that a wound dramatically alters the normal metabolic state and that increased nutrients must be provided to the wound for healing (1–6). Hunter in 1794 (5), followed later by Cuthbertson and Moore (3) in the 1950s, identified the fact that an acute wound takes priority for nutrients in order to heal. As a result, some degree of body protein loss occurs to obtain the necessary amino acids and energy. In general, it was felt that normal healthy man could tolerate some loss of body protein or more specifically lean body mass without complication in order to heal an acute wound. Nutritional support was not emphasized (2–6).

It is now clear that optimum nutrition is essential for wound healing, especially in the increasing populations of patients who are also catabolic or who have established protein-energy malnutrition (PEM). These processes correspond with poorly healing or nonhealing wounds.

There is a known cause-and-effect relationship between malnutrition and poor healing (13–16). In addition, the once-considered adaptive host response to a wound is now considered maladaptive, especially in the severely traumatized or compromised host (Tables 1 and 2) (16–22). The injury-induced hypermetabolic, catabolic state leads to losses of body protein which greatly exceed the 10% of total body protein safety area (20–22). These increased losses of lean body mass and body protein

Table 1 Major Metabolic Abnormalities with Response to Injury "Stress Response"

Marked increase in metabolic rate
Sustained increase in body temperature
Marked increase in glucose demands and a marked stimulus to liver gluconeogenesis
Rapid skeletal muscle breakdown caused by a demand for amino acid substrate for use as a direct energy source, for gluconeogenesis, and for hepatic acute-phase protein production
Lack of ketosis, indicating that fat is not the major calorie source
Unresponsiveness of the rate of gluconeogenesis and catabolism to substrate
Decreased endogenous anabolic hormone activity

Table 2 Effect of Injury on Metabolic Demands

Illness	Increase above basal (%)
Starvation	−10–0
Elective operation	0–10
Major infection	25–50
Long bone fracture	25–50
Multiple blunt trauma	50–70
Infection, head injury	—
Thermal injury	—
10% BSA	25
20% BSA	50
40% BSA	75
50% BSA	100

result in both severe systemic complications and local wound compromise (Table 3) (18–26).

Of importance is the fact that the initial diversion of nutrients from the lean mass compartment to the wound cannot occur with losses of lean mass exceeding 15–20% of normal, as there exists an intense competition for these nutrients to restore lean body mass (Fig. 1). Therefore, the wound ceases to heal (28–30). Early provision of nutritional support and improved anabolism is necessary to correct the catabolism-induced local wound impairment, especially in populations already at risk for impaired healing (22–30) (Table 4).

It is therefore essential to reassess the early studies on wound healing where the use of host protein stores to heal a wound was considered to be adaptive as this process is only adaptive in normal healthy man.

2. NUTRITIONAL ASSESSMENT

The presence of any significant wound increases energy demands by 30–50% and protein demands by at least 50% above normal needs. These increased demands are the result of the systemic metabolic changes associated with an injury and the increased nutrient demands of the wound (33–37). The presence of a hypercatabolic state, as described in Table 1, results in a further increase in nutrient demands. The

Table 3 Complications Relative to Loss of Lean Body Mass[a]

Lean body mass (% loss of total)	Complications (Related to lost lean mass)	Associated mortality (%)
10	Impaired immunity, increased infection	10
20	Decreased healing, weakness, infection	30
30	Too weak to sit, pressure sores, pneumonia, no healing	50
40	Death, usually from pneumonia	100

[a] Loss relative to normal or ideal lean body mass.

PRIORITY FOR PROTEIN INTAKE
VS.
%LOSS OF LEAN TISSUE

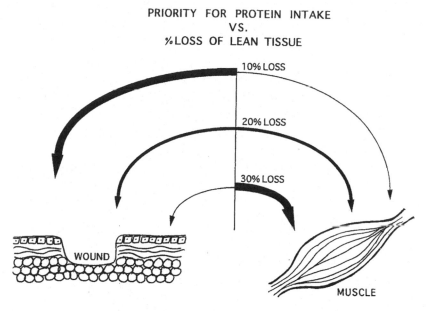

Figure 1 As lean mass decreased, more consumed protein is used to restore LBM, with less being available to the wound. Wound healing rate decreases until lean mass is restored. With a loss of lean mass exceeding 20% of total, spontaneous wounds can develop due to the thinning of skin from lost collagen.

management of PEM also requires at least a 50% increase in calories and doubling of protein intake to restore lost lean mass.

Assessment tools include a variety of standard nutritional formulas and also indirect calorimetry which can be readily performed by a nutritionist. Of course, anyone managing wounds should also be able to make these assessments (33–38).

Assessment, of the degree of PEM, if present, is outlined in Table 5. A prealbumin level is considered to be the most sensitive biochemical indication (33–38).

3. GENERAL NUTRITIONAL SUPPORT

Optimum nutrition should be initiated immediately, in the presence of any hypercatabolic state, e.g., trauma or infection, and also in an already compromised host with pre-existing malnutrition or with chronic illness, especially in the frail elderly.

The standard caloric and protein intake guidelines are presented in Table 6. The guidelines are based on increases over and above the recommended daily allowance (RDA), used for the normal healthy population. It is important to recognize

Table 4 Conditions Associated with Development of Protein-Energy Malnutrition and Impaired Healing

Catabolic illness: the stress response e.g., trauma, surgery, wounds, infection, corticosteroids
Involuntary weight loss exceeding 10% of ideal body weight
Chronic illnesses: e.g., diabetes, cancer, mental impairment, arthritis, renal failure

Table 5 Markers of Malnutrition

Index	Mild	Moderate	Severe
% ideal body weight	80–90	70–80	≤ 70
% weight loss	5–15	15–25	≥ 25
Albumin (g/dL)	2.6–3.5	2.1–2.7	≤ 2.1
Prealbumin (mg/dL)	10–15	5–10	≤ 5

that inadequate nutrition-induced impaired healing can be readily corrected with refeeding (15,39–41). The ideal distribution of calories is shown in Table 7 (31,32,40).

Protein intake corresponds best with wound healing. An intake of 1.5 g/kg/day appears to be the ideal value (40–44). Proteins with increased concentrations of essential and conditionally essential amino acids have a higher biologic value (Table 8) (42–44).

Clearly, there are other systemic reasons for impaired healing besides nutrition but its correction and maintenance is likely the most correctable (30–32).

4. SPECIFIC NUTRIENT NEEDS

The wound, in addition to requiring energy and protein, has specific nutrient needs both macro- and micronutrient. The micronutrients used by the wound are especially important as added provision is often needed to avoid a deficiency state. These specific nutrients will be discussed (45–50).

4.1. Arginine and Glutamine

Arginine and glutamine are nitrogen-rich amino acids, which are important in wound healing. Both are used in a variety of aspects of healing as described in Tables 9 and 10. In addition, the levels of both these amino acids rapidly decrease with injury (45–47). Supplementation has been recommended by many experts although a deficiency-induced impairment in wound healing has not been well documented. Both arginine and glutamine are considered to be conditionally essential amino acids as endogenous production does not appear to be sufficient to keep up with demands during the "stress response" (45–50).

4.2. Carbohydrates and Lactate

Carbohydrates are utilized in a number of aspects of healing besides being used as energy. Matrix is composed of proteoglycans and glycosaminoglycans, which are

Table 6 Daily Nutritional Requirements

Condition	Calories (cal/kg)	Protein (g/kg)
Normal	25–30	0.6
Wound alone	30–35	1.3
Hypercatabolic	35–40	1.5–2.0
PEM and wound	35–40	1.5

Table 7 Caloric Mix

Macronutrient	% calories
Carbohydrate (complex form)	55–60%
Fat (Polyunsaturated)	25%
Protein (High biologic value)	20%

Table 8 Protein

Essential macronutrient for all healing phases
Deficiency leads to impairment in all healing phases
Certain amino acids are more important, namely cysteines, the essential and conditionally essential amino acids, glutamine and arginine
Recommended dose is 1.5 g/kg/day for injured or compromised man, especially with a significant wound

Table 9 Arginine

Promotes wound healing
Precursor for proline in collagen
Precursor for nitric oxide
Increases hydroxyproline production
Stimulates release of anabolic hormones, insulin, and human growth hormone and insulin-like growth factor
Local immune stimulant of lymphocytes
Considered a conditionally essential amino acid
Large doses recommended 15–25 g/day

Table 10 Glutamine

Direct fuel for epithelial cells, fibroblasts, and macrophages
Lymphocyte fuel
Improves neutrophils killing
Anticatabolic agent, preserving lean mass
Stimulates release of growth hormone
Potent antioxidant in form of glutathione
Considered a conditionally essential amino acid
Large doses recommended 10–30 g/day in divided doses, b.i.d. to t.i.d.

Table 11 Wound Lactate

Produced by wound cells especially macrophages
Required for macrophage release of angiogenesis factors
Stimulates collagen synthesis by fibroblasts
Energy source

made from polysaccharide chains linked to protein. Glucose is also used to glycosy-late hydroxyproline (51,52).

Lactate is a metabolic byproduct of glucose. This 2-carbon compound appears to have many very important wound healing effects (Table 11).

The increase in lactate which is produced by all wound cells activates the genetic expression of many key healing pathways (53,54).

4.3 Fatty Acids

The essential omega-6 fatty acids, linoleic and linolenic acid, are required for both cell membrane formation and prostaglandin production. A deficiency is difficult to produce unless using a fat-free diet. Recent data would also indicate that the replacing of these fatty acids, with omega-3 fatty acids, can impair healing (55).

4.4. Vitamin C (Ascorbic Acid)

The water-soluble ascorbic acid has long been known to be essential for healing, and a severe deficiency state leads to symptoms of scurvy (56).

Description of the markedly abnormal wound healing in sailors suffering from scurvy is evident in the writings of physicians and explorers beginning in the 16th century.

A number of investigators have reported ascorbic acid to be essential for over-all collagen synthesis (57–59). A deficiency leads to a decrease in total collagen. Others have clearly shown that the hydroxylation of proline and lysine is dependent on molecular oxygen, ascorbic acid, and $Fe++$. Ascorbic acid appears to activate prolyl and lysyl hydroxylase. This process is required to stabilize the triple helix structure of collagen. A vitamin C deficiency state impairs immune function. Vitamin C is also an important intracellular antioxidant (Table 12) (15).

The recommended daily allowance in normal man to maintain body vitamin C levels is 30–60 mg/day. However, after injury, vitamin C levels rapidly decrease. The process is felt to be due to increased usage in the injured area. An intake of 2 g/day

Table 12 Vitamin C—Ascorbic Acid

Collagen synthesis
Hydroxylation of proline and lysine
Neutrophils antibacterial activity
Complement activation
Water-soluble intracellular antioxidant
An essential micronutrient
Increased losses after injury
Recommended dose with wounds—200 mg/day

Table 13 Vitamin A

Promotes the early inflammatory reaction to wounding
Increases angiogenesis
Increases hydroxyproline and collagen accumulation
Involved in cell differentiation, especially epithelial keratinization
Necessary for cell-mediated and humoral immune defenses
An essential micronutrient
Increased losses of vitamin A seen with injury
Recommended daily dose with injury or malnutrition is 10,000–25,000 IU

was necessary to maintain plasma levels after severe burns. However, for a moderate wound, an intake of 200 mg/day is recommended (57–60).

4.5. Vitamin A

The fat-soluble vitamin A is also recognized as an essential prohealing agent. Like all vitamins, it has multiple actions. The most important appears to be the promotion of the key early inflammatory reaction to wounding. In fact, vitamin A supplementation, systemically or topically, has been shown to reverse the anti-inflammatory impairment of healing by corticosteroids (61–64).

Vitamin A is also involved in angiogenesis and cell differentiation, especially keratinocytes. Supplemental vitamin A has also been reported to increase wound collagen content. One theory, as to the mechanism of action, is the influence on cellular phenotypes by directly affecting gene expression. Vitamin A also affects cell surface glycoproteins involved in cell adherence, intracellular communication, and interaction with growth factors (Table 13).

Vitamin A is also important for immune function with a deficiency leading to infection. Both cell-mediated immunity and humoral defense mechanisms depend on vitamin A. Like vitamin C, vitamin A levels decrease after injury. Increased metabolism and increased urinary losses are known to occur (65,66).

Since large amounts of vitamin A are stored in the liver, rapid depletion is not likely in healthy man. However, malnourished patients are likely already deficient and injured patients have increased losses. Replacement therapy in these groups is indicated at a daily dose of 10,000–25,000 IU (65,66).

4.6. Vitamin E

There is currently no evidence that vitamin E has a specific role in normal wound healing (67). There is also not a recognized deficiency state of this fat-soluble vitamin

Table 14 Zinc

An essential component of DNA, RNA polymerase, metalloproteinase activity
Involved with DNA synthesis, protein synthesis, mitosis, cell proliferation
Cell membrane stability by inhibition of lipid peroxidation
Host defenses
An essential micronutrient
Increased losses after injury in urine
Dose for wounds 5–15 mg/day although higher doses are usually used

with injury. Its potent antioxidant values make this compound systemically highly important. In addition, vitamin E affects a variety of host defenses and is often supplemented in critical illness for these effects but not for wound healing. Excess vitamin E appears to retard scar formation.

4.7. Microminerals: Zinc, Copper, Iron

4.7.1. Zinc

Although zinc has been considered an essential micromineral for centuries, its specific importance, especially in wound healing, has only been recognized in the last 50 years. If zinc levels are low, healing is slowed and with replacement healing is restored.

Zinc has many metabolic roles. Zinc is a critical cofactor for many metalloenzymes, including DNA and RNA polymerase, protein synthesis, and matrix metalloproteinase activity. Zinc stimulates cell proliferation, thereby stabilizing cell membranes. Zinc has an important role in immune function recognized by the fact that a deficiency leads to increased infection. Its specific role is not yet clear (68–72).

There is an increased loss of zinc in the urine after injury. As with other micronutrients, the proper replacement therapy is undefined. The recommended dose for a stable wound patient is 3–4 mg/day and for the catabolic patient 5–6 mg/day. As zinc is quite insoluble and difficult to absorb, a standard replacement is in the form of zinc sulfate 220 mg/b.i.d. (Table 14) (73,74).

4.7.2. Copper

Copper is also a key micromineral involved in collagen cross-linking thru hydroxylation of proline and hydroxyproline. Copper is essential for erythropoesis and for the action of the antioxidant superoxide dismitase. The recommended intake is 1–1.5 mg/day.

4.7.3. Iron

Iron, especially $Fe++$, is required for hydroxylation of lysine and proline a fundamental step in collagen synthesis. An iron deficiency also leads to anemia and impaired leukocyte killing both factors which could affect healing (21,74). Standard iron replacement is used to prevent or correct a deficiency.

5. USE OF ANABOLIC AGENTS

Increasing anabolic activity has been demonstrated to decrease the catabolic response to injury, thereby preserving lean body mass which improves all aspects of wound healing. These agents can be seen as providing added benefit to nutritional support. Anabolic hormones also directly increase wound healing most notably human growth hormone (HGH), insulin-like growth factors (IGF-1), and the synthetic testosterone analogs.

5.1. Human Growth Hormone (HGH)

Human growth hormone increases total body protein synthesis (75–78). Unfortunately, HGH levels decrease with severe injury.

A large number of studies have demonstrated the wound healing properties of HGH as well as its anticatabolic properties. Skin is a target tissue for HGH both directly by its growth factor effect on human fibroblasts and indirectly through increasing circulating IGF-1, a known wound growth factor (75–78).

Side effects include hyperglycemia and an overall stimulation of inflammation and metabolic rate (79,80). Its anti-insulin properties and the need to give HGH parenterally limit its use in the wound population.

5.2. Insulin-Like Growth Factor (IGF-1)

Insulin-like growth factor is a known wound growth factor acting on all phases of healing. A number of clinical trials have demonstrated its anabolic properties. The IGF-1 levels also decrease in severely injured or infected patients (81–83). Hypoglycemia is a complication of IGF-1 making glucose monitoring essential. The IGF-1 is usually provided parenterally. However, there is an increasing interest in topical use, which would limit systemic complications (83).

5.3. Anabolic Steroid (Oxandrolone)

Anabolic steroids have been recognized to be potent anabolic agents for decades (84). Currently, the safest such agent and the only steroid FDA approved to treat weight loss and catabolism is oxandrolone (85,87). This anabolic steroid is given orally, is excreted by the kidney, and has no effects on metabolism other than protein synthesis.

Oxandrolone acts on androgenic receptors in lean mass, especially on the skin fibroblast. A number of studies have demonstrated its ability to preserve lean mass after injury thereby improving local healing. In addition, several recent studies have demonstrated direct wound healing properties. One mechanism is the increase in the messenger RNA for collagen synthesis (87,88). However, in other studies, all aspects of healing appear to be increased. Like all other anabolic agents, oxandrolone is to be used only when optimum nutrition has been achieved.

REFERENCES

1. Cuthbertson D. Inter-relationships of metabolic changes consequent to injury. Br Med Bull 1954; 10:33–37.
2. Moore FD. Getting well. The biology of surgical convalescence. Am N Y Sci 1958; 73:387–390.
3. Hunter J. Treatise on the blood, inflammation and gunshot wounds. London Nicol 1923: 17–94.
4. Moore FD, Brennan M. Surgical injury, body composition, protein metabolism and neuro-endocrinology. In: Ballinger W, Collins J, eds. Manual of Surgical Nutrition. Philadelphia: Saunders W, 1975:169–202.
5. Kobak M. Benditt E, Wissler B, et al. The relationship of protein deficiency to experimental wound healing. Surg Gynecol Obstet 1947; 85:751–756.
6. Levinson S, Parani C, Braasch J. The effect of thermal burns on wound healing. Surg Gynec Obstet 1954; 99:77–82.
7. Haines E, Briggs H, Shea R, et al. Effect of complete and partial starvation on the rate of fibroplasias in the healing wound. Arch Surg 1933; 27:846–858.

8. Thompson W, Randin I, Frank I. Effect of hypoproteinemia on wound disruption. Arch Surg 1938; 36:500–518.
9. Wallace JI, Schwartz RS, LaCroix AZ, Uhlmann RF, Pearlman RA. Involuntary weight loss in older outpatients: incidences and clinical significance. J Am Geriatr Soc 1995; 43:329–337.
10. McCamsh M. Malnutrition and nutrition support interventions: costs, benefits, outcomes. Nutrition 1993; 4:556–557.
11. Lipschitz D. Malnutrition in the elderly. Semin Dermatol 1991; 10:273–281.
12. EK A, Unosson M, Larsson J, et al. The development and healing of pressure sores related to the nutritional slate. Clin Nutr 1991; 10:245–250.
13. Warren M, Morgan D. Malnutrition in surgical patients: an unrecognized problem. Lancet 1977; 1:689–692.
14. Coats K, Morgan S, Bartolucci A. Hospital associated malnutrition: a re-evaluation 12 years later.
15. Haydock D, Hill G. Impaired wound healing in surgical patients with varying degrees of malnutrition. J Parenter Enteral Nutr 1986; 10:550–554.
16. Pinchcofsky-Devin G, Kaminski M. Correlation of pressure sores and nutritional status. J Am Geriatr Soc 1986; 39:435–440.
17. Demling R. Endocrine changes with illness: in current surgical therapy. J Cameron Ed Mosby 1998; 3:113–114.
18. Bessy J. Stress response to injury: endocrinologic and metabolic current practice of surgery. L Greenfield Ed Churchill 1995; 1–12.
19. Wolfe R. Relation of metabolic studies to clinical nutrition: the example of burn injury. Am J Clin Nutr 1996; 64:800–808.
20. Wolfe R. An integrated analysis of glucose, fat and protein metabolism in severely traumatized patients. Ann Surg 1989; 209:63–72.
21. Demling R. Anticatabolic and anabolic strategies in critical illness: a review of current treatment modalities. Shock 1998; 10:155–160.
22. Bissey PQ. Metabolic response to critical illness. In: Wilmore D, ed. Pre- and Post Operative Care of the Surgical Patient. Vol. 1. Critical Care. New York: Scientific American, 1996:11.
23. Bergstrom N. Lack of nutrition: in AHCPR preventive guidelines. Decubitus 1993; 6: 4–6.
24. Weingarten M. Obstacles to wound healing. Wounds 1993; 5:238–244.
25. Shizgal H. Nutritional assessment and skeletal muscle function. Am J Clin Nutr 1986; 44:761–771.
26. Levenson S, Serfter E. Dynutrition, wound healing and resistance to infection. Clin Plast Surg 1977; 4:375–385.
27. Kotler D, Tierney AR, Wang J, Pierson RN Jr. Magnitude of cell body mass depletion and timing of death from wasting in AIDS. Am J Clin Nutr 1989; 40:444–447.
28. Windsor J, Hill GL. Weight loss with physiologic impairment—a basic indication of surgical risk. Ann Surg 1988; 207:290–296.
29. Wallace JL, Schwartz RS. Involuntary weight loss in elderly outpatients: recognition, etiologies and treatment. Clin Geriatr Med 1997; 113:717–735.
30. Torun B, Cherv F. Protein-energy malnutrition. In: Shels M, ed. Modern Nutrition in Health and Disease. Philadelphia, PA: Lea and Felguan, 1994:950.
31. DeBiasse M, Wilmore D. What is Optimum Nutritional Support? in New Horizons Vol 53. Philadelphia: Williams Wilkins, 1994:122–135.
32. Lipschitz D. Approaches to the nutritional support of the older patient. Clin Geriatr Med 1995; 11:715–730.
33. American Dietetic Association. Nutrition assessment in the adult. In: Manual of Clinical Dietetics. Chicago ILL: The American Dietetic Association, 1996:3.
34. Klipstein-Grobusch K, Reilly J. Energy intake and expenditure in elderly patients admitted to the hospital with acute illness. Br J Nutr 1995; 73:323–324.

35. Rodriguez D. Nutrition in patients with severe burns: state of the art. J Burn Care Rehab 1996; 17:62–70.
36. Barrocas A. Nutritional assessment. Practical approaches. Clin Geriatr Med 1995; 11:675–683.
37. Evans W, Campbell D. Nutrition, exercise and healthy aging. J Am Diet Assoc 1997; 97:632 638.
38. Lukaski H. Methods for the assessment of human body composition. Am J Clin Nutr 1987; 46:163–175.
39. Haydock D, Hill G. Improved wound healing response to surgical patients receiving intravenous nutrition. Brit J Surg 1987; 74:320–323.
40. Demling RH, Stasik L, Zagoren AJ. Protein-energy malnutrition and wounds: nutritional intervention. Treatment of Chronic Wounds Number 10. Hauppauge, NY: Curative Health Services, 2000.
41. Bergstrom N, Bennett MA, Carlson CE, et al. Treatment of pressure ulcers. Clinical Practice Guideline, No. 15. AHCPR Publication No. 95-0652. Rockville, MD: Agency for Health Care Policy and Research, December, 1994.
42. Demling R, DeSanti L. Increased protein intake during the recovery phase after severe burns increases body weight gain and muscle function. J Burn Care Rehab 1998; 17:151–168.
43. Breslow R, Hallfrisch J. The importance of dietary protein in healing pressure ulcers. J Am Geriatr Soc 1993; 41:357–362.
44. Volpi E, Ferrando A, Yeckel W, et al. Exogenous amino acids stimulate net muscle protein synthesis in the elderly. J Clin Invest 1998; 101:2000–2007.
45. Barbel A, Lazarou S, Efron B, et al. Arginine enhances wound healing and lymphocyte immune responses in humans. Surgery 1990; 108:331–337.
46. Furst P, Abers S, Stehle P. Evidence for nutritional need for glutamine in catabolic patients. Kidney Int 1989; 36:287–291.
47. Caldwell M. Local glutamine metabolism in wounds and inflammation. Metabolism 1989; 38:34–39.
48. Roth E, Karner J, Collenschlager G. Glutamine: an anabolic effector. JPEN 1990; 14:130–136.
49. Barbol A. Arginine: biochemistry, physiology and therapeutic implications. JPEN 1986; 10:227–237.
50. Visek W. Arginine and disease states. J Nutr 1985:532–541.
51. Linker A. Structure of heparin sulfate oligosaccharides and their degradation by exo-enzymes. J Biochem 1979; 183:711–720.
52. Weitzhander M, Bernfield M. In: Cohen C, ed. Proteoglycan Glycoconjungates in Wound Healing: Biochemical and Clinical Aspects. Philadelphia: W. B. Saunders, 1992:195.
53. Jensen J, Hunt TK. Effect of lactate, pyruvate and pH on secretion of angiogenesis and mitogenesis factors by macrophages. Lab Invest 1986; 54:574–578.
54. Hunt TK, Hussain Z. In: Cohen C, ed. Wound Microenvironment in Wound Healing: Biochemical and Chemical Aspects. Philadelphia: W. B. Saunders, 1992:274.
55. Halsey T, O'Neill J, Nebleth W. Experimental wound healing in essential fatty acid deficiency. J Pediatr Surg 1980; 15:505–508.
56. Lanman T. Vitamin C deficiency and wound healing. Ann Surg 1937; 165:616–622.
57. Schorah C. Total vitamin C and dehydroascorbic acid concentration in plasma of critically ill patients. Am J Clin Nutr 1996; 63:760–765.
58. Hornig D, et al. Ascorbic acid. In: Modern Nutrition in Health and Disease. Philadelphia: Lea and Febiger, 1988:417.
59. Gross R. The effect of ascorbate on wound healing. Int Opthalmol Clin 2000; 40:51–57.
60. Lund C, Levenson S, Green R. Ascorbic acid, thiamine, riboflavin and nicotinic acid in relation to acute burns in man. Arch Surg 1947; 55:557–583.

61. Erlich H. Effect of beta carotene, vitamin A and glucocarotenoids on collagen synthesis in wounds. Proc Soc Exp Biol Med 1971; 137:936–938.
62. Kinsky N. Antioxidant functions of carotenoids. Free Rad Biol Med 1989; 7:617–635.
63. Weinzwieg J, Weinzweig B, Levenson S. Supplemental vitamin A prevents the tumor induced defect in wound healing. Ann Surg 1990; 211:269–276.
64. Olson J. Vitamin A, retinoids and carotinoids. In: Shils M, Young V, eds. Modern Nutrition in Health and Disease. Philadelphia: Lea and Febiger, 1988:328.
65. Durin M, Tannock I. Influence of vitamin A on immunologic response. Immunology 1972; 23:283–287.
66. Cohen B, Gell G, Cullen P. Reversal of postoperative immunosuppression in man by vitamin A. Surg Gynec Obstet 1979; 179:658–662.
67. Erhlich P, Tarver H, Hunt TK. Inhibiting effects of vitamin E on collagen synthesis and wound repair. Ann Surg 1972; 175:235–240.
68. Demling R. Micronutrients in critical illness. Crit Care Clin 1995; 11:651–670.
69. Gottschlich M. Vitamins supplementation in the patient with burns. J Burn Care and Rehabil 1996; 12:273–280.
70. Chesters J: Biochemistry of Zinc in Cell Division and Tissue Growth in Zinc in Human Biology. International Life Science Institute London, 1989:109–118.
71. Prasad A. Zinc: an overview. Nutrition 1995; 11:93–100.
72. Berger M, et al. Copper, zinc, and selenium balances and status after major trauma. J Trauma 1996; 40:103–109.
73. Berger M, Cavadine C, Cheolero R, et al. Influence of large intakes of trace elements on recovery after major burns. Nutrition 1994; 10:327–334.
74. Demling R, De Santi L. Use of anticatabolic agents for burns. Curr Opin Crit Care 1996; 2:482–491.
75. Ziegler T, Wilmore D. Strategies for attenuating protein-catabolic responses in the critically ill. Am Rev Med 1994; 45:459–463.
76. Sherman S, Demling R, et al. Growth hormone enhances re-epithelialization of human split thickness skin graft donor sites. Surg Forum 1989; 40:37.
77. McManson J, Smith R, Wilmore D. Growth hormone stimulation protein synthesis during hypocaloric parenteral nutrition. Ann Surg 1988; 208:136–149.
78. Gatzen C, Scheltinga MR, Kimbrough TDD, Jacobs DO, Wilmore DW. Growth hormone attenuates the abnormal distribution of body water in critically ill surgical patients. Surgery 1992; 112:181.
79. MacGorman L, Rizza R, Gerich P. Physiologic concentration of growth hormone exerts insulin like and insulin antagonistic effect on both hepatic and extrahepatic tissues in man. J Clin Endocrin Metab 1981; 53:556–559.
80. Kappel M, Hansen M, Diamant M, Pedersen B. In vitro effects of human growth hormone on the proliferative responses and cytokine production of blood mononuclear cells. Horm Metab Res 1994; 26:612–614.
81. Lieberman S, Butterfield G, Harrison D, Hoffman A. Anabolic effects of insulin like growth factor-1 in cachectic patients with acquired immunodeficiency syndrome. J Clin Endocrin Metab 1999; 78:404–410.
82. Bondy C, Underwood L, Clemmons D. Clinical uses of insulin like growth factor-1. Ann Internal Med 1994; 120:593–601.
83. Abribat T, Brazeau P, Davingnon L, Gurrel P. Insulin like growth factor-1 blood levels in severely burned patients: effect of time post injury, age of patient and burn severity. Clin Endocrin 1993 1993; 39:583–589.
84. Tennenbaum R, Shkear G. Effect of anabolic steroid on wound healing. Oral Surg 1970; 30:834–835.
85. Karim A, Ranney E, Zagarella BA, et al. Oxandrolone disposition and metabolism in man. Clin Pharmacol Ther 1973; 14:862–866.
86. Fox M, Minot A. Oxandrolone, a potent anabolic steroid. J Clin Endocrinol 1962; 22:921–926.

87. Demling R, Orgill D. The anticatabolic and wound healing effects of the testosterone analog, oxandrolone after severe burn injury. J Crit Care 2000; 15:12–18.
88. Demling R, DeSanti L. Oxandrolone, an anabolic steroid significantly increases the rate of weight gain in the recovery phase after burn injury. J Trauma 1997; 43:47–50.
89. Demling R. Oxandrolone, an anabolic steroid enhances the healing of a cutaneous wound in the rat. Wound Rep Regen 2000; 8:97.
90. Erlich P. Thr influence of the anabolic agent oxandrolone upon the experssion of procollagen types I and II in RNA in human fibroblasts cultured on collagen or plastic. Wounds 2001; 13:66–70.

51
Physical Agents in Wound Repair

Joseph McCulloch
School of Allied Health Professions, Louisiana State University Health Sciences Center, Shreveport, Louisiana, U.S.A.

1. INTRODUCTION

Physical agents, also termed therapeutic modalities, have been a part of the medical armamentarium for centuries. In writings of Hippocrates in 410 BC, and in earlier works of the Babylonians, note is made of the use of potions and bandages (1). Many of these treatments employed heat as a therapeutic agent.

Many healthcare providers prescribe and use modalities such as heat and cold in routine practice. Physical therapists have extensive education in the physics and therapeutic application of a broad array of physical agents. In recent years, knowledge gained from the use of physical agents in treatment of musculoskeletal disorders has lead to an increased interest in their use facilitating wound repair.

One of the most researched and supported agents for the acceleration of repair is electrical stimulation. The body of knowledge, of this agent alone, warrants separate discussion elsewhere in this text. We will focus here on other forms of electromagnetic, acoustical, and physical energy.

2. ELECTROMAGNETIC RADIATION

Diathermy, infrared, ultraviolet, and low power LASERs are physical agents that emit energy with wavelengths and frequencies that are termed electromagnetic radiation (2). These are demonstrated in a range termed the electromagnetic spectrum (Table 1).

Radiation is the process by which energy is propagated through space or matter. In electromagnetic radiation, rays travel at the speed of light and exhibit both magnetic and electrical properties. One of the most common forms of radiant energy is sunlight. Radiant energy from the sun travels through space at around 300 million m/sec. Within the sun's rays, we receive two therapeutic forms of energy, infrared and ultraviolet, both of which have utility in wound care.

2.1. Infrared

Infrared is a form of radiant energy that produces heat. This can occur by heating or cooling an object to a temperature different than the surrounding environment.

Table 1 Portion of Electromagnetic Spectrum That Includes
Physical Agents Frequently Used in Wound Healing

Source	Wavelength in Angstroms[a]
Ultraviolet	
UVC	2000–2900 Å
UVB	2900–3200 Å
UVA	3200–4000 Å
Visible spectrum	Violet to red lies between the ultraviolet and infrared sources
Infrared	
Nonluminous	14,430 Å
Luminous	28,860 Å
Hot whirlpool (99 F)	93,097 Å

[a] Angstrom unit (Å)—An internationally adopted unit of length equal
to 10^{-10} m or 0.1 nm.
Source: Modified from Ref. 2.

For this reason, both heat and cold are considered to be infrared modalities. From
a physical therapy perspective, this would include physical agents such as cold
packs, whirlpools, paraffin baths, hot packs, and luminous and nonluminous forms
of infrared. However, most of these agents are not used in wound care.

In the early to mid-1900s, infrared lamps were used to produce vasodilation
and thereby attempt to aid in tissue perfusion. While there may have been some
physiological benefit from this, more often than not, what occurred was wound
desiccation and resultant eschar formation. At the time, this was thought to be desirable as it minimized wound exudation. As more evidence supporting moist wound
healing emerged, infrared use began to wane.

Conductive moist heat, such as occurs from hot packs, has been demonstrated
to facilitate healing by increasing tissue saturation with oxygen (3). The problem with
heat from a hot pack however is the potential for a burn secondary to the 170 F heat
of the pack. Even though the pack is wrapped in insulation prior to being placed on
the patient, persons with poor circulation or insensitivity could easily sustain a burn.

2.2. Ultraviolet

The second therapeutic form of radiation supplied by the sun is ultraviolet (UV).
Long before there was an understanding of the electromagnetic energy of the sun,
sun baths were prescribed as a therapy for patients. Hippocrates (460–370 B.C.)
and Galen (131–201 A.D.) routinely directed their patients to lie in the sun (11).
Developments in the last century resulted in an ability for UV to be generated by
artificial sources. It has been used to treat a variety of skin conditions, most notably
psoriasis, acne vulgaris, and ectopic dermatitis (12).

The effectiveness of UV at producing biological changes in tissues is wavelength dependent. By example, UVA radiation from the sun or from UV lamps with
a wavelength between 315 and 400 nm results in pigmentation changes such as mild
erythema or tanning. UVB from the sun or from lamps with a wavelength between
280 and 315 nm may result in marked erythema or blistering. Neither of these forms
of UV have much utility in wound care. Instead, UVC radiation with wavelengths

between 200 and 280 nm is more beneficial. Radiation from the sun at this wavelength gets absorbed in the ozone layer and therefore does not reach the earth. We therefore must rely on therapeutic generators to produce UVC (Fig. 1).

While UVC radiation can produce some erythema in the skin, it is mainly known for its bactericidal properties (13). Several theories on how UVC works have been suggested. Gates (14) studied the effects of UVC on *Escherichia coli* and noted that the bacteria were maximally effected at a wavelength of 260 nm. He concluded that the absorption of radiation by the nucleic acids was lethal to the bacteria. Further work by Kellner (15) resulted in a proposed model relating a series of events that followed radiation. He felt that irradiation resulted in inhibition of bacterial nuclear function and that DNA synthesis ceased to occur. Other studies have implicated interruption of DNA synthesis as a means of action, but negative effects of UVC on RNA have also been suggested (16).

Despite the lack of consensus on the exact mechanism of action, recent studies have provided further evidence of the effectiveness of the bactericidal action of UVC (17). Conner-Kerr et al. (18,19) provided evidence that UVC may be effective against several commonly found wound pathogens. They observed that when MRSA was exposed to a 5-sec irradiation with UVC, there was a 99.9% kill rate. When the treatment time was increased to 45 sec, there was a 100% kill rate. Similar results were found with treatment of *Enterococcus faecalis*. These results were all in vitro however and clinical application, at these treatment levels, has not been as effective.

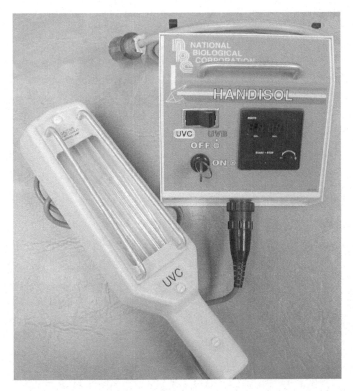

Figure 1 The Dermawand UVC unit. (Courtesy of National Biological Corporation, Twinsburg, OH.)

A recent study by Thai et al. (20) found that in order to obtain the same type of in vivo results with UVC as seen in Conner-Kerr's earlier in vitro work, treatment time needed to be lengthened. While the exact clinical treatment time and length necessary to obtain a 100% kill rate in human chronic wounds is still not known, the authors found that a single 180-sec dose of UVC could eliminate MRSA from lightly colonized chronic wounds. Wounds that were heavily colonized required additional treatments over the course of a month.

If UVC is to be considered as a treatment option, great care must be taken in application to avoid inadvertent damage to viable tissue (21). UVC dosage should be determined at each session based on wound appearance and response to the previous treatment. Generally, when a person is first begun on UV therapy, exposure time should be about 15 sec at a distance of 2.5 cm. This is based on an individual having rather fair skin. Individuals with greater pigmentation can tolerate longer initial treatment times. Periwound tissue or areas in the wound that do not require radiation should be shielded with a layer of paper towel or by application of petroleum jelly.

3. ULTRASOUND

Ultrasound (US) is another physical agent that had its initial start in the treatment of soft tissue injuries of the musculoskeletal system. Knowledge gained in this area has made US a natural modality for use in wound management since much of the mode of action deals with its proinflammatory effects. The term ultrasound refers to high frequency ($f > 20,000$ cycles per sec) mechanical vibrations produced when electrical energy is converted to sound waves. The term "ultra" implies that the sound waves are beyond the range of human hearing.

Therapeutic US (Fig. 2) has both thermal and nonthermal properties. Most of the physiological changes, that have an effect on wound healing, can be attributed to the nonthermal effects. At thermal intensities ($1-1.5 \, W/cm^2$) US is effective in providing deep heat through tissues of high water content. In addition, US at

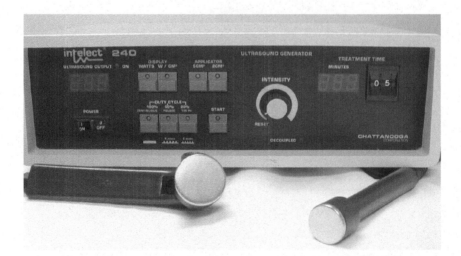

Figure 2 Clinical Ultrasound unit with two sound heads. The smaller sound head is useful in treating smaller surface areas. (Courtesy of Intelect 240®, Chattanooga Group, A Division of Encore Medical, LP, Hixson, TN.)

thermal levels has been used to increase metabolism and enzyme activity to a limited degree (22).

The nonthermal effects of US are primarily the result of a process termed acoustic streaming which produces an enhanced flow of fluid in response to ultrasonic forces. The fluid movements produced are of microscopic proportions and are termed microstreaming. Microstreaming causes high-velocity fluid movement gradients to occur next to cell membranes. This in turn is thought to result in the cell membranes becoming physically altered thereby changing cell permeability and ion transport. One example of this is the demonstrated effect of US on collagen-secreting fibroblasts. Therapeutic levels of US have been demonstrated to temporarily increase the uptake of calcium ions by the fibroblasts (23,24).

Nonthermal US involves either the delivery of continuous mode US at low intensities ($< 0.3 \, W/cm^2$) or by pulsing the US at about $1 \, W/cm^2$. The pulsing is typically set at 2 ms on/8 ms off. This is referred to as a 20% duty cycle.

Being an acoustic and not an electromagnetic energy, US responds differently than other physical agents. Unlike electromagnetic energy that travels well through a vacuum, US energy relies on molecular collision for effective transmission (25). For this reason, some type of coupling medium such as an amorphous hydrogel or water must be used. In shallow wounds, it is often possible to deliver US through a sterile sheet hydrogel dressing. A coupling medium must still be placed on the hydrogel sheet to minimize friction between the sound head and the dressing.

Ultrasound effectiveness is also frequency dependent. The higher the frequency of US emitted, the less the sound will diverge. In the body, the lower the frequency, the greater the penetration of the sound. Conversely, at higher frequencies, sound waves are more superficially absorbed.

While there is extensive basic science research on US, relatively little has been done in the clinical area. Most of the clinical trials in wound healing have focused on treatment of venous and pressure ulcers.

Dyson et al. (26) studied 25 patients divided into two groups. One group ($n = 13$) received 3 MHz pulsed-mode (20% duty cycle) US applied to the periwound skin for 5–10 min at $1.0 \, W/cm^2$. The other group ($n = 12$) served as a control and received only sham US treatment. After 4 weeks of treatment, three times per week, wound size was measured and compared to baseline measurements. Those receiving the active US were at $66.4\% \pm 8.8\%$ of baseline size while the control group wounds were at $91.6\% \pm 8.9\%$ of baseline. While there was a statistically significant difference in the results ($p < 0.05$), there was no analysis to indicate if the groups were statistically similar in starting size.

Roche and West (27) conducted a similar study on 26 patients with venous ulcers. There were two groups of equal size. One group received standard care (control) for 8 weeks while the other received standard care plus 3 MHz US (treatment). Those receiving US healed at a statistically significant faster rate ($p < 0.001$) than the control subjects. It is of note that even though subjects were randomized to group, the treatment group ended up with a greater proportion of the larger wounds. Given that small wounds generally heal faster than larger ones, the findings of this study deserve attention.

In a larger study involving 108 patients, Callum et al. (28) evaluated the effect of US on the healing of chronic ulcers (87% venous). Treatment subjects ($n = 52$) received standard care and pulsed US while the control group ($n = 56$) received only standard care. The US given was 1 MHz at an intensity of $0.5 \, W/cm^2$. At the end of 12 weeks, the percentage of healed ulcers was 20% greater in the US than the control group. The difference between the groups was statistically significant ($p < 0.05$).

Forty patients with pressure ulcers were evaluated in a double-blind study by McDiarmid et al. (29) The patients all had partial-thickness (stage II) wounds and were randomized into two groups treated three times weekly with either 3 MHz pulsed US at 0.8 W/cm² for 5–10 min (treatment) or with sham US (control). At the end of the study, 10 patients remained in the US group and eight in the sham group. Though statistical significance was not reported, the authors did indicate that US therapy appeared to improve the healing rate of infected, but not clean, ulcers.

While Nussbaum et al. (30) looked at US in pressure ulcer healing, it is hard to assess US influence alone since the study involved nursing care alone, nursing care with LASER and nursing care alternated with US or UVC. They studied 16 patients with 18 wounds. While it was reported that US/UVC treatment had a greater effect on healing than did nursing care with or without LASER, it is not possible to determine if the same results could have been obtained with either of the modalities alone or was it the cumulative effect.

Another randomized trial of US in the treatment of pressure ulcers was performed by ter Riet (31). This was a multicenter, placebo-controlled study involving 88 patients with pressure ulcers. Subjects in the treatment group ($n = 45$) received US therapy while the control subjects ($n = 43$) received sham therapy. At the conclusion of the 12-week trial, the authors noted that a significant treatment effect with US failed to be demonstrated.

4. INTERMITTENT PNEUMATIC COMPRESSION

Intermittent pneumatic compression (IPC) is a mechanical method of delivering compression to edematous extremities. While this form of therapy has been available clinically for decades, most of its use has centered around management of lymphatic and venous swelling. The use of IPC in facilitating repair in venous ulcerations first appeared in the literature in 1981 (32). Pilot testing demonstrated the potential value of IPC in healing venous ulcers when combined with Unna boot therapy. These findings were later supported in a randomized-controlled trial of 22 patients (33). Patients in this study were randomized into a treatment group ($n = 12$) that received standard wound care along with twice weekly IPC and Unna boot application and a control group ($n = 10$) that received only standard care and Unna boot therapy. Subjects who received IPC healed at a statistically faster rate ($p < 0.05$) than individuals receiving only Unna boot compression.

Intermittent pneumatic compression is available in two forms. Units either deliver compression via a single inflatable sleeve that fits over the limb or by a segmented sleeve designed to give sequential compression. Coleridge-Smith et al. (34), in a randomized study of 55 subjects, examined the effects of sequential IPC on ulcer healing. Subjects in the control group received standard wound care and gradient support stockings while treatment subjects additionally received home treatment with sequential IPC. Patients reported using the device 3–4 hr/day. The median ulcer healing rate was 19.8% for the treatment subjects as compared to 2.1% for the control subjects.

A recent Cochrane review (35) of IPC in treatment of venous ulcers indicated that further trials are required to determine whether IPC increases the healing of venous ulcers. The randomized-controlled trials reviewed had small sample sizes and some revealed positive effects while others did not.

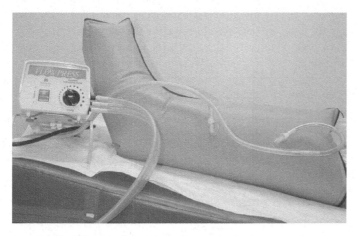

Figure 3 Patient receiving intermittent pneumatic compression. (Courtesy of Flow Press®, Huntleigh Healthcare, Inc., Eatontown, NJ.)

Should it be decided that IPC is to be used in the management of a venous ulcer, clinicians should first assess whether there is significant lymphatic involvement. The lymphatic system is a low pressure system and the higher pressures (40–60 mmHg) typically used in venous management can collapse the lymphatic system and lead to further problems. True lymphedema responds much better to manual lymphatic drainage, a technique that involves very light massage of the lymphatic collectors. If lymphatic disease is deemed to be a minimal contributor to the lower extremity swelling, then IPC may be of value. Treatment is generally performed by placing the patient supine, elevating the leg slightly and applying a plastic bag then the compressive sleeve to the extremity (Fig. 3). Compression is delivered at less than diastolic pressure (generally at 40–50 mmHg) at a cycling of 120 sec of compression to 30 sec of relaxation. Treatment duration is about 1 hr and is best if performed at least three times per week. Following each treatment session with IPC, the extremity should be wrapped with a compression bandage to maintain the benefits gained from the treatment and to prevent the leg from swelling again. Once there is evidence that the extremity has reduced in volume to the desired level, patients can generally be maintained with custom support stockings. Measuring a patient for a custom stocking before the leg volume has been effectively reduced is a waste of money since gravity will always encourage the leg to swell and fill any available space in the garment.

5. WHIRLPOOL

Quite often, when one thinks of the role of physical therapy in wound care, whirlpool comes to mind. For years, whirlpool was a preferred form of mechanical debridement for burns and most wounds. During the past 10 years, a great deal has been learned about the potential negative effects of whirlpool including cross-contamination, high irrigation pressures, and the tendency to promote dependent edema.

While full body submersion in a whirlpool might provide a quick means to cleanse a large surface area, the risk of fecal contamination to surgical sites and other wounds must be considered. Despite thorough cleansing of equipment between patients, it is also possible for pieces of tissue to become trapped within the mechanical systems of tanks and promote cross contamination between patients. Such problems have been minimized in newer hydrotherapy systems on the market today.

Irrigation pressure from the whirlpool turbines at highest settings, while unknown, likely far exceeds the recommendations of the Agency for Health Care Policy and Research in its pressure ulcer guidelines (36). These guidelines state that pressures greater than 15 psi should not be used over healthy granulation tissue. For this reason, pulsatile lavage systems have been fashioned after the jet lavage typically used in surgery. The newer lavage systems available for use in wound care are sterile, single use units that provide for low pressure irrigation of wounds. Most units also come equipped with suction units to aid in removing wound irrigant and debris as well as stimulating the granulation tissue. One study by Haynes et al. (37) noted that pulsatile lavage with suction caused wounds to granulate two and on-half times faster than wounds treated with whirlpool.

Clinicians should think twice before using whirlpool therapy for treatment of venous ulcers. While dependency and warmth may facilitate blood flow in an ischemic extremity, it most certainly will complicate an already edematous extremity in patients with venous insufficiency. McCulloch and Boyd (38) studied the effects of whirlpool and the dependent position on 40 normal subjects. Limb volume measurements were made with subjects lying supine, sitting with the limb dependent and sitting with the limb in a whirlpool bath at 40°C (104 F). There was a statistically significant difference in limb volume between all groups with the most pronounced increase in limb volume being seen when the whirlpool was utilized ($p < 0.01$).

6. SUMMARY

Many benefits can be seen from the diligent use of physical agents in wound management. Care must be taken however to select the appropriate modality and apply it with the requisite skill. The high energy sources of agents such as infrared, ultraviolet, and ultrasound predispose these agents to causing potential harm, if not used according to manufacturer guidelines. Likewise, the inappropriate use of agents such as intermittent pneumatic compression and whirlpool, while likely not having devastating consequences, can cause wound repair to be delayed. Physical therapists should be considered as resources for any wound care team that would like to integrate physical agents in wound healing.

REFERENCES

1. Nutton V. The rise of medicine. In: Porter R, ed. Cambridge Illustrated History of Medicine. Cambridge: Cambridge University Press, 2000:52–81.
2. Prentice W. The science of therapeutic modalities. In: Prentice W, ed. Therapeutic Modalities for Allied Health Professionals. New York: McGraw Hill, 1998:3–12.
3. Rabkin J, Hunt T. Local heat increases blood flow and oxygen tension in wounds. Arch Surg 1987; 122:221–225.

4. Santilli S, Valusek P, Robinson C. Use of a noncontact radiant heat bandage for the treatment of chronic venous stasis ulcers. Adv Wound Care 1999; 12:89–93.

5. Cherry G, Wilson J. The treatment of ambulatory venous ulcer patients with warming therapy. Ostomy Wound Manage 1999; 45:65–70.

6. Kloth L, Berman J, Dumit-Minkel S, Sutton C, Papanek P, Wurzel J. Effects of a normothermic dressing on pressure ulcer healing. Adv Skin Wound Care 2000; 45:69–74.

7. Kloth L, et al. Effects of heated and unheated warm-up dressings on full thickness pressure ulcers. In: Ryan T, ed. Warming and Wound Healing: Warm-Up Active Wound Therapy. London: Royal Society of Medicine Press, 2000:43–48.

8. Kloth L, et al. A randomized controlled clinical trial to evaluate the effects of noncontact normothermic wound therapy on chronic full thickness pressure ulcers. Adv Skin Wound Care 2002; 15:270.

9. Price P, Bale S, Crook H, Harding K. The effect of a radiant heat dressing on pressure ulcers. J Wound Care 2000; 9.

10. McCulloch J, Knight C. Noncontact normothermic wound therapy and offloading in the treatment of neuropathic foot ulcers in patients with diabetes. Ostomy Wound Manage 2002; 48:38–44.

11. Stillwell G. Ultraviolet therapy. In: Krusen F, ed. Handbook of Physical Medicine and Rehabilitation. 2nd ed. Philadelphia: WB Saunders, 1971:350–351.

12. Fischer E, Solomon S. Physiologic effects of ultraviolet radiation. In: Licht S, ed. Therapeutic Electricity and Ultraviolet Radiation. Baltimore: Waverly Press, 1959: 273–275.

13. High A, High J. Treatment of infected skin wounds using ultraviolet radiation: an in vitro study. Physiotherapy 1983; 41:55–57.

14. Gates F. Discussion and correspondence on nuclear derivatives and the lethal action of ultraviolet light. Science 1928; 68:479.

15. Kellner A. Growth, respiration and nuclear acid synthesis in ultraviolet-irradiated and in photoactivated *Escherichia coli*. J Bacteriol 1953; 65:252.

16. Painter R. The action of ultraviolet light on mammalian cells. In: Giese A, ed. Photophysiology. New York: Academic Press, 1970:177–179.

17. Sullivan P, Conner-Kerr T, Smith S. The effects of UVC irradiation on group A streptococcus in vitro. Ostomy Wound Manage 1999; 45:50–54,56–58.

18. Conner-Kerr T, Sullivan P, Gaillard J, Franklin M, Jones R. The effects of ultraviolet radiation on antibiotic-resistant bacteria in vitro. Ostomy Wound Manage 1998; 44: 50–56.

19. Conner-Kerr T, et al. UVC reduces antibiotic-resistant bacterial numbers in living tissue. SAWC Selected Abstracts. Ostomy Wound Manage 1999; 45:84.

20. Thai T, Houghton P, Deast D, Campbell K, Woodbury M. Ultraviolet light C in the treatment of chronic wounds with MRSA: a case study. Ostomy Wound Manage 2002; 48:52–60.

21. Kloth L. Physical modalities in wound management: UVC, therapeutic heating and electrical stimulation. Ostomy Wound Manage 1995; 41:18–27.

22. Dyson M, Pond J, Warwick J, et al. The stimulation of tissue regeneration by means of ultrasound. Clin Sci 1995; 35.

23. Mummery C. The Effect of Ultrasound on Fibroblasts in vitro. London: University of London, 1978.

24. Mortimer A, Dyson M. The effect of therapeutic ultrasound on calcium uptake in fibroblasts. Ultrasound Med Biol 1988; 14:499–506.

25. Draper D, Prentice W. Therapeutic ultrasound. In: Prentice W, ed. Therapeutic Modalities for Allied Health Professionals. New York: McGraw Hill, 1998:264.

26. Dyson M, et al. Stimulation of healing of varicose ulcers by ultrasound. Ultrasonics 1976; 14:232.

27. Roche C, West J. A controlled trial investigating the effect of ultrasound on venous ulcers referred from general practitioners. Physiotherapy 1984; 70:745.

28. Callum M, et al. A controlled trial of weekly ultrasound therapy in chronic leg ulceration. Lancet 1987; 8:204.

29. McDiarmid T, et al. Ultrasound and the treatment of pressure sores. Physiotherapy 1985; 71:66.

30. Nussbaum E. Comparison of ultrasound/ultraviolet-C and laser for treatment of pressure ulcers in patients with spinal cord injury. Phys Ther 1994; 74:812.

31. ter Riet G. A randomized clinical trial of ultrasound in the treatment of pressure ulcers. Phys Ther 1996; 76:1301.

32. McCulloch J. Intermittent compression for the treatment of a chronic stasis ulcer. Phys Ther 1981; 91:1452.

33. McCulloch J, Marler K, Neal M, Phifer T. Intermittent pneumatic compression improves venous ulcer healing. Adv Wound Care 1994; 7:22–26.

34. Smith PC, Sarin S, Hasty J, Scurr J. Sequential gradient pneumatic compression enhances venous ulcer healing: a randomized trial. Surgery 1990; 108:871–875.

35. Mani R, Vowden K, Nelson E. Intermittent pneumatic compressin for treating venous leg ulcers (Cochrane Review). Issue 4. Oxford: The Cochrane Library, 2002.

36. Bergstrom N, et al. US Department of Health and Human Services. Public Health Service, Agency for Health Care Policy and Research. Clinical Practice Guidelines No. 15. AHCPR Publication No. 95–0652, 1994.

37. Haynes L, et al. Comparison of pulsavac and sterile whirlpool regarding the promotion of tissue granulation [abstr]. Phys Ther 1994; 74(suppl 5).

38. McCulloch J, Boyd V. The effects of whirlpool and the dependent position on lower extremity volume. JOSPT 1992; 16:169–173.

52

Objective Assessment in Wound Healing

Marco Romanelli and Antonio Magliaro
Department of Dermatology, University of Pisa, Pisa, Italy

1. INTRODUCTION

Imaging cutaneous ulcers to detect the progression of a disease is a routine part of medical practice. Although imaging technology has continuously evolved over the years in all fields of medicine, its direct application to cutaneous disorders has increased only in recent years. In fact, only over the past decade has significant research been undertaken to further develop techniques for specifically examining the skin. Advances in both the technology of imaging and computer systems have greatly supported this process and brought it closer to the clinical area (1). Assessment of any wound should begin with the determination of the extent of the wound. Because the extent of a wound is a dynamic process, it requires repeated systematic assessment. The total wound extent is based on the wound dimensions and the tissue level involved. The clinical evaluation of the extent of the tissue involvement due to a skin lesion and, moreover, the way a lesion evolves over time are often assessed according to the common sense and memory of the clinician. Evaluations are, in general, performed on the basis of clinical experience and using very basic, low-tech equipments to make objective measurements. The determination of the extent of a wound may also be accomplished by noninvasive and invasive technologies. Noninvasive wound assessment includes the measurement of perimeter, maximum dimensions of length and width, surface area, volume, amount of undermining, and determination of tissue viability (2). Invasive methods may be necessary to quantify the extent of a wound. The tissue involvement in a wound must be defined from its surface to its depth and may vary depending on the organs involved. The total wound extent should be determined by means of the integration of the maximum possible amount of available data.

A wound can be further described through the use of various parameters, which include the following: duration, blood flow, oxygen, infection, edema, inflammation, repetitive trauma and/or insult, innervation, wound metabolism, nutrition, previous wound manipulation, and coexisting systemic factors. These parameters are clues to the definition of the cause, pathophysiology, and status of the wound, but we consider also fundamental a complete and careful history and physical examination.

The use of skin imaging techniques to improve the management of wounds remains a novel area for most practitioners, as the traditional approach continues to be used for clinical inspection. The techniques used to obtain an effective wound assessment are currently based on the use of transparent acetate sheets, which are applied to the ulcer so as to measure its perimeter manually. The depth of the lesion is measured by positioning a q-tip inside it or by filling the lesion cavity with hypoallergenic material to produce a cast, which is then measured to obtain the volume of the lesion. The main goal of current research is to create a system that monitors the qualitative and quantitative evolution of wounds with an easy-to-use technological system, which is able to produce an objective evaluation of the wound status and which allows the evolution of the wound to be monitored by means of measurable attributes (3). Dedicated wound photography, high-frequency ultrasound assessment, laser Doppler perfusion imaging (LDPI), confocal microscopy (CM), transcutaneous oxymetry, pH measurement, and magnetic resonance imaging are some of the techniques that are currently available and being used to specifically examine different types of wounds.

This chapter reviews current noninvasive technology and the relevance of such methods to clinical practice in wound healing.

2. WOUND PHOTOGRAPHY

The visual nature of wounds lends itself well to surface imaging. Illustrative documentation of wounds has been an established practice in dermatology over the years. Innovations in photographic techniques have greatly improved the capacity to create and record images of wounds, which can be used for a wide variety of goals—in some cases, increasing the amount of information that is derived from naked-eye inspection.

Traditional film photography can give an accurate and objective representation of the condition of a wound and is a relatively inexpensive and an easy method for visually documenting a wound's condition. Serial photography can be particularly useful in monitoring patients affected by acute and chronic wounds with images taken at different times allowing comparison and helping detect early changes, thereby reducing unnecessary therapies. These images provide a visual record of changes in the appearance of the surface of the wound during the healing process but gives no indication as to the dimensional changes occurring deep within the wound (4).

Digital photography uses a film-free digital camera that captures an image and then stores it in an electronic memory (5,6). The ability to store images in this format allows them to be easily displayed on a computer monitor or transferred to other storage media. The versatility of digital imaging has made it ideal for recording and storing images of the skin (7,8).

Clinical applications are numerous, and changes in skin lesions can readily be documented and monitored through serial imaging. Digital photography is also useful in the relatively new area of telemedicine (9). High-quality images of the skin can be sent via Internet to a distant center of excellence for advice on management, without the need for the center experts to physically examine the patients.

3. ULTRASONOGRAPHY

Although introduced in the 1950s in many medical fields, diagnostic ultrasonography (US) has only recently been used for dermatological studies. The US equipment available up to 15 years ago did not have sufficient resolution to achieve satisfactory results in skin studies because of low-frequency probes, but present-day units, with their improved technical characteristics, permit a specific application in dermatology (10). Electronic linear probes of 7.5–13 MHz, mostly equipped with color Doppler, sometimes need the interposition of a synthetic separator of 1.5 cm maximum thickness to include the region of interest within the best focal range (0.5–3 cm). These probes may prove effective in the study of flat and regular surfaces and provide a wider field of view than sectorial probes (11). Water-bath sectorial mechanical probes with 10–20 MHz frequency have very superficial focalization and are excellent in the study of irregular surfaces, particularly the wound volume, thanks to their small size and small support. The main advantages of this method of imaging include its noninvasiveness, safety, high patient tolerability, and relatively low cost.

The technique of US involves the detection of reflected sound waves through tissues that have inherently different acoustic properties. Images of the skin can be displayed in one-dimensional A mode (adequate for skin-thickness measurements), two-dimensional B mode (which produces a vertical cross-section of the tissue being scanned), or C mode (which produce images horizontal to the skin surface). Computer processing can create three-dimensional images (12). Generally, a higher ultrasound frequency provides a better resolution of the image. Resolution is defined as either axial resolution, which refers to the smallest thickness of a structure that can be measured and is directly dependent on the ultrasound frequency, or lateral resolution, which refers to the width of the smallest structures that can be resolved and depends mainly on the geometric shape of the ultrasound beam.

Most common ultrasound units used in imaging abdominal organs use a frequency of 7.5 MHz, which provides an axial resolution of only 3–5 mm. Units used in dermatology need to achieve much greater resolution to be able to visualize the skin and usually operate at a 20–25 MHz range, providing an axial resolution of 50–80 μm and a lateral resolution of 200–300 μm. Higher-frequency ultrasound imaging operating at frequencies between 40 and 100 MHz can provide an axial resolution of 17–30 μm and a lateral resolution of 33–94 μm (13–15). Although this improvement in resolution allows more detailed visualization of the upper skin layers, the higher-frequency ultrasound waves penetrate tissues poorly and, therefore, do not provide clear images of deeper skin layers and subcutaneous regions.

When ultrasound waves penetrate through the skin, they are partially reflected at the boundaries between adjacent structures, and "echoes" of various amplitudes are generated. The resulting ultrasound image that is produced consists of regions of varying echogenicity, which correlate to different histological regions of the skin. Generally, with 20 MHz ultrasound, the dermis and hypodermis can be distinguished easily, but the epidermis over most of the body, except on the palm and sole, cannot be visualized as a separate structure because it is too thin to be resolved. Purpose-built 100 MHz high-frequency ultrasound units allow more detailed visualization of the upper skin layers and in palmar skin can detect distinct structures such as the stratum corneum, hair follicles, and eccrine sweat-gland ducts. Ultrasonic frequencies in excess of 500 MHz have been used on skin biopsy specimens to produce images of great detail; however, such high frequencies require high intensities that can damage living tissue and, therefore, are not useful in vivo. The main clinical value of US has been in the objective monitoring of disease progression, with serial measurements allowing the effectiveness of treatment in patients to be assessed more accurately.

One of the main uses of cutaneous US is in the measurement of skin thickness, which has been shown to be reliable and accurate. The actual method of evaluating skin thickness is very easy, painless, and safe and can be applied to any part of the body.

   This function has been used to assess skin-thickness changes in a variety of skin diseases such as scleroderma and morphea, photodamaged and chronologically aged skin, and psoriasis. High-frequency ultrasound is used to analyze the ultrastructure in chronic wounds, hypertrophic scars, keloids, and normal surrounding skin (16). The parameters investigated are the depth between skin surface and the inner limit of the dermis and the tissue density. The depth measurement, expressed in millimeters, gives an estimate of wound volume and scar thickness. Compared with photography, US can be applied to easily monitor the progression of wound repair giving indications on dimensional changes related to wound volume (17). Ultrasonography is characterized by the high echogenicity of the dermis, which is sharp compared to a hypoechogenicity of subcutaneous fat. This technique allows an accurate determination of granulation, sloughy/necrotic tissue, and the physical dimensions of ulcers while also providing an index to the structural components of the ulcer (18).

4. LASER DOPPLER SYSTEMS

Skin microcirculation is known to consist of two functionally different networks: (a) the superficial, nutritive and (b) the deeper, mainly thermoregulatory vascular bed. For examination of each network, different techniques have been established. The nutritional network of the skin can be examined by capillary microscopy, which has a short penetration depth of a few microns. The number of visible capillaries in the skin correlates with the degree of compensation of peripheral arterial occlusive disease. In chronic critical limb ischemia, the number of capillaries is reduced and, in severe cases, even avascular fields are found. A laser Doppler can be used for investigation of the mainly thermoregulatory bed, which is located in deeper layers of the skin. Nutritive circulation is also partly determined by this method. If this technique is combined with capillary microscopy, the thermoregulatory portion of the laser Doppler signal can be estimated. Signals measured with the laser Doppler are calculated values of the product of blood cell average speed and concentration. Directional effects are usually not considered, except in flux measurements of single vessels. In 1993, a further development of this technique was introduced: the laser Doppler imager. This device makes it possible to map the local distribution of the laser Doppler flux without direct contact, thus producing a two-dimensional, color-coded image (19).

4.1 Laser Doppler Flowmetry

Laser Doppler flowmetry is commonly used because it is a noninvasive, simple, objective measurement, which evaluates cutaneous blood flow 1–2 mm under the skin surface and gives a continuous or near-continuous record. Monochromatic, coherent laser light is conducted by glass fibers to a probe, attached to the skin by means of adhesive discs. The movement of blood cells leads to a scattering of the laser light, generated by a low-powered helium–neon source, inducing a Doppler shift. The backscattered signal containing data on flux, cell concentration, and cell velocity is displayed on screens and the data may be recorded by a computer (20,21). This technique is useful in the evaluation of wound healing and it is used in stage 2 and stage 3 pressure ulcers for the constant evaluation of local skin microcirculation. It has been shown that local blood flow increased at the ulcer edge at rest and after stress at 44°C when compared with surrounding skin.

4.2 Laser Doppler Perfusion Imaging

Laser Doppler perfusion imaging is a technique that has been finding increasing utility in skin research. It measures cutaneous perfusion by scanning a low-power laser beam over a region of skin (22,23). When monochromatic light interacts with a moving object such as a blood cell, a slight change in the frequency of the scattered light is induced according to the Doppler effect, whereas the light backscattered from nonmoving tissue structures remains at the same frequency. The frequency shift is dependent on the average speed of the blood cells. At each measurement site, the backscattered laser light is detected by a photodetector, and the resulting signal is used to calculate the degree of tissue perfusion, which is expressed in arbitrary units. The scanning laser beam can penetrate to an average depth of 0.2 mm below the surface of the skin. An important feature of this technique is the fact that the instrument is positioned at 50 cm distance from the area under investigation, allowing an easy and reproducible assessment inside the wound bed (24).

The images obtained by LDPI are displayed on a computer monitor using various colors to depict the variations in perfusion that occur in different regions of the skin (25). The measurements obtained are objective and reproducible. The instrument has been used to evaluate the effects of postural changes on blood flow (26), as well as postural vasoregulation and mediators of reperfusion injury in venous ulceration (27). It has also been used to monitor changes in experimental skin wounds and island flaps (28) and to assess burn wound depth (29).

5. TRANSCUTANEOUS OXYMETRY

Transcutaneous oxymetry is a valid technique widely used in the evaluation of local skin microcirculation, nutrition, and tissue ischemia (30). Many methods for noninvasive measurements of tissue O_2 are available. One of these is the tcP_{O2} technique, based on the electrochemical reduction of oxygen, which is measured on the skin surface with a calibrated Clark electrode (31). The tcP_{O2} measurement provides information about the tissue oxygenation in superficial skin layers. The postheating reactive hyperemia responses of tcP_{O2} can be used as a relative index of the vasodilatory capacity of skin microvessels. The tcP_{O2} values depend on skin microcirculation, arterial P_{O2}, oxygen consumption in skin tissue, and oxygen diffusion through the skin itself. The values evaluated represent the partial pressure of oxygen diffusing from the capillaries and give data on the oxygenation of superficial skin layers (32). The tcP_{O2} and tcP_{CO2} values have been used for monitoring the evolution of leg ulcers and improving their management, but we have to consider that these values can be determined by many local factors such as blood flow, thickness of epidermis, conductivity of the gases, and the production and consumption of such gas in situ. Other perfusion analyses such as arteriography, capillaroscopy, plethysmography, and videomicroscopy are considered difficult to perform and too invasive (33).

6. pH MEASUREMENT

pH measurement is defined as the negative logarithm of the activity of hydrogen ions in aqueous solution, used to express acidity and alkalinity on a scale of 0–14. The pH value of normal skin ranges from about 4.8 to 6.0 in relation to the presence of the so-called "acid mantle" while the interstitial fluid shows neutral values (34). Several studies have shown that the acid mantle plays an important role as a regulating factor in stratum corneum homeostasis in maintaining the integrity of barrier function. The role of pH in wound healing has proven to be of fundamental importance, and prolonged chemical acidification of the wound bed has been shown to increase the healing rate in chronic venous leg ulcers. The mechanism of interaction between acidic pH and the wound-healing process is related to the potential to increase tissue-oxygen availability through oxygen dissociation and to reduce the histotoxicity of bacterial end products, thus stimulating the wound's healing process. pH values in chronic venous leg ulcers and in pressure ulcers were found to be alkaline or neutral if compared with the normal surrounding skin (35). The change of value is in accordance with the stage of the ulcer, moving to an acidic state during the healing process. Two significant methods are widely used for measuring cutaneous pH: the colorimetric technique and the glass electrode potentiometric measurement. The most common pH instrument is a flat glass electrode connected to a meter and applied to the skin, with one or two drops of bidistillated water interposed between the electrode and the skin. The use of a flat electrode is important in order to provide appropriate contact with the skin surface. The electrode is applied onto the skin at intervals of 10 sec until stabilization of the reading. Measurements are performed at a room temperature that is below 23°C and a relative humidity of <65%, because sweat can influence the results. Readings should be taken 12 hr after the application of detergents or creams to the skin.

Measurement of pH is a noninvasive technique, simple, easy to use, and provides important information about changes in wounds.

7. CONFOCAL MICROSCOPY

Confocal microscopy has recently become quite commonly used in the dermatological field. The basic principle uses a light source and a lens to focus on a specific plane within the sample of tissues. The returning light from this focal point is detected by the instrument and used to create an image that is a composite of a large number of imaged points. The final image acquired is clear, because the system is trained to detect mainly the light that is directly backscattered from the focal point and to exclude any scattered and reflected light from out-of-focus planes, thus minimizing image blur. The light source used can be either intense-visible light or near-infrared light, as used with the video-rate laser-scanning confocal microscope.

The main advantage of CM is that it can allow the skin to be evaluated in its native state either in vivo or when freshly biopsied (ex vivo) without the fixing, sectioning, and staining that is necessary for routine histology.

Confocal microscope imaging of normal skin in vivo gives clear images of the cellular layers of the epidermis and upper dermal region. Beyond the dermoepidermal junction, at a depth of 100–150 μm, blood flow in the capillary loops within each dermal papilla can be evaluated at the highest resolution; erythrocytes, leucocytes, and platelets can be distinguished in relation to their relative sizes and shapes. Further, imaging at depths of 100–350 μm below the stratum corneum can show a network of fibers and bundles in the papillary dermis and superficial reticular network that represent the collagen network. Skin appendages such as sebaceous glands, hair shafts, and sweat-gland ducts can also be seen (36).

The quality of images obtained by CM can depend on the type of confocal microscope used and the ability of the operator. Traditional confocal microscopes require the use of fluorescent dyes in order to achieve adequate tissue contrast in creating a clear image. For in vivo skin examination, some commercially available confocal microscopes can achieve image contrast entirely through the detection of reflected light from within the skin, whereas others require an intradermal injection of a fluorescent contrast agent, before different skin-cell layers can be clearly visualized.

The completely noninvasive nature and high-resolution capability of CM have made it a useful instrument in skin research. Some skin conditions that have been studied in vivo with CM and have been reported in the literature include solar keratoses, psoriasis, amelanotic melanoma, and allergic contact dermatitis, where dendritic cells resembling activated Langerhans cells have been directly visualized (37,38). Confocal microscopy has been shown to characterize the pattern of neovascularization and reinnervation in a model of human skin equivalent grafted in a pig (39), confirming that angiogenesis occurs first and acts as an influencing and guiding factor on innervation in experimental wound healing (40).

Currently, confocal microscopes are costly instruments and, although available commercially, their use is mainly confined to research. However, as the technology of CM improves and smaller, more affordable instruments become available, the technique could have immense potential as a diagnostic tool in wound healing, enabling clinicians to characterize wound parameters, image skin lesions, and diagnose them without the need for biopsy, and to define the margins of skin lesions prior to any intended excision (41).

8. MAGNETIC RESONANCE IMAGING

Magnetic resonance imaging is a valuable diagnostic technique that can be used to image a variety of body tissues (42). The basis of the MRI technique is the varying response of different molecules when they are perturbed within a magnetic field. Atoms with an odd number of protons will respond strongly to the presence of a magnetic field. A radio-frequency pulse is used to knock spinning protons out of alignment with the magnetic field. When the pulse is turned off, the proton will return to its previous state at a rate dependent on its interaction with its environment. Magnetic resonance imaging utilizes the abundance of hydrogen in the human body as its signal source (43). A series of encoded radio-frequency pulses are transmitted, and the returning signals from the excited atoms are collected. A magnitude image of these signal intensities is then displayed by the computer after data processing. Depending on the timing of the sequence used, the strength of the signal received from a given tissue will vary because of the different molecular relaxation times.

Initial research in the dermatological field of MRI involved the study of cutaneous melanocytic lesions. Subsequent trials demonstrated that clinically useful MRI scans of any skin lesion, whether or not it contains melanin, could be obtained with excellent resolution (44,45). Tumor depths measured by MRI correlate well with postoperative histologic measurements (46). Thus, MRI should be of help to dermatologic, plastic, hand, and ear, nose, and throat surgeons in the preoperative determination of tumor size, underlying tissue involvement, and exact location of the tumor. In addition, postoperatively, MRI can define and possibly detect skin cancer recurrences under skin flaps and grafts. Magnetic resonance imaging procedures can plan surgical intervention or perform closed drainage of poorly localized abscess cavities. The MRI procedures may accelerate the decision for surgery or closed drainage in patients with signs of severe infected lesions and significantly improve survival. In infected wounds, MRI provided excellent anatomoradiologic correlations by precisely defining the extent of infection (47). The results of this study confirmed the correlation of MRI parameters with histologic and physiologic data on the wound-healing process, demonstrating again more the usefulness of MRI in monitoring and assessing the time-dependent changes of angiogenesis during the wound-healing process. One important aspect of the wound-healing phases is represented by angiogenesis, which is a process characterized by new vessel growth toward and into the tissue. Without new vessels, which ensure an adequate supply of blood, oxygen, and nutrients to the wound area, wound healing cannot proceed. Although MRI imaging of the skin is mainly a research tool, we consider MRI to be a noninvasive, safe procedure that can be used in vivo to assess wound-healing process. Magnetic resonance imaging provides a noninvasive quantitative assay for the wound-healing process, but its use in clinical settings requires further development.

9. CONCLUSIONS

Wound-healing assessment is becoming a more and more sophisticated section in wound management due to the introduction of different types of equipment, which are able to monitor noninvasively the various phases of tissue repair. With the availability of biomedical engineering technologies, wound-measurement instruments are rapidly evolving, as evidenced by the considerable amount of data produced in recent literature. The wide range of clinical and biochemical parameters to be assessed represents the main challenge for the years to come, although caregivers will hopefully be provided with user-friendly tools to be used routinely and safely. A better reproducibility on the part of the various devices and a reduction in costs is to be expected in the near future, allowing widespread diffusion of the techniques in question among end users. In clinical use, applications of these technologies will be differentiated from basic research and particular emphasis will be placed on therapeutic control and the prevention of recurrences.

REFERENCES

1. Corcuff P, Pierard GE. Skin imaging: state of art at the dawn of year 2000. Curr Prob Dermatol 1998; 26:1–11.
2. van Rijswijk L. Wound assessment and documentation. Wounds 1996; 8(2):57–69.
3. Romanelli M, Gaggio G, Coluccia M, Rizzello F, Piaggesi A. Technological advances in wound bed measurements. Wounds 2002; 14(2):58–66.
4. Perednia DA. What dermatologists should know about digital imaging. J Am Acad Dermatol 1991; 25:89–108.
5. Ratner D, Thomas CO, Bickers D. The uses of digital photography in dermatology. J Am Acad Dermatol 1999; 41:749–756.
6. Bittorf A, Fartasch M, Schuler G, Diepgen TL. Resolution requirements for digital images in dermatology. J Am Acad Dermatol 1999; 37:195–198.
7. Kvedar JC, Edwards RA, Menn ER, Mofid M, Gonzalez E, Dover J, Parrish JA. The substitution of digital images for dermatological physical examination. Arch Dermatol 1997; 133:161–170.

8. Price MA, Goldstein GD. The use of a digital imaging system in a dermatologic surgery practice. Dermatol Surg 1997; 23:31–32.

9. Krupinski EA, LeSueur B, Ellsworth L, Levine N, Hansen R, Silvis N, et al. Diagnostic accuracy and image quality using a digital camera for teledermatology. Telemed J 1999; 5:257–263.

10. Gropper CA, Stiller MJ, Shupack JL, Driller J, Rorke M, Lizzi F. Diagnostic high-resolution ultrasound in dermatology. Int J Dermatol 1993; 32:243–262.

11. Tumball DH, Starkoski BG, Harasiewicz KA, Semple JL, From L, Gupta AK, Sander N, Goster FS. A 40–100 MHz B-scan ultrasound backscatter microscope for skin imaging. Ultrasound Med Biol 1995; 21:79–88.

12. Stiller MJ, Drilller MD, Shupack JL, Gropper CG, Rorke MC, Lizzi FL. Three-dimensional imaging for diagnostic ultrasound in dermatology. J Am Acad Dermatol 1993; 29:171–175.

13. Fornage BD, McGavran MR, Duvic M, Waldron CA. Imaging of the skin with 20 MHz US. Radiology 1993; 189:69–76.

14. Harland CC, Bamber JC, Gusterson BA, Mortimer PS. High frequency, high resolution B-scan ultrasound in the assessment of skin tumours. Br J Dermatol 1993; 128:525–532.

15. Gniadecka M, Quistorff B. Assessment of dermal water by highfrequency ultrasound: comparative studies with nuclear magnetic resonance. Br J Dermatol 1996; 135:218–224.

16. Whiston RJ, Melhuish J, Harding KG. High resolution ultrasound imaging in wound healing. Wounds 1993; 5(3):116–121.

17. Dyson M, Moodley S, Verjee L, Verling W, Weinman J, Wilson P. Wound healing assessment using 20 MHz ultrasound and photography. Skin Res Technol 2003; 9: 116–121.

18. Rippon MG, et al. Ultrasound assessment of skin and wound tissue: comparison with histology. Skin Res Technol 1998; 4:147–154.

19. Wardell K, Nilsson G. Laser Doppler imaging of skin. In: Serup J, Jemec BE, eds. Handbook of Non-invasive Methods and the Skin. London: CRC Press, 1995:421–428.

20. Bircher A, De Boer EM, Agner T, Wahlberg JE, Serup J. Guidelines for measurement of cutaneous blood flow by laser Doppler flowmetry. Contact Dermatitis 1994; 30:65–72.

21. Wardell K, Andersson T, Anderson C. Analysis of laser Doppler perfusion images of experimental irritant skin reactions. Skin Res Technol 1996; 2:149–157.

22. Moller H, Bjorkner B, Bruze M, Lundqvist K, Wollmer P. Laser Doppler perfusion imaging for the documentation of flare-up in contact allergy to gold. Contact Dermatitis 1999; 41:131–135.

23. Sommer A, Veraart J, Neumann M, Kessels A. Evaluation of the vasoconstrictive effects of topical steroids by laser Doppler perfusion imaging. Acta Derm Venereol 1998; 78:15–18.

24. Vongsavan N, Mattews B. Some aspects of the use of laser Doppler flow meters for recording tissue blood flow. Exp Physiol 1993; 78:11–18.

25. Bray R, Forrester K, Leonard C, Mc Arthur R, Tulip J, Lindsay R. Laser Doppler imaging of burn scars: a comparison of wavelength and scanning methods. Burns 2003; 29: 199–206.

26. Svedman C, Cherry GW, Ryan TJ. Postural changes in the circulation of venous leg ulcer patients studied with the laser Doppler imager. J Invest Dermatol 1992; 98:640a.

27. He CF, Cherry GW, Arnold F. Postural vasoregulation and mediators of reperfusion injury in venous ulceration. J Vasc Surg 1997; 25:647–653.

28. Arnold F, He CF, Jia CY, Cherry GW. Perfusion imaging of skin island flap blood flow by a scanning laser-Doppler technique. Br J Plast Surg 1995; 48:280–287.

29. Niazi ZBM, Essex TJH, Papini R, et al. New laser Doppler scanner: a valuable adjunct in burn depth assessment. Burns 1993; 19:485–489.

30. Sheffield PJ. Measuring tissue oxygen tension: a review. Undersea Hyper Med 1998; 25:179–184.

31. Nemeth AJ, Falanga V. Clinical parameters and transcutaneous oxygen measurements for the prognosis of venous ulcer. J Am Acad Dermatol 1989; 20:186–194.
32. Romanelli M, Katz MH, Alvarez AF, Eaglstein WH, Falanga V. The effect of topical nitroglycerin on transcutaneous oxygen. Br J Dermatol 1991; 124:354–357.
33. Takiwaki H, Nakanishi H, Shono Y, Arase S. The influence of cutaneous factors on transcutaneous PO_2 and PCO_2 at various body sites. Br J Dermatol 1991; 125:243–247.
34. Dikstein S, Zlogorski A. Skin surface hydrogen ion concentration (pH). In: Leveque JL, ed. Cutaneous Investigation in Health and Disease: Noninvasive Methods and Instrumentation. New York/Basel: Marcel Dekker, 1988:59–78.
35. Glibbery AB, Mani R. pH in leg ulcers. Int J Microcirc Clin Exp 1992; 2:109.
36. Rajadhyaksha M, Gonzalez S, Zavislan JM, Anderson RR, Webb R. In vivo confocal scanning laser microscopy of human skin. Advances in instrumentation and comparison with histology. J Invest Dermatol 1999; 113:293–301.
37. Aghassi D, Anderson RR, Gonzalez S. Confocal laser microscopic imaging of actinic keratoses in vivo: a preliminary report. J Am Acad Dermatol 2000; 43:42–48.
38. Gonzalez S, Rajadhyaksha M, Rubinstein G, Anderson RR. Characterization of psoriasis in vivo by reflectance confocal microscopy. J Med 1999; 30:337–356.
39. Ferretti A, Boschi E, Stefani A, Saturnino S, Romanelli M, Lemmi M, Giovannetti A, Longoni B, Mosca F. Angiogenesis and nerve regeneration in a model of human skin equivalent transplant. Life Sci 2003; 73:1985–1994.
40. Gu XH, Terenghi G, Kangesu T, Navsaria HA, Springaal DR, Leigh IM, Green CJ, Polka JM. Regeneration pattern of blood vessels and nerves in cultured keratinocyte grafts assessed by confocal laser scanning microscopy. Br J Dermatol 1995; 132:376–383.
41. Vardaxis NJ, Brans TA, Boon ME, Kreis RW, Marres LM. Confocal laser scanning microscopy of porcine skin: implications for human wound healing. J Anat 1997; 190:601–611.
42. Conolly S, Macovski A, Pauly J, Schenck J, Kwong K, Chesler D, Hu X, Chen W, Patel M, Ugurbil K. Magnetic resonance imaging. In: Bronzino JD, ed. The Biomedical Engineering Handbook. Florida: CRC Press, 1995:1006–1014.
43. Bittoun J, Saint-Jalmes H, Querleux BG, Darrasse L, Jolivet O, Idy-Peretti I, Wartski M, Richard SB, Leveue J. In vivo high resolution MR imaging of the skin in a whole-body system at 1.5 T. Radiology 1990; 176:457–460.
44. Richards S, Querleux B, Bittoun J, Jolivet O, Idy-Peretti I, de Lacharriere O, Leveque JL. Characterisation of the skin in-vivo by high resolution magnetic resonance imaging: water behaviour and age-related effects. J Invest Dermatol 1993; 100:705–709.
45. Idy-Peretti I, Bittoun J, Alliot F, Richard SB, Querleux BG, Cluzan RV. Lymphedematous skin and subcutis: in vivo high resolution magnetic resonance imaging evaluation. J Invest Dermatol 1998; 110:782–787.
46. El-Gammal S, Hartwig R, Aygen S, Bauermann T, EI-Gammal C, Altmeyer P. Improved resolution of magnetic resonance microscopy in examination of skin tumors. J Invest Dermatol 1996; 106:1287–1292.
47. Helbich TH, Roberts TPL, Rollins MD, Shames DM, Turetschek K, Hopf H, Muhler M, Hunt TK, Brasch RC. Noninvasive assessment of wound healing angiogenesis with contrast-enhanced MRI. Acad Radiol 2002; 9(suppl 1):S145–S147.

53

Tissue Adhesives: Advances in Wound Therapies

S. C. Davis and A. L. Cazzaniga
Department of Dermatology and Cutaneous Surgery, University of Miami School of Medicine, Miami, Florida, U.S.A.

1. INTRODUCTION

Tissue adhesives are materials that are designed to polymerize upon application. Biological tissue adhesives, also referred to as tissue sealants and glues, have been used as adjunct therapies to promote wound healing since the 1900s. Over the years, they have been used for a variety of surgical applications including hemostasis, tissue welding, grafting, and sealing. More recently, tissue adhesives have been used as topical delivery systems for growth factors (1,2), cell lines (3), and as liquid occlusive dressings to cover open superficial wounds (4,5).

Tissue adhesives can be natural or synthetic based and include fibrin sealants, albumin-based compounds such as glutaraldehydes glues, polyethylene glycol (PEG) polymers, collagen-based adhesives, and cyanoacrylates (CAS) glues.

BioGlue (CryoLife, Inc.) is a synthetic albumin-glutaraldehyde-based tissue adhesive approved by the Food and Drug Administration (FDA) in December 2001 for use as an adjunct in open surgical repair of large vessels. Glutaraldehyde exposure causes lysine molecules of bovine serum albumin, extracellular matrix proteins, and cell surfaces to bind to each other creating a strong scaffold. Animals treated with BioGlue showed a significant decrease in seroma formation compared to control groups (6). Although BioGlue has been successfully used for repair of acute aortic dissections and as an adjunct to suture repair in large-vessel anastomoses, it has been shown to have an adverse effect on nerve function (7).

For tissue adhesion, PEG polymers have been used; however, since they are activated by light, their use is time consuming and complicated. The latest tissue adhesives to be developed are collagen-based adhesives. They are a combination of bovine collagen and bovine thrombin and have the capacity of creating a matrix which assists in coagulation and delivery of fibrinogen to the wounded area.

Initially, tissue adhesives were derived from the natural materials, fibrinogen and thrombin, which are designed to enhance the body's natural clotting mechanism. The first fibrin emulsion was described almost a century ago by Bergel (8); however, it was not until 1944 when the earliest clinical use of a fibrinogen and thrombin agent was reported (9). One of the major problems with early fibrin sealants was that the human fibrinogen was found to be a source of hepatitis and many of the patients that were treated with the early formulations became infected. In the 1970s additional refinement in the fibrin sealant allowed for the first commercially available fibrin sealant in Europe in 1982 (10). Spotnitz et al. in 1987 (11) reported an inexpensive and efficient method for local blood bank preparation of fibrin sealants that greatly reduced the risk of blood-borne disease transmission, including acquired immune deficiency syndrome. However, there was still the concern of hepatitis transmission in the United States and in 1977 the Food and Drug Administration revoked the licenses for commercial fibrin sealants that had pooled human fibrin. Therefore, during the 1980s and 1990s, many surgeons had to result in preparing their own fibrin sealants. This resulted in many of these "home-made" products not being standardized or virally inactivated. In 1998, the FDA finally approved the first fibrin sealant to help control bleeding.

Over the years, fibrin sealants have been widely used as an adjunct to surgical operations to control bleeding as well as controlling the leakage of body fluids. Various delivery methods have been used including a spray technique and the use of cellulose sponges soaked in fibrinogen which is then activated with thrombin. Desired characteristics of fibrin sealants include: excellent hemostatic properties, good adherence capacity of the material, biodegradable, easily applied, favorable to tissue repair, and cost effective.

Tissue adhesives have been used extensively to close uncomplicated lacerations as an option to standard wound closure techniques, e.g., staples and sutures. Tissue adhesives have various advantages over standard wound closure methods including ease of application which requires less time to apply as well as the elimination of a follow-up visit for removal of the sutures or staples. Although there are many uses for tissue adhesives for wound care, this chapter will focus only on two. The first is the use of tissue adhesives for graft take and the second is their use as an occlusive dressing.

2. TISSUE ADHESIVES: GRAFT TAKE

Survival of skin grafts is highly dependent on hemostasis and graft stabilization. Two of the most common reasons for skin graft loss are poor hemostasis which leads to the development of a hematoma and seroma formation beneath the graft. These conditions create a physical barrier between the wound bed and graft which leads to a reduction in nutritional factors. Other reasons for graft loss include an infected and/or inadequate vascularized recipient bed. It is important to properly secure the graft in place since any subsequent shearing or lifting destroys the fragile graft–wound bed interface.

Tissue adhesives can provide several benefits to tissue skin grafting, such as hemostasis, improve adherence, and take of the donor skin and as an antibacterial barrier. Of all tissue sealants, fibrin-based adhesives are one of the materials of choice for improving skin graft take. It is essential for graft take that fibrin be present in the skin graft–wound bed interface. Fibrin glue prevents the formation of hematomas beneath the grafts and provides a cross-linked fibrin network for support and nutrition between the skin graft and the recipient wound bed by providing a scaffold for fibroblasts migration and increase revascularization. The method of application is important on the resultant graft take. O'Grady et al. (12) reported that the graft needs to be applied within a few minutes after the application of the fibrin glue in order to maximize its effect and graft take is improved by a thin application of fibrin glue rather than a thick layer, regardless of the fibrin concentration.

Fibrin glues to secure skin grafts were first reported by Tidrick and Warner in 1944 (13). Since then, the use of tissue adhesives in promoting graft take has been described for split-thickness graft on chronic wounds (14) and burns (15). Even though fibrin glue on donor sites does not appear to be completely homeostatic (16), they has been shown to be very effective in reducing blood loss during skin graft anchoring. In a study on 20 patients, Vibe and Pless (17) were able to show a significant enhancement in split skin graft area take using fibrin glue, especially if grafts were located on difficult-to-graft body regions, such as on skin folds. Animal studies have shown that fibrin glue may even be helpful in reducing scar formation by reducing inflammation and skin graft contraction (18). After grafting, it is important to note that survival is also dependent upon occlusion of the graft (19). Keeping the graft initially moist and preventing dehydration provides an optimal environment for graft–wound bed interface.

In addition to improving skin graft adhesion and take, tissue sealants have been shown to act as antimicrobial barriers protecting the grafts by invading micro-organisms and reducing the rate the infection. In a clinical study, Vedung and Hedlung (20) demonstrated the benefit of fibrin glue when it was applied on graft-infected burn wounds. One postulated mechanism of action is that fibrin glue may provide a better microenvironment for phagocyte motility and a detrimental environment for bacteria growth. The inclusion of antibiotics to tissue adhesives has also been reported. Van der Ham et al. (21) studied the addition of cefotaxime and clindamycin in fibrin glue to seal colonic anastomoses in rats. They concluded that fibrin glue antibiotic combinations resulted in stronger bowel anastomoses. However, greater adhesion formation, an undesirable occurrence in bowel surgery, was also observed.

3. TISSUE ADHESIVES: LIQUID DRESSINGS

Cyanoacrylates were first produced in 1949 (22). The surgical use of these compounds was initially proposed by Coover et al. (23) in 1959. They are liquids that polymerize in the presence of moisture to form an adhesive film. The short chain CAs such as methyl- and ethyl-CAs "super glue" are not used clinically since they have been found to be toxic to tissues (24). The intermediate length CA, butylcyanoacrylate, has been used for a variety of indications, e.g. incisions, lacerations, skin graft adherence, etc. (25) More recently, a longer chain CA, octyl-2-cyanoacrylate, has been used to close lacerations instead of staples or sutures. This product is now marketed as DERMABOND® topical skin adhesive. It has been shown to produce good cosmetic results, allow faster wound closure, and avoids the need for future staple or suture removal (26). 2-Octylcyanoacrylates (2-OCA) are less toxic than the lower homologues of 2-OCAs, (41) making them an excellent candidate for use as a tissue adhesive. In addition to their use as tissue adhesives (glues) and film formers, CAs are good hemostatic agents (27) and may have antimicrobial activities (28) and reduce infection rates (29).

A modified, more flexible but weaker formulation of DERMABOND™ was recently evaluated by our group for treating partial thickness wounds, i.e., minor cuts and abrasions. It was anticipated that, when exposed to the moist wound surface and skin proteins, the liquid would rapidly polymerize into a film, which would offer the advantages of an occlusive dressing. Since the first controlled documentation in pigs by Winter in 1962 (30) and in humans by Hindman and Maibach in 1963

(31), occlusive dressings have been known to speed epithelization in acute wounds. Many controlled studies in animals and in man have confirmed that occlusive dressings speed resurfacing of acute wounds by up to 30% compared to wounds left open to the air (1,2,32–35). The occlusive dressing effect on epithelization is most strongly linked to creating and keeping a moist wound environment. A wide range of occlusive materials with moisture vapor transmission rates varying from 0 to 35 g/m^2/hr are all able to speed epithelization (36). Studies have also shown that, to obtain the optimal occlusive dressing effect on epithelization, the occlusive dressing must be placed on the wounds within 6 hr and may be discontinued after 2 days (34). Generally, dressing studies in pig and human wounds have given the same results: hydrocolloid (33,37–40) and polyurethane (35,41–43) dressings speed healing in both pig and man. In a recently published study, we compared the effect on partial thickness wounds of a flexible and thin film forming version of the octyl-2-cyanoacrylate-based product, a liquid bandage (Liquid Bandage: Johnson & Johnson) to two over the counter bandage products, standard bandage (Sheer quality Band-Aid® brand adhesive bandages, Johnson & Johnson), a new hydrocolloid bandage (Advanced Healing quality Band-Aid® brand adhesive bandages, Johnson and Johnson), and open air treatment (4). We used an acute partial thickness wound healing pig model to assess the healing properties of all these products. The liquid bandage was instantly hemostatic and no bleeding was observed in the wounds after treatment. Wounds treated with the liquid bandage healed statistically faster than all hydrocolloid bandage, standard bandage or untreated control wounds (Fig. 1).

Tissue adhesives decrease the likelihood of infection as compared to suturing due to the noninvasive application procedure (44,45). It is easy to imagine that

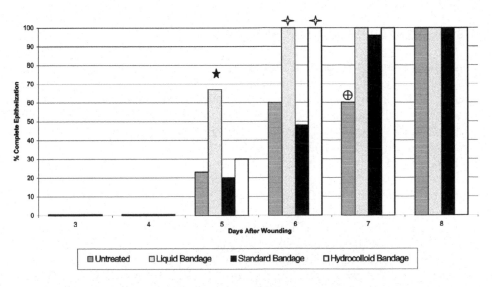

★ p < 0.02 significance compared to all other treatment groups.
✧ p < 0.005 significance compared to untreated and standard bandage.
◎ p < 0.001 significance compared to all other treatment groups.

Figure 1 Epithelization results. Data are presented as the number of wounds completely epithelized over the number of wounds assessed multiplied by 100 then plotted against days after healing.

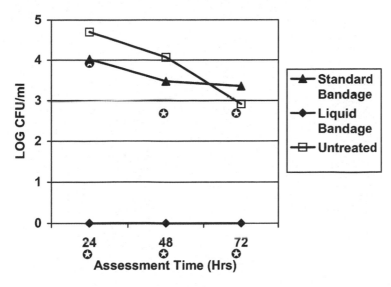

○ p < 0.02 significance compared to all other treatment groups.

Figure 2 Barrier study: *P. aeruginosa* recovery. Similar results were seen with *S. aureus*.

punctures made by suturing may allow micro-organisms to enter the wound area thus increasing the possibility of bacterial colonization. In addition, cyanoacrylate films may reduce wound infection through an inherent antimicrobial property that kills microbes at the wound site or by acting as a physical microbial barrier that prevents the entrance of microbes from the surrounding environment to the wound (46–48).

Our group has evaluated the barrier and antimicrobial properties of a cyanoacrylate bandage against *Staphylococcus aureus* and *Pseudomonas aeruginosa* on partial thickness wounds in swine (44). For the barrier study, we used our porcine model where we covered partial thickness wounds with the various treatments then inoculated the surface and perimeter of the test materials to see if the bacteria could enter the wound site. We found that no bacteria were able to gain entrance into the wounds when treated with the liquid bandage as compared to standard gauze bandage (Fig. 2). For the antimicrobial study where we first inoculated wounds then treated with the liquid bandage, we found that the liquid bandage was able to significantly reduce the number of inoculated bacteria as compared to standard gauze bandage and hydrocolloid bandage (Fig. 3). From these studies, we concluded that the cyanoacrylate bandage was effective in protecting wounds from external bacterial invasion and also reducing bacterial contamination.

4. CONCLUSION

One of the major benefits of tissue adhesives is hemostasis control. These materials were originally developed to stop bleeding by improving focal coagulation by mimicking the body's own coagulation mechanisms. Other common uses of tissue adhesives include tissue welding or sealing, enhancement of graft take and liquid bandage. Tissue adhesives can improve the survival of donor tissues by sealing the

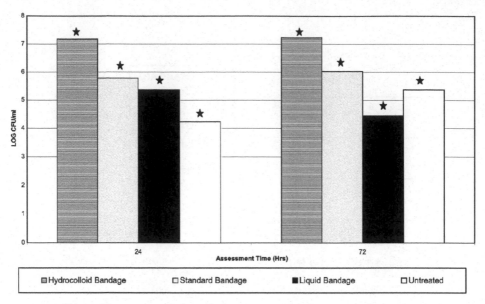

* p< 0.004 significance compared to all other treatment groups.

Figure 3 Antimicrobial results: *P. aeruginosa* recovery. Similar results were seen with *S. aureus*.

edges of skin grafts and providing an optimal graft–wound base interface. Thanks to technological advances, tissue adhesives are being developed to deliver medications, pharmaceutical compounds, growth factors, and cell lines. The possible use of tissue adhesives as drug delivery systems will be an exciting contribution to the area of wound care.

REFERENCES

1. Zarge JI, Husak V, Huang P, Greisler HP. Fibrin glue containing fibroblast growth factor type I and heparin decreases platelet deposition. J Surg 1997; 174:188–192.
2. Fasol R, Schemacher B, Schaudraff K, et al. Experimental use of a modified fibrin glue to induce the site directed angiogenesis from the aorta to the heart . J Thorac Cardiovasc Surg 1994; 107:1432–1439.
3. Kaiser HW, Stark GB, Kopp J, et al. Cultured autologous keratinocytes in fibrin glue suspension, exclusively and combined with STS-allograft (preliminary clinical and histological report of a new technique). Burn 1994; 20:23–29.
4. Davis SC, Eaglstein WH, Cazzaniga AL, Mertz PM. An octyl-2- cyanoacrylate formulation speeds healing of partial thickness wounds. Dermatol Surg 2001; 27:783–788.
5. Eaglstein WH, Sullivan TP, Giordano PH, Miskin BM. A liquid bandage for the treatment of minor cuts and abrasions. Dermatol Surg 2002; 28:263–267.
6. Menon NG, Downing S, Goldber NH, Silverman RP. Seroma prevention using an albumin-glutaraldehyde-based tissue adhesive in the rat mastectomy model. Ann Plast Surg 2003; 50:639–643.
7. LeMaire SA, Schmittling ZC, Undar A, et al. A new surgical adhesive (BioGlue) causes acute phrenic nerve injury and diaphragmatic paralysis. Presented at the Association for Academic Surgery, Tampa, FL, November 3, 2002.
8. Bergel S. Über wirkungen des fibrins. Dtsch Med Wochenschr 1909; 35:633.

9. Cronkite EP, Lozner EL, Deaver JM. Use of thrombin and fibrinogen in skin grafting. J Am Med Assoc 1944; 124:976–978.

10. Jackson MR. Fibrin sealants in surgical practice: An overview. A J Surg 2001; 182:1s–7s.

11. Spotnitz WE, Mintz PD, Avery N, et al. Fibrin glue from stored plasma. An in expensive and efficient method for local blood band preparation. Am Surg 1987; 53:460–462.

12. O'Grady, et al. An evaluation of fibrin tissue adhesive concentration and application thickness on skin graft survival. Laryngoscope 2000; 110:1931–1935.

13. Tidrick RT, Warner ED. Fribrin fixation of skin transplants. Surgery 1944; 15:90–95.

14. Dalstrom KK, Weis-Fogh US, Medgyese S, Rostgaad J, Sorensen H. The use autologous fibrin adhesive in skin transplnatation. Plast Reconstr Surg 1992; 90:968.

15. Stuart JD, et al. Application of single-donor fibrin glues to burn. 1988 J Burn Care Rehabil 1988; 9(6):619–622.

16. Achauer BM, Miller SR, Lee TE. The hemostatic effect of fibrin glue on graft donor sites. J Burn Care Rehabil 1994; 15:24.

17. Vibe P, Pless J. A new method of skin graft adhesion. Scand J Plast Reconstr Surg 1983; 17:263.

18. Bornemisza G, Tarsoly E, Miko I. Restoration of skin defects with fibrin glue. Acta Chir Hung 1986; 27:249.

19. Carver N, Navsaria A, Green CJ, Leigh IM. The effect of backing materials on keratinocyte autograft take. B J Plastic Surg 1993; 46:228–234.

20. Vedung S, Hedlung A. Fibrin glue: Its use for skin grafting of contaminated burn wounds in areas difficult to immobilize. J Burn Care Rehabil 1993; 14:356.

21. Van der Ham AC, Kort WJ, Weijma IM, et al. Effect of antibiotics in fibrin sealant on healing colonic anastomoses in the rat. Br J Surg 1992; 79:525–528.

22. Ardis AE. U.S. Patent No. 2467926 and 2467927, 1949.

23. Coover HW, Joyner FB, Shearer NH, Wicker TH. Chemistry and performance of cyanoacrylate adhesives. J Soc Plast Eng 1959; 15:413–417.

24. Toriumi DM, Raslan WF, Friedman M, Tardy ME. Histotoxicity of Cyanoacrylate tissue adhesives. A comparative study. Arch Otolaryngol Head Neck Surg 1990; 116(5): 546–550.

25. Galil KA, Schofield I, Wright GZ. Effect of n-2butyl cyanoacrylate (histoacryl blue) on the healing of skin wounds. J Can Dent Assoc 1984; 50:565–569.

26. Quinn J, Wells G, Sutcliffe T, et al. A randomized trial comparing octylcyanoacrylate tissue adhesive and sutures in the management of lacerations. J Am Med Assoc 1997; 277(19):1527–1530.

27. Bhaskar SN, Jacoway JR, Margetis PM, et al. Oral tissue response to chemical adhesives (cyanoacrylate). Oral Surg 1966; 22:394–404.

28. Quinn JV, Osmond MH, Yurack JA, Moir PJ. N-2-butylcyanoacrylate: Risk of bacterial contamination with an appraisal of its antimicrobial effects. J Emerg Med 1995; 13(4): 581–585.

29. Noordzij JP, Foresman PA, Rodeheaver GT, Quinn JV, Edlich RF. Tissue Adhesive Wound Repair Revisited. J Emerg Med 1994; 12(5):645–649.

30. Winter GD. Formation of scab and the rate of epithelization of superficial wounds in the skin of the young domestic pig. Nature 1962; 193:293–294.

31. Hindman CD, Maibach HI. Effect of air exposure and occlusion on experimental human skin wounds. Nature 1963; 200:377–378.

32. Eaglstein WH, Mertz PM. New method for assessing epidermal wound healing: the effect of triamcinolone acetonide and polyurethene film occlusion. J Invest Dermatol 1978; 71:382–384.

33. Nemeth AJ, Eaglstien WH, Taylor JR, et al. Faster healing and less pain in skin biopsy sites treated with an occlusive dressing. Arch Dermatol 1991; 127:1679–1683.

34. Bolton LL, Johnson CL, Rijswijk LV. Occlusive dressings: therapeutic agents and effects on drug delivery. Clin Dermatol 1992; 9:573–583.

35. Eaglstein WH, Davis SC, Mehle AL, Mertz PM. Optimal use of an occlusive dressing to enchance healing. Arch Dermatol 1988; 124(3):392–395.
36. Bolton LL, Monte K, Pirone LA. Moisture and Healing: Beyond the Jargon. Ostomy Wound Manage 2000; (suppl 1A):51s–62s.
37. Alvarez OM, Mertz PM, Eaglstein WH. The effect of occlusive dressings on collagen synthesis and re-epithelialization in superficial wounds. J Surg Res 1983; 35:142–148.
38. Champsaur A, Amanon R, Nefzi Marichy J. Use of DuoDerm on skin graft donor sites: comparative study with tulle gras. Ann Chir Plast Esthet 1986; 31:273.
39. Madden MR, Nolan E, Finkelstein JL, et al. Comparison of an occlusive and semi-occlusive dressing and the effect of the wound exudate upon keratinocyte proliferation. J Trauma 1989; 29:924–930.
40. Smith DJ, Thomson PD, Bolton LL, Hutchinson JJ. Microbiology and healing of the occluded skin-graft donor site. Plast Reconstr Surg 1993; 91:1094–1097.
41. Barnett A, Berkowitz RL, Mills R, Vistnes LM. Comparison of synthetic adhesive moisture vapor permeable and fine mesh gauze dressings for split-thickness skin graft donor sites. Am J Surg 1983; 145:379–381.
42. Stair TO, Dorta J, Altieri MF, Lippe MS. Poly urethane and silver sulfadiazine dressings in treatments of partial-thickness burns and abrasions. Am J Emerg Med 1986; 4: 214–217.
43. James JH, Watson AC. The use of OpSite a permeable–permeable dressing on skin graft donor sites. Br J Plast Surg 1975; 28:107–110.
44. Quinn JV, Maw J, Ramotar K, Wenckebach G, Wells G. Octylcyanoacrylate tissue adhesive vs. suture wound repair in a contaminated wound model. Surgery 1997; 69–72.
45. Hirko MK, Lin PH, Greisler HP, Chu CC. Biological properties of suture materials. In: Chu CC, von Fraunhofer JA, Greisler HP, eds. Wound Closure Biomaterials. Florida: CRC Press, 1997:271–273.
46. Quinn JV, Osmond MH, Yurack JA, Moir PJ. N-2-butylcyanoacrylate: Risk of contamination with an appraisal of its antimicrobial effects. J Emerg Med 1995; 13:581–585.
47. Eiferman RA, Snyder JW. Antibacterial effect of cyanoacrylate glue. Arch Opthalmol 1983; 101:958–960.
48. Mertz PM, Davis SC, Cazzaniga AL, Drosou A, Eaglstien WH. Barrier and antibacterial properties of 2-octyl cyanoacrylate-derived wound treatment films. J Cutan Med Surg 2002; 7(1):1–6.

54

Cutaneous Wound Healing Models in Swine

Anna Drosou and Patricia M. Mertz
Department of Dermatology and Cutaneous Surgery, University of Miami School of Medicine, Miami, Florida, U.S.A.

The astounding progress in the field of wound care could not have been achieved without the contribution of research conducted at the preclinical level. Human research, albeit the ultimate way of determining the efficacy and safety of a therapeutic modality, presents a number of practical and ethical limitations. Several of the techniques used to evaluate wound healing and reveal the mechanisms of the tested treatments, such as frequent histologic examination of the wound or measurement of the tensile strength, are not readily acceptable in patients. Difficulties also exist in finding patients with similar wounds or having a control wound in the same patient in order to avoid intrapersonal variations in healing. Animal research offers greater wound homogeneity without compliance issues. Information derived from animal research contributes to revealing the mechanisms of normal and delayed healing and excessive scar formation, designing advanced wound treatment agents and dressings, and avoiding unnecessary human testing.

Numerous animal wound healing models have been developed. Rabbits, rats, mice, guinea pigs, and domestic pigs are frequently used. Swine, a tight-skinned animal, is considered preferable to loose-skinned small mammals, because of closer anatomical and physiological similarities to human wound healing process (1–3) (Fig. 1). Pig skin has similar dermal–epidermal thickness ratio, number and distribution of adnexal structures, epidermal turnover time, and lipid composition of stratum corneum as human skin and is characterized by the presence of an underlying adipose rather than muscle layer. Moreover, pigs, like humans, heal mainly through re-epithelialization, while in loose-skinned animals, contraction is the principal healing mechanism. Additionally, in small mammals, the wound size is small and the number of wounds that can be created on the same animal is limited so that different treatments cannot easily be compared on the same animal. On a pig, numerous wounds can be created and the same animal serves as its own control, while the larger size of wounds allows easier survey of the healing process. As a result, swine has been extensively used in preclinical cutaneous wound healing research.

A variety of wound models in pigs described in the literature are reviewed in this chapter, including partial and full-thickness excisional wounds, partial and

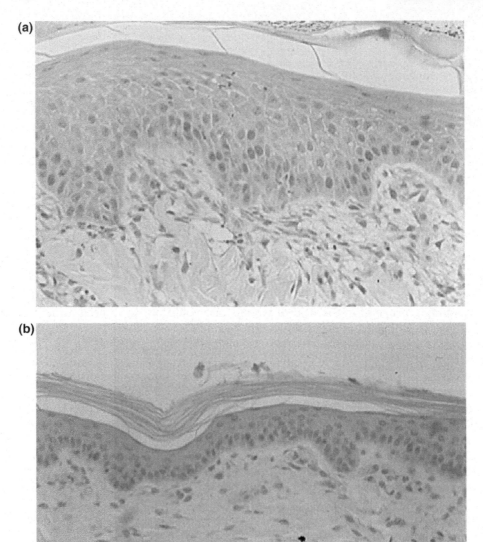

Figure 1 Histological comparison of hemotoxin and eosin stained back skin from pig (a) and man (b).

full-thickness burns, incisional, chemically induced necrotic wounds, bacterial contaminated, laser-induced, ischemic, pressure, and irradiation wound models. Additionally, the most commonly performed techniques for evaluation of epidermal and dermal regeneration are reviewed, including methods for assessment of re-epithelialization, epidermal proliferation, basement membrane re-establishment, restoration of epithelial barrier function, granulation tissue formation, collagen production, wound breaking strength, wound contraction, neovascularization, and scar formation. The role of antimicrobials in bacterial inoculated wounds will also be reviewed.

1. MODELS OF NORMAL WOUND HEALING

Partial thickness excisional wounds are frequently used in wound healing studies. Before wounding, the experimental animals are clipped and skin is washed with a nonantibiotic soap. Several researchers use antiseptic solutions to ensure that bacterial proliferation will not influence the results of the study. However, our group considered it preferable not to use antiseptic solutions because of their potential effect on the healing process. Moreover, in the majority of the clinical situations, wounds are not created in aseptical conditions, with the exception of surgically induced wounds. Rectangular wounds are made with a dermatome, mainly in the paravertebral and thoracic areas, where the underlying bones provide the necessary resistance in order to use the dermatome efficiently (Fig. 2). Chvapil et al. (4), in order to avoid jamming of the excised epidermis and formation of an uneven wound edge, cut the lateral edges of all wounds with a scalpel prior to the dermatome excision. The size and exact depth (usually 0.2–0.4 mm) of wounds can be adjusted depending on the researcher's preferences and the dermatome available. A wound drainage collector placed over each wound may be used to prevent cross-contamination from adjacent wounds (5). Hemostasis is usually performed by direct pressure but may also be performed with the application of topical agents. Treatments are applied after wounding and removal of any blood or fluid present. One technique that has been useful for delivery of liquid treatment agents is wound chambers. They have also been useful for collection of the wound fluid and evaluation of its composition (6). In this type of wounds, the epidermis and upper dermis are removed. The lower dermis, which contains the epithelial appendages, is spared. Re-epithelialization occurs quickly from both the keratinocytes of the adjacent skin and the ones lying in the hair follicles and apocrine glands. There is no lag phase; wound repair starts immediately after wounding. Partial thickness wounds heal in approximately 7 days without scarring. This model is frequently used to test the effects of various treatment agents and dressings on re-epithelialization and imitates closely a variety of superficial human wounds, like a child's scrapped knee or a surgical skin graft donor site.

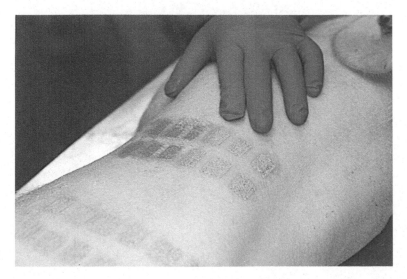

Figure 2 Dermatone wounds of $3 \times 7 \times 0.3$ mm on the parathorax of a domestic pig.

In *full-thickness excisional wounds* both epidermis and dermis are removed. Punch biopsies or excision with scalpel can be used to produce the wounds. In the case when scalpel excision is chosen, the outline of each wound can be made with a scalpel with the aid of a template in order to assure uniformity of the wounds (7). After removal of the template, the incision can be increased to the desired depth. Alternatively, the borders of the area to be wounded can be tattooed to facilitate the excision, and the measurement of wound surfaces and of contraction (8,9) (Fig. 3) Wound chambers can be used for the delivery of liquid treatments. In these models, re-epithelialization occurs only from the wound edges, and the role of granulation tissue formation and wound contraction is more pronounced in full thickness than in partial thickness wounds. Wounds heal with obvious scarring. Full-thickness wounds have also been studied in the Yucatan Mini-pigs and the relationship of age and growth factor expression correlated (10). Full-thickness wounds are an excellent model in cases in which the investigation of the effect of an agent on wound contraction, tensile strength, or scarring is the goal.

Incisional wounds are usually full-thickness wounds extending to the muscular fascia. Incisional models resemble closely human wounds after scalpel incision. Healing occurs quickly, mainly with re-epithelialization. They are easy to make and commonly used to evaluate effects of different treatments on tensile strength and collagen formation or to investigate the mechanism of wound healing process (11,12). Incisional wounds may also be made with biopsy punches of various sizes (Fig. 4).

Burn wound models: second degree or full thickness have been developed in order to study the mechanism of healing after burns and determine the effect of topical and antibacterial agents on burn wound healing (13). Standardized burns may be produced with heated metallic rods of specific weight left for a few seconds on the

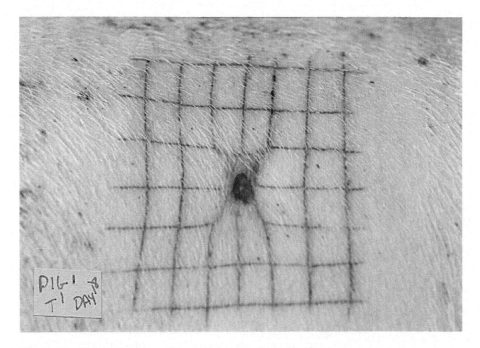

Figure 3 Tattooed area and wound contraction over time.

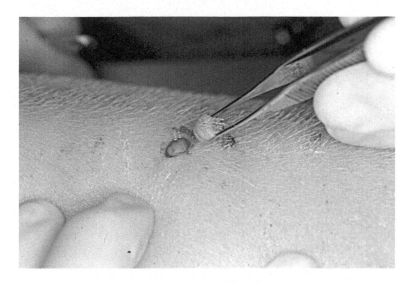

Figure 4 Four millimeter punch used to make a full-thickness wound.

skin or by exposure of skin to hot steam or water and scalding. (13,14). In a model described by Davis et al. (13), brass rods (385 g) are heated in boiling water and wiped dry to prevent water droplets from creating a steam burn on the skin. Then, they are placed for 6 sec at a vertical position perpendicular to the skin's surface with all pressure applied by gravity. The burn epidermis is then removed and treatments are applied (Fig. 5). Different water temperatures and application times have been used by different researchers. The role of early debridement has been investigated and has been shown to enhance re-epithelialization in second degree burn wounds (14). Macroscopically, after burn wounding, there is no obvious blister formed on the pig skin because there is no fluid-accumulation and the numerous hair follicles hold the denaturized skin in place. However, histologic examination reveals separation of the epidermis similar to human blisters. Full-thickness epidermal wound model, that causes necrosis of the epidermis sparing the dermis, has also been created and are useful in evaluating the epidermal healing process without involvement of dermal repair (15). Burns, albeit an acute injury, heal differently than other acute wounds. The thermal injury produces a zone of tissue damage and tissue injury continues even after the removal of the heat. In burn wounds, there is a lag phase, lasting up to 48 hr, during which re-epithelialization does not begin. Once re-epithelialization begins, the rate is usually similar to the re-epithelialization rate of other acute wounds. These models provide useful information for the management of burn wounds since treatments that accelerate wound healing in knife wounds may behave differently in burn wounds (13). Chemical burn wound models also are used and evaluated, providing a better understanding of the mechanisms of similar burns in humans (16).

Laser wound models have also been developed in order to compare the different postoperative wound care regimens and their effect on the quality and rate of healing after laser resurfacing or to evaluate wound healing after laser-induced incisions. In the model described by Davis et al. (17), a short-pulsed CO_2 laser was used, with settings similar to those used clinically for human skin resurfacing (Fig. 6). Short-pulsed CO_2 lasers employ selective photothermolysis and vaporize tissue.

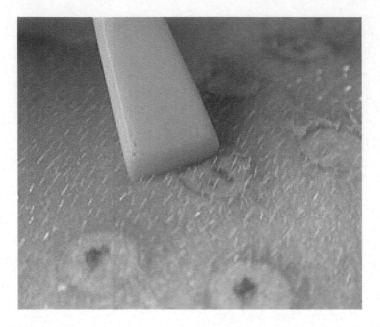

Figure 5 The burned epidermis is removed from a deep second degree burn wound.

Laser-induced wounds have a different pattern of injury and results from knife wounds or burns may not be predictive of the effect of an agent on laser wounds. Several authors have compared wound healing among incision wounds or dermal ablation made with CO_2 or other surgical modalities (18–20). Laser wounds were found to be weaker than knife wounds and re-epithelialized at a slower rate.

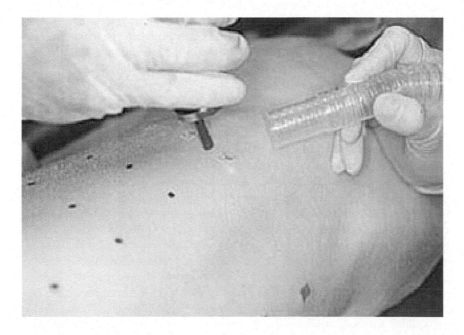

Figure 6 CO_2 laser injury.

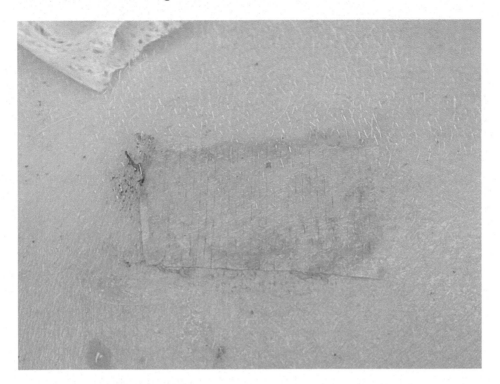

Figure 7 Skin graft in swine.

Graft take models have also been described and are used to evaluate the acceleration of re-epithelialization, and the graft take after transplantation of autologous or bioengineered skin, or keratinocyte suspension (21,22). The recipient sites are usually full-thickness excisional wounds, but could be any wound type. Graft take models can also be used to investigate the effects of different dressings or treatment on the survival of diverse kinds of grafts (Fig. 7).

Mekkes et al. (23). developed a *necrotic full-thickness wound model* by excising the epidermis and upper dermis with an electrokeratome and then applying 20% trichloroacetic acid for a few minutes on the wound bed to cause necrosis until full-thickness depth. Treatments are applied three days later to ensure that trichloroacetic acid will not influence the results. This model results in full-thickness wounds containing necrotic dermal connective tissue and subcutaneous fat and can be useful in examining the debriding effect of a diversity of enzymes and other treatments.

1.1. Bacteria-Challenged Wound Models

Infection is an important parameter that negatively influences wound healing. The need to evaluate the efficacy of antimicrobial and antiseptic agents in vivo and to investigate the effects of different dressings on bacterial proliferation led to the development of wound models that are challenged by inoculating known amounts of pathogens. In *bacteria-challenged partial thickness or second degree burn wound models* (24,25), wounds are inoculated with a pathogen such as *Pseudomonas aeruginosa* or *Staphylococcus aureus* (Fig. 8). The number of pathogens inoculated is usually more than 10^5 CFU/mL. After wounding, treatments are applied, either immediately or

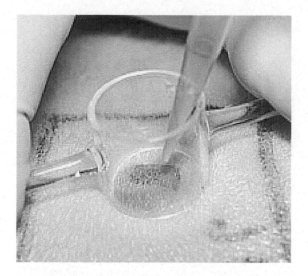

Figure 8 Bacterial inoculation of wounds.

after a 24-hr colonization time. In the first case, the bacteria could be more susceptible to the antimicrobials, since they do not have time to attach, invade the wound bed and form a bacterial biofilm, depending on the species. Bacterial biofilm formation, which greatly increases bacterial resistance, has been identified in animal and human wounds (26,27). So, it appears that a delay on the application of treatments may imitate more closely the clinical situation. At specific time points after the application of treatments, the bacteria are recovered from the wounds and quantitated. Scrubbing, washing, swabbing, or biopsy can be used for bacterial recovery (28). Although tissue biopsy was the former gold standard for bacterial quantitation, rigorous scrubbing with a surfactant may be preferable, since it gives reproducible results, removes attached bacteria, gives comparable results to tissue biopsy and is more convenient. Moreover, it seems that there is a concentration gradient of bacteria within wound tissue, with the higher bacterial concentration in the superficial layers and the lowest in the hypodermal level (29). Scrubbing successfully removes the superficial bacterial population in addition to the bacteria in the lower tissue.

Likewise, in order to determine the efficacy of wound dressings as barriers against bacterial invasion, a *bacteria-challenged barrier wound model* has been developed by Mertz et al. (30). Here, partial thickness wounds are made, the tested dressings are applied. Then, the dressings and the surrounding area are challenged with a high inoculum of pathogenic bacteria. A polyurethane dressing is used to cover the entire challenged area and keep the inoculated bacteria outside. After a few days, the number of bacteria that invaded the wound is determined following the removal of the dressing.

1.2. No Chronic Wounds/Delayed Healing Models

Chronic wounds, such as venous, arterial, diabetic, and pressure ulcers, are commonly encountered in the clinical practice and there is need for the development of experimental models mimicking these kinds of wounds. To date, no wound model successfully simulating human chronic wounds has been described. However, several models which heal at a slower rate than normal wounds and may bear some similarities to human chronic wounds have been developed.

A few *pressure wound models* have been described. Daniel et al. (31) caused paraplegia of pigs after spinal cord transection and created grade III pressure sores on the atrophic hind limb of the paralyzed pigs by applying 600 mmHg of pressure for 7 hr or longer. Kambic et al. (32) created a pressure sore model in monoplegic pigs, reducing thereby the complications, and the mortality associated with the previous model. Monoplegia is induced by surgical resection of unilateral lumbar nerve roots. After a 5–14 day waiting period for muscle atrophy, a pressure applicator is inserted percutaneously on the area over the trochanteric area and left there for several hours. General anesthesia is not required during the pressure period. Depending on the magnitude and the duration of the pressure, grade I–grade IV sores can be created (33). The required pressure is 800 mmHg for 48 hr for full-thickness sores in this model.

An *ischemic wound model* has been described by Sullivan et al. (34) providing the possibility of studying the ability of various topical agents and dressings to facilitate the healing of wounds with compromised arterial supply. Flaps were created, on the dorsum of a pig, and polyurethane dressing was placed between the wound bed and under the flap to prevent rapid revascularization (Fig. 9). Subsequently, partial thickness wounds were created on the flaps. Impaired healing occurs in the wounds located distally in the flap, while the proximal wounds (close to the flap pedicle) heal at a normal rate.

Irradiation is a frequent cause of impaired wound healing in patients. *Post-irradiation wound models* have been described in the literature and various irradiation protocols have been compared (35). The irradiation protocol used by Bernatchez et al. (36). (1500 Rad from a Cobalt-60 source, at a distance of 100 cm, on a

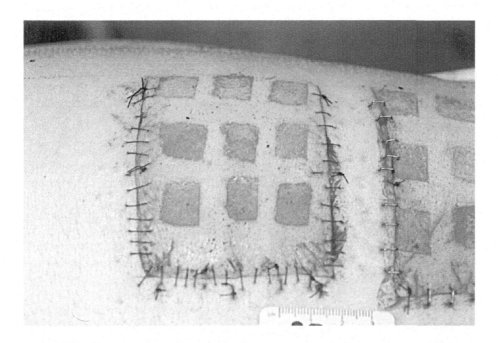

Figure 9 Ischemic wound model.

7×30 cm surface, with 2 cm target depth) caused a 50% delay of re-epithelialization of wounds on the irradiated site of the experimental animals, while the wounds of the nonirradiated site healed at the same rates with control animals. This model could be used to compare the effects of different treatments on wounds with impaired healing. However, it is important to take into consideration that in clinical practice, small multiple doses are used instead of a single large dose, so results might be different in a clinical setting.

2. EVALUATION OF THE WOUND HEALING PROCESS

During cutaneous wound healing, epidermal and dermal components are restored through a complex process that involves a dynamic interaction between many cell types, diverse mediators, and extracellular matrix. Keratinocytes, fibroblasts, endothelial cells, platelets, and white blood cells are activated, secrete multiple cytokines and growth factors, migrate and proliferate resulting in the reestablishment of the pre-wounding stage. The complexity of this multiphase process gave rise to multiple methods for evaluation of wound healing. Each step, such as inflammation, production and secretion of growth factors and cytokines, re-epithelialization, neovascularization, fibroblast proliferation, collagen production and granulation tissue formation, contraction, restoration of the tensile strength of the wound, and scar formation, can be quantitated and important information about the effects of various interventions on the wound healing process is derived. The most common methods to evaluate cutaneous healing used in swine models of wound healing are reviewed.

2.1. Evaluation of Epidermal Repair

Histological assessment and morphometric analysis, after hematoxylin–eosin staining, is most frequently used to evaluate the degree of re-epithelialization of wounds. Wound biopsies are taken, including surrounding uninjured tissue, and the *percentage of wound epithelialized* is calculated by dividing the length of the wound surface covered with at least one epithelial layer to the original wound length. In the technique described by Winter (37), the area of regenerated epidermis is estimated by examining every fifth section in a series cut at 10 μm and measurement of the separate lengths of regenerated epidermis and the total lengths of the section within 0.01 mm. The results can also be expressed as the *proportion of wounds that are completely re-epithelialized* at a specific time point. Additional information deriving from the histologic assessment is the measurement of the *epithelial thickness* (38), or number of epidermal cell layers. *Computerized morphometric analysis* can also be used in order to provide more precise measurements (5,39).

Planimetry determines wound dimension by calculating wound surface based on wound tracings. *Image analysis* can also be used to calculate the remaining wound area. Ozturk et al. (40) compare two methods of image analysis. In the first, wound areas are calculated by pixel counting and corrected with perspective scaling. In the second, a three-dimensional image reconstruction from a single camera is made by projecting a structured light pattern onto the skin. Price et al. (41) also used an *image analysis system* to calculate re-epithelialization. Acetate sheets with sized circles were held against the wound area and tracings of the epithelialized areas were made. The images were then scanned, edited to give a solid area by pixel counting and compared with a control area consisting with a completely filled circle.

Another method for macroscopic determination of wound re-epithelialization is the *epidermal migration assay*, developed by eaglstein and colleagues (42,43). The entire wound area, including surrounding unwounded skin, is excised using a dermatome. The excised specimens are incubated for three or more hours in 2N NaBr to allow separation of the epidermis of the dermis. Following separation, the integrity of the epidermal portion is evaluated macroscopically and graded as healed, if no defect is detected, or nonhealed (with a defect) (Fig. 10). The newly formed epithelium must be at least five cells thick to allow for successful separation from the dermis without defects. Results are expressed as the percentage of wounds healed at a specific time point. Moreover, the time needed for 50% of the wounds in each treatment group to heal (HT50) is calculated and compared.

The *epidermal proliferation activity* can be calculated by in vivo incorporation of the thimidine analog 5-bromo-2-deoxyuridine (BrdU) in epithelial cells and subsequent immunodetection (44). The measurement of BrdU positive cells per millimeter length of epithelium can be done from the margins of the wounds, since epidermal proliferation activity from the wound edges correlates well with the epithelial proliferation over the entire wound length. Another immunohistochemical technique, using PC10, a monoclonal antibody against proliferating cell nuclear antigen (PCNA), can be used to assess epidermal proliferation during epidermal healing (45).

Assessment of the *re-establishment of the basement membrane* can be done by electron microscopy, while immunohistochemical markers (laminin, chondroitin sulfate basement membrane protein, collagen VII and IV, bullous pemphigoid antigen, fibronectin, and others) can be used to provide more precise information about maturation of basement membrane and wound healing mechanism.

Measurement of wound fluid total protein has been found to be a reliable noninvasive marker of the *epithelial barrier function* and decrease of epidermal protein leakage can be used for comparison of the restoration of epithelial integrity (46). The wound fluid can be collected in wound chambers placed over the wounds and the volume and total protein concentration of wound fluid are calculated. The restoration of the barrier function of the new epidermis coincides histologically with a three- or four-layer epithelium, a stratum corneum, and rete ridges formation on the basement membrane (6). *Evaporimetry* quantitates the transepidermal water loss and can be used as a marker of re-establishment of epidermal barrier function (47).

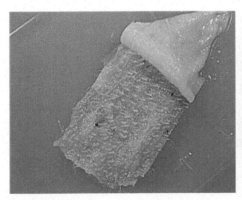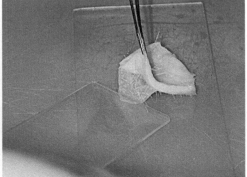

Figure 10 Picture of separated skin.

2.2. Evaluation of Dermal Repair

Granulation tissue formation is commonly assessed histopathologically. Mertz et al. (48) quantified granulation tissue formation by projecting the section on a grid paper, tracing the granulation tissue area and subsequently performing computer image analysis on this area. Bennet et al. (5) assessed newly formed dermis by computerized morphometric analysis of section stained with Gomori trichrome, since neodermal tissue stains brilliant red, while preexisting dermis stains green with Gomori stain. Lamme et al. (8) used staining with antibodies against α-smooth muscle actin to detect myofibroblasts presence as an indicator of dermal regeneration. Proliferation of fibroblasts can be assessed immunohistochemically using antibodies against PCNA and calculating the positively stained cells located   below the epidermal–dermal junction (5,45).

The *wound content of collagen*, main product of fibroblasts during cutaneous healing, is frequently used as a marker of dermal repair. Hydroxyproline, an aminoacid found mainly in collagen, is commonly quantitated and used as a measure of wound collagen. Immunohistochemical techniques allow for more accurate measurements, and have the advantage of providing additional information regarding the location and distribution patterns of collagen in the dermis. Histology, using Masson's trichrome stain and morphometric analysis, can also provide information about collagen content. Changes in collagen stainability (from blue to red) in burn wounds have been shown by Chvapil et al. (49) to reflect collagen denaturation and can be used as an indicator of the depth of thermal injury. Methods to evaluate *collagen biosynthesis assays*, such as measurement of the incorporation of [^{14}C] proline into [^{14}C] hydroxyproline in dermal specimens (50), are also frequently used to assess the biosynthetic properties of the injured dermis. Measurement of procollagen mRNA is valuable as an indicator of fibroblasts biosynthetic activity.

Wound breaking strength does not always correlate with collagen content of wounds, as increased breaking strength could result from increased cross-linking or different orientation of collagen fibers, or deposition of more mature type of collagen (10). Several techniques have been developed for assessment of breaking strength (11,21,51). Byl et al. (11) attached alligator clamps, gripped at the excised wound tissue, to a container into which water was titrated at a controlled speed. The required tension to cause separation of the wound edges was recorded. The maximum tension generated by this technique is 10,000 g. Converse et al. (20) used the Instron 5552 tensiometer, measured peak breaking forces and converted them to tensile strength values (kilogram force per cm^2). Maximum tensile strength is determined by measuring the tensile strength of intact skin.

Wound contraction and epithelialization are independent processes. Hinrichsen et al. (52) measured wound contraction in full-thickness wounds by outlining the tattooed wound area immediately after wounding and 5 months later. Contraction was calculated as area reduction. Correction for the animal growth is done in order to avoid overestimation of wound contraction.

Neovascularization occurs during the proliferative phase of wound healing. Histology is helpful for qualitative comparisons of angiogenesis in the wounded area. Roesel and Nanney (53) used Von Willebrand factor immunostaining of histological sections to facilitate the identification of blood vessels. Then, they performed quantitative assessment by computerized morphometric analysis of the percentage of capillary area and the mean diameter of vessels. Laminin has been used by others for staining of blood vessels (37).

OI(degrees)

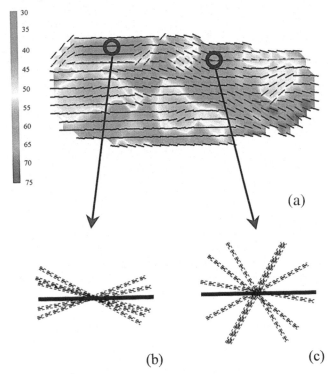

Figure 11   Comparsion of collagen fiber alignment using the Small Angle Light Scattering (SALS) technique.

Collagen fibers have random orientation in normal skin, while in scar tissue they appear to have a greater degree of alignment. Measurement of *collagen fiber alignment* can be used as a *marker of scar formation*. Small angle light scattering, a HeNe continuous unpolarized laser device, permits quantitative structural characterization of collagen and can be used to quantify and compare collagen fiber alignment between wounds of different treatment groups (51) (Fig. 11). Other researchers have evaluated scar formation by calculating the percentage of wounds with scar tissue through the histopathological finding of poorly organized bundles of collagen observed under polarized light (35,54.) However, this technique does not provide accurate quantitative measurements and is not able to detect small differences in collagen orientation. Alternatively, clinical evaluation of scar formation, using the Vancouver Scar Assessment or other visual analog grading systems, can be performed.

2.3. Other Measurements

Clinical evaluation can be used for grading overall healing, granulation tissue formation, eschar formation, necrosis, edema, exudation, erythema, re-epithelialization, inflammation, and irritation in the different treatment groups. As a rule, clinical evaluation is more subjective and less sensitive than other methods.

Histological evaluation is frequently used to determine among others the degree of inflammation by measuring the mixed leukocytic infiltrate. White blood cell morphology and anatomic abnormalities can be detected better with electron microscopy. In case interstitial dermal neutrophils contain intracellular bacteria, wound is considered infected by some authors (38). Electron microscopy and confocal laser scanning microscopy are useful additional methods to conventional light microscopy for cytomorphological studies (3).

Immunohistochemistry is very helpful in unlocking wound healing mechanisms, by allowing us to determine the effects of the tested therapeutic modalities on diverse cytokines, growth factors, and numerous dermal and epidermal antigens.

Moreover, various *additional molecular biology techniques*, such as Western Blot analysis, radiometric enzyme assays, enzyme-linked immunosorbent assay (ELISA), and substrate gel electrophoresis, are performed to assess growth factor, cytokine, and enzyme content of the wound fluid or tissue.

3. SUMMARY

Swine has been extensively used in wound healing research and various wound models have been created, imitating the diverse types of human wounds. In this article, the most widely used wound models and techniques to study wound healing in swine have been outlined.

ACKNOWLEDGMENTS

We wish to thank Stephen C. Davis, Assistant Professor and Alejandro Cazzaniga, Research Associate for their help with this chapter.

REFERENCES

1. Sullivan TP, Eaglstein WH, Davis SC, Mertz PM. The pig as a model for human wound healing. Wound Rep Reg 2001; 9:66–76.
2. Montagna W, Yun JS. The skin of the domestic pig. J Invest Dermatol 1994; 43:11–21.
3. Vardaxis NJ, Brans TA, Boon ME, Kreis RW, Marres LM. Confocal laser scanning microscopy of porcine skin: implications for human wound healing studies. J Anat 1997; 190:601–611.
4. Chvapil M, Gaines JA, Chvapil TA, Benson D, Tellez C. An optimal morphometric method for quantitating wound epithelialization. J Surg Res 1988; 44:266–276.
5. Bennett LL, Rosenblum RS, Perlov C, Davidson JM, et al. An in vivo comparison of topical agents on wound repair. Plast Reconstr Surg 2001; 108(3):675–685.
6. Breuing K, Andree C, Helo G, Slama J, et al. Growth factors in the repair of partial thickness porcine skin wounds. Plast Reconstr Surg 1997; 100(3):657–664.
7. Dyson M, Young S, Pendle L, Webster DF, Lang SM. Comparison of the effects of moist and dry conditions on dermal repair. J Invest Dermatol 1988; 91(5):434–439.
8. Lamme EN, Gustafsson TO, Middelkoop E. Cadexomer-iodine ointment shows stimulation of epidermal regeneration in experimental full thickness wounds. Arch Dermatol Res 1998; 290:18–24.
9. Svenjo T, Pomahac B, Yao F, Slama J, Eriksson E. Accelerated healing of full thickness skin wounds in a wet environment. Plast Reconstr Surg 2000; 106(3):602–614.
10. Yao F, Visvatti S, Johnson CS, Chen M, Siama J, Wenger A, Erriksson, E. Age and growth factors in porcine full thickness wound healing. Wound Repair Regen 2001; 9:371–377.

11. Byl NN, McKenzie A, Wong T, West J, Hunt TK. Incisional wound healing: a controlled study of low and high ultrasound. JOSPT 1993; 18(5):619–628.

12. Robinson JK, Garden JM, Taute PM, Leibovich SJ, et al. Wound healing in porcine skin following low-output carbon dioxide laser irradiation of the incision. Ann Plast Surg 1987; 18(6):499–505.

13. Davis SC, Mertz PM, Eaglstein WH. Second degree burn healing: the effect of occlusive dressings and a cream. J Surg Res 1990; 48:245–248.

14. Davis SC, Bilevich ED, Cazzaniga AL, Eaglstein WH, Mertz PM. Early debridement of second-degree burn wounds enhances the rate of epithelialization/an animal model to evaluate burn wound therapies. J Burn Care Rehabil 1996; 17:558–561.

15. Rigal C, Pieraggi MT, Serre G, Bouissou H. Optimization of a model of full-thickness epidermal burns in the pig and immunohistochemical study of epidermodermal junction regeneration during burn healing. Dermatology 1992; 184:103–110.

16. Reid FM, Graham J, Niemuth NA, Singer AW, et al. Sulfur mustard-induced skin burns in weanling swine evaluated clinically and histopathologically. J Appl Toxicol 2000; 20(suppl 1):S153–S160.

17. Davis SC, Badiavas E, Rendon-Pellerano MI, Pardo RJ. Histological comparison of postoperative wound care for laser resurfacing in a porcine model. Dermatol Surg 1999; 25(5):387–393.

18. Molgat YM, Pollack SV, Hurwitz JJ, Bunas SJ, et al. Comparative study of wound healing with CO_2 laser and other surgical modalities: preliminary findings. Int J Dermatol 1995; 34(1):42–47.

19. Ben-Baruch G, Fidler JP, Wessler T, Bendick P, Schellhas HF. Comparison of wound healing between chopped mode-superpulse mode CO_2 laser and steel knife incisions. Lasers Surg Med 1988; 8:596–599.

20. Converse GM, Ries WR, Reinisch L. Comparison of wound healing using the CO_2 laser at 10.6 μm and 9.55 μm. Laryngoscope 2001; 111:1231–1236.

21. Andree C, Reimer C, Page CP, Slama J, et al. Basement membrane formation during wound healing is dependent on epidermal transplants. Plast Reconstr Surg 2001; 107(1):97–104.

22. Yamagushi Y, Hosokawa K, Kawai K, Inoue K, et al. Involvement of keratinocyte activation phase in cutaneous graft healing: comparison of full-thickness to split-thickness grafts. Dermatol Surg 2000; 26(5):463–468.

23. Mekkes JR, Poole CL, Das PK, Bos JD, Westerhof W. Efficient debridement of necrotic wounds using proteolytic enzymes derived from Antarctic krill: a double blind, placebo-controlled study in a standardized animal wound model. Wound Repair Regen 1998; 6(1):50–57.

24. Marshall DA, Mertz PM, Eaglstein WH. Occlusive wound dressings: does dressing type influence the growth of common wound pathogens? Arch Surg 1990; 125:1136–1139.

25. Oliveria-Gandia M, Davis SC, Mertz PM. Can occlusive composition influence proliferation of bacterial pathogens?. Wounds 1998; 10(1):4–11.

26. Serralta VW, Harrison-Balestra C, Cazzaniga A, Davis SC, Mertz PM. Lifestyles of bacteria in wounds: presence of Biofilms. Wounds 2001; 13(1):29–34.

27. Bello YM, Fallabella AF, Cazzaniga AL, Harrison-Balestra C, Mertz PM. Are biofilms present in chronic wounds? Symposium of Advanced Wound Care, Las Vegas, 2001.

28. Gaspari AA. Techniques for sampling the bacterial flora of skin. Rietschel RL, Spencer TS, eds. Methods of Cutaneous Investigation. Marcel Dekker, 1990:143–170.

29. Barnett A, Dave B, Ksander GA, Vistnes LM. A concentration gradient of bacteria within wound tissues and scab. J Surg Res 1986; 41:326–332.

30. Mertz PM, Marshall DA, Eaglstein WH. Occlussive dressings to prevent bacterial invasion and wound infection. J Am Acad Dermatol 1985; 12(4):662–666.

31. Daniel RK, Priest DL, Wheatley DC. Etiologic factors in pressure sores: an experimental model. Arch Phys Med Rehabil 1981; 62:492–498.

32. Kambic HE, Reyes E, Manning T, et al. Influence of ac and dc electrical stimulation on wound healing in pigs: a biomechanical analysis. J Invest Surg 1993; 6:535–543.

33. Hyodo A, Reger SI, Negami S, Kambic H, Reyes E, Browne EZ. Evaluation of a pressure sore model using monoplegic pigs. Plast Reconstr Surg 1995; 96(2):421–428.

34. Sullivan T, Davis SC, Cazzaniga AL, Mertz PM. A new model for studying re-epithelialization of partial thickness wounds in hypoxic skin. Wounds 2001; 13(1):24–28.

35. Cvapil M, Chvapil TA. Wound healing models in the miniature Yucanan pig. Swindle MM, Moody DC, Phillips LD, eds. Swine as Models in Biochemical Research. Iowa State University Press, 1992:265–289.

36. Bernatchez SF, Parks PJ, Grussing DM, Matalas SL, Nelson GS. Histological characterization of a delayed wound healing model in pig. Wound Repair Regen 1998; 6(3):223–233.

37. Winter GD. Formation of the scab and the rate of epithelialization of superficial wounds in the skin of young domestic pigs. Nature 1962; 193:293–294.

38. Mertz PM, Davis SC, Brewer LD, Franzen L. Can antimicrobials be effective without impairing wound healing? The evaluation of a cadexomer iodine ointment. Wounds 1994; 6(6):184–193.

39. Reagan BJ, Madden MR, Huo J, et al. Analysis of cellular and decellular allogeneic dermal grafts for the treatment of full thickness wounds in a porcine model. J Trauma Inj Infect Crit Care 1997; 43(3):458–466.

40. Ozturk C, Nissannov J, Dubin S, et al. Measurement of wound healing by image analysis. Biomed Sci Instrum 1995; 31:189–193.

41. Price RD, Das-Gupta V, Frame JD, Navsaria HA. A study to evaluate primary dressings for the application of cultured keratinocytes. Br J Plast Surg 2001; 54:687–696.

42. Eaglstein WH, Mertz PM. New method for assessing epidermal wound healing: the effects of triamcinolone acetonide and polyethelene film occlusion. J Invest Dermatol 1978; 71:382–384.

43. Mertz PM, Hedba PA, Eaglestein WH. A porcine model for evaluating epidermal wound healing. In: Tumbleson ME, ed. Swine in Biomedical Research. Vol. 1. Plenum Publishing Corporation, 1986.

44. Agren MS. Matrix metalloproteinases are required for re-epithelialization of cutaneous wounds. Arch Dermatol Res 1999; 291:583–590.

45. Levine R, Agren MS, Mertz PM. Effect of occlusion on cell proliferation during epidermal healing. J Cutan Med Surg 1998; 2(4):193–198.

46. Breuing K, Eriksson E, Liu PY, Miller DR. Healing of partial thickness porcine skin wounds in a liquid environment. J Surg Res 1992; 52:50–58.

47. Sawchuk WS, Friedman KJ, Manning T, Pinnell SR. Delayed healing in full thickness wounds treated with aluminum chloride solution. J Am Acad Dermatol 1986; 15(5): 982–989.

48. Mertz PM, Davis SC, Franzen L, et al. Effects of an arginine-glucine-aspartic acid peptide-containing artificial matrix on epithelial migration in vitro and experimental second degree burn wound healing in vivo. J Burn Care Rehabil 1996; 17(3):199–206.

49. Chvapil M, Speer DP, Owen JA, Chvapil TA. Identification of the depth of burn injury by collagen stainability. Plast Reconstr Surg 1984; 73(3):438–441.

50. Alvarez OM, Mertz PM, Eaglstein WH. The effect of occlusive dressings on collagen synthesis and reepithelialization in superficial wounds. J Surg Res 1983; 35:142–148.

51. Charney J, Williamson MB, Bernhart FW. An apparatus for the determination of the tensile strength of healing wounds. Science 1947; 105:396–397.

52. Hinrichsen N, Birk-Sorensen L, Gottrup F, Hjortdal V. Wound contraction in an experimental porcine model. Scand J Plast Reconstr Hand Surg 1998; 32:243–248.

53. Roesel JF, Nanney LB. Assessment of different cytokine effects on angiogenesis using an in vivo model of cutaneous wound repair. J Surg Res 1995; 58:449–459.

54. Bowes LE, Jimenez MC, Hiester ED, Sacks MS, Brahmatewari J, Mertz P, Eaglstein WH. Collagen fiber orientation as quantified by small angle light scattering in wounds treated with transforming growth factor-beta2 and its neutralizing antibody. Wound Repair Regen 1999; 7(3):179–188.

55

Human Models in Wound Healing Research

Jonathan Kantor and David J. Margolis

Departments of Dermatology and Biostatistics and Epidemiology, University of Pennsylvania School of Medicine, Philadelphia, Pennsylvania, U.S.A.

1. INTRODUCTION

Despite significant advances over the past 40 years in areas of immunology, biochemistry, and genetics, the ways in which disease processes and their therapies are studied in patients have changed little. Traditionally, patient-based research has been oriented around the drug approval process which, in the case of the United States, is mediated largely through phase I, II, and III trials for FDA approval of new therapies.

Over the past decade or so, there has been an increasing stress on developing novel techniques to better estimate the efficacy of therapies in actual patients. One technique, prognostic modeling, has been used for some time in order to determine what patients are at risk of developing disease (or, alternatively, healing from disease). Prognostic models, as well as explanatory models, have been used in several areas in dermatologic research, including melanoma prognosis and, more recently, wound healing prognosis.

Another method of modeling wound healing in people involves the use of surrogate markers of disease, or response to disease. This technique has been used extensively in areas such as cardiology, where following blood pressure—rather than other more definitive endpoints, such as death or hospitalization—has become increasingly popular. One of the major advantages of this technique, as will be elaborated further below, is the potential time- and cost-savings that could be gleaned in a clinical trial setting.

This chapter will address both prognostic models and surrogate endpoints individually and will conclude with a section outlining the advantages (as well as the pitfalls) of using these techniques in concert.

2. PROGNOSTIC MODELS

In the 17th century, medical texts included sections on the prognosis of disease, and for many years physicians' minds were valued more for their prognostic knowledge than their therapeutic acumen (1). However, adopting an evidence-based approach to prognosis is a relatively recent development. Rather than attempting to predict prognosis based on anecdote and limited experience, evidence-based prognostic modeling utilizes statistical techniques to analyze the impact of multiple factors on prognosis. Potential prognostic factors are generally gleaned not from individual clinicians' experiences, but from large pooled sets of patient data. Much of the following section is based on an article that we published several years ago on the use of prognostic models for dermatologic research (2).

Population-based statistics often provides a broad idea of the prognosis of a disease. For example, let us say we wish to predict the chances of a venous leg ulcer healing. Studies have shown that approximately 50% of venous leg ulcers heal after 24 weeks of standard therapy. It is also known, however, that smaller wounds are more likely to heal quickly than larger wounds and that patients with other complicating medical conditions, such as diabetes, may take longer to heal. The 50% figure takes all of these patients into account. It would therefore be less than ideal to present the 50% healing rate figure to two patients, one a young healthy woman with a small venous ulcer and the other a malnourished gentleman with diabetes who is on chronic steroid therapy. In order to effectively estimate the probability that an *individual* wound will heal within a given time frame, we need to form a prognostic model that would include these types of variables that may affect disease prognosis.

We recently studied the use of a novel marker of wound healing, percentage change in ulcer area over the first 4 weeks of therapy, as a marker of wound healing within the first 24 weeks of therapy. This technique reflected essentially a single-variable prognostic model with the variable being the percentage change in wound area over the first few weeks of standard therapy (3).

2.1. Explanatory and Prognostic Models

An explanatory or causal model expresses inferences regarding an exposure's effect on the development of an outcome. More formally, it is defined as the conditional probability of disease with respect to an exposure divided by the conditional probability of disease with respect to the absence of the exposure. The exposure in an explanatory model is evaluated with regard to whether it "causes" the outcome (4). When developing causal models, investigators often attempt to mitigate the effects of confounding variables—variables associated with both the disease and the exposure. These variables may mask or augment the measured association between the exposure of interest and the disease (or outcome of interest).

In contrast to an explanatory model, a prognostic model must be able to describe the relationship or probability that the presence of a certain group of risk factors will result in an outcome. The relationship of the prognostic factor to the outcome does not have to be based on biologic plausibility or causality. The inclusion of a variable into this model depends only on its ability to improve the prediction of the outcome. The clinical utility of a model is closely related to its ease of use by clinicians. Therefore, clinically useful models often simply count the presence or absence of the fewest variables needed to predict the outcome accurately. This is one of the reasons we included only a single variable in our model of venous leg ulcer healing.

2.2. Techniques
2.2.1. Regression Techniques

The basic techniques underlying prognostic modeling involve determining what quantifiable factors affect outcome and their relative contribution to the outcome. Logistic regression is commonly used to model diseases, and can be used to create a model of the probability of the occurrence of a dichotomous outcome variable, such as healing at 24 weeks (5,6). This method uses one dependent variable, which is a mathematical transformation of the probability function. The odds ratio in a logistic model is developed via further mathematical transformation. Both unadjusted (from a single variable logistic model) and fully adjusted (from a multiple variable logistic model) odds ratios are generally reported with 95% confidence intervals. Fully adjusted odds ratios may be estimated by adjusting for factors a priori considered to be clinically important, statistically important variables (based on a *p*-value of <0.05 in the single variable model), and demographic variables (such as insurance status, age, gender, and ethnicity). In a prognostic model, the exposure variables are then used to calculate the probability of the dependent (outcome) variable.

2.2.2. Neural Net Analysis

Neural networks are nonparametric algorithms that are coarsely patterned to simulate the perceived biologic processes involved in human learning (7). They contain a series of mathematical equations that are used to simulate biological process of learning and memory. They have been used as a method to create prognostic and diagnostic models for several biomedical problems including myocardial infarction and pulmonary embolism (8,9). This method is used for less frequently than logistic regression.

2.2.3. Recursive Partitioning (CART)

Recursive partitioning is an alternative way to formulate a prognostic rule. It is computer intensive but requires little assistance from the analyst (10). It is a nonparametric multivariable technique that first determines the best predictor of the outcome (i.e., healing at 24 weeks) among all of the punitive prognostic factors. The presence or absence of this predictor is used to split the modeling sample into two groups. The process is repeated in a sequential stepwise fashion until further partitioning is not possible, thereby yielding a step-by-step branching tree based on the presence or absence of specific variables. The result is a tree diagram, with final groupings (terminal nodes) representing subgroups of patients with a specific pattern of predictors and a certain probability of the outcome of interest. This technique has been used for medical application in the past and the utility of this approach was recently compared to logistic regression (11–13). One study has compared the relative merits of logistic regression, neural networks, and CART for developing prognostic models and found that all three methods may be used effectively (14).

2.3. Evaluation

Prognostic models may be evaluated in terms of calibration (goodness-of-fit) and discrimination (6,15–17). Calibration is the degree to which the predicted probability agrees with the actual event. Discrimination is the degree to which a prediction from the model can separate those who will have the outcome from those who will not. For example, a well-calibrated model can correctly predict that an individual has a 70% chance of healing within 24 weeks, while a discriminating model correctly distinguishes between who will heal within 24 weeks and who will not.

The generalizability of a model should also be assessed. The generalizability of a model is an estimate of how well the model works in populations (data sets) other than the population used to create the model. This is best estimated by determining both the calibration and discrimination of a model using data from many sites (18,19). A prognostic model can also be understood as a diagnostic test. Therefore, many of the techniques used to evaluate the discrimination of diagnostic tests such as sensitivity, specificity, positive and negative predictive values, and receiver–operator characteristic (ROC) curves may be applied to prognostic models as well (20,21).

The sensitivity (or true positive rate) of a prognostic model is the proportion of those that truly experienced the event (such as wound healing within 24 weeks) who are identified as such by the prognostic model. The specificity (or false positive rate) of a prognostic model is the proportion of those that truly did not experience the event being tested for (i.e., those that were not healed at 24 weeks) who were so identified by the prognostic model (22). The positive predictive value of a prognostic model is the probability that a person with a positive result is a true positive (i.e., healed by 24 weeks). The negative predictive value is the probability that a person with a negative result did not experience the event (in our case, not healed at 24 weeks). The negative predictive value is the probability that a person with a negative result did not experience the event (in our case, not healed at 24 weeks) (22). Positive and negative predictive values are thus clinically useful measures of the value of a prognostic model.

An ROC curve is a graphical representation of sensitivity (true positive rate) vs. 1-specificity (false positive rate) (21). The ROC curve provides a measure of the accuracy of a test. A useless test would have an equal number of true positive and false positive results, and hence an area under the curve of 0.5. The better the test, the closer the area under the curve is to 1. Area under the ROC curve of >0.7 can be thought of as acceptable, >0.8 can be thought of as good, and >0.9 can be thought of as excellent (23).

Brier scores are commonly used by atmospheric scientists to summarize the forecast performance of their models, and have been used by epidemiologists to measure goodness-of-fit (24–26). A Brier score is the average of the mean squared error of the predicted and the observed event for any data set. Scores can vary between 0 and 1. A more accurate model has a Brier score closer to 0. A model that agrees with the known outcome 50% of the time and disagrees with it 50% of the time would have a Brier score of 0.25 (26). The greatest advantage of the Brier score is that it is a measure of both discrimination and calibration. It can be decomposed to express estimates of discrimination and calibration, and it has been used in the past to make comparisons between study samples (26,27).

2.4. Generalizability and Validation

One limitation of all statistical models is that the external validity or generalizability of a model cannot be described in conclusive terms (28). However, if a prognostic model is to be appropriately clinically applied in a different population of inference, its performance must be tested in an external (validation) data set. External validity refers to the extent to which the results of the model represent events seen in a referent population of interest (4). Lack of external validity cannot be corrected for statistically, so it is essential for a clinician to evaluate and understand the generalizability of a prognostic model to his or her clinical setting (4). In practical terms, this means that prognostic models must be validated on patient data that were not used to test the model. Ideally, external validation should also examine data on a diverse and varied set of patients, culled from a population other than the one used to formulate the model. For example, a model developed by using patient data from an academic medical center would ideally be validated on a set of patient data from patients seen at small clinical practices.

Despite the value of prognostic models, several potential limitations should be noted. First, even if a model has been externally validated, it may not be generalizable to all populations. For example, a melanoma prognostic model that accurately predicts death from melanoma in several different regions in the United States may not be applicable in central Africa. Second, the model may yield information that is not clinically useful. Third, over-reliance on any model may be dangerous, since few if any prognostic models discriminate 100% between outcomes. Indeed, flipping a coin provides a model which correctly predicts a binary (yes/no) outcome 50% of the time. Finally, like any tool, a prognostic model is only useful when used in combination with a complete clinical understanding of the patient. Despite the potential drawbacks of prognostic models, if created and used correctly, they can be a very clinically useful and reliable method of determining the prognosis of individuals with disease.

3. SURROGATE ENDPOINTS

A surrogate endpoint or marker is a measured endpoint that may be used in lieu of the definitive endpoint. From a statistical perspective, the surrogate endpoint represents a response variable for which a test of the null hypothesis of no relationship to treatment would also be a valid test of the corresponding null hypothesis based on the true endpoint (29). By definition, then, the surrogate endpoint needs to correlate to the true outcome and captures the effect of treatment (30). The definitive endpoint is usually (but not always) the endpoint of actual clinical interest. A perfect surrogate marker is one which mediates the effect of the therapy on the outcome. For example, a surrogate marker for disease progression to death in HIV is the CD4+ cell count.

In general, endpoints should be able to be measured reliably and accurately, since ultimately the strength of any downstream data (such as clinical trial results) are dependent on the strength of the (surrogate) endpoint used.

Let us say that we wish to predict early on which patients are unlikely to heal using standard care for their wounds. One way to select the appropriate surrogate markers for the endpoint of complete healing is to utilize the techniques discussed earlier in this chapter in order to determine whether there are any surrogate markers that could be used appropriately in lieu of the definitive endpoint (complete healing).

Several years ago, we published a study looking at markers for failure to heal in patients with venous leg ulcers (4). In this study, we found that if a wound did not decrease in size after the first 4 weeks of standard therapy, it was unlikely to heal after 24 weeks of standard care. If this is indeed the case, could improvement in the first 4 weeks of therapy be used as a surrogate marker for wound healing?

The question, then, from the perspective of clinical trial design is can we simply extend clinical trials for a duration of only 4 weeks in lieu of 24 weeks—in other words, can we directly extrapolate the percentage change in wound area to the percentage healed after 24 weeks of care? Is percentage change in area after 4 weeks of therapy enough of a prognostic factor alone that it can be used not only to *predict* the outcome, but also as a *surrogate* for this outcome of interest? In theory, yes. At this point, however, further research is needed in order to develop surrogate markers that can be reliably used in wound healing trials.

An National Institutes of Health workshop recently addressed the use of surrogate endpoints in clinical trials (31). In this article, the authors pointed out some of the advantages of surrogate markers—the potential for cost savings, time savings, and increasing the sample size of clinical trials—while also highlighting the potential shortcomings of this technique. The central limitation of surrogates is that in theory they need to reflect a point in the progression from disease to resolution (or from wound to healed wound). As another article has pointed out (32), this is a significant limitation and in many cases surrogates fail to provide an effective substitute for the definitive endpoint. This may be because the disease process progresses in ways that were not anticipated—that is, the surrogate may not represent the "recovery" process from disease to cure. If the disease progresses or recovers in a way that is not mediated through the surrogate, then potentially the surrogate may not serve a useful purpose. These and other limitations mean that surrogate endpoints must only be used and adopted with care and with an eye to the limitations of these techniques (33,34).

A surrogate endpoint need not be a single factor, and indeed may be composed of a combination of variables (similar to a prognostic model). Since simplicity is one of the main advantages of using surrogate endpoints, including too many variables as part of the surrogate design may ultimately make the surrogate marker too cumbersome for practical use. Including both CD4+ cell count and viral load, for example, may make a better surrogate marker than one or the other alone.

One of the main advantages of surrogate endpoints is the time- and cost-savings that can be incurred in clinical trial design. A trial of a novel therapy for wound healing could be run faster, and at a far lower cost, if a surrogate endpoint were used rather than waiting until several months have passed and looking for complete healing. Including only patients that are unlikely to heal with standard care (as determined using a prognostic model) could further reduce the cost of this trial.

As an example, a study was recently completed that examined the use of surrogate markers for venous ulcer healing (35). In this large cohort study of approximately 30,000 patients, the authors examined surrogate markers of venous ulcer healing in 4 weeks. The authors demonstrated that wound parameters including the log healing rate, log wound area ratio, and percentage change in wound area over the first 4 weeks of care can be valid surrogate markers of complete healing in 12 or 24 weeks of care. This was demonstrated using a number of techniques including the area under the ROC curve as discussed above. These surrogates were further validated by demonstrating that established risk factors for not healing such as wound size and wound duration are also important risk factors for not achieving the surrogate endpoint. As noted above, these findings could be used to better design future clinical trials and to better tailor treatment to patients who are unlikely to heal with standard care alone.

This chapter has addressed some of the useful models of wound healing that are currently being explored in patient-oriented research. Prognostic models can be used to predict which patients will do well, and are useful both in informing patients of their prognosis as well as in better designing research trials. Surrogate endpoints—which are currently an area of active research—may be used to develop faster and less costlier clinical trials, a potential boon to patients, clinicians, and pharmaceutical companies. Despite the many advantages of these techniques, they have significant limitations. As noted above, a trial is only as strong as the surrogate endpoint that is used. Therefore, further research is needed on large generalizable populations before surrogate endpoints for wound healing can be appropriately used in practice.

REFERENCES

1. Sennert D. The Art of Chirurgery. London, 1661.
2. Kantor J, Margolis DJ. Prognostic models: evidence based approach to predicting disease outcome. J Cutan Med Surg 1999; 3:157–161.
3. Kantor J, Margolis DJ. A multicentre study of percentage change in venous leg ulcer area as a prognostic index of healing at 24 weeks. Brit J Dermatol 2000; 142:960–964.
4. Rothman KJ, Greenland S. Modern Epidemiology. 2nd ed. Philadelphia: Lippincott-Raven, 1998.
5. Watson JH, Sox HC, Neff RK, et al. Clinical prediction rules: applications and methodological standards. N Engl J Med 1985; 313:793–799.
6. Hosmer DW, Lemeshow S. Applied Logistic Regression. New York: John Wiley & Sons, 1989.
7. Tu JV. Advantages and disadvantages of using artificial neural networks versus logistic regression for predicting medical outcomes. J Clin Epidemiol 1996; 49:1225–1231.
8. Baxt WG. Use of an artificial neural network for the diagnosis of myocardial infarction. Ann Intern Med 1991; 115:843–848.
9. Patil S, Henry JW, Rubenfire M, et al. Neural network in the clinical diagnosis of acute pulmonary embolism. Chest 1993; 104:1685–1689.
10. Breiman L, Friedman JH, Olshen RA, et al. Classification and Regression Trees. Belmont, CA: Wadsworth International, 1984.
11. Crichton NJ, Hindle JP, Marchini J. Models for diagnosing chest pain: is CART helpful? Stat Med 1997; 16:717–727.
12. Yarnold PR, Soltysik RC, Bennett CL. Predicting in-hospital mortality of patients with AIDS-related *Pneumocystis carinii* pneumonia: an example of hierarchically optimal classification tree analysis. Stat Med 1997; 16:1451–1463.
13. Pilote L, Miller DP, Califf RM, et al. Determinants of the use of coronary angiography and revascularization after thrombolysis for acute myocardial infacrtion. N Engl J Med 1996; 335:1198–1205.
14. Selker HP, Griffith JL, Patil S, et al. A comparison of performance of mathematical predictive methods for medical diagnosis: identifying acute cardiac ischemia among emergency department patients. J Investig Med 1995; 43:468–476.
15. Hosmer DW, Lemeshow S. Goodness of fit tests for multiple logistic regression model. Commun Statist Theor Math 1980; 10:1043–1069.
16. Hlatky MA, Califf RM, Harrell FE Jr, et al. Clinical judgement and therapeutic decision making. J Am Coll Cardiol 1990; 15:1–14.
17. Hlatky MA, Mark DB, Harrell FE Jr, et al. Rethinking sensitivity and specificity. Am J Cardiol 1987; 59:1195–1198.
18. Harrell FE Jr, Lee KL, Mark DB. Multivariable prognostic models: issues in developing models, evaluating assumptions and adequacy, and measuring and reducing errors. Stat Med 1996; 15:361–387.
19. Harrell FE Jr, Lee KL, Califf RM, et al. Regression modeling strategies for improved prognostic prediction. Stat Med 1984; 3:143–152.
20. Clarke JR, Hayward CZ. A scientific approach to surgical reasoning. I. Diagnostic accuracy—sensitivity, specificity, prevalence, and predictive value. Theor Surg 1990; 5:129–132.

21. Clarke JR, O'Donnell TF Jr. A scientific approach to surgical reasoning. III. What is abnormal? Test results with continuous values and receiver operating characteristic (ROC) curves. Theor Surg 1991; 6:45–51.

22. Last JM, ed. A Dictionary of Epidemiology. 3rd ed. New York: Oxford University Press, 1995.

23. Murphy-Filkins R, Teres D, Lemeshow S, et al. Effect of changing patient mix on the performance of an intensive care unit severity-of-illness model: how to distinguish a general from a specialty intensive care unit. Critical Care Med 1996; 24:1968–1973.

24. Arkes HR, Dawson NV, Speroff T, et al. The covariance decomposition of the probability score and its use in evaluating prognostic estimates. SUPPORT investigators. Med Decis Making 1995; 15:120–131.

25. Dolan JG, Bordley DR, Mushlin AI. An evaluation of clinicians' subjective prior probability estimates. Med Decis Making 1986; 6:216–223.

26. Yates FJ. External correspondence: decompositions of the mean probability score. Organ Behav Hum Performance 1982; 30:132–156.

27. Redelmeirer DA, Bloch DA, Hickam DH. Assessing predictive accuracy: how to compare Brier scores. J Clin Epidemiol 1991; 44:1141–1146.

28. Campbell DT, Stanley JC. Experimental Design and Quasi-Experimental Designs for Research. Boston: Houghton Miffin Company, 1963.

29. Prentice, RL. Surrogate endpoints in clinical trials: definition and operational criteria. Stat Med 1989; 8:431–440.

30. Freedman LS, Graubard BI. Statistical validation of intermediate endpoints for chronic diseases. Stat Med 1992; 11:167–178.

31. De Gruttola VG, Clax P, DeMets DL, et al. Considerations in the evaluation of surrogate endpoints in clinical trials: summary of a National Institutes of Health workshop. Controlled Clin Trials 2001; 22:485–502.

32. Fleming TR, DeMets DL. Surrogate end points in clinical trials: are we being misled? Ann Intern Med 1996; 125:606–613.

33. Buyse M. Statistical validation of surrogate endpoints: problems and proposals. Drug Inf J 2000; 34:447–454.

34. Lesko LJ, Atkinson, AJ. Use of biomarkers and surrogate endpoint in drug development and regulatory decision making: criteria, validation, strategies. Annu Rev Pharmacol Toxicol 2001; 41:347–366.

35. Gelfand JM, Hoffstad O, Margolis DJ. Surrogate endpoints for the treatment of venous leg ulcers. J Invest Dermatol 2002; 119:1420–1425.

Index